Neuroimaging: Brain Networks and Connectivity

Neuroimaging: Brain Networks and Connectivity

Editor: Nubia Cartman

AMERICAN
MEDICAL PUBLISHERS
www.americanmedicalpublishers.com

AMERICAN
MEDICAL PUBLISHERS
www.americanmedicalpublishers.com

Cataloging-in-Publication Data

Neuroimaging : brain networks and connectivity / edited by Nubia Cartman.
p. cm.
Includes bibliographical references and index.
ISBN 979-8-88740-310-6
1. Brain--Imaging. 2. Nervous system--Imaging. 3. Diagnostic imaging. 4. Nervous system--Radiography.
I. Cartman, Nubia.
RC386.6.D52 N48 2023
616.804 754--dc23

American Medical Publishers,
41 Flatbush Avenue,
1st Floor, New York,
NY 11217, USA

ISBN 979-8-88740-310-6 (Hardback)

Contents

Preface VII

Chapter 1 **The potential of the human connectome as a biomarker of brain disease** 1
Marcus Kaiser

Chapter 2 **Functional diffusion tensor imaging at 3 Tesla** 5
René C.W. Mandl, Hugo G. Schnack, Marcel P. Zwiers, René S. Kahn and Hilleke E. Hulshoff Pol

Chapter 3 **Interpreting the effects of altered brain anatomical connectivity on fMRI functional connectivity: A role for computational neural modeling** 14
Barry Horwitz, Chuhern Hwang and Jeff Alstott

Chapter 4 **A review of attention-deficit/hyperactivity disorder from the perspective of brain networks** 25
Angelica De La Fuente, Shugao Xia, Craig Branch and Xiaobo Li

Chapter 5 **Imaging structural and functional brain networks in temporal lobe epilepsy** 31
Boris C. Bernhardt, SeokJun Hong, Andrea Bernasconi and Neda Bernasconi

Chapter 6 **Development of functional brain connectivity in the young brain** 45
G. E. Anna-Jasmijn Hoff, M. P. Van den Heuvel, Manon J. N. L. Benders, Karina J. Kersbergen and L. S. De Vries

Chapter 7 **Graph theoretical analysis of developmental patterns of the white matter network** 52
Zhang Chen, Min Liu, Donald W. Gross and Christian Beaulieu

Chapter 8 **A systematic investigation of the invariance of resting-state network patterns: Is resting-state fMRI ready for pre-surgical planning?** 65
K. Kollndorfer, F. Ph. S. Fischmeister, G. Kasprian, D. Prayer and V. Schöpf

Chapter 9 **Task vs. rest—different network configurations between the coactivation and the resting-state brain networks** 79
Xin Di, Suril Gohel, Eun H. Kim and Bharat B. Biswal

Chapter 10 **Parcellation of the cingulate cortex at rest and during tasks: A meta-analytic clustering and experimental study** 88
Diana M. E. Torta, Tommaso Costa, Sergio Duca, Peter T. Fox and Franco Cauda

Chapter 11 **Extraversion and neuroticism relate to topological properties of resting-state brain networks** 102
Qing Gao, Qiang Xu, Xujun Duan, Wei Liao, Jurong Ding, Zhiqiang Zhang, Yuan Li, Guangming Lu and Huafu Chen

Chapter 12 **Decreased small-world functional network connectivity and clustering across resting state networks in schizophrenia: An fMRI classification tutorial** 116
Ariana Anderson and Mark S. Cohen

Chapter 13 **GroupICA dual regression analysis of resting state networks in a behavioral variant of frontotemporal dementia** 134
Riikka Rytty, Juha Nikkinen, Liisa Paavola, Ahmed Abou Elseoud, Virpi Moilanen, Annina Visuri, Osmo Tervonen, Alan E. Renton, Bryan J. Traynor, Vesa Kiviniemi and Anne M. Remes

Chapter 14 **Graph theory reveals dysconnected hubs in 22q11DS and altered nodal efficiency in patients with hallucinations** 144
Marie-Christine Ottet, Marie Schaer, Martin Debbané, Leila Cammoun, Jean-Philippe Thiran and Stephan Eliez

Chapter 15 **Age-related changes in brain structural covariance networks** 154
Xinwei Li, Fang Pu, Yubo Fan, Haijun Niu, Shuyu Li and Deyu Li

Chapter 16 **PANDA: A pipeline toolbox for analyzing brain diffusion images** 166
Zaixu Cui, Suyu Zhong, Pengfei Xu, Yong He and Gaolang Gong

Chapter 17 **A longitudinal study of structural brain network changes with normal aging** 181
Kai Wu, Yasuyuki Taki, Kazunori Sato, Haochen Qi, Ryuta Kawashima and Hiroshi Fukuda

Chapter 18 **Dysregulated but not decreased salience network activity in schizophrenia** 193
Thomas P. White, James Gilleen and Sukhwinder S. Shergill

Chapter 19 **Disparity between dorsal and ventral networks in patients with obsessive-compulsive disorder: Evidence revealed by graph theoretical analysis based on cortical thickness from MRI** 205
Seung-Goo Kim, Wi Hoon Jung, Sung Nyun Kim, Joon Hwan Jang and Jun Soo Kwon

Chapter 20 **Modular reorganization of brain resting state networks and its independent validation in Alzheimer's disease patients** 223
Guangyu Chen, Hong-Ying Zhang, Chunming Xie, Gang Chen, Zhi-Jun Zhang, Gao-Jun Teng and Shi-Jiang Li

Permissions

List of Contributors

Index

Preface

This book was inspired by the evolution of our times; to answer the curiosity of inquisitive minds. Many developments have occurred across the globe in the recent past which has transformed the progress in the field.

Neuroimaging is a branch of medical imaging that employs imaging technology to investigate the anatomy and function of the nervous system in a non-invasive manner. With the help of neuroimaging, the doctors and researchers can explore how the CNS, more specifically, the brain function is affected in states of health and disease. Conditions such as stroke and head injury may affect the normal brain functions related to cognition and information processing. Neuroimaging studies two major aspects of the brain. First, neuroimaging studies how the brain and the brain network works. Second, neuroimaging studies how different activities affect the brain. The essential tasks for neuroimaging are the refinement of preoperative differential diagnosis, precise anatomical localization for operational planning, detection of response to therapy, detection of tumor development, and recognition of treatment-related adverse effects. Major neuroimaging techniques include, computed tomography scan (CT), magnetic resonance imaging (MRI), positron emission tomography scan (PET), and diffusion tensor imaging (DTI). This book discusses the fundamentals as well as the recent developments in the field of neuroimaging. It presents researches and studies on brain networks and connectivity performed by experts across the globe. This book is a resource guide for experts as well as students.

This book was developed from a mere concept to drafts to chapters and finally compiled together as a complete text to benefit the readers across all nations. To ensure the quality of the content we instilled two significant steps in our procedure. The first was to appoint an editorial team that would verify the data and statistics provided in the book and also select the most appropriate and valuable contributions from the plentiful contributions we received from authors worldwide. The next step was to appoint an expert of the topic as the Editor-in-Chief, who would head the project and finally make the necessary amendments and modifications to make the text reader-friendly. I was then commissioned to examine all the material to present the topics in the most comprehensible and productive format.

I would like to take this opportunity to thank all the contributing authors who were supportive enough to contribute their time and knowledge to this project. I also wish to convey my regards to my family who have been extremely supportive during the entire project.

Editor

1

The potential of the human connectome as a biomarker of brain disease

Marcus Kaiser[1,2,3]*

[1] School of Computing Science, Newcastle University, Newcastle upon Tyne, UK
[2] Institute of Neuroscience, Newcastle University, Newcastle upon Tyne, UK
[3] Department of Brain and Cognitive Sciences, Seoul National University, Seoul, South Korea

***Correspondence:**
Marcus Kaiser, School of Computing Science, Newcastle University, Claremont Tower, Newcastle upon Tyne, NE1 7RU, UK
e-mail: m.kaiser@ncl.ac.uk

The human connectome at the level of fiber tracts between brain regions has been shown to differ in patients with brain disorders compared to healthy control groups. Nonetheless, there is a potentially large number of different network organizations for individual patients that could lead to cognitive deficits prohibiting correct diagnosis. Therefore changes that can distinguish groups might not be sufficient to diagnose the disease that an individual patient suffers from and to indicate the best treatment option for that patient. We describe the challenges introduced by the large variability of connectomes within healthy subjects and patients and outline three common strategies to use connectomes as biomarkers of brain diseases. Finally, we propose a fourth option in using models of simulated brain activity (the dynamic connectome) based on structural connectivity rather than the structure (connectome) itself as a biomarker of disease. Dynamic connectomes, in addition to currently used structural, functional, or effective connectivity, could be an important future biomarker for clinical applications.

Keywords: brain connectivity, network disease, brain disorders, classification, diagnosis

The study of how different components of the brain, may they be neurons or brain regions, are connected has become an emerging field within the neurosciences (Sporns et al., 2004; Bullmore and Sporns, 2009; Kaiser, 2011). The analysis of physical connections within neural systems gained momentum around 20 years ago with the availability of information on the nematode *Caenorhabditis elegans*' nervous system (White et al., 1986; Achacoso and Yamamoto, 1992) and the rhesus monkey's visual system of cortico-cortical connections (Felleman and van Essen, 1991; Young, 1992). Now called connectomics, the field aims to discover the structure of brain networks, representing physical connections such as axons or fiber tracts. As a next milestone, the first data sets of the Human Connectome Project are being released. What will the next 20 years bring? Like for genomics, the hopes are that features of the connectome of a patient can be a biomarker for diseases and an indicator for therapeutic interventions. Identifying biomarkers for diseases based on large-scale genome studies has been challenging. Is the link between connectivity and brain disease also over-weighted? What could a structural connectome in principle tell us about the brain organization in health and disease?

In analogy to genetics, we may distinguish a genotype and a phenotype of brain organization. The genotype is given by the structural connectivity either observed at the level of individual synapses (microconnectome) or at the level of fiber tracts between brain regions (macroconnectome) (DeFelipe, 2010) and we will refer to this as connectome. As for every novel field, the underlying techniques are still under development (Jbabdi and Johansen-Berg, 2011). Diffusion tensor and diffusion spectrum imaging can give us information on potential structural connections of the macroconnectome. The phenotype represents activity, as seen in functional Magnetic Resonance Imaging (fMRI) or EEG, or behavior, as for cognitive clinical scores. We refer to these patterns as consequences on dynamics or behavior due to changed brain connectivity.

The problem of diagnosing a disease, as in genetics, is due to the fact that several mutations of the genotype might result in the same phenotype (disease). Observing brain connectivity, there might be several combinations of changes in fiber tracts leading to hallucinations or seizures, for example. Also, the same connectome organization might lead to different dynamics for changes that affect the internal anatomy and activity of network nodes but not the nodes' topology (**Figure 1**). The idea that many pathways can lead to similar behavior is linked to the concept of degeneracy (Tononi et al., 1999; Price and Friston, 2002), "the ability of elements that are structurally different to perform the same function or yield the same output." If the output (phenotype) is cognitive deficits in patients, the number of connectome (genotype) patterns that lead to such behavior can be seen as the degeneracy of a brain disease. Also, a higher degeneracy, meaning that more connectome patterns are linked to a disease, might result in a higher incidence in a population. A related observation has been made in the field of genetics when linking genetic changes to diseases: multiple genotypes might lead to the same phenotype (heterogeneity) (Addington and Rapoport, 2012). Therefore, detecting one connectivity pattern linked to a disease might only relate to a fraction of all patients. Moreover, many connectome changes will be

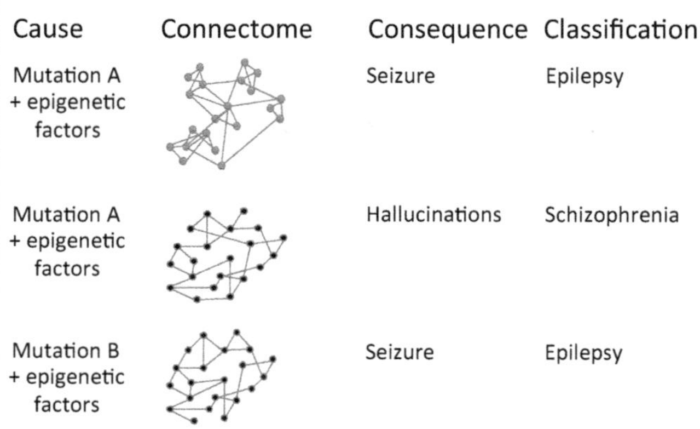

FIGURE 1 | Mapping between underlying developmental causes of connectome changes, ranging from genetic factors to spatiotemporal epigenetic factors, to resulting brain connectivity ("connectome"), observable network behavior ("consequence"), and final disease classification. Similar patterns within each of the four categories are shown in red. Note that both genetic patterns and network features alone may be insufficient to inform the clinical diagnosis of a disease: first, the same genetic mutation A might lead to a different connectivity due to different epigenetic factors. Second, different genetic mutations A and B could lead to the same connectivity due to additional factors. Third, the same connectivity might lead to different behavior and disease classification due to changes that solely affect the anatomical organization within individual nodes.

neutral in that they do not lead to a brain disorder; thus variability in the healthy population is expected to be large as well. As for genetics, connectomics is currently moving to large-scale studies, e.g., the 1,200-subject Human Connectome Project or the 1,000-subject Functional Connectomes study, to address this underlying variability.

Another problem besides large connectome variability ("noise") is that cognitive deficits might arise from small changes ("signal"). Development can be seen as a system of nonlinear dynamics (Turing, 1952). It has become clear that genetic encoding (Kendler et al., 2011) and self-organization shape the formation of neural systems in health and disease. For self-organization, the interaction with the environment (external factors) or physical constraints (internal factors) can influence the establishment and survival of axonal connections. Consequently, small changes during development might lead to a different connectome and as a result to a different resulting consequence for cognition and behavior of human subjects. As the dynamics in the brain are also non-linear, a small change in structural connectivity might be sufficient to lead to changes in cognition and behavior. Relatively small changes in connectivity might be sufficient to lead to a brain disorder. Therefore, some connectivity patterns seen in patients might be quite close to the organization of healthy subjects.

Let us look at some cases of how brain diseases could be linked to brain connectivity. Also, let us only use two cases of how a network structure (edge or node) in a patient could differ from that of a control group: a significant increase or a significant decrease of a network measure. We will only look at a single measure here, say number of streamlines for edges and total strength of its connections for nodes, but our general observations also hold for a combination of network measures (Costa et al., 2007; Kaiser et al., 2009; van den Heuvel et al., 2012).

First, a disease might affect a single brain region which could have an effect on brain dynamics by changing its own activity pattern, the pattern of directly connected neighbors of the region, and, indirectly, the activity in the rest of the brain mediated by intermediate brain regions. As a simplification, let us assume that only structural connections from that brain region will be altered. As each brain region (for a parcellation in humans of 110 cortical and subcortical regions including both hemispheres) is connected to around 10 other brain regions, there are $2^{10} = 1{,}024$ possible changes assuming that each connection could either be significantly increased or decreased in a patient. Thus even at the local scale, only affecting a single brain region, many variations of a disease are possible.

Second, a disease could affect a set of network nodes. For example, regions of the neocortex mature at different times during development: medial regions before lateral regions and posterior before anterior regions. A change in the maturation of the frontal lobe could affect multiple regions at the same time and might affect a whole network module (Nisbach and Kaiser, 2007). Say that 10 regions show a different internal structure that also manifests itself in altered fiber tracts between them and other brain regions. Therefore, assuming 10 fiber tracts per brain region, or $10^2 = 100$ fiber tracts for all 10 affected regions, show changes leads to $2^{100} = 1.3*10^{30}$ variants. Let us look at a simpler model where an increase (or a reduction) in at least 10 of those 100 fiber tracts is sufficient to lead to the behavioral features of a disease. There are $\binom{100}{10} = 1.7*10^{13}$ ways to choose 10 out of 100 connections. Given that 10 is the lower bound for disease onset, choosing 11, 12, 13, etc. connections leads to even more variations at this regional level.

Third, a disorder could lead to changes of a set of edges at the global level as a result of widely distributed changes. If there are 500 bidirectional connections (fiber tracts) between our 110 brain regions, there are $2^{500} = 3.3*10^{150}$ possible changes compared to a benchmark brain based on a population of healthy subjects.

We know that there is huge variability not only in the surface shape of human brains but also in its related connectivity pattern (Van Essen, 1997; Hilgetag and Barbas, 2006). Clearly, only a small fraction of connectome patterns is linked to a brain disorder. Even if we assume that there are thousands of subtypes of brain disorders, e.g., different kinds of epilepsy, and that many diseases change synaptic efficacy without changing structural connectivity, there might still be billions of connectome changes that could lead to the clinical patterns observed in patients with one type of a disease. Clearly, no two patients are the same (neither are no two control subjects).

If there is a multitude of ways how connectome changes could lead to a disease, how can we use brain connectivity information to inform the diagnosis and treatment of clinical patients? First, some links between connectome and consequential brain dynamics might manifest themselves through changes of global network features despite the variability in the changes of individual connections. Examples are global topological changes, observed through diffusion tensor imaging, in remitted geriatric depression and amnestic mild cognitive impairment (Bai et al., 2012). However, the same global changes, say a deviation from the brain's small-world organization towards random or regular connectivity (Reijneveld et al., 2007), could be observed across diseases and therefore limit their use as a classifier for brain diseases.

Second, some changes might be so widespread that they affect the majority or all of the brain regions leaving fewer degrees of freedom for variability in connectomes. The overall pattern of altered structural connectivity in schizophrenia patients (Skudlarski et al., 2010), along with resulting functional connectivity changes (Fornito et al., 2012), would be one example for this case.

Third, changes that are linked to a brain disease might only affect specific circuits in the network. In that way, while the strength of most connections also varies in healthy controls, more consistent changes to specific fiber tracts would be expected for patients. As a consequence, changes in selected circuits would be common for a group of patients but a consistent change for all fiber tracts of a circuit would not occur in control subjects. While this is a potentially powerful approach it does need *a priori* knowledge about the affected circuit. Such circuits might be identified by large-cohort studies in patients or through "knock-out" studies, e.g., using transcranial magnetic stimulation (Hilgetag et al., 2001), in healthy subjects.

Finally, I would propose a novel approach to deal with the variability in brain disorders, which is the use of computer simulations of brain activity, based on the connectivity in individual patients. Such simulations are already emerging as a way to understand the structural correlates of dynamical changes and disease progression (Deco et al., 2011; Cabral et al., 2012; Raj et al., 2012). As shown above, multiple structural connectivity changes might lead to the same changes in brain dynamics, patient behavior, or clinical test scores. Simulating the activity in the brain of individual patients can inform us about the expected behavioral features and thus about the presence or absence of one sub-type of brain disorder. These models can go beyond the observation of patterns in the recordings of brain activity as simulated dynamics could include more complex models. For example, a model based on structural connectivity might include simulated activity of individual neurons or local circuits, which cannot be observed by non-invasive neuroimaging.

Using simulations in a clinical setting has several benefits. First, simulated behavioral features can be mapped to brain activity in patients that is available through fMRI, Positron Emission Tomography (PET), Magnetoencephalography (MEG), EEG, Electrocorticography (ECoG), or recordings in resected tissue (Roopun et al., 2010), depending on the disease. Second, the simulated behavior can be compared with the experimentally obtained behavior to validate and constrain a model: simulated activity can be compared with the clinical recordings of a patient. Third, observing dynamics in networks opens up the possibility to use the tools of nonlinear dynamics and time series analysis to find patterns that could be biomarkers for a given disease. Importantly, changes in brain dynamics might be visible even in cases where the structural connectivity is not significantly different from that of a healthy control group. Such simulations are becoming available both at the local (Blue Brain Project, Markram, 2006) and global level (Virtual Brain Project, Jirsa et al., 2010) and will be support through the Human Brain Project and other initiatives.

In conclusion, there is a large number of underlying structural connectome changes that might lead to the same functional and behavioral changes in healthy subjects and patients. This variety makes the detection of a brain disorder—not just the classification of the type of disorder (Hyman, 2010)—difficult. We propose the use of computer models to use the simulated dynamics (dynamic connectome) based on structural connectivity, rather than the directly measured structural connectivity alone, as a biomarker. In the same way that biology has moved from genes to gene expression data, the use of dynamic connectomes, observing or simulating activity in neural circuits, opens up future potential for clinical applications.

ACKNOWLEDGMENTS

I would like to thank Drs Simon Eickhoff (Düsseldorf) and Stephen Jackson (Nottingham) for inspiring me to work on this question following a discussion at the Fusion Workshop at Korea University. This work was supported by the WCU program through the National Research Foundation of Korea funded by the Ministry of Education, Science and Technology (R32-10142), the CARMEN e-science project[1] as well as another project funded by EPSRC (EP/ K026992/1).

[1] http://www.carmen.org.uk

REFERENCES

Achacoso, T. B., and Yamamoto, W. S. (1992). *AY's Neuroanatomy of C. Elegans for Computation*. Boca Raton, FL: CRC Press.

Addington, A. M., and Rapoport, J. L. (2012). Annual research review: impact of advances in genetics in understanding developmental psychopathology. *J. Child Psychol. Psychiatry* 53, 510–518. doi: 10.1111/j.1469-7610.2011.02478.x

Bai, F., Shu, N., Yuan, Y., Shi, Y., Yu, H., Wu, D., et al. (2012). Topologically convergent and divergent structural connectivity patterns between patients with remitted geriatric depression and amnestic mild cognitive impairment. *J. Neurosci.* 32, 4307–4318. doi: 10.1523/JNEUROSCI.5061-11.2012

Bullmore, E., and Sporns, O. (2009). Complex brain networks: graph theoretical analysis of structural and functional systems. *Nat. Rev. Neurosci.* 10, 186–198. doi: 10.1038/nrn2575

Cabral, J., Hugues, E., Kringelbach, M. L., and Deco, G. (2012). Modeling the outcome of structural disconnection on resting-state functional connectivity. *Neuroimage* 62, 1342–1353. doi: 10.1016/j.neuroimage.2012.06.007

Costa, L. d. F., Rodrigues, F. A., Travieso, G., and Villas Boas, P. R. (2007). Characterization of complex networks: a survey of measurements. *Adv. Phys.* 56, 167–242. doi: 10.1080/00018730601170527

Deco, G., Jirsa, V. K., and McIntosh, A. R. (2011). Emerging concepts for the dynamical organization of resting-state activity in the brain. *Nat. Rev. Neurosci.* 12, 43–56. doi: 10.1038/nrn2961

DeFelipe, J. (2010). From the connectome to the synaptome: an epic love story. *Science* 330, 1198–1201. doi: 10.1126/science.1193378

Felleman, D. J., and van Essen, D. C. (1991). Distributed hierarchical processing in the primate cerebral cortex. *Cereb. Cortex* 1, 1–47. doi: 10.1093/cercor/1.1.1

Fornito, A., Zalesky, A., Pantelis, C., and Bullmore, E. T. (2012). Schizophrenia, neuroimaging and connectomics. *Neuroimage* 62, 2296–2314. doi: 10.1016/j.neuroimage.2011.12.090

Hilgetag, C. C., and Barbas, H. (2006). Role of mechanical factors in the morphology of the primate cerebral cortex. *PLoS Comput. Biol.* 2:e22. doi: 10.1371/journal.pcbi.0020022

Hilgetag, C. C., Theoret, H., and Pascual-Leone, A. (2001). Enhanced visual spatial attention ipsilateral to rTMS-induced 'virtual lesions' of human parietal cortex. *Nat. Neurosci.* 4, 953–957. doi: 10.1038/nn0901-953

Hyman, S. E. (2010). The diagnosis of mental disorders: the problem of reification. *Annu. Rev. Clin. Psychol.* 6, 155–179. doi: 10.1146/annurev.clinpsy.3.022806.091532

Jbabdi, S., and Johansen-Berg, H. (2011). Tractography: where do we go from here? *Brain Connect.* 1, 169–183. doi: 10.1089/brain.2011.0033

Jirsa, V. K., Sporns, O., Breakspear, M., Deco, G., and McIntosh, A. R. (2010). Towards the virtual brain: network modeling of the intact and the damaged brain. *Arch. Ital. Biol.* 148, 189–205.

Kaiser, M. (2011). A tutorial in connectome analysis: topological and spatial features of brain networks. *Neuroimage* 57, 892–907. doi: 10.1016/j.neuroimage.2011.05.025

Kaiser, M., Hilgetag, C. C., and van Ooyen, A. (2009). A simple rule for axon outgrowth and synaptic competition generates realistic connection lengths and filling fractions. *Cereb. Cortex* 19, 3001–3010. doi: 10.1093/cercor/bhp071

Kendler, K. S., Aggen, S. H., Knudsen, G. P., Roysamb, E., Neale, M. C., and Reichborn-Kjennerud, T. (2011). The structure of genetic and environmental risk factors for syndromal and subsyndromal common DSM-IV axis I and all axis II disorders. *Am. J. Psychiatry* 168, 29–39. doi: 10.1176/appi.ajp.2010.10030340

Markram, H. (2006). The blue brain project. *Nat. Rev. Neurosci.* 7, 153–160. doi: 10.1038/nrn1848

Nisbach, F., and Kaiser, M. (2007). Developmental time windows for spatial growth generate multiple-cluster small-world networks. *Eur. Phys. J. B* 58, 185–191. doi: 10.1140/epjb/e2007-00214-4

Price, C. J., and Friston, K. J. (2002). Degeneracy and cognitive anatomy. *Trends Cogn. Sci.* 6, 416–421. doi: 10.1016/S1364-6613(02)01976-9

Raj, A., Kuceyeski, A., and Weiner, M. (2012). A network diffusion model of disease progression in dementia. *Neuron* 73, 1204–1215. doi: 10.1016/j.neuron.2011.12.040

Reijneveld, J. C., Ponten, S. C., Berendse, H. W., and Stam, C. J. (2007). The application of graph theoretical analysis to complex networks in the brain. *Clin. Neurophysiol.* 118, 2317–2331. doi: 10.1016/j.clinph.2007.08.010

Roopun, A. K., Simonotto, J. D., Pierce, M. L., Jenkins, A., Nicholson, C., Schofield, I. S., et al. (2010). A nonsynaptic mechanism underlying interictal discharges in human epileptic neocortex. *Proc. Natl. Acad. Sci. U S A* 107, 338–343. doi: 10.1073/pnas.0912652107

Skudlarski, P., Jagannathan, K., Anderson, K., Stevens, M. C., Calhoun, V. D., Skudlarska, B. A., et al. (2010). Brain connectivity is not only lower but different in schizophrenia: a combined anatomical and functional approach. *Biol. Psychiatry* 68, 61—69. doi: 10.1016/j.biopsych.2010.03.035

Sporns, O., Chialvo, D. R., Kaiser, M., and Hilgetag, C. C. (2004). Organization, development and function of complex brain networks. *Trends Cogn. Sci.* 8, 418–425. doi: 10.1016/j.tics.2004.07.008

Tononi, G., Sporns, O., and Edelman, G. M. (1999). Measures of degeneracy and redundancy in biological networks. *Proc. Natl. Acad. Sci. U S A* 96, 3257–3262. doi: 10.1073/pnas.96.6.3257

Turing, A. M. (1952). The chemical basis of morphogenesis. *Philos. Trans. R. Soc. Lond. B Biol. Sci.* 237, 37–72.

van den Heuvel, M. P., Kahn, R. S., Goni, J., and Sporns, O. (2012). High-cost, high-capacity backbone for global brain communication. *Proc. Natl. Acad. Sci. U S A* 109, 11372–11377. doi: 10.1073/pnas.1203593109

Van Essen, D. C. (1997). A tension-based theory of morphogenesis and compact wiring in the central nervous system. *Nature* 385, 313–318. doi: 10.1038/385313a0

White, J. G., Southgate, E., Thomson, J. N., and Brenner, S. (1986). The structure of the nervous system of the nematode *Caenorhabditis elegans*. *Philos. Trans. R. Soc. Lond. B Biol. Sci.* 314, 1–340. doi: 10.1098/rstb.1986.0056

Young, M. P. (1992). Objective analysis of the topological organization of the primate cortical visual system. *Nature* 358, 152–155. doi: 10.1038/358152a0

2

Functional diffusion tensor imaging at 3 Tesla

René C. W. Mandl[1]*, Hugo G. Schnack[1], Marcel P. Zwiers[2], René S. Kahn[1] and Hilleke E. Hulshoff Pol[1]

[1] *Department of Psychiatry, Brain Center Rudolf Magnus, University Medical Center Utrecht, Utrecht, Netherlands*
[2] *Radboud University Nijmegen, Donders Institute for Brain, Cognition and Behaviour Centre for Cognitive Neuroimaging, Nijmegen, Netherlands*

Correspondence:
René C. W. Mandl, Department of Psychiatry, Brain Center Rudolf Magnus, University Medical Center Utrecht, A01.126, Heidelberglaan 100, 3584CX Utrecht, Netherlands
e-mail: r.mandl@umcutrecht.nl

In a previous study we reported on a non-invasive functional diffusion tensor imaging (fDTI) method to measure neuronal signals directly from subtle changes in fractional anisotropy along white matter tracts. We hypothesized that these fractional anisotropy changes relate to morphological changes of glial cells induced by axonal activity. In the present study we set out to replicate the results of the previous study with an improved fDTI scan acquisition scheme. A group of twelve healthy human participants were scanned on a 3 Tesla MRI scanner. Activation was revealed in the contralateral thalamo-cortical tract and optic radiations during tactile and visual stimulation, respectively. Mean percent signal change in FA was 3.47% for the tactile task and 3.79% for the visual task, while for the MD the mean percent signal change was only −0.10 and −0.09%. The results support the notion of different response functions for tactile and visual stimuli. With this study we successfully replicated our previous findings using the same types of stimuli but on a different group of healthy participants and at different field-strength. The successful replication of our first fDTI results suggests that the non-invasive fDTI method is robust enough to study the functional neural networks in the human brain within a practically feasible time period.

Keywords: white matter, DTI, activation, MRI imaging, task performance and analysis

INTRODUCTION

Neurobehavioral functions depend on a dynamic flow of information between different gray matter brain regions that are interconnected via white matter pathways (Catani and Ffytche, 2005; Mesulam, 2005). Imaging techniques such as diffusion tensor imaging (DTI; Le Bihan et al., 1986; Basser et al., 1994) in combination with fiber tracking (Conturo et al., 1999; Jones et al., 1999; Mori and van Zijl, 2002) allow us to non-invasively study the anatomy of these pathways – but not their activity.

Numerous studies examined the various aspects of using diffusion-weighted MRI in a functional setup (DfMRI) to measure activation in gray matter, using weak (Le Bihan et al., 1986, 1988) or strong diffusion weighting (Boxerman et al., 1995; Prichard et al., 1995; Gulani et al., 1999; Darquie et al., 2001; Jin et al., 2006; Le Bihan et al., 2006; Jin and Kim, 2008; Stroman et al., 2008; Yacoub et al., 2008; Aso et al., 2009; Flint et al., 2009; Kershaw et al., 2009; Autio et al., 2011; Baslow et al., 2012; Branzoli et al., 2013; Tirosh and Nevo, 2013). In our first fDTI study (Mandl et al., 2008) we proposed a non-invasive functional diffusion tensor imaging (fDTI) method that has the potential to detect the white matter fibers that are active during neurobehavioral functioning. In that study, eight healthy participants were scanned on a 1.5 MRI Tesla scanner during a tactile experiment and a visual experiment to assess the validity of the fDTI method. The results of these experiments revealed activation in the contralateral thalamo-cortical tract and optic radiations during tactile and visual stimulation, respectively. Furthermore, these results not only suggested a slowly varying response function for both the tactile and visual stimuli but also that these response functions are different for the different types of stimuli. We speculated that the differences between the response functions could be due differences in perceived intensity of the different stimuli used – the checkerboard stimulus being perceived more intense than the tactile stimulus. **Figure 1A** shows the response functions for a single tactile and a single visual stimulus. In the current study we set out to replicate our previous findings using the same types of stimuli but on a different group of healthy participants with a new fDTI acquisition scheme using a 3 Tesla MRI scanner.

Functional diffusion tensor imaging is based on the assumption that task-related changes in fractional anisotropy (Basser and Pierpaoli, 1996; FA) are a sign of local fiber activity. The principle of the fDTI method as applied in this study is outlined in **Figure 2**. In our first fDTI study (Mandl et al., 2008) the conservative non-parametric sign-test formed the statistical basis to test for tract activation. Note that in the present study we used the more familiar parametric t-test because the findings from our first fDTI study suggested that the usage of the t-test instead of the sign-test produces very similar results. We hypothesized that morphological changes of glial cells (e.g., oligodendrocytes) induced by activity-related increases in extracellular potassium concentrations could lead to shape changes of the extra-cellular space (ECS; Ransom et al., 1985; Sykova, 2004; Beshay et al., 2005) and, in turn, lead to a measurable increase in FA. Indeed, changes in the diffusion profile due to changes in the ECS in white matter have been shown *in vitro* using diffusion weighted imaging in the rat optic nerve (Anderson et al., 1996). An earlier study (Prichard et al., 1995) reported that electrical stimulation induced significant changes in the diffusion properties of brain tissue in rats. Using intrinsic optical imaging (MacVicar et al., 2002) slowly varying activity-related signal changes were measured in the rat optical nerve, which were attributed to glial cell swelling. However, a

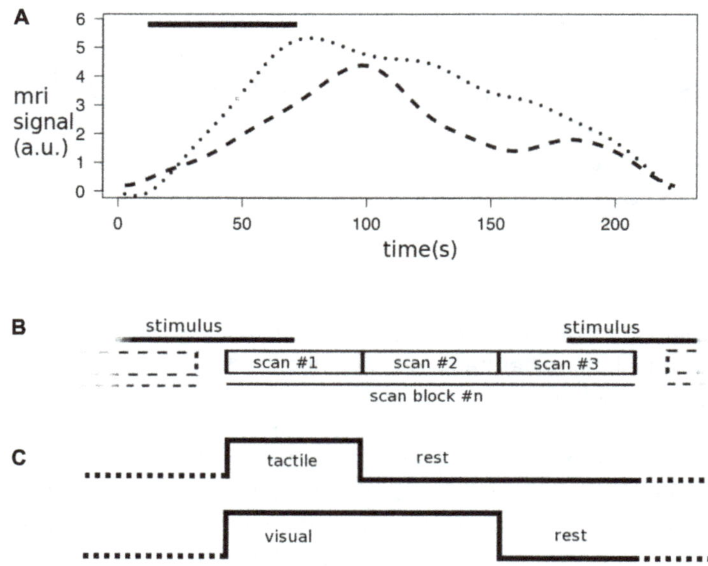

FIGURE 1 | Response functions and task encoding. The graphs represent the time course of the measured diffusion weighted MRI signal for a single tactile stimulus (dots) or visual stimulus (dashes; adapted from Mandl et al., 2008) and the scan in combination with a scan block as used in the fDTI experiment. **(A)** Both the tactile stimulus and visual stimulus (bar) started after 12 s with a duration of 60 s. **(B)** The results of the response function experiment show that the maximum of the response function (dotted line) for the tactile stimulus (bar) falls within the first scan of a scan block while the maximum of the response function (dashed line) of the visual stimulus is found between the first and second scan. **(C)** Therefore in the fDTI experiment the tactile task the first scan is contrasted against the second and third scan, while for the visual task the first and second scan are contrasted against the third scan. The signal during the stimulus is constantly increasing (reflecting a reduction in diffusivity in the transverse direction of the tract).

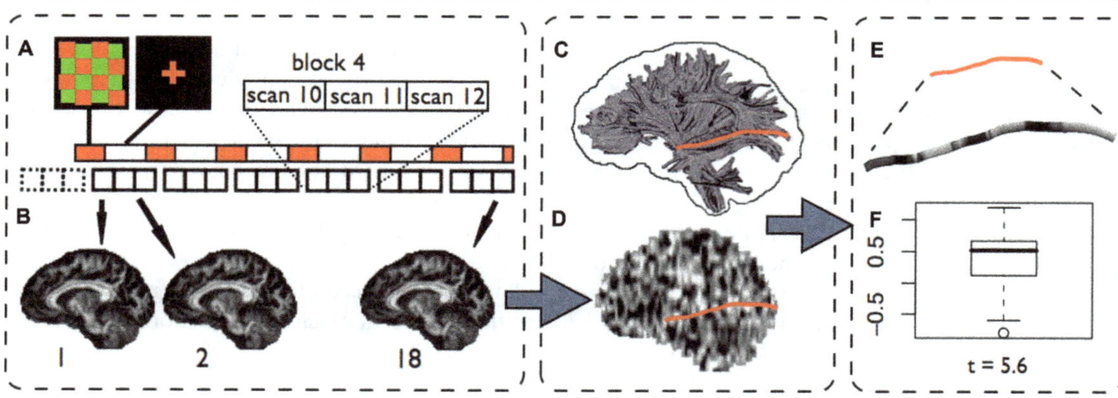

FIGURE 2 | The fDTI method (visual experiment). (A) In the fDTI experiment 1+6 blocks of 3 DTI scans are acquired. The first block (dashed lines) is a dummy block added to correct for possible scanner onset effects and is disregarded in the further analysis. The necessity for the lag between task and scans is explained in **Figure 2**. For each of the 18 DTI scans an FA map is computed **(B)**. A statistical parameter map (SPM) is computed **(D)** on the FA maps using a general linear model. Fiber tracts are reconstructed for the complete brain **(C)** and, for each tract, the *t*-values found in the SPM along that tract were grouped into a single set of *t*-values **(E)**. For each tract a statistical test (student's *t*-test) is done **(F)** on the set of *t*-values to test if the average *t*-value found along the tract is significantly ($t > 5$) greater then zero.

study using the real-time tetramethylammonium (TMA^+) iontophoretic method in combination with intrinsic optical imaging (Sykova et al., 2003) showed that the concentration of TMA+ in the ECS did not change although similar changes in the intrinsic optical imaging signal were measured. Therefore the authors concluded that it was unlikely that glial cell swelling was the primary mechanism for these intrinsic optical signal changes and they suggested that a more plausible explanation may be found in morphological changes of glial cells. Our first fDTI results (Mandl et al., 2008) support this conclusion as the FA-signal changes in the active fibers measured in that study were due to opposite changes in parallel and transverse diffusion coefficients which (for a large part) cancel each other out leading to only small changes in mean diffusivity (MD). If cell swelling was the underlying mechanism for the measured FA-signal changes then an overall reduction in MD is expected because cell swelling would result in a decrease in both transverse and parallel diffusivity in the active conditions. More recent studies (Stroman et al., 2008; Flint et al., 2009) showed that increased levels of potassium lead to changes in both intrinsic optical signal values and MRI proton density measurements for gray and subcortical white matter in rats, suggesting that activity-related changes in the ECS of gray matter as well as white matter can be measured using MRI. In addition, Tirosh and Nevo (2013) showed, using ultra-high field MRI, that neuronal activation results in a 19.5% reduction of the ADC in excised and vital newborn rat spinal cord and concluded that this reversible drop in ADC was due to a reduction in water displacement and could not be related to any hemodynamic effect because the tissue samples were blood-free. Indeed, the contribution of hemodynamic effects to diffusion-weighted functional imaging in gray matter is a topic of extensive research. Various hypercapnia challenge studies show that in gray matter changes in ADC can be measured even when strong diffusion weighting is used. Hypercapnia induces a strong vascular response but no neuronal activity. Because of the strong diffusion weighting, changes in cerebral blood flow and/or cerebral blood volume are not expected to pay a major contribution to the measured change in ADC (Yacoub et al., 2008). However, it was shown that gradient coupling between changes in extravascular susceptibility gradients (i.e., BOLD effect) and the diffusion gradients can result in substantial changes in ADC (Zhong et al., 1991; Hong and Dixon, 1992). These results implicate that DfMRI is not immune to possible hemodynamic effects and posed the question whether or not the reported DfMRI activity-related ADC changes can be fully explained by this gradient coupling effect (Song et al., 1996; Does et al., 1999; Goerke and Moller, 2007; Miller et al., 2007; Lu et al., 2009; Ding et al., 2012; Rudrapatna et al., 2012). Although the results presented in (Stroman et al., 2008; Flint et al., 2009; Tirosh and Nevo, 2013) do provide important evidence that neuronal activation significantly reduces water displacement that can be measured using DfMRI it does not provide information on the relative contributions of the different contrast mechanisms to the measured ADC changes in gray matter. In our first fDTI study we also could not rule out the influence of hemodynamic effects on the measured task-related FA changes in white matter. Indeed, two recent vascular challenge studies (Ding et al., 2012; Rudrapatna et al., 2012) in adult Spraque-Dawley rats using strong diffusion gradients (b-values equal or higher than 1000) showed signal changes in white matter ranging between 1 and 2% both in MD and FA. Similar to these results the absolute percent signal change for FA reported in our first fDTI study ranged between 0.98 and 1.45% but in contrast to these results the absolute percent signal change for MD was much lower (between 0.03 and 0.21%) suggesting that the measured ADC changes cannot be readily explained by hemodynamic effects alone and are more in line with possible shape changes of the ECS.

Normal activity-induced ECS changes, however, are expected to be very small as compared to the physiological noise (Gulani et al., 1999) and a reliable detection of the signal change would require a large number of measurements. In the proposed fDTI method we assume that these activity-related glial shape changes extend over the entire active fiber so that a substantial increase in signal-to-noise ratio (SNR) can be achieved by pooling the signal changes over the complete fiber. It is the adoption of a fiber-based statistics -rather than a voxel-based statistics- that enables us to measure the signal within a practically feasible time period.

In our first fDTI study a tactile experiment and a visual experiment were selected for their expected lack of overlap in activated fibers, which allowed us to study both the specificity and sensitivity of the fDTI method. Also the chance of task related motion artifacts was reduced because a subject's response was not required in either of the tasks. In the present study we used the same types of stimuli but with a new acquisition scheme on a 3 Tesla MRI scanner. For white matter voxels that are part of an *active* fiber, we expected that the FA was higher during the active condition than during the rest condition, thus showing a positive correlation with the task. For the tactile task, activation was expected for the afferent fibers of the thalamo-cortical tracts that connect the thalamus and the contralateral primary sensory area (Kandel et al., 2000). For the visual task, activation was expected mainly for fibers that are bilaterally part of the optic radiation (Kandel et al., 2000).

MATERIALS AND METHODS

Twelve healthy subjects participated in this study. All experiments presented in this study were approved by the medical ethical committee for human subjects of the University Medical Center Utrecht, the Netherlands, and all subjects signed written informed consent prior to participation. For the tactile stimulus experiment the participants were instructed to keep their eyes closed for the duration of the whole experiment. During the active condition, the palm and fingers of the subject's right hand were brushed in a random fashion (approximately 1 Hz) by an investigator. In the visual response function experiment the subjects were instructed to look at a red fixation cross that was projected on the center of a screen visible from inside the scanner at all times. During the active condition a red and green checkerboard was shown that alternated at a frequency of 8 Hz.

IMPROVEMENTS OF THE fDTI ACQUISITION

In the present study we utilized an fDTI acquisition scheme that was improved in several ways to increase specificity by further excluding possible confounding factors (the time settings of this acquisition scheme are detailed in **Figure 1**). (1) We optimized the time settings separately for the tactile stimulus and the visual stimulus because the results of the previous study suggested a considerable time lag in the order of tens of seconds for the visual stimulus, which was not found for the tactile stimulus (**Figure 1A**).

(2) For each type of stimulus, scan slice directions were chosen perpendicular to the expected active tracts in order to minimize the effects of possible motion artifacts that may introduce false positives. If a slice is corrupted because of motion artifacts then for a tract that runs completely through that slice, all points are affected. In contrast, for a tract that runs in the direction perpendicular to that slice only one point is affected. Therefore, the scan slice direction was set in the transverse direction for the tactile stimulus, which is perpendicular to the thalamo-cortical tracts and for the visual stimulus the scan slice direction was set in the coronal direction, which is perpendicular to the optic radiations. (3) The voxel size was set to be anisotropic pointing into the direction of the tracts that are expected to become active in order to reduce partial voluming. (4) In the fDTI experiment 6 blocks of

3 DTI scans were acquired (**Figure 2A**) where stimulus periods (60 s) alternated with resting periods (120 s). Thus, instead of a simple on/off task-design each stimulus period was now followed by two resting periods. In this way possible effects of any periodic signal changes that are not related to the task such as cerebrospinal fluid pulsations (Kao et al., 2008) were minimized.

(5) For both tactile and visual fDTI experiments the stimulus period was shifted with respect to the corresponding acquisition. Now a stimulus period starts at the middle of the last scan of a block and stops at the middle of the first scan of the consecutive block. This shift between the start of the stimulus period and the start of the DTI scan(s) associated with activation was added for two reasons.

First, the time-course experiment described in our first fDTI study showed a slowly varying response function for both the tactile and the visual stimulus (see **Figure 2A**), which was later also reported for gray matter (Baslow et al., 2012). Because of the slowly varying response function the expected signal maximum now falls in the first DTI scan period for tactile stimulus and in the middle of the first and second DTI scans for the visual stimulus. Second, effects of possible faster varying signal changes (such as signal changes due to task-related head motion or blood oxygen-level dependent, BOLD signal) now affect activation and rest DTI scans equally, thereby canceling each other out. Because both activation and rest DTI scans were acquired partially during an activation period (**Figure 1A**).

(6) Rudrapatna et al. (2012) argued that measures derived from the diffusion tensor (e.g., FA) may be devoid of their usual meaning rendering interpretation difficult because the signal is slowly varying during the acquisition of all 7 scans (that is, 1 scan without diffusion weighting and 6 diffusion-weighted scans). To determine if this non-stationarity of the signal would substantially affect the fDTI measurements we circular shifted the diffusion gradient scheme by one for each subsequent epoch. This "round robin" diffusion gradient scheme is detailed in **Table 1**.

SCAN ACQUISITION PARAMETERS

For each experiment a separate T1-weighted scan, two conventional high-resolution DTI scans, and an fDTI scan were acquired. All scans were acquired on a Philips Achieva 3 Tesla whole-body MR scanner (Intera Achieva, Philips, Best, The Netherlands) using an eight-channel head coil.

A sagittal 3D T1-weighted whole brain scan was acquired for anatomical reference, inter-subject registration, the creation of a white matter mask and visualization of the results (acquisition matrix 304 × 299 × 200; FOV = 240 mm × 240 mm × 160 mm; TR = 10 ms; TE = 4.6 ms; flip angle = 8 degrees; SENSE parallel imaging in both phase encoding directions = 1.5; total scan duration 602 s). Next, two conventional transverse Stejskal-Tanner diffusion weighted single shot spin-echo, echo planar imaging (SS-EPI) DTI scans were acquired (FOV = 240 mm × 240 mm; acquisition matrix 128 × 128; reconstruction matrix 128 × 128; slice thickness 2 mm; 75 consecutive slices; flip angle = 90 degrees; TE = 68 ms; TR = 7047 ms; parallel imaging SENSE factor = 3; total scan duration 268 s, no cardiac gating; Mandl et al., 2008; van den Heuvel et al., 2008). The second conventional DTI scan differs from the first one in that the k-space readout direction (anterior–posterior) is reversed. These conventional DTI-scans were used for reconstruction of the fibers (**Figure 2C**). The functional time series of DTI scans (the fDTI set) were acquired during the execution of an alternating sequence of a neurobehavioral task and a resting condition. For the tactile experiment a total of seven sets of three transverse SS-EPI DTI scans (acquisition matrix = 96 × 96; FOV = 240 mm; 30 slices; slice-thickness = 7 mm; no gap; TE = 78 ms; TR = 6000 ms; parallel imaging SENSE factor = 3; 90 degrees flip angle; 6 non-collinear diffusion gradient directions with b-factor = 1000 s/mm^2 and 2 scans without diffusion gradients; scan duration per DTI scan = 60 s) were collected. No cardiac gating was used as it would lengthen the experiments. For the visual experiment the fDTI scans were acquired in coronal direction with otherwise identical parameter settings. The first set is a dummy set that was added to eliminate possible scanner onset effects (e.g., gradient heating). Per set the order of the diffusion gradient directions was circular shifted (**Table 1**). For the dummy set the same ordering of the diffusion gradients was used as for the first real set. For each set one stimulus period was presented. A stimulus period started at the middle of the acquisition period of the last DTI scan of the previous block and stopped at the middle of the acquisition period of the first scan of the current block (**Figure 2A**). The subjects left the scanner room for at least 15 min to rest between the two experiments. The order of the fDTI experiments (first tactile then visual or vice versa) was balanced and randomized.

Table 1 | Gradients settings used in the visual and tactile fDTI experiments.

	Scan block #1	Scan block #2	Scan block #3	Scan block #4	Scan block #5	Scan block #6
Gradient #1	G(1, 0, 0)	G(0, 1/2√2, 1/2√2)	G(1/2√2, 0, 1/2√2)	G(1/2√2, 1/2√2, 0)	G(0, 0, 1)	G(0, 1, 0)
Gradient #2	G(0, 1, 0)	G(1, 0, 0)	G(0, 1/2√2, 1/2√2)	G(1/2√2, 0, 1/2√2)	G(1/2√2, 1/2√2, 0)	G(0, 0, 1)
Gradient #3	G(0, 0, 1)	G(0, 1, 0)	G(1, 0, 0)	G(0, 1/2√2, 1/2√2)	G(1/2√2, 0, 1/2√2)	G(1/2√2, 1/2√2, 0)
Gradient #4	G(1/2√2, 1/2√2, 0)	G(0, 0, 1)	G(0, 1, 0)	G(1, 0, 0)	G(0, 1/2√2, 1/2√2)	G(1/2√2, 0, 1/2√2)
Gradient #5	G(1/2√2, 0, 1/2√2)	G(1/2√2, 1/2√2, 0)	G(0, 0, 1)	G(0, 1, 0)	G(1, 0, 0)	G(0, 1/2√2, 1/2√2)
Gradient #6	G(0, 1/2√2, 1/2√2)	G(1/2√2, 0, 1/2√2)	G(1/2√2, 1/2√2, 0)	G(0, 0, 1)	G(0, 1, 0)	G(1, 0, 0)

G(x, y, z) is the gradient direction vector where x points in the subjects right–left direction, y points in anterior–posterior direction and z points in the inferior–superior direction. For each subsequent scan block the set of six gradients is rotationally shifted by one.

FIBER TRACKING

The two conventional DTI scans were combined to remove susceptibility-induced distortions (Andersson et al., 2003). After correction (Andersson and Skare, 2002) of the gradient-induced distortions and subject motion the diffusion tensors were computed using robust tensor estimation (Chang et al., 2005) based on M-estimators yielding a single DTI volume. The DTI volume was used to reconstruct the fiber tracts for the whole brain with the FACT algorithm (Mori et al., 1999). Parameter settings: minimum FA > 0.15, maximum angle between current major eigenvector and previous major eigenvector <37 degrees, average maximum angle between current major eigenvector and major eigenvectors of neighboring voxels (R-value) < 37 degrees, minimum fiber length 50 mm, number of fiber starting points per voxel $= 8$. The fiber tracking was constrained within the white matter by using a white matter mask that was created on the T1-weighted scan using SPM2 (Wellcome Department of Cognitive Neurology, London, UK) and overlaid on the conventional DTI set. The rigid transformation needed to align the T1-weighted scan with the conventional DTI volume was computed between the T1-weighted image and the diffusion unweighted scan from the (susceptibility corrected) conventional DTI image with the ANIMAL software package (Collins et al., 1995) using mutual information as a similarity metric.

STATISTICAL ANALYSIS

Because the measured FA values and noise characteristics may vary considerably at different positions along a fiber, the effect size of a task-related signal change is not constant for all voxels that are part of the fiber tract. Therefore statistical tests that assume equal effect sizes for all parts of the fiber are not suited to test for fiber activation. In the fDTI method the comparison between active and rest FA values is performed *per voxel* using a general linear model (GLM). The resulting t-value then represents the difference between activation and rest independent of the effect size. The results for all voxels together form a statistical parameter map (SPM) that is used to test for task-related fiber activation (**Figure 2D**). The computation of the SPM is described below. For each of the reconstructed fibers (**Figure 2C**) the set of t-values in the SPM that coincides with the fiber is selected (**Figure 2E**) and tested whether its mean t-value is significantly greater than zero (here we used a fixed threshold of $t > 5$, uncorrected; **Figure 2F**). Because of the differences in response functions for tactile and visual stimuli, different task encoding regressors for the reconstruction of the SPM were used in the tactile and visual experiment (**Figure 1**). The first DTI scan (activation) was compared with the second and third DTI scan (rest) of the set for the tactile stimulus, while for the visual stimulus the first and second DTI scan (activation) were compared to the third DTI scan (rest).

STATISTICAL PARAMETER MAP CREATION

To correct for inter-scan subject motion all different diffusion weighted (and unweighted) volumes were rigidly aligned (using cross-correlation as similarity metric) with their counterparts from the first DTI scan. Next, the FA maps were computed for each of the 18 registered DTI scans. For each FA time series (i.e., the FA value of a single voxel followed over time) a t-statistic was computed using a GLM with two regressors. The first regressor encoded for activation (activation $= 1$, rest $= 0$). The second regressor (with linear increasing values between 0 and 1) was added to correct for effects of possible scanner drift. The results of the first regressor form the SPM that is used to test for activation of the entire fiber tracts (**Figure 2D**). Realignment of the SPM with the reconstructed tracts was done using a linear transformation that was computed between the average diffusion unweighted scan of the conventional DTI scan and the fDTI set using cross-correlation as a similarity metric.

ACCUMULATED RESULTS

The accumulated results here were created analog to accumulated results presented in (Mandl et al., 2008). In short, for each subject a binary map of the complete set of voxels that coincides with the active fibers found is placed in one common space using the linear transformation that registers the subject's anatomy scan with the Montreal Neurological Institute MNI-305 template. Each of the transformed sets is then blurred with a 3-dimensional Gaussian kernel with a full width at half maximum of 7 mm followed by a threshold at a value of 0.1 yielding a second binary map. Finally these binary maps of the subjects are accumulated and overlaid on the subjects' average anatomy. Thus the value of a (colored) voxel represents the minimum number of subjects for which an active fiber can be associated with that voxel.

RESULTS

Figure 3 shows the active fibers found for a single subject in the tactile fDTI experiment and the visual fDTI experiment. For

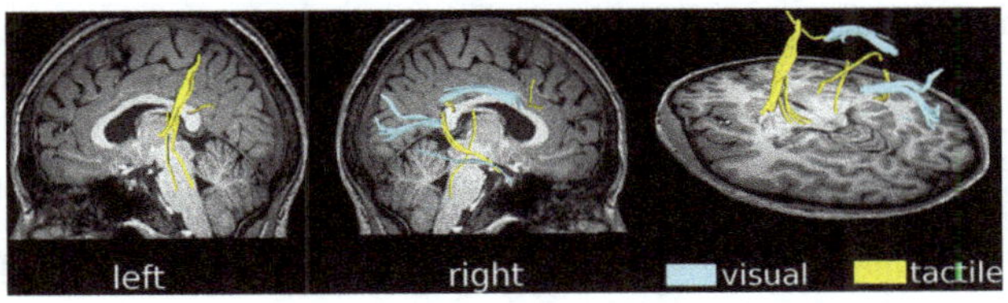

FIGURE 3 | fDTI results for a single subject. Tracts that were found active during the visual task (blue) and the tactile task (yellow) using the fDTI method. During the tactile task, activation was found predominantly contra-laterally for the thalamo-cortical tracts running from the thalamus to the primary sensory cortical area. Activation during the visual task was found, amongst others, for tracts that are part of the optic radiation and the genu of the corpus callosum.

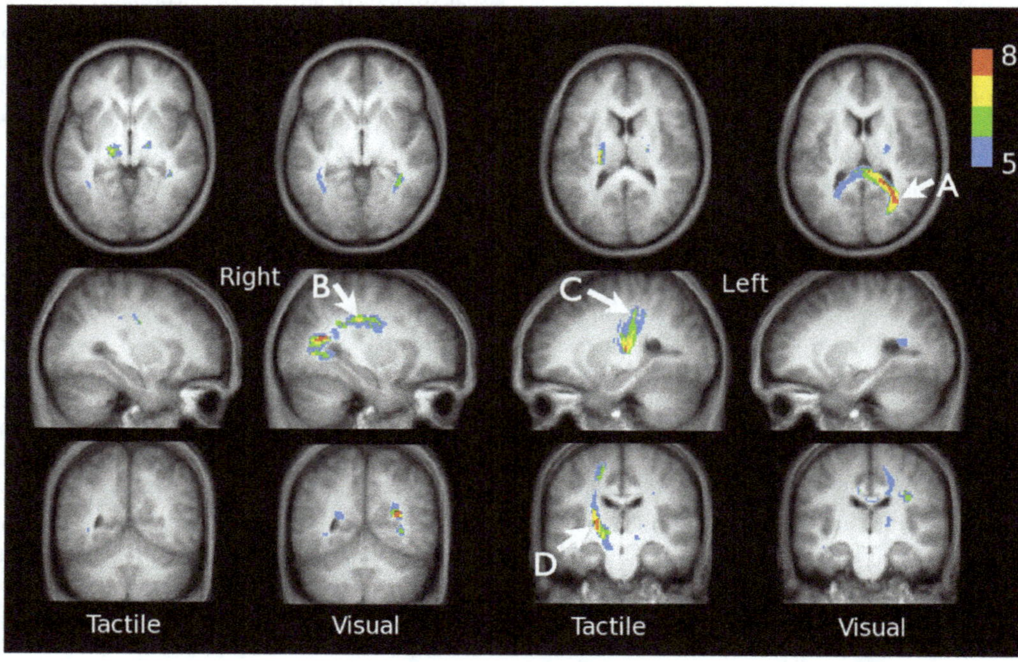

FIGURE 4 | Accumulated fDTI results of all 12 individuals for the tactile and visual tasks. For both tasks the cumulative fDTI results were computed and overlaid on the subjects' average anatomy. The value of a (colored) voxel represents the minimum number of subjects for which active fibers are found at that position. Visual activation is found for tracts that are part of the forceps major **(A)** MNI-coordinate (31, −58, 16), superior longitudinal fasciculus **(B)** MNI-coordinate (31, −24, 34), and at positions that correspond with the optic radiations. The results show that the majority of the tactile activation is found in the contralateral tracts connecting the thalamus and sensory cortex. Maximum cumulative values are found at MNI-coordinates (−27, −30, 34; **C**) and (−19, −22, −3; **D**).

each task, the results of all individuals were placed in a common space to study the cumulative activation patterns (**Figure 4**). For the tactile experiment contralateral activation of the left sensory thalamo-cortical tract was found. A maximum cumulative value 7 of 12 (indicating the number of subjects that had an active fiber running through that voxel) for the superior part of the left thalamo-cortical tract was found at (−27, −30, 34) in MNI space. The maximum cumulative value 8 (of 12) for the inferior part of the left thalamo-cortical tract was found at MNI coordinate (−19, −22, −3).

For the visual experiment bilateral activation was found predominantly in the optic radiations. The maximum cumulative value 8 (of 12) for the visual task was found at MNI coordinate (31, −58, 16), which is located in the forceps major (according to the JHU white matter tractography atlas; Hua et al., 2008). More superior, a local maximum cumulative value 7 (of 12) was found at MNI location (31, −24, 34), in the right superior longitudinal fasciculus.

The mean percent signal change found for the voxels part of the active fibers for the tactile task was 3.47% (SD = 1.86), −0.10% (0.44), −0.65% (2.01), 0.09% (0.57) and 0.10% (0.18) computed for the FA, MD, transverse diffusivity, parallel diffusivity and the diffusion-unweighted signal (B0), respectively. For the visual task the mean percent signal change was 3.79% (1.79) for the FA, −0.09% (0.70) for the MD, −0.35% (1.03) for transverse diffusivity, 0.63% (0.86) for parallel diffusivity and 0.14% (0.25) for the B0 signal.

DISCUSSION

Here we report activation measured along white matter tracts in the brains of healthy volunteers during tactile and visual stimulation using fDTI on an MRI scanner operating at 3 Tesla. This replication of our previous fDTI results on a different group of healthy participants using a different MRI scanner operating at 3 Tesla can be seen as a further indication that the fDTI method can successfully be applied to measure white matter activation. The white matter activation patterns that we found are very similar to the activation patterns found in our first fDTI study. For the tactile stimulus, task-related changes in FA-values were found in the contralateral sensory thalamo-cortical tract. A maximum cumulative value 7 was found for the superior part of the left thalamo-cortical tract at MNI coordinate (−27, −30, 34) which is in good agreement the results of a recent fMRI study that used a tactile stimulus similar to the one we used (Jang et al., 2013). That study reported that for stimulation applied to the palm of the right hand of 15 healthy volunteers the peak activation value was found at MNI coordinate (−38, −24, 60), which is located in the primary sensory motor cortex.

For the visual stimulus task-related changes in FA-values were predominantly found in the optic radiations and forceps major. The latter contains fibers that connect homotopic visual regions. Interestingly, activation was also found in the right superior longitudinal fasciculus – a major fiber bundle that connects to the intraparietal sulcus (Uddin et al., 2010). The intraparietal sulcus is a structure that has been associated with perceptual motor-coordination, visuo-spatial working memory and visual attention (Swisher et al., 2007). Structural changes in white matter adjacent to this structure that were induced by training of a complex visuo-motor skill have been reported previously (Scholz et al., 2009). In that study no significant correlation was found between these structural FA changes and training progress or performance level, and it was therefore suggested that these FA changes could be more related to the amount of time spend training. Our results suggest that visual attention may also play a role in the reported structural FA changes because in our visual task no learning was involved.

The aim of our first fDTI study was to demonstrate that it was possible to non-invasively measure task-related activation in the brains' white matter. Based on the results from that study we hypothesized that subtle task-related morphological changes of glial cells resulted in measurable FA changes. However, we could not exclude possible hemodynamic contributions to the measured signal. Indeed, two recent vascular challenge studies (Ding et al., 2012; Rudrapatna et al., 2012) showed measurable changes in the order of 1–2% for the both FA and MD in white matter. Their results showed that the changes for MD where of the same size (or higher) than the changes in FA. Also, changes in the diffusion-unweighted signal (B0) were even more pronounced (this was also reported in humans; Kershaw et al., 2009). In contrast, the results from our first fDTI showed that the mean percent signal change in MD computed for all voxels part of the active fibers was much smaller then the mean percent signal change in FA. The same pattern was found in our current study with the mean percent signal change in FA for the tactile task being 3.47% and for the visual task 3.79% while for the MD the mean percent signal change was only −0.10% for the tactile task and −0.09% for the visual task. In addition, for the B0 signal the corresponding mean percent signal change was 0.10% for the tactile task and 0.14% for the visual task. This pattern of a relatively large mean percent signal change for FA compared with the mean percent signal change in MD and B0 is more in line with the hypothesized activity-related morphological glial cell changes and suggests that the observed signal changes cannot be explained by hemodynamics alone (Song et al., 1996; Does et al., 1999; Goerke and Moller, 2007; Miller et al., 2007; Lu et al., 2009). Thus, a possible hemodynamic contribution (and if present by itself a valid and interesting contrast mechanism for measuring activation in white matter) may not fully explain the measured fDTI signal. Other confounding factors that are not directly related to neuronal activation may also have contributed to the measured changes in FA. For instance, fMRI studies showed that changes in respiration patterns can introduce magnetic susceptibility changes leading to artificial activation patterns found in white matter (Windischberger et al., 2002). In our approach, however, the role of this type of magnetic susceptibility changes is probably quite limited because of the introduction of the temporal shift for the stimulus onset (**Figure 1A**). Because of this shift, this type (and other types) of fast varying task-related signal changes (e.g., BOLD contrast) are largely canceled out. Furthermore, the stimulus design used in this study (1 stimulus period followed by 2 rest periods) reduces the possibility that any type of sinusoid signal fluctuations could interfere with task-related signal changes and therefore contribute to the measured changes in FA-signal.

Diffusion-weighted MR acquisitions are known to be very sensitive to motion artifacts (e.g., cardiac pulsation, voluntary subject motion). In our first fDTI study we used the same 2-dimensional axial DTI acquisition for both the tactile and visual experiment. In a 2-dimensional sequence, motion artifacts typically affect the quality of the scan at a slice level. For tracts running in parallel with the slice direction (such as optic radiations) the sensitivity to motion artifacts is therefore relatively high because large parts of the tract run trough one single slice. This in contrast to tracts running perpendicular to the slice direction (such as the thalamo-cortical tracts) because here each slice only contains a small part (1 or 2 voxels) of the complete tract. In the current experiments we used a coronal slice direction for the visual experiment to eliminate this difference in sensitivity to motion artifacts. The fact that the results of the current study are similar to the results of our first fDTI study suggests that the chosen slice direction is not a dominant factor in the experimental setup.

Despite the application of the temporal lag to maximize the measured signal change and the increased SNR due to the increased main magnetic field strength the bilateral activation predominantly found for the visual experiment in the optic radiations appears to be less pronounced at 3 Tesla than the activation found for the visual experiment in the optic radiations at 1.5 Tesla (Mandl et al., 2008). This difference in sensitivity may be explained by the lower number of stimulus periods (6) in the 3 Tesla experiment as compared to the number of stimulus periods (12) in the 1.5 Tesla experiment. Moreover, due to the smaller voxel size at 3 Tesla (43.75 mm^3) compared to the voxel size at 1.5 Tesla (64 mm^3) the SNR between a single fDTI scan 1.5 Tesla is comparable to a single fDTI scan at 3 Tesla because the expected increase in SNR with a factor of $\sqrt{2}$ due to a doubling of the main magnetic field strength (3 Tesla vs 1.5 Tesla) cancels out. Also, because of the thick slices used in the 3 Tesla experiments (7 mm) internal dephasing may contribute to a reduction of the SNR.

In the current study we applied a circular shift to the gradient direction settings for subsequent fDTI scans to determine if the non-stationarity of the response function during acquisition (Rudrapatna et al., 2012) would substantially alter the results. The successful replication of the results of our first fDTI study suggests that the effect of a non-stationary signal on the detection of white matter activation is limited although we cannot exclude that additional variation introduced by the use of this circular shift lowered the sensitivity of the fDTI method.

Both 1.5 and 3 Tesla experiments were specifically designed to maximize the specificity of the fDTI method to minimize the change of spurious fiber activation because the main purpose of these experiments was to assess the feasibility of the fDTI method. Further experiments are needed to determine the optimal stimulus and MRI parameter scanner settings to optimize the sensitivity of the fDTI method.

In conclusion, we replicated the results of our previous fDTI study using the same types of stimuli but with an improved scan acquisition scheme on a different group of healthy participants using a 3 Tesla MRI scanner. This replication of our previous fDTI results suggests that the fDTI method can be applied within feasible time period and is robust enough to become a valuable tool that can help us to get a better understanding of the dynamics of functional neural networks in the human brain.

ACKNOWLEDGMENTS

This work was supported by a grant from the Dutch Science Organization for Medical Research NWO ZON-MW VIDI Program (Hilleke E. Hulshoff Pol, 917.46.370).

REFERENCES

Anderson, A. W., Zhong, J., Petroff, O. A., Szafer, A., Ransom, B. R., Prichard, J. W., et al. (1996). Effects of osmotically driven cell volume changes on diffusion- weighted imaging of the rat optic nerve. Magn. Reson. Med. 35, 162–167. doi: 10.1002/mrm.1910350206

Andersson, J. L., and Skare, S. (2002). A model-based method for retrospective correction of geometric distortions in diffusion-weighted EPI. Neuroimage 16, 177–199. doi: 10.1006/nimg.2001.1039

Andersson, J. L., Skare, S., and Ashburner, J. (2003). How to correct susceptibil- ity distortions in spin-echo echo-planar images: application to diffusion tensor imaging. Neuroimage 20, 870–888. doi: 10.1016/S1053-8119(03)00336-7

Aso, T., Urayama, S., Poupon, C., Sawamoto, N., Fukuyama, H., and Le Bihan, D. (2009). An intrinsic diffusion response function for analyz- ing diffusion functional MRI time series. Neuroimage 47, 1487–1495. doi: 10.1016/j.neuroimage.2009.05.027

Autio, J. A., Kershaw, J., Shibata, S., Obata, T., Kanno, I., and Aoki, I. (2011). High b-value diffusion-weighted fMRI in a rat forepaw electrostimulation model at 7 T. Neuroimage 57, 140–148. doi: 10.1016/j.neuroimage.2011.04.006

Baslow, M. H., Hu, C., and Guilfoyle, D. N. (2012). Stimulation-induced decreases in the diffusion of extra-vascular water in the human visual cortex: a window in time and space on mechanisms of brain water transport and economy. J. Mol. Neurosci. 47, 639–648. doi: 10.1007/s12031-011-9700-6

Basser, P. J., Mattiello, J., and LeBihan, D. (1994). Estimation of the effective self- diffusion tensor from the NMR spin echo. J. Magn. Reson. B 103, 247–254. doi: 10.1006/jmrb.1994.1037

Basser, P. J., and Pierpaoli, C. (1996). Microstructural and physiological features of tissues elucidated by quantitative-diffusion-tensor MRI. J. Magn. Reson. B 111, 209–219. doi: 10.1006/jmrb.1996.0086

Beshay, J. E., Hahn, P., Beshay, V. E., Hargittai, P. T., and Lieberman, E. M. (2005). Activity-dependent change in morphology of the glial tubular lattice of the crayfish medial giant nerve fiber. Glia 51, 121–131. doi: 10.1002/glia.20192

Boxerman, J. L., Hamberg, L. M., Rosen, B. R., and Weisskoff, R. M. (1995). MR contrast due to intravascular magnetic susceptibility perturbations. Magn. Reson. Med. 34, 555–566. doi: 10.1002/mrm.1910340412

Branzoli, F., Techawiboonwong, A., Kan, H., Webb, A., and Ronen, I. (2013). Functional diffusion-weighted magnetic resonance spectroscopy of the human primary visual cortex at 7 T. Magn. Reson. Med. 69, 303–309. doi: 10.1002/mrm.24542

Catani, M., and Ffytche, D. H. (2005). The rises and falls of disconnection syndromes. Brain 128, 2224–2239. doi: 10.1093/brain/awh622

Chang, L. C., Jones, D. K., and Pierpaoli, C. (2005). RESTORE: robust estima-tion of tensors by outlier rejection. Magn. Reson. Med. 53, 1088–1095. doi: 10.1002/mrm.20426

Collins, D. L., Holmes, C. J., Peters, T. M., and Evans, A. C. (1995). Automatic 3-D model-based neuroanatomical segmentation. Hum. Brain Mapp. 3, 190–208. doi: 10.1002/hbm.460030304

Conturo, T. E., Lori, N. F., Cull, T. S., Akbudak, E., Snyder, A. Z., Shimony, J. S., et al. (1999). Tracking neuronal fiber pathways in the living human brain. Proc. Natl. Acad. Sci. U.S.A. 96, 10422–10427. doi: 10.1073/pnas.96.18.10422

Darquie, A., Poline, J. B., Poupon, C., Saint-Jalmes, H., and Le Bihan, D. (2001). Transient decrease in water diffusion observed in human occipital cor- tex during visual stimulation. Proc. Natl. Acad. Sci. U.S.A. 98, 9391–9395. doi: 10.1073/pnas.151125698

Ding, A. Y., Chan, K. C., and Wu, E. X. (2012). Effect of cerebrovascular changes on brain DTI quantitation: a hypercapnia study. Magn. Reson. Imaging 30, 993–1001. doi: 10.1016/j.mri.2012.02.012

Does, M. D., Zhong, J., and Gore, J. C. (1999). In vivo measurement of ADC change due to intravascular susceptibility variation. Magn. Reson. Med. 41, 236–240. doi: 10.1002/(SICI)1522-2594(199902)41:2<236::AID-MRM4>3.0.CO;2-3

Flint, J., Hansen, B., Vestergaard-Poulsen, P., and Blackband, S. J. (2009). Diffusion weighted magnetic resonance imaging of neuronal activity in the hippocampal slice model. Neuroimage 46, 411–418. doi: 10.1016/j.neuroimage.2009. 02.003

Goerke, U., and Moller, H. E. (2007). Transient signal changes in diffusion-weighted stimulated echoes during neuronal stimulation at 3T. J. Magn. Reson. Imaging 25, 947–956. doi: 10.1002/jmri.20891

Gulani, V., Iwamoto, G. A., and Lauterbur, P. C. (1999). Apparent water diffusion measurements in electrically stimulated neural tissue. Magn. Reson. Med. 41, 241–246. doi: 10.1002/(SICI)1522-2594(199902)41:2<241::AID-MRM5>3.0.CO;2-E

Hong, X., and Dixon, W. T. (1992). Measuring diffusion in inhomogeneous systems in imaging mode using antisymmetric sensitizing gradients. J. Magn. Reson. 99, 561–570.

Hua, K., Zhang, J., Wakana, S., Jiang, H., Li, X., Reich, D. S., et al. (2008). Tract probability maps in stereotaxic spaces: analyses of white mat- ter anatomy and tract-specific quantification. Neuroimage 39, 336–347. doi: 10.1016/j.neuroimage.2007.07.053

Jang, S. H., Seo, J. P., Ahn, S. H., and Lee, M. Y. (2013). Comparison of cortical activation patterns by somatosensory stimulation on the palm and dorsum of the hand. Somatosens. Mot. Res. 30, 109–113. doi: 10.3109/08990220.2013.775117

Jin, T., and Kim, S. G. (2008). Functional changes of apparent diffusion coefficient during visual stimulation investigated by diffusion-weighted gradient-echo fMRI. Neuroimage 41, 801–812. doi: 10.1016/j.neuroimage.2008.03.014

Jin, T., Zhao, F. Q., and Kim, S. G. (2006). Sources of functional apparent diffusion coefficient changes investigated by diffusion-weighted spin-echo fMRI. Magn. Reson. Med. 56, 1283–1292. doi: 10.1002/mrm.21074

Jones, D. K., Simmons, A., Williams, S. C., and Horsfield, M. A. (1999). Non-invasive assessment of axonal fiber connectivity in the human brain via diffusion tensor MRI. Magn. Reson. Med. 42, 37–41. doi: 10.1002/(SICI)1522-2594(199907)42:1<37::AID-MRM7>3.0.CO;2-O

Kandel, E. R., Schwartz, J. H., and Jessell, T. M. (2000). Principles of Neural Science, 4th Edn. New York: McGraw-Hill Inc.

Kao, Y. H., Guo, W. Y., Liou, A. J., Hsiao, Y. H., and Chou, C. C. (2008). The respiratory modulation of intracranial cerebrospinal fluid pulsation observed on dynamic echo planar images. Magn. Reson. Imaging 26, 198–205. doi: 10.1016/j.mri.2007.07.001

Kershaw, J., Tomiyasu, M., Kashikura, K., Hirano, Y., Nonaka, H., Hirano, M., et al. (2009). A multi-compartmental SE-BOLD interpretation for stimulus-related signal changes in diffusion-weighted functional MRI. NMR Biomed. 22, 770–778. doi: 10.1002/nbm.1391

Le Bihan, D., Breton, E., Lallemand, D., Aubin, M. L., Vignaud, J., and Laval-Jeantet, M. (1988). Separation of diffusion and perfusion in intravoxel incoherent motion MR imaging. Radiology 168, 497–505.

Le Bihan, D., Breton, E., Lallemand, D., Grenier, P., Cabanis, E., and Laval-Jeantet, M. (1986). MR imaging of intravoxel incoherent motions: application to diffusion and perfusion in neurologic disorders. Radiology 161, 401–407.

Le Bihan, D., Urayama, S. I., Aso, T., Hanakawa, T., and Fukuyama, H. (2006). Direct and fast detection of neuronal activation in the human brain with diffusion MRI. Proc. Natl. Acad. Sci. U.S.A. 103, 8263–8268. doi: 10.1073/pnas.0600644103

Lu, J., Dai, G., Egi, Y., Huang, S., Kwon, S. J., Lo, E. H., et al. (2009). Characterization of cerebrovascular responses to hyperoxia and hypercapnia using MRI in rat. Neuroimage 45, 1126–1134. doi: 10.1016/j.neuroimage.2008.11.037

MacVicar, B. A., Feighan, D., Brown, A., and Ransom, B. (2002). Intrinsic optical signals in the rat optic nerve: role for K+ uptake via NKCC1 and swelling of astrocytes. Glia 37, 114–123. doi: 10.1002/glia.10023

Mandl, R. C. W., Schnack, H. G. S., Zwiers, M. P., van der Schaaf, A., Kahn, R. S., and Hulshoff Pol, H. E. (2008). Functional diffusion tensor imaging: measuring task-related fractional anisotropy changes in the human brain along white matter tracts. PLoS ONE 3:e3631. doi:10.1371/journal.pone.0003631

Mesulam, M. (2005). Imaging connectivity in the human cerebral cortex: the next frontier? Ann. Neurol. 57, 5–7. doi: 10.1002/ana.20368

Miller, K. L., Bulte, D. P., Devlin, H., Robson, M. D., Wise, R. G., Wool- rich, M. W., et al. (2007). Evidence for a vascular contribution to diffusion FMRI at high b value. Proc. Natl. Acad. Sci. U.S.A. 104, 20967–20972. doi: 10.1073/pnas.0707257105

Mori, S., Crain, B. J., Chacko, V. P., and van Zijl, P. C. (1999). Three-dimensional tracking of axonal projections in the brain by magnetic resonance imaging. Ann. Neurol. 45, 265–269. doi: 10.1002/1531-8249(199902)45:2<265::AID-ANA21>3.0.CO;2-3

Mori, S., and van Zijl, P. C. (2002). Fiber tracking: principles and strategies – a technical review. NMR Biomed. 15, 468–480. doi: 10.1002/nbm.781

Prichard, J. W., Zhong, J., Petroff, O. A., and Gore, J. C. (1995). Diffusion-weighted NMR imaging changes caused by electrical activation of the brain. NMR Biomed. 8, 359–364. doi: 10.1002/nbm.1940080709

Ransom, B. R., Yamate, C. L., and Connors, B. W. (1985). Activity-dependent shrinkage of extracellular space in rat optic nerve: a developmental study. J. Neurosci. 5, 532–535.

Rudrapatna, U. S., van der Toorn, A., van Meer, M. P., and Dijkhuizen, R. M. (2012). Impact of hemodynamic effects on diffusion-weighted fMRI signals. Neuroimage 61, 106–114. doi: 10.1016/j.neuroimage.2012.02.050

Scholz, J., Klein, M. C., Behrens, T. E., and Johansen-Berg, H. (2009). Training induces changes in white-matter architecture. Nat. Neurosci. 12, 1370–1371. doi: 10.1038/nn.2412

Song, A. W., Wong, E. C., Tan, S. G., and Hyde, J. S. (1996). Diffusion weighted fMRI at 1.5 T. Magn. Reson. Med. 35, 155–158. doi: 10.1002/mrm.1910350204

Stroman, P. W., Lee, A. S., Pitchers, K. K., and Andrew, R. D. (2008). Magnetic resonance imaging of neuronal and glial swelling as an indicatior of function in cerebral tissue slices. Magn. Reson. Med. 59, 700–706. doi: 10.1002/mrm.21534

Swisher, J. D., Halko, M. A., Merabet, L. B., McMains, S. A., and Somers, D. C. (2007).

Visual topography of human intraparietal sulcus. J. Neurosci. 27, 5326–5337. doi: 10.1523/JNEUROSCI.0991-07.2007

Sykova, E. (2004). Extrasynaptic volume transmission and diffusion param- eters of the extracellular space. Neuroscience 129, 861–876. doi: 10.1016/j.neuroscience.2004.06.077

Sykova, E., Vargova, L., Kubinova, S., Jendelova, P., and Chvatal, A. (2003). The relationship between changes in intrinsic optical signals and cell swelling in rat spinal cord slices. Neuroimage 18, 214–230. doi: 10.1016/S1053-8119(02)00014-9 Tirosh, N., and Nevo, U. (2013). Neuronal activity significantly reduces water displacement: DWI of a vital rat spinal cord with no hemodynamic effect. Neuroimage 76, 98–107. doi: 10.1016/j.neuroimage.2013.02.065

Uddin, L. Q., Supekar, K., Amin, H., Rykhlevskaia, E., Nguyen, D. A., Greicius, M. D., et al. (2010). Dissociable connectivity within human angular gyrus and intraparietal sulcus: evidence from functional and structural connectivity. Cereb. Cortex 20, 2636–2646. doi: 10.1093/cercor/bhq011

van den Heuvel, M., Mandl, R., Luigjes, J., and Hulshoff Pol, H. (2008). Microstruc- tural organization of the cingulum tract and the level of default mode functional connectivity. J. Neurosci. 28, 10844–10851. doi: 10.1523/JNEUROSCI.2964- 08.2008

Windischberger, C., Langenberger, H., Sycha, T., Tschernko, E. M., Fuchsjager- Mayerl, G., Schmetterer, L., et al. (2002). On the origin of respiratory artifacts in BOLD-EPI of the human brain. Magn. Reson. Imaging 20, 575–582. doi: 10.1016/S0730-725X(02)00563-5

Yacoub, E., Uludag, K., Ugurbil, K., and Harel, N. (2008). Decreases in ADC observed in tissue areas during activation in the cat visual cortex at 9.4 T using high dif- fusion sensitization. Magn. Reson. Imaging 26, 889–896. doi: 10.1016/j.mri.2008. 01.046

Zhong, J., Kennan, R. P., and Gore, J. C. (1991). Effects of susceptibility variations on NMR measurements of diffusion. J. Magn. Reson. 95, 13.

3

Interpreting the effects of altered brain anatomical connectivity on fMRI functional connectivity: A role for computational neural modeling

Barry Horwitz[1]*, Chuhern Hwang[1,2,3] and Jeff Alstott[4,5]

[1] Brain Imaging and Modeling Section, National Institute on Deafness and Other Communication Disorders, National Institutes of Health, Bethesda, MD, USA
[2] National Institute of Biomedical Imaging and Bioengineering, National Institutes of Health, Bethesda, MD, USA
[3] Department of Biomedical Engineering, University of Virginia, Charlottesville, VA, USA
[4] Section on Critical Brain Dynamics, National Institute of Mental Health, National Institutes of Health, Bethesda, MD, USA
[5] Brain Mapping Unit, Behavioural and Clinical Neuroscience Institute, University of Cambridge, Cambridgeshire, UK

***Correspondence:**
Barry Horwitz, Brain Imaging and Modeling Section, National Institute on Deafness and Other Communication Disorders, National Institutes of Health, 10 Center Drive, Room 5D39, MSC 1402, Bethesda, MD 20892, USA
e-mail: horwitzb@nidcd.nih.gov

Recently, there have been a large number of studies using resting state fMRI to characterize abnormal brain connectivity in patients with a variety of neurological, psychiatric, and developmental disorders. However, interpreting what the differences in resting state fMRI functional connectivity (rsfMRI-FC) actually reflect in terms of the underlying neural pathology has proved to be elusive because of the complexity of brain anatomical connectivity. The same is the case for task-based fMRI studies. In the last few years, several groups have used large-scale neural modeling to help provide some insight into the relationship between brain anatomical connectivity and the corresponding patterns of fMRI-FC. In this paper we review several efforts at using large-scale neural modeling to investigate the relationship between structural connectivity and functional/effective connectivity to determine how alterations in structural connectivity are manifested in altered patterns of functional/effective connectivity. Because the alterations made in the anatomical connectivity between specific brain regions in the model are known in detail, one can use the results of these simulations to determine the corresponding alterations in rsfMRI-FC. Many of these simulation studies found that structural connectivity changes do not necessarily result in matching changes in functional/effective connectivity in the areas of structural modification. Often, it was observed that increases in functional/effective connectivity in the altered brain did not necessarily correspond to increases in the strength of the anatomical connection weights. Note that increases in rsfMRI-FC in patients have been interpreted in some cases as resulting from neural plasticity. These results suggest that this interpretation can be mistaken. The relevance of these simulation findings to the use of functional/effective fMRI connectivity as biomarkers for brain disorders is also discussed.

Keywords: neural modeling, fMRI, functional connectivity, brain disorders, human brain

INTRODUCTION

In the past few years, brain connectivity analyses have become important tools in the investigation of brain disorders [besides the articles in this Special Issue, see, for example, the Frontiers in Systems Neuroscience Special Issue on Brain Connectivity Analysis: Investigating Brain Disorders (Horovitz and Horwitz, 2012; Horwitz and Horovitz, 2012)] [1]. Probably the most common connectivity studies have used diffusion tensor imaging (DTI) [2] to investigate brain anatomical connectivity and functional magnetic resonance imaging (fMRI) to examine functional and/or effective connectivity. Although there still exists some confusion in the literature as to the definition of the latter two terms (Horwitz, 2003), for the purposes of this article we follow Friston (1994) and take functional connectivity to denote a statistical relationship between the functional neuroimaging signals in two or more brain regions (e.g., a correlation coefficient or a regression coefficient), and effective connectivity to mean the direct effect of one brain region's activity on another during a specified experimental condition (e.g., the functional strength of the directed anatomical link from one region to another during a particular task).

[1] Please note that we use the term "brain disorder" quite loosely. In particular, because there are both structural and functional changes during normal development and normal aging, studies of either of these processes can be considered here, since many of the issues that come about when comparing patients and healthy subjects would also be present when comparing subjects in different age groups.

[2] See Appendix for a list of all abbreviations used in this paper.

The earliest functional connectivity neuroimaging studies that used positron emission tomographic (PET) data were acquired during the so-called resting state (e.g., Horwitz et al., 1984), but gave way a few years later to task-based studies (Horwitz et al., 1992), especially when fMRI became available (e.g., Friston et al., 1997; Bokde et al., 2001). Thus, there developed a substantial literature on activation studies of patients with brain disorders employing functional/effective brain connectivity analysis methods (e.g., Horwitz et al., 1995; Bokde et al., 2006; Just et al., 2007; Rytsar et al., 2011). However, during the past decade or so, there has been an explosion in the number of studies using resting state fMRI (rsfMRI) to characterize functional brain connectivity in normal subjects (e.g., Biswal et al., 1995; Yeo et al., 2011) and in patients with a variety of neurological, psychiatric, and developmental disorders (e.g., Cherkassky et al., 2006; Wang et al., 2006; Alexander-Bloch et al., 2010; Lynall et al., 2010; Damoiseaux et al., 2012; Venkataraman et al., 2012; Lynch et al., 2013). The literature on functional neuroimaging connectivity studies in brain disorder patients is now huge, and obviously difficult to summarize. It is possible to generalize, however, and say that almost all published studies have found differences in functional (or effective) connectivity between patients and healthy control subjects. Often, the differences correspond to a decreased connectivity in the patients, although in many instances, increased interregional connectivity has been reported; sometimes, both types of differences are found together (e.g., Horwitz et al., 1995; Damoiseaux et al., 2012; Venkataraman et al., 2012). Note also that it has become widely appreciated that neuroimaging studies of brain connectivity, both functional and structural, have the potential for generating useful biomarkers for the detection and diagnosis of brain disorders and for the assessment of their treatment [for example, for Alzheimer's disease (AD), see (Horwitz and Rowe, 2011; Damoiseaux, 2012)].

Nonetheless, the question does arise as to how these alterations in functional/effective connectivity should be interpreted. For example, some researchers have suggested that an increased functional/effective connectivity may reflect some type of compensatory change that helps maintain normal function in spite of aberrant function in other parts of the brain. Also, can one attribute, as is often done, a reduced functional/effective connectivity to a decreased structural link between two brain regions? A decreased structural link may manifest itself as a reduced axonal input (either fewer axons or less effective synaptic inputs) from one neural population to another. How can we determine if these interpretations of functional brain connectivity analyses are justified? With respect to human brain disorders, it is obviously hard (indeed impossible at present) to actually do this using experimental data, since invasive techniques cannot be employed. Furthermore, the complexity of the mammalian brain mostly precludes any sort of direct comparison between measures of interregional neuronal connectivity and fMRI based measures in non-human animals, although some recent efforts in this direction (Logothetis, 2012), including using optogenetic approaches (Lee, 2011), show some promise. Rather, these issues have started to be addressed using computational neural modeling.

In this paper, we will discuss a few of these neural modeling efforts in the section entitled Simulated fMRI Data and Functional/Effective Connectivity, focusing especially on what has been learned about how to interpret differences in functional/effective connectivity between patients and healthy subjects in Simulating the Effect of Altered Anatomical Connectivity on Functional/Effective Connectivity. We will conclude in The Role of Simulation in the Development of fMRI Biomarkers with some thoughts on the role that neural modeling can play in developing fMRI functional/effective connectivity based biomarkers for various aspects related to the detection and treatment of brain disorders.

SIMULATED fMRI DATA AND FUNCTIONAL/EFFECTIVE CONNECTIVITY

There have been a number of investigators who have developed multi-region network models that can simulate functional neuroimaging data. These models vary with respect to how "biologically realistic" are the elements that comprise each model. Efforts of this sort that deal with the kind of task-related flow/metabolic neuroimaging data generated by PET and fMRI began in the mid-to-late 90s (Arbib et al., 1995; Tagamets and Horwitz, 1998; Horwitz and Tagamets, 1999), and have increased dramatically since then (e.g., Corchs and Deco, 2004; Deco et al., 2004, 2008; Husain et al., 2004; Edin et al., 2007; Marreiros et al., 2008; Smith et al., 2013). Recently, a number of groups have developed modeling platforms for examining simulated rsfMRI data (for instance, Alstott et al., 2009; Honey et al., 2009; Cabral et al., 2011, 2012b; Smith et al., 2011; Ritter et al., 2013). Although some of these modeling efforts have focused on examining differences between healthy subjects and patients, others have used the computational models to address how specific tasks are implemented at the neural level. Relevant to the discussion that will follow, we will illustrate three of these modeling efforts.

The model developed by Tagamets and Horwitz (1998), although initially applied to regional cerebral blood flow (rCBF) PET data, was soon extended to blood oxygenation level dependent (BOLD) fMRI (Horwitz and Tagamets, 1999). The model was designed to simulate a short-term memory task for visual objects. It consisted of a number of distinct neuronal populations along the ventral visual processing stream arranged in the following brain regions (see **Figure 1**): primary and secondary visual cortex (V1), extrastriate visual cortex (V4 and IT), and prefrontal cortex (PFC). The visual feature that was modeled was object shape, and thus the V1 neurons were configured to respond to line orientation (for simplicity, the orientations were restricted to horizontal and vertical). The basic neuronal element in each module was a modified Wilson–Cowan unit (Wilson and Cowan, 1972), which consists of an excitatory-inhibitory pair that can be thought of as representing an extremely simplified cortical column. Each model population contained 81 basic elements. The populations were connected together based, as much as possible, on known primate neuroanatomy. For example, connectivity was such that the spatial receptive field increased as one moved down the object processing pathway. The PFC region contained four distinct simulated neuronal populations whose activities were designed to correspond to the experimental data of Funahashi et al. (1990), obtained from monkeys during the performance of a delayed response task. The model simulated

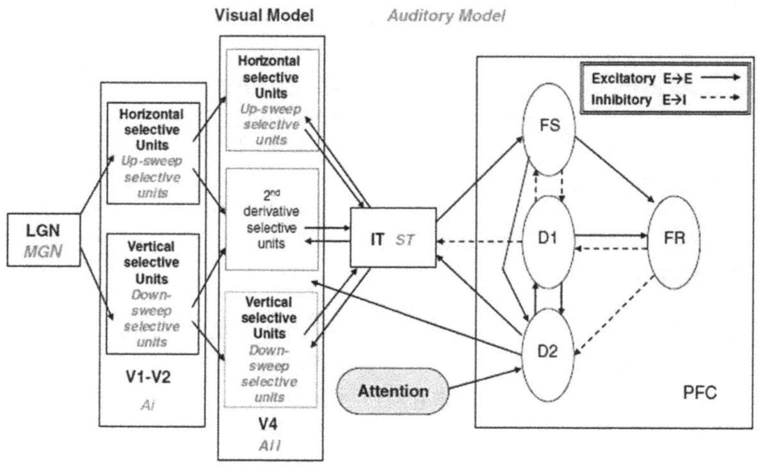

FIGURE 1 | Large-scale neural network models of the visual and auditory object processing pathways (Tagamets and Horwitz, 1998; Husain et al., 2004). Shown are the modules specific to the visual model (LGN, V1-V2, V4, IT) in black-bold and those specific to the corresponding auditory model (MGN, Ai, Aii, ST, PFC) in gray-italics. Within each module are sub-modules. The PFC module is common to both models and shown are its sub-modules. Each sub-module contains 81 basic neural elements consisting of an interacting pair of excitatory and inhibitory units (Wilson and Cowan, 1972). Connections between modules are display (solid: excitatory-to-excitatory; dashed: excitatory to inhibitory). Models perform a delayed match-to-sample task for either visual objects (combinations of horizontal and vertical lines) or auditory objects (combinations of pure tones and up- and down-frequency sweeps. Abbreviations: LGN, lateral geniculate nucleus; MGN, medial geniculate nucleus; V1-V2, primary and secondary visual cortex; V4, extrastriate visual cortex; IT, inferior-temporal cortex; Ai, primary auditory cortex; Aii, secondary auditory cortex; ST, superior temporal gyrus-sulcus; PFC, prefrontal cortex. Taken from Horwitz and Smith (2008).

a delayed match-to-sample task, in which a simulated object is presented for a short period of time, there is a delay period, and a second object is presented. The goal was to determine if the second object was the same as the first. An intertrial interval then occurred, and another trial began. The entire simulation corresponded to multiple trials, as would occur during an actual PET or fMRI study. The properties of the simulated neurons were configured so that their firing patterns were similar to those obtained from electrophysiological monkey studies. The spatiotemporal integrated synaptic activities (absolute value of the excitatory and inhibitory neuronal inputs) were assumed to represent the rCBF in each area for PET (Tagamets and Horwitz, 1998). For fMRI, the integrated synaptic activities were calculated for a time period of about 50 ms (the time needed to acquire a single MRI slice), convolved with a function representing the hemodynamic response, and then downsampled each TR (e.g., $TR = 2$ s) to represent simulated BOLD-fMRI (Horwitz and Tagamets, 1999). Good agreement was obtained between the simulated PET data and the experimental PET data of Haxby et al. (1995) (see Tagamets and Horwitz, 1998 for details). This model was later modified by Husain et al. (2004) to produce a simulation model for auditory object processing. Both the visual and auditory models were subsequently employed to simulate fMRI-functional connectivity data (time-series correlations) (Horwitz et al., 2005; Kim and Horwitz, 2008).

It is important to notice that these kinds of multiregion large-scale simulations require a combination of three component models. The first component is a structural model that indicates how the simulated brain regions are anatomically linked, and what are the strengths of the linkages. The second component is a neuronal model. The third component is a hemodynamic response model that converts the neural activity into a neuroimaging signal. In the simulations just discussed, the structural model was based on primate neuroanatomy, the neuronal model was the Wilson-Cowan unit, and the hemodynamic model was a simple Poisson convolution function acting on the integrated synaptic activity.

An example of simulating human rsfMRI data was provided by Honey et al. (2009). They used a structural model based on diffusion spectrum imaging (DSI) data obtained from five normal human participants originally described by Hagmann et al. (2008) (see **Figure 2A**)[3]. The structural connections were evaluated from streamline tractography values between each pair of 998 cortical regions. The neural model assigned to each of these regions employed the neural mass model of Breakspear et al. (2003), which represents an ensemble of excitatory and inhibitory neurons possessing both ligand-gated and voltage-gated membrane channels. A non-linear hemodynamic model was used to convert simulated neural activity into simulated BOLD fMRI data (Friston et al., 2000) (see **Figure 2B**). Honey et al. (2009) used this formulation to compare simulated rsfMRI data against actual fMRI data obtained in the same subjects from whom the DSI data were acquired. Their main conclusion was that in both the simulated and experimental data, the underlying structural connectivity constrained the pattern of resting state functional connectivity, although some functional connectivity between non-anatomically connected regions was also present. These

[3]The two matrices shown in **Figure 2** were generated by the current authors using the structural, neural, and hemodynamic models originally employed by Honey et al. (2009) and Alstott et al. (2009).

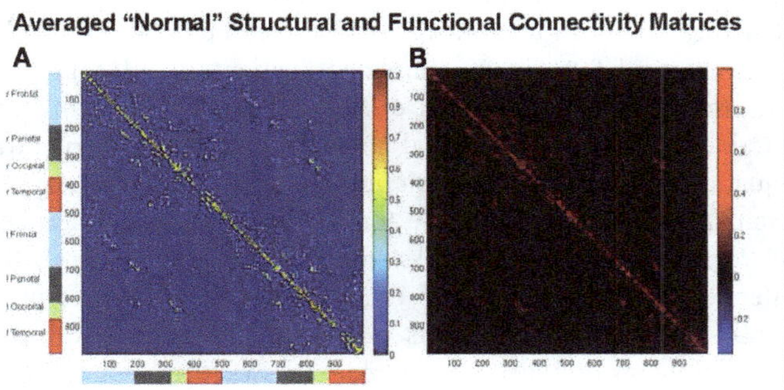

FIGURE 2 | Brain connectivity matrices. (A) Structural connectivity matrix among the set of 998 ROIs of the average of the DSI data of five normal subjects of Hagmann et al. (2008). **(B)** Functional connectivity matrix of Pearson correlations from the computational model used by Honey et al. (2009) and Alstott et al. (2009) for the averaged structural matrix of **(A)**, showing relatively high simulated rsfMRI-FC within lobes, and lower rsfMRI-FC between hemispheres.

findings were supported by a resting state fMRI functional connectivity (rsfMRI-FC) study in monkey by Adachi et al. (2012), who also performed a simulation study employing the modeling framework of an earlier Honey et al. paper (2007).

Gustavo Deco and his colleague have used a comparable modeling approach to that of Honey et al. (2009) to investigate other aspects of rsfMRI data (Deco et al., 2009; Cabral et al., 2011). For instance, Cabral et al. (2011) found that slow power fluctuations in gamma (60 Hz) oscillations at the local neural level could result in long-range interregional resting state synchrony at very low frequencies (<0.1 Hz), indicating that local neural dynamics can have an important effect on network connectivity patterns [see Hlinka and Coombes (2012) for a similar finding]. Cabral and colleagues employed the same structural model as used by Honey et al. [although downsampled to 66 regions of interest (ROIs) from the full set of 998 of the original], as well as the same hemodynamic model. However, they utilized a simpler neural model: the Kuramoto oscillator (Kuramoto, 1984), which has been used extensively to examine the behavior of coupled oscillatory systems. Other component models were employed in other studies by this group. For example, in Deco et al. (2009), the structural model was that of the macaque monkey obtained using anatomical connectivity values from the CoCoMac database (Kotter, 2004), and the neural model utilized the Wilson-Cowan formulation (Wilson and Cowan, 1972). An important insight they found was the critical role that conduction delays between connected brain regions play in allowing synchrony to emerge.

It is worth noting that the main reason different component models are used in different studies is because each study is attempting to understand just a few aspects of the data. So, a neural oscillator model was used when the goal of the study was to relate high frequency neural activity to low frequency BOLD activity, as was the case in the Cabral et al. paper (2011). Some of the other studies that were mentioned placed more emphasis on neural realism, and so models more directly inspired by neurons were employed. In all cases, because there are so many interacting neural units in these large-scale simulations, the simplest neural model that embodied the crucial features of the data was chosen. As more such studies appear in the future, it will be important to determine the degree to which the simulated results depend on the exact nature of the component models that are used. For example, resting state studies may well be somewhat insensitive to the exact neural and metabolic models that are employed, whereas task-based studies may show a strong dependence on the composition of the neural model that is used.

An important issue to mention here is that because these large-scale models can produce multiregional simulated fMRI data that are comparable to experimental data, many of the same analysis techniques that are applied to the experimental data can be applied as well to the simulated data. This is important, given that network analysis techniques, especially graph theory, are commonly employed in MRI studies of structural and functional connectivity (Achard et al., 2006; Bassett and Bullmore, 2006; Bullmore and Sporns, 2009; Sporns, 2012), and as we shall see, these network metrics can be utilized for investigating brain disorders.

Finally, even though the current paper is focused on fMRI functional/effective connectivity, it is worth noting that there also is a vast literature in which brain connectivity analyses are performed on EEG/MEG data (e.g., Gevins and Bressler, 1988; Gross et al., 2001; Daunizeau et al., 2009; Brookes et al., 2011; Rong et al., 2011), and large-scale neural modeling has been employed to help interpret experimental findings (for example, see Wendling et al., 2009; Banerjee et al., 2012).

SIMULATING THE EFFECT OF ALTERED ANATOMICAL CONNECTIVITY ON FUNCTIONAL/EFFECTIVE CONNECTIVITY

One important application of these large-scale simulation models has been the investigation of the effects of various types of brain alterations on functional/effective connectivity. As we pointed out in the Introduction, interpreting the results of a brain alteration in real experimental data is difficult because of the complexity of the underlying neural architecture, coupled with neuroplasticity that can occur in real brains subsequent to the alteration. In a large-scale simulation, however, everything is under the control of the researcher, and, in principle, everything that goes on during a simulation can be tracked and evaluated.

Cabral and colleagues published a study that nicely illustrates what can be learned about bran disorders from simulations of rsfMRI (Cabral et al., 2012b). In this investigation, the effects of structural disconnection on rsfMRI-FC was examined using a large-scale neural modeling framework. The structural model that was employed consisted of 90 ROIs derived from DTI data acquired from 21 healthy participants; the neural model for each ROI, based on the dynamical equations of Mattia and Del Giudice (2002), generated spontaneous neural activity; and the hemodynamic model that the authors used was the Balloon-Windkessel model of Friston et al. (2000). The simulated rsfMRI-FC was evaluated as the temporal correlation between ROI time series, and graph theoretic measures (Bassett and Bullmore, 2006; Bullmore and Sporns, 2009) were employed to characterize the pattern of connectivity among all the ROIs. Two types of structural disconnection were simulated—global and local. In the equations relating the change in neural activity (firing rate) in one region (region n) to that in other regions, there exists a term kC_{np}, where k is the global excitatory coupling between all regions and C_{np} is the structural coupling strength from region p to region n. For the global disconnection simulations, k was uniformly reduced. It was found that a number of the graph theoretic metrics changed, resulting in a less globally correlated and globally integrated set of BOLD values. The second kind of structural disconnection that they simulated was a more localized type, in which Cabral and colleagues successively removed randomly 1% of the possible links (what they termed "pruning the matrix"). The results for this case were similar to that for the global disconnection case—a reduction in functional connectivity leading to reduced global integration.

Cabral et al. (2012a) went on to explicitly compare simulated rsfMRI-FC with experimental data acquired from patients with schizophrenia (Lynall et al., 2010). The experimental data showed that, compared to healthy control subjects, the schizophrenia patients had weakened functional connectivity and an increased diversity of functional connections. Cabral and colleagues tested the hypothesis that these disrupted functional networks in the patients could be explained by a global decrease in structural coupling between cortical regions. They found that a small decrease in the global structural coupling parameter, k, yielded a reduced functional connectivity that resulted in graph theoretic changes similar to those documented by Lynall et al. (2010).

Other simulation studies have examined the effects of focal lesions on rsfMRI-FC, including investigations that employed structural models based on macaque connectivity (Honey and Sporns, 2008) and those that used structural data from humans (Alstott et al., 2009). We will discuss the latter of these. The structural, neural, and hemodynamic models used by Alstott et al. (2009) were the same ones as those employed by Honey et al. (2009): a DSI data set from 5 healthy human participants (Hagmann et al., 2008), the neural model of Breakspear et al. (2003) and the Friston et al. balloon model (Friston et al., 2000). A number of important findings were reported, including one showing that lesions along the cortical midline, in the temporo-parietal junction and in frontal cortex resulted in large and widely distributed reductions in rsfMRI-FC; some of these alterations involved regions outside the lesion site. In contrast, lesions of sensory and motor regions produced functional connectivity changes that were more localized to the area of the lesion (see **Figure 3**).

The studies involving alterations in anatomical connectivity that we have so far mentioned involved simulating rsfMRI data. Task-based fMRI also has been examined using large-scale modeling, and one such paper by Kim and Horwitz (2009) investigated the effect of decreased structural connectivity on task-related effective connectivity. The general question that this study asked was: how should one interpret a significant difference between patients and controls in the effective connectivity between two nodes? In particular, does such a difference imply that there is a corresponding alteration in the underlying structural connectivity between the nodes? Kim and Horwitz used the large-scale neural model of Tagamets and Horwitz (1998), discussed in Simulated fMRI Data and Functional/Effective Connectivity, to address these questions. They reduced the strength of the structural connection from IT to PFC (see **Figure 4**, upper) by an average of 80% in 20 simulated "patients," and compared the simulated fMRI obtained during the DMS task with comparable data from 20 "normal control" simulations. Structural equation modeling (SEM) (McIntosh et al., 1994) was used to evaluate effective connectivity for all the connections between all regions in the network. As shown in **Figure 4** (lower), the effective connection from IT to PFC (FS) indeed was significantly reduced in the patients relative to the controls. So, this simulation result suggests that reduced structural connectivity can be reflected as reduced fMRI effective connectivity. **Figure 4** also shows that the effective connectivity downstream from the induced structural disconnection (i.e., the connectivity within the PFC) also was generally reduced. This result is not unexpected: the disruption in the IT-FS connection leads to incorrect neural processing in downstream parts of the PFC network. The third result from this simulation is, at first glance, unexpected: the increased effective connectivity "upstream" (e.g., the V1–V4 effective linkage) in patients relative to controls. As mentioned in Introduction, numerous groups have reported increased patient functional/effective connectivity (e.g., for AD, Horwitz et al., 1995; Damoiseaux et al., 2012), and in many cases, this increase is attributed to some type of neural plasticity. The simulation produced by Kim and Horwitz (2009) indicates that this interpretation may not always be warranted. In the simulation, no structural alteration in the V1–V4 connections weights took place. Rather, the increased effective connectivity resulted from a reduced feedback effective connection from PFC to V4, which in turn led to V4 being more influenced by V1 activity than was the case in the normal subjects. A major conclusion from the Kim and Horwitz study was that interpretation of fMRI functional/effective connectivity changes in patients relative to controls requires a careful consideration of the entire network mediating the task under study.

What about the situation for rsfMRI-FC? Would similar findings as illustrated by the Kim–Horwitz study (Kim and Horwitz, 2009) occur, or are those interpretational problems found only in task-based fMRI studies? As Alstott et al. (2009) showed, both increases and decreases in rsfMRI-FC occurred following cortical lesions. For example, as illustrated in **Figure 3B**, a lesion centered in the left temporo-parietal junction resulted in strengthened rsfMRI-FC in the contralesional hemisphere. Some of these increases are due to direct loss of inputs from the lesioned area, resulting in greater functional connectivity between right hemisphere nodes. As was the case with the Kim-Horwitz example, these increases are not the result of any change in the strength of the anatomical connection weights.

The studies discussed above obviously did not consider all the complexities that are likely to be found in investigations of brain disorders. Future neural modeling efforts will be needed to address such issues as how the various kinds of neuroplasticity, which can operate over multiple time scales, even ones whose duration are within the time frame of a single scan, affect the functional/effective connectivity of relevant networks. Some of these neuroplastic changes may occur due to changes in anatomical connectivity.

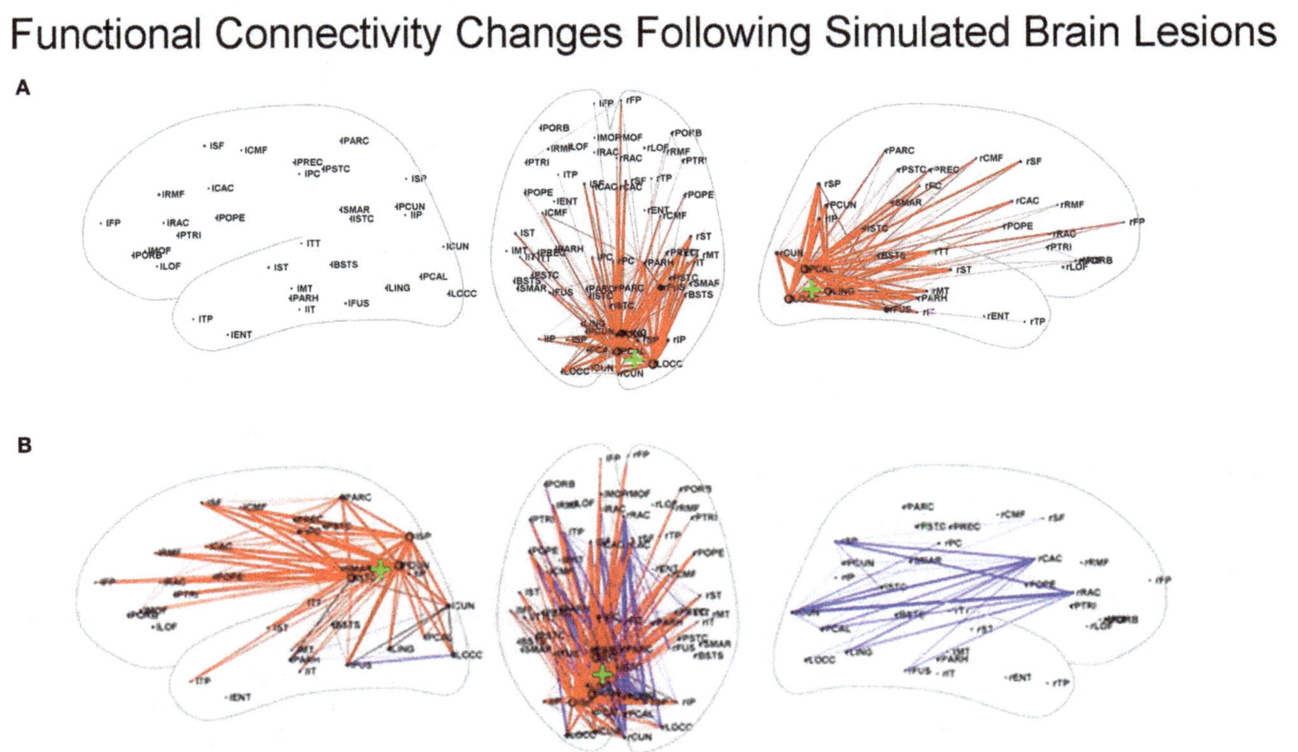

FIGURE 3 | Functional connectivity changes following simulated brain lesions (Alstott et al., 2009). Dorsal (middle) and left and right hemisphere views of significant changes between lesioned and normal groups in simulated resting state functional connectivity (all in the dorsal view; hemisphere specific in the lateral views) between 66 anatomical areas constructed from the 998 ROIs used by Alstott et al. Red (blue) lines indicate a decreased (increased) correlation for the lesioned brains. Center of the lesion site indicated by the green "+." **(A)** Lesion in sensory cortex; **(B)** lesion in temporo-parietal junction. Slightly modified from Alstott et al. (2009); [**(A)** is from Supplementary. Figure 1A; **(B)** is from Figure 4B].

It is worth noting, by the way, that we have oversimplified things by assuming that there is a clear distinction between anatomical and function/effective connectivity. At the level of neuron and synapse, however, this distinction breaks down: in which category does one place axonal sprouting and the formation of new synapses, or even the strengthening of a single synaptic contact? Indeed, one kind of connectivity change can lead to a change in the other—Hebbian learning would be an obvious example. These issues will need to be confronted in future neural modeling studies.

THE ROLE OF SIMULATION IN THE DEVELOPMENT OF fMRI BIOMARKERS

An important issue that was alluded to in the Introduction was the utilization of neuroimaging for generating assorted biomarkers for brain disorders. Horwitz and Rowe (2011) have discussed the various uses for which such biomarkers could be employed[4]. These include detection or prediction of a disorder, differential diagnosis, and staging a disorder and investigating treatment efficacy.

A significant and obvious point related to biomarker development is that such markers are meant to be used on individual patients (or potential patients). As such, an important issue is how likely is it that fMRI will be able to provide sufficient signal-to-noise ratio to be usable in single subjects (Horwitz and Rowe, 2011; Damoiseaux, 2012; Vemuri et al., 2012). Most of the experimental studies we have mentioned were group studies, and although these investigations are important for discerning signal patterns that have the potential to discriminate between patients (actual or potential) and non-affected individuals (or between different types of patients), clinically useful fMRI biomarkers are still a future goal, not a present reality. Two areas of fMRI research that are likely to lead to improvements are in hardware development and in advances in the use of multivariate signal processing techniques (e.g., Smith et al., 2010); for a review, see Smith, 2012.

A second issue, implicit in our previous discussion, concerns what kind of fMRI technique (i.e., resting state fMRI or task-based fMRI) is better to use for a particular brain disorder. The answer depends on two things: which brain disorder is the focus of interest, and which question is the biomarker attempting to address. In some cases, it may be that rsfMRI will be more appropriate. For example, getting small children to do a specific set of tasks could lead to compliance problems of one sort or another. In other cases, task-based fMRI might have a significant advantage. Specifically, task-based fMRI provides the opportunity to record behavioral measures during scanning, and thus, these behavioral measures can be correlated with the changes in connectivity. This

[4]The Horwitz-Rowe article focused on neurodegenerative disorders; however, many of the points made are relevant for numerous brain disorders.

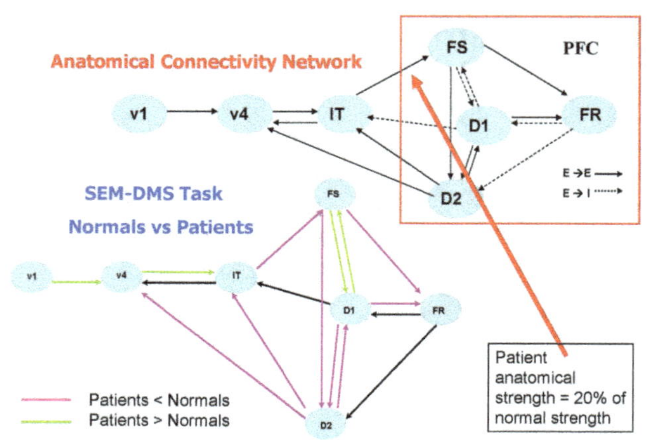

FIGURE 4 | Comparison of fMRI effective connectivity differences between simulated patients and normal subjects for a delayed match-to-sample task for visual shape (Kim and Horwitz, 2009). The top part of the figure shows the nodes and connections of the neural net model used (Tagamets and Horwitz, 1998) (it is the same model shown in **Figure 1**, which should be consulted for abbreviations). Simulated patients' data were obtained by reducing the connection weight between the IT and FS modules an average of 20% of its normal value. The lower part of the figures shows the results of applying an effective connectivity analysis (structural equation modeling) to the normal and patient networks. Significant reductions in patients relative to controls are in violet, significant increases are in green. Modified from Kim and Horwitz (2009).

is a powerful method for determining which connectivity changes are aiding the person being scanned and which are reducing their performance. Similar behavioral correlations have been used with resting state connectivity changes, but the behavioral measure is on a subject by subject basis, not on a trial by trial basis. For example, Venkataraman et al. (2012) found two co-existing patterns of connectivity in their schizophrenia patients: increased frontal-parietal connectivity that was associated with severity of positive symptoms, and decreased parietal-temporal connectivity that was related to negative symptoms.

As an illustration of the task vs. resting issue, consider AD. We know that the pathology of AD can be found in individuals' brains decades before clinical symptoms appear (Reiman et al., 1996; Hampel et al., 2011), and young adults at risk for developing late-onset AD show default mode network (DMN) alterations (Filippini et al., 2009). Given this situation, if an appropriate therapy were available, when should it be given? One might want to start it before a patient demonstrates cognitive deficiency (in which case there may be a significant reduction in viable brain tissue), but perhaps not years or decades before, given the likely costs of the treatment and the potential side-effects of the therapy. In analogy with cardiovascular disease, a "cognitive stress test" during fMRI scanning might provide a way to assess neural integrity. However, one study (Fleisher et al., 2009) has been used to argue against task-based fMRI studies and in favor of rsfMRI in AD. Fleisher et al. showed that rsfMRI of the DMN had a larger effect size than did an fMRI encoding task for distinguishing AD high-risk from low-risk groups. However, it should be noted that although functional connectivity was utilized for the rsfMRI portion of the study, the researchers only used differences in regional BOLD deactivation in DMN nodes during the encoding part of the investigation. As Horwitz and Rowe (2011) have suggested, a task-base network analysis, targeting a network that shows early impairment in AD (such as memory), might be more sensitive compared to examining individual region of interests, since network analysis is intrinsically multivariate. One would determine if the at-risk subject's data fit the network defined by healthy control subjects performing the same task. If the fit is bad, that would suggest that therapy might be warranted. This scheme is based on the notion that neuroplasticity enables behavioral performance to be maintained during the many years during which brain pathology builds up.

As we have just seen, progress has been slow in developing fMRI based biomarkers. Among the reasons for this are the difficulty in performing neuroimaging studies on patients, and importantly, not being able to actually "know the answer." Of the patients at risk for a given disorder, how many will actually get the disorder, and when will they get it? Patient variability is often huge, and different individuals could have different amounts of neuroplasticity over the years during which a disorder may have gone undiagnosed. How do we know that a group difference in some fMRI metric will be large enough in individuals to be able to distinguish a single subject with a high sensitivity and specificity? Note that the problem is not just scanner signal-to-noise, as was mentioned earlier. Rather, the additional problem is that there is large subject-to-subject variability in humans, even in healthy subjects—structural brain differences (e.g., see Amunts and Zilles, 2001), and functional differences (e.g., see Kanwisher and Yovel, 2006).

Computational neural modeling may provide a method to circumvent some of these issues in attempting to determine if an fMRI based metric can serve as a biomarker for detecting a brain abnormality. As an illustration, how weak can a brain structural disconnection be so that it is undetectable using rsfMRI-FC analysis? In our review of the simulation studies of Deco, Cabral and their group and Alstott, Honey, Sporns and their colleagues, the extent of the structural damage was quite large in many cases. For example, Alstott et al. (2009) found in one of their analyses many significant differences in functional connectivity in 5 subjects when they deleted 50 ROIs from an anatomical area (see **Figure 3** for two examples). Using the same set of models (structural, neural, and hemodynamic) as Alstott and collaborators, we targeted two anatomical areas for modification: the left precuneus (LPr) and the left medial frontal cortex (LMPF). All modifications were performed on the 25 ROIs closest in Euclidean distance to the center of the targeted areas. Specifically, the structural connectivities in a targeted area were scaled by 0.5 from the normal values. We examined focal, unidirectional, and bidirectional modifications. In focal alterations, connections among the 25 ROIs in a single anatomical area were scaled by 0.5, but connections between these targeted ROIs and all other ROIs in the cortex were left unmodified. Bidirectional and unidirectional structural alterations were only applied to the two separate anatomical regions—LPr and LMPF. In bidirectional modifications, the connections from one set of 25 target ROIs to and from the second set of 25 target ROIs were scaled by the specified amount of 0.5. In unidirectional modifications, the connections from one set of ROIs in LMPF to the

LPr set of ROIs were scaled, but the connections from the latter set of ROIs to the former set were left intact.

Simulations were run for 10 "normals" subjects and 10 "patients." Variation in the subjects was introduced by adding or subtracting to all the structural connection weights random numbers from a Gaussian distribution with a standard deviation of 0.01. Pearson correlations between the time series of the simulated BOLD activity from each anatomical area for each "normal" subject and for each "patient" were evaluated. Given the small number of "subjects" (10 in each group), and the relatively weak reduction of structural connectivity between just two brain areas, it is not surprising that there were few robust group differences. Indeed, no significant group differences in rsfMRI-FC between the two targeted areas LPr and LMPF were found in any of the cases (focal, unidirectional, bidirectional). These simulation results thus indicate the relative insensitivity of simple rsfMRI-FC to detecting the presence of structural modifications that are weak and of restricted extent, even if one knows where to look. That is, not much change occurs when one input is reduced to areas that have inputs from multiple other areas. Simulations could be used to see if the situation is different when the modification affects a connection between nodes engaged in a task, as was the case for the Kim-Horwitz simulation (Kim and Horwitz, 2009) that was discussed earlier, but that would require adjusting the structural and neural models so that a specific task can be performed. Moreover, newer experimental and data analysis procedure could arise to improve the situation. For instance, high spatial resolution MRI may be able to find mild abnormalities in either structural or functional connectivity in the future.

CONCLUSIONS

In this paper we reviewed some recent efforts at using neural modeling to help understand and interpret human neuroimaging data comparing patients with brain disorders to healthy subjects. Experimental neuroimaging data provide macroscopic measures of brain structure and function. In the case of fMRI, these data are indirect measures of function; the signals are those of the metabolic/hemodynamic consequences of neural activity. Among the factors confounding the interpretation of such data in patients are the sheer complexity of neural anatomy and connectivity and the immense plasticity of the brain. Large-scale neural modeling provides a way to study such a system and investigate how the size and extent of various modifications translate into alterations in neuroimaging signals. Furthermore, because we know what alterations actually took place in the modeled brains, potential interpretations of actual data can be checked against the simulated data.

Our review of several studies that explored the fMRI consequences of alterations in anatomical connectivity lead to several conclusions. First, interpretation of changes in either functional or effective connectivity is not as straightforward as one might first suppose. Although a weakening of the structural connection strength between brain areas can appear as a decreased functional/effective connection, decreases and increases in functional/effective connectivity between areas not directly affected by the brain alteration are also found. Essentially, one must keep in mind that in a functional network, one cannot just change one link; functional networks are such that changes in one part of the network result in changes everywhere else (although not all these changes will be large enough to be statistically significant). Moreover, some of the changes in parts of a network unaffected by the structural alterations may result in a strengthening of the functional/effective connectivity, but these changes are not necessarily the result of neuroplasticity. Task-based fMRI may be a better choice than rsfMRI to deal with this issue, since it is often possible in task-based fMRI to acquire performance data during the scanning. Such data can then be correlated with the measured functional/effective connectivity, and the results of such an analysis may strengthen a claim for neuroplasticity mediating the altered connection. The net conclusion from all this is that the reverse inference—that a change in functional/effective connectivity in a patient means that there is a corresponding change in the underlying structural connectivity—is unwarranted.

We also discussed utilizing large-scale neural modeling as a tool for helping to develop fMRI resting state and/or task-based biomarkers for brain disorders. This is an area that is just beginning, but it does have potential advantages, especially in terms of cost and time. It is cheaper and less time consuming to run a large number of simulations than it is to find subjects and run fMRI experiments. But little work has been done in this area, so it will be a while before one can assess whether or not modeling can provide significant help in deciding which potential biomarkers are viable.

ACKNOWLEDGMENTS

This work was supported by the Intramural Research Programs of the National Institute on Deafness and Other Communication Disorders, the National Institute of Mental Health, and the National Institute of Biomedical Imaging and Bioengineering, all part of the National Institutes of Health. The simulations performed for this paper utilized the high-performance computational capabilities of the Biowulf Linux cluster at the National Institutes of Health, Bethesda, MD. The authors wish to thank the two reviewers for a number of useful comments and suggestions.

REFERENCES

Achard, S., Salvador, R., Whitcher, B., Suckling, J., and Bullmore, E. (2006). A resilient, low-frequency, small-world human brain functional network with highly connected association cortical hubs. *J. Neurosci.* 26, 63–72. doi: 10.1523/JNEUROSCI.3874-05.2006

Adachi, Y., Osada, T., Sporns, O., Watanabe, T., Matsui, T., Miyamoto, K., et al. (2012). Functional connectivity between anatomically unconnected areas is shaped by collective network-level effects in the macaque cortex. *Cereb. Cortex* 22, 1586–1592. doi: 10.1093/cercor/bhr234

Alexander-Bloch, A. F., Gogtay, N., Meunier, D., Birn, R., Clasen, L., Lalonde, F., et al. (2010). Disrupted modularity and local connectivity of brain functional networks in childhood-onset schizophrenia. *Front. Syst. Neurosci.* 4:147. doi: 10.3389/fnsys.2010.00147

Alstott, J., Breakspear, M., Hagmann, P., Cammoun, L., and Sporns, O. (2009). Modeling the impact of lesions in the human brain. *PLoS Comput. Biol.* 5:e1000408. doi: 10.1371/journal.pcbi.1000408

Amunts, K., and Zilles, K. (2001). "Advances in cytoarchitectonic mapping of the human cerebral cortex," in *Anatomical Basis of Functional Magnetic Resonance Imaging,* Vol. 11, eds T. P. Naidich, T. A. Yousry, and V. P. Mathews

(Philadelphia, PA: Harcourt), 151–169.

Arbib, M. A., Bischoff, A., Fagg, A. H., and Grafton, S. T. (1995). Synthetic PET: analyzing large-scale properties of neural networks. *Hum. Brain Mapp.* 2, 225–233. doi: 10.1002/hbm.460020404

Banerjee, A., Pillai, A. S., and Horwitz, B. (2012). Using large-scale neural models to interpret connectivity measures of cortico-cortical dynamics at millisecond temporal resolution. *Front. Syst. Neurosci.* 5:102. doi: 10.3389/fnsys.2011.00102

Bassett, D. S., and Bullmore, E. (2006). Small-world brain networks. *Neuroscientist* 12, 512–523. doi: 10.1177/1073858406293182

Biswal, B., Yetkin, F. Z., Haughton, V. M., and Hyde, J. S. (1995). Functional connectivity in the motor cortex of resting human brain using echo-planar MRI. *Magn. Reson. Med.* 34, 537–541. doi: 10.1002/mrm.1910340409

Bokde, A. L., Lopez-Bayo, P., Meindl, T., Pechler, S., Born, C., Faltraco, F., et al. (2006). Functional connectivity of the fusiform gyrus during a face-matching task in subjects with mild cognitive impairment. *Brain* 129, 1113–1124. doi: 10.1093/brain/awl051

Bokde, A. L., Tagamets, M.-A., Friedman, R. B., and Horwitz, B. (2001). Functional interactions of the inferior frontal cortex during the processing of words and word-like stimuli. *Neuron* 30, 609–617. doi: 10.1016/S0896-6273(01)00288-4

Breakspear, M., Terry, J. R., and Friston, K. J. (2003). Modulation of excitatory synaptic coupling facilitates synchronization and complex dynamics in a biophysical model of neuronal dynamics. *Network* 14, 703–732. doi: 10.1088/0954-898X/14/4/305

Brookes, M. J., Hale, J. R., Zumer, J. M., Stevenson, C. M., Francis, S. T., Barnes, G. R., et al. (2011). Measuring functional connectivity using MEG: methodology and comparison with fcMRI. *Neuroimage* 56, 1082–1104. doi: 10.1016/j.neuroimage.2011.02.054

Bullmore, E., and Sporns, O. (2009). Complex brain networks: graph theoretical analysis of structural and functional systems. *Nat. Rev. Neurosci.* 10, 186–198. doi: 10.1038/nrn2575

Cabral, J., Hugues, E., Sporns, O., and Deco, G. (2011). Role of local network oscillations in resting-state functional connectivity. *Neuroimage* 57, 130–139. doi: 10.1016/j.neuroimage.2011.04.010

Cabral, J., Kringelbach, M. L., and Deco, G. (2012a). Functional graph alterations in schizophrenia: a result from a global anatomic decoupling? *Pharmacopsychiatry* 45(Suppl. 1), S57–S64. doi: 10.1055/s-0032-1309001

Cabral, J., Hugues, E., Kringelbach, M. L., and Deco, G. (2012b). Modeling the outcome of structural disconnection on resting-state functional connectivity. *Neuroimage* 62, 1342–1353. doi: 10.1016/j.neuroimage.2012.06.007

Cherkassky, V. L., Kana, R. K., Keller, T. A., and Just, M. A. (2006). Functional connectivity in a baseline resting-state network in autism. *Neuroreport* 17, 1687–1690. doi: 10.1097/01.wnr.0000239956.45448.4c

Corchs, S., and Deco, G. (2004). Feature-based attention in human visual cortex: simulation of fMRI data. *Neuroimage* 21, 36–45. doi: 10.1016/j.neuroimage.2003.08.045

Damoiseaux, J. S. (2012). Resting-state fMRI as a biomarker for Alzheimer's disease? *Alzheimers Res. Ther.* 4, 8. doi: 10.1186/alzrt106

Damoiseaux, J. S., Prater, K. E., Miller, B. L., and Greicius, M. D. (2012). Functional connectivity tracks clinical deterioration in Alzheimer's disease. *Neurobiol. Aging* 33, 828.e19–828.e30. doi: 10.1016/j.neurobiolaging.2011.06.024

Daunizeau, J., Kiebel, S. J., and Friston, K. J. (2009). Dynamic causal modelling of distributed electromagnetic responses. *Neuroimage* 47, 590–601. doi: 10.1016/j.neuroimage.2009.04.062

Deco, G., Jirsa, V., McIntosh, A. R., Sporns, O., and Kotter, R. (2009). Key role of coupling, delay, and noise in resting brain fluctuations. *Proc. Natl. Acad. Sci. U.S.A.* 106, 10302–10307. doi: 10.1073/pnas.0901831106

Deco, G., Jirsa, V. K., Robinson, P. A., Breakspear, M., and Friston, K. (2008). The dynamic brain: from spiking neurons to neural masses and cortical fields. *PLoS Comput. Biol.* 4:e1000092. doi: 10.1371/journal.pcbi.1000092

Deco, G., Rolls, E. T., and Horwitz, B. (2004). "What" and "where" in visual working memory: a computational neurodynamical perspective for integrating fMRI and single-cell data. *J. Cogn. Neurosci.* 16, 683–701. doi: 10.1162/089892904323057380

Edin, F., Macoveanu, J., Olesen, P., Tegner, J., and Klingberg, T. (2007). Stronger synaptic connectivity as a mechanism behind development of working memory-related brain activity during childhood. *J. Cogn. Neurosci.* 19, 750–760. doi: 10.1162/jocn.2007.19.5.750

Filippini, N., MacIntosh, B. J., Hough, M. G., Goodwin, G. M., Frisoni, G. B., Smith, S. M., et al. (2009). Distinct patterns of brain activity in young carriers of the APOE-epsilon4 allele. *Proc. Natl. Acad. Sci. U.S.A.* 106, 7209–7214. doi: 10.1073/pnas.0811879106

Fleisher, A. S., Sherzai, A., Taylor, C., Langbaum, J. B., Chen, K., and Buxton, R. B. (2009). Resting-state BOLD networks versus task-associated functional MRI for distinguishing Alzheimer's disease risk groups. *Neuroimage* 47, 1678–1690. doi: 10.1016/j.neuroimage.2009.06.021

Friston, K. J. (1994). Functional and effective connectivity in neuroimaging: a synthesis. *Hum. Brain Mapp.* 2, 56–78. doi: 10.1002/hbm.460020107

Friston, K. J., Buechel, C., Fink, G. R., Morris, J., Rolls, E., and Dolan, R. J. (1997). Psychophysiological and modulatory interactions in neuroimaging. *Neuroimage* 6, 218–229. doi: 10.1006/nimg.1997.0291

Friston, K. J., Mechelli, A., Turner, R., and Price, C. J. (2000). Nonlinear responses in fMRI: the balloon model, volterra kernels, and other hemodynamics. *Neuroimage* 12, 466–477. doi: 10.1006/nimg.2000.0630

Funahashi, S., Bruce, C., and Goldman-Rakic, P. S. (1990). Visuospatial coding in primate prefrontal neurons revealed by oculomotor paradigms. *J. Neurophysiol.* 63, 814–831.

Gevins, A. S., and Bressler, S. L. (1988). "Functional topography of the human brain," in *Functional Brain Imaging*, eds G. Pfurtscheller and F. H. Lopes da Silva (Bern: Hans Luber Publishers), 99–116.

Gross, J., Kujala, J., Hämäläinen, M., Timmermann, L., Schnitzler, A., and Salmelin, R. (2001). Dynamic imaging of coherent sources: studying neural interactions in the human brain. *Proc. Natl. Acad. Sci. U.S.A.* 98, 694–699. doi: 10.1073/pnas.98.2.694

Hagmann, P., Cammoun, L., Gigandet, X., Meuli, R., Honey, C. J., Wedeen, V. J., et al. (2008). Mapping the structural core of human cerebral cortex. *PLoS Biol.* 6:e159. doi: 10.1371/journal.pbio.0060159

Hampel, H., Wilcock, G., Andrieu, S., Aisen, P., Blennow, K., Broich, K., et al. (2011). Biomarkers for Alzheimer's disease therapeutic trials. *Prog. Neurobiol.* 95, 579–593. doi: 10.1016/j.pneurobio.2010.11.005

Haxby, J. V., Ungerleider, L. G., Horwitz, B., Rapoport, S. I., and Grady, C. L. (1995). Hemispheric differences in neural systems for face working memory: a PET-rCBF study. *Hum. Brain Mapp.* 3, 68–82. doi: 10.1002/hbm.460030204

Hlinka, J., and Coombes, S. (2012). Using computational models to relate structural and functional brain connectivity. *Eur. J. Neurosci.* 36, 2137–2145. doi: 10.1111/j.1460-9568.2012.08081.x

Honey, C. J., Kotter, R., Breakspear, M., and Sporns, O. (2007). Network structure of cerebral cortex shapes functional connectivity on multiple time scales. *Proc. Natl. Acad. Sci. U.S.A.* 104, 10240–10245. doi: 10.1073/pnas.0701519104

Honey, C. J., and Sporns, O. (2008). Dynamical consequences of lesions in cortical networks. *Hum. Brain Mapp.* 29, 802–809. doi: 10.1002/hbm.20579

Honey, C. J., Sporns, O., Cammoun, L., Gigandet, X., Thiran, J. P., Meuli, R., et al. (2009). Predicting human resting-state functional connectivity from structural connectivity. *Proc. Natl. Acad. Sci. U.S.A.* 106, 2035–2040. doi: 10.1073/pnas.0811168106

Horovitz, S. G., and Horwitz, B. (2012). Introduction to special topic - brain connectivity analysis: investigating brain disorders. Part 2: original research articles. *Front. Syst. Neurosci.* 6:4. doi: 10.3389/fnsys.2012.00004

Horwitz, B. (2003). The elusive concept of brain connectivity. *Neuroimage* 19, 466–470. doi: 10.1016/S1053-8119(03)00112-5

Horwitz, B., Duara, R., and Rapoport, S. I. (1984). Intercorrelations of glucose metabolic rates between brain regions: application to healthy males in a state of reduced sensory input. *J. Cereb. Blood Flow Metab.* 4, 484–499. doi: 10.1038/jcbfm.1984.73

Horwitz, B., Grady, C. L., Haxby, J. V., Ungerleider, L. G., Schapiro, M. B., Mishkin, M., et al. (1992). Functional associations among human posterior extrastriate brain regions during object and spatial vision. *J. Cogn. Neurosci.* 4, 311–322. doi: 10.1162/jocn.1992.4.4.311

Horwitz, B., and Horovitz, S. G. (2012). Introduction to special topic - brain connectivity analysis: investigating brain disorders. Part 1: the review articles. *Front. Syst. Neurosci.* 6:3. doi: 10.3389/fnsys.2012.00003

Horwitz, B., McIntosh, A. R., Haxby, J. V., Furey, M., Salerno, J. A., Schapiro, M. B., et al. (1995). Network analysis of PET-mapped visual pathways in Alzheimer type dementia. *Neuroreport* 6, 2287–2292. doi: 10.1097/00001756-199511270-00005

Horwitz, B., and Rowe, J. B. (2011). Functional biomarkers for neurodegenerative disorders based on the network paradigm. *Prog. Neurobiol.* 95, 505–509. doi: 10.1016/j.pneurobio.2011.07.005

Horwitz, B., and Smith, J. F. (2008). A link between neuroscience and informatics: large-scale modeling of memory processes. *Methods* 44, 338–347. doi: 10.1016/j.ymeth.2007.02.007

Horwitz, B., and Tagamets, M.-A. (1999). Predicting human functional maps with neural net modeling. *Hum. Brain Mapp.* 8, 137–142. doi: 10.1002/(SICI)1097-0193(1999)8:2/3<137::AID-HBM11> 3.0.CO;2-B

Horwitz, B., Warner, B., Fitzer, J., Tagamets, M.-A., Husain, F. T., and Long, T. W. (2005). Investigating the neural basis for functional and effective connectivity: application to fMRI. *Philos. Trans. R. Soc. Lond. B Biol. Sci.* 360, 1093–1108. doi: 10.1098/rstb.2005.1647

Husain, F. T., Tagamets, M.-A., Fromm, S. J., Braun, A. R., and Horwitz, B. (2004). Relating neuronal dynamics for auditory object processing to neuroimaging activity. *Neuroimage* 21, 1701–1720. doi: 10.1016/j.neuroimage.2003.11.012

Just, M. A., Cherkassky, V. L., Keller, T. A., Kana, R. K., and Minshew, N. J. (2007). Functional and anatomical cortical underconnectivity in autism: evidence from an fMRI study of an executive function task and corpus callosum morphometry. *Cereb. Cortex* 17, 951–961. doi: 10.1093/cercor/bhl006

Kanwisher, N., and Yovel, G. (2006). The fusiform face area: a cortical region specialized for the perception of faces. *Philos. Trans. R. Soc. Lond. B Biol. Sci.* 361, 2109–2128. doi: 10.1098/rstb.2006.1934

Kim, J., and Horwitz, B. (2008). Investigating the neural basis for fMRI-based functional connectivity in a blocked design: application to interregional correlations and psycho-physiological interactions. *Magn. Reson. Imaging* 26, 583–593. doi: 10.1016/j.mri.2007.10.011

Kim, J., and Horwitz, B. (2009). How well does structural equation modeling reveal abnormal brain anatomical connections? An fMRI simulation study. *Neuroimage* 45, 1190–1198. doi: 10.1016/j.neuroimage.2009.01.006

Kotter, R. (2004). Online retrieval, processing, and visualization of primate connectivity data from the CoCoMac database. *Neuroinformatics* 2, 127–144. doi: 10.1385/NI:2:2:127

Kuramoto, Y. (1984). *Chemical Oscillations, Waves, and Turbulence.* Berlin: Springer-Verlag. doi: 10.1007/978-3-642-69689-3

Lee, J. H. (2011). Tracing activity across the whole brain neural network with optogenetic functional magnetic resonance imaging. *Front. Neuroinform.* 5:21. doi: 10.3389/fninf.2011.00021

Logothetis, N. K. (2012). Intracortical recordings and fMRI: an attempt to study operational modules and networks simultaneously. *Neuroimage* 62, 962–969. doi: 10.1016/j.neuroimage.2012.01.033

Lynall, M. E., Bassett, D. S., Kerwin, R., McKenna, P. J., Kitzbichler, M., Muller, U., et al. (2010). Functional connectivity and brain networks in schizophrenia. *J. Neurosci.* 30, 9477–9487. doi: 10.1523/JNEUROSCI.0333-10.2010

Lynch, C. J., Uddin, L. Q., Supekar, K., Khouzam, A., Phillips, J., and Menon, V. (2013). Default mode network in childhood autism: posteromedial cortex heterogeneity and relationship with social deficits. *Biol. Psychiatry* 74, 212–219. doi: 10.1016/j.biopsych.2012.12.013

Marreiros, A. C., Kiebel, S. J., and Friston, K. J. (2008). Dynamic causal modelling for fMRI: a two-state model. *Neuroimage* 39, 269–278. doi: 10.1016/j.neuroimage.2007.08.019

Mattia, M., and Del Giudice, P. (2002). Population dynamics of interacting spiking neurons. *Phys. Rev. E Stat. Nonlin. Soft Matter Phys.* 66, 051917. doi: 10.1103/PhysRevE.66.051917

McIntosh, A. R., Grady, C. L., Ungerleider, L. G., Haxby, J. V., Rapoport, S. I., and Horwitz, B. (1994). Network analysis of cortical visual pathways mapped with PET. *J. Neurosci.* 14, 655–666.

Reiman, E. M., Caselli, R. J., Yun, L. S., Kewei, C., Bandy, D., Minoshima, S., et al. (1996). Preclinical evidence of Alzheimer's disease in persons homozygous for the e4 allele for apolipoprotein E. *N. Engl. J. Med.* 334, 752–758. doi: 10.1056/NEJM199603213341202

Ritter, P., Schirner, M., McIntosh, A. R., and Jirsa, V. K. (2013). The virtual brain integrates computational modeling and multimodal neuroimaging. *Brain Connect.* 3, 121–145. doi: 10.1089/brain.2012.0120

Rong, F., Holroyd, T., Husain, F. T., Contreras-Vidal, J. L., and Horwitz, B. (2011). Task-specific modulation of human auditory evoked response in a delayed-match-to-sample task. *Front. Psychol.* 2:85. doi: 10.3389/fpsyg.2011.00085

Rytsar, R., Fornari, E., Frackowiak, R. S., Ghika, J. A., and Knyazeva, M. G. (2011). Inhibition in early Alzheimer's disease: an fMRI-based study of effective connectivity. *Neuroimage* 57, 1131–1139. doi: 10.1016/j.neuroimage.2011.05.029

Smith, J. F., Chen, K., Pillai, A. S., and Horwitz, B. (2013). Identifying effective connectivity parameters in simulated fMRI: a direct comparison of switching linear dynamic system, stochastic dynamic causal, and multivariate autoregressive models. *Front. Neurosci.* 7:70. doi: 10.3389/fnins.2013.00070

Smith, J. F., Pillai, A., Chen, K., and Horwitz, B. (2010). Identification and validation of effective connectivity networks in functional magnetic resonance imaging using switching linear dynamic systems. *Neuroimage* 52, 1027–1040. doi: 10.1016/j.neuroimage.2009.11.081

Smith, S. M. (2012). The future of FMRI connectivity. *Neuroimage* 62, 1257–1266. doi: 10.1016/j.neuroimage.2012.01.022

Smith, S. M., Miller, K. L., Salimi-Khorshidi, G., Webster, M., Beckmann, C. F., Nichols, T. E., et al. (2011). Network modelling methods for FMRI. *Neuroimage* 54, 875–891. doi: 10.1016/j.neuroimage.2010.08.063

Sporns, O. (2012). From simple graphs to the connectome: networks in neuroimaging. *Neuroimage* 62, 881–886. doi: 10.1016/j.neuroimage.2011.08.085

Tagamets, M.-A., and Horwitz, B. (1998). Integrating electrophysiological and anatomical experimental data to create a large-scale model that simulates a delayed match-to-sample human brain imaging study. *Cereb. Cortex* 8, 310–320 doi: 10.1093/cercor/8.4.310

Vemuri, P., Jones, D. T., and Jack, C. R. Jr. (2012). Resting state functional MRI in Alzheimer's disease. *Alzheimers Res. Ther.* 4, 2. doi: 10.1186/alzrt100

Venkataraman, A., Whitford, T. J., Westin, C. F., Golland, P., and Kubicki, M. (2012). Whole brain resting state functional connectivity abnormalities in schizophrenia. *Schizophr. Res.* 139, 7–12. doi: 10.1016/j.schres.2012.04.021

Wang, L., Zang, Y., He, Y., Liang, M., Zhang, X., Tian, L., et al. (2006). Changes in hippocampal connectivity in the early stages of Alzheimer's disease: evidence from resting state fMRI. *Neuroimage* 31, 496–504. doi: 10.1016/j.neuroimage.2005.12.033

Wendling, F., Ansari-Asl, K., Bartolomei, F., and Senhadji, L. (2009). From EEG signals to brain connectivity: a model-based evaluation of interdependence measures. *J. Neurosci. Methods* 183, 9–18. doi: 10.1016/j.jneumeth.2009.04.021

Wilson, H. R., and Cowan, J. D. (1972). Excitatory and inhibitory interactions in localized populations of model neurons. *Biophys. J.* 12, 1–24. doi: 10.1016/S0006-3495(72)86068-5

Yeo, B. T., Krienen, F. M., Sepulcre, J., Sabuncu, M. R., Lashkari, D., Hollinshead, M., et al. (2011). The organization of the human cerebral cortex estimated by intrinsic functional connectivity. *J. Neurophysiol.* 106, 1125–1165. doi: 10.1152/jn.00338.2011

APPENDIX

Abbreviations:

AD	Alzheimer's Disease
BOLD	Blood oxygenation level dependent
DMN	Default mode network
DSI	Diffusion spectrum imaging
DTI	Diffusion tensor imaging
fMRI	Functional magnetic resonance imaging
LPr	Left precuneus area
LMPF	Left medial prefrontal area
PET	Positron emission tomography
PFC	Prefrontal cortex
rCBF	Regional cerebral blood flow
ROI	Region of interest
rsfMRI	Resting state fMRI
rsfMRI-FC	Resting state fMRI functional connectivity
SEM	Structural equation modeling
TR	Repetition time

4

A review of attention-deficit/hyperactivity disorder from the perspective of brain networks

Angelica De La Fuente*[1], *Shugao Xia*[2], *Craig Branch*[2,3] and *Xiaobo Li*[2,3,4,5]**

[1] *Ferkauf Graduate School of Psychology, Albert Einstein College of Medicine, Yeshiva University, Bronx, NY, USA*
[2] *Gruss Magnetic Resonance Research Center, Albert Einstein College of Medicine, Yeshiva University, Bronx, NY, USA*
[3] *Department of Radiology, Albert Einstein College of Medicine, Yeshiva University, Bronx, NY, USA*
[4] *Department of Neuroscience, Albert Einstein College of Medicine, Yeshiva University, Bronx, NY, USA*
[5] *Department of Psychiatry and Behavioral Sciences, Albert Einstein College of Medicine, Yeshiva University, Bronx, NY, USA*

Correspondence:
Xiaobo Li, Department of Radiology, Albert Einstein College of Medicine, Yeshiva University, 1300 Morris Park Avenue, Gruss 204, Bronx, NY 10461, USA.
e-mail: xli.aecom@gmail.com; xiaobo.li@einstein.yu.edu

Attention-deficit/hyperactivity disorder (ADHD) is the most commonly diagnosed neurodevelopmental disorder in childhood, which affects more than 5% of the population worldwide. ADHD is characterized by developmentally inappropriate behaviors of inattention, and/or impulsivity and hyperactivity. These behavioral manifestations contribute to diminished academic, occupational and social functioning, and have neurobiological bases. Neuronal deficits, especially in the attention and executive function processing networks, have been implicated in both children and adults with ADHD by using sophisticated structural and functional neuroimaging approaches. These structural and functional abnormalities in the brain networks have been associated with the impaired cognitive, affective, and motor behaviors seen in the disorder. The goal of this review is to summarize and integrate emerging themes from the existing neuroimaging connectivity studies based on advanced imaging techniques, applied in data of structural magnetic resonance imaging (MRI), functional MRI (fMRI), diffusion tensor imaging, electroencephalography and event related potential: and to discuss the results of these studies when considering future directions for understanding pathophysiological mechanisms and developmental trajectories of the behavioral manifestations in ADHD. We conclude this review by suggesting that future research should put more effort on understanding the roles of the subcortical structures and their structural/functional pathways in ADHD.

Keywords: ADHD, brain networks, structural MRI, fMRI, DTI, EEG/ERP

INTRODUCTION

Attention deficit/hyperactivity disorder (ADHD) is the most commonly diagnosed neurodevelopmental disorder in childhood. Diagnoses of ADHD are made based on developmentally inappropriate behavioral symptoms, which have been categorized into three subtypes: inattentive, impulsive and hyperactive, and combined type. These core behavioral symptoms must be pervasive across situations, persistent for more than 6 months and observed before the age of 7 years, defined by the diagnostic and statistical manual of mental disorders (DSM-IV-TR) issued by the American Psychiatric Association (2000). The DSM-IV-TR reported that 3–7% of school-aged children have ADHD. However, most recent surveys have estimated significantly increased prevalence rates, from 6.9% in 1998 to 9.0% in 2009, shown in children aged 5–17 years (Akinbami et al., 2011).

Attention deficit/hyperactivity disorder is considered one of the most hereditable disorders with an estimated mean heritability of 75% (Faraone, 2005). Besides the genetic component, ADHD also has neurobiological and environmental underpinnings. The etiology of this highly inhomogeneous disorder is still unknown. Apart from the behavioral symptoms that are used for diagnostic measurements, both children and adults with ADHD have been found to have impairments in neural networks associated with sensory and cognitive processing functions. For instance, neuronal deficits in attention and executive function processing networks have been frequently reported in both children and adults with ADHD, by using sophisticated structural and functional neuroimaging approaches (Bush, 2005; Konrad and Eickhoff, 2010). And these structural and functional abnormalities in the brain have been associated with impaired cognitive, affective, and motor behaviors seen in ADHD approaches (Bush, 2005; Konrad and Eickhoff, 2010). In addition, spontaneous low-frequency functional activities have been reported in multiple brain regions, which formed the default mode network (DMN), during wakeful resting-state functional magnetic resonance imaging (fMRI) acquisition (Bartels and Zeki, 2005). Patients with ADHD have been reported to have both structural and functional abnormalities associated with the DMN (Konrad and Eickhoff, 2010; Castellanos, 2012).

In this study, we will review and summarize these existing studies, which have assessed the regional features and systems-level patterns of the structural and functional brain networks in ADHD, based on advanced computational techniques applied to data of structural MRI, diffusion tensor imaging (DTI), fMRI, electroencephalography (EEG), and event related potential (ERP). We will also discuss the results of these studies when considering future directions for understanding pathophysiological mechanisms and developmental trajectories of the behavioral manifestations in ADHD.

STRUCTURAL MRI-BASED BRAIN NETWORKS IN ADHD

Structural MRI is the primary imaging tool used for studying brain anatomy and identifying changes in brain structures. Commonly used structural MRI measures include volume and density of the gray (GM) or white matter (WM) of the whole brain or sub-regions, as well as the regional and whole brain cortical GM thickness (Vaidya, 2012). Techniques for investigating the topological and structural features of the anatomical brain networks have also been developed by using regional volume or thickness as basic metric (Lerch et al., 2006; He and Evans, 2007; Zielinski et al., 2010).

The early estimations showed approximately 4–5% overall cerebral and cerebellar volumetric reductions in children and adolescents with ADHD, compared to that of typically developing controls (TDC; Castellanos, 2002; Carmona et al., 2005). Other structural MRI studies have reported volumetric reductions in the frontal lobe, [including orbitofrontal (OFC), superior frontal (SFC), and dorsolateral prefrontal (DLPFC) cortices], posterior and anterior cingulate gyri, precentral gyrus, caudate nuclei, corpus callosum (CC), as well as the cerebellum (Seidman et al., 2005; Shaw et al., 2006; Bush, 2011). Significantly reduced whole brain cortical GM thickness has also been found in children with ADHD when compared to TDC (Shaw et al., 2006, 2007; Makris et al., 2007). Studies also showed significantly thinner cortical thickness in regions including bilateral DLPFC and OFC, anterior and posterior cingulate cortex (PCC) and the temporo-occipito-parietal junction, in adults with ADHD when compared to controls (Makris et al., 2007; Proal et al., 2011). The rate of cortical thinning in these regions has been shown to be inversely associated with the severity of hyperactivity and impulsiveness in normal development (Shaw, 2011).

Basal ganglia regions, such as the globus pallidus, putamen, and caudate have been reported to have structural abnormalities in children with ADHD. Structural MRI studies have detected reduced globus pallidus, putamen, and caudate volumes in voxel-based studies (Frodl and Skokauskas, 2012), and in manual tracing region of interest (ROI)-based deformation analysis (Qiu et al., 2009) in children with ADHD. Interestingly, they did not find any regional volumetric differences of the basal ganglia in adults with ADHD when compared to age-matched controls (Qiu et al., 2009; Frodl and Skokauskas, 2012). However, clinical studies found that the hyperactive/impulsive symptoms, observed in children with ADHD, significantly decline over time, whereas the inattentive symptoms rarely vanish (Lahey et al., 2005). Thus, the similar striatal volumes shown in the adults with ADHD and age-matched control may explain the vanished hyperactivity/impulsivity symptoms during the adulthood in many of the clinical cases. More cross-sectional and longitudinal investigations need to be done, to clarify the relationships among the striatum, its associated brain pathways, and the developmental trajectories of the disorder.

By now, most replicated findings from the voxel-based and ROI-based structural MRI studies have suggested significant decrease of the whole brain GM and WM volumes and significant regional underdevelopment in the prefrontal cortex (PFC), including the OFC, DLPFC, and SFC, basal ganglia substructures (striatum and globus pallidus), and cerebellum, in patients with ADHD (Frodl and Skokauskas, 2012). Structural changes, in the brain networks encompassing PFC and its connections to the striatum and cerebellum, have been found to be associated cognitive impairments, such as distractibility, forgetfulness, impulsivity, poor planning, and locomotor hyperactivity, in both children and adults with ADHD (Seidman et al., 2005; Arnsten, 2006).

From literature, structural MRI-based techniques for constructing the anatomical brain networks, such as in (Lerch et al., 2006; He and Evans, 2007; Zielinski et al., 2010), have not yet been implemented in cohorts with ADHD. Investigations of the topological features and pair-wise nodal communication patterns of the anatomical networks, and their relationships with the clinical and behavioral manifestations are important future directions in the research field related to ADHD.

FUNCTIONAL BRAIN NETWORKS IN ADHD

Functional MRI techniques provide a way to understand normal brain functions and to test for regional brain dysfunctions associated with disorders (Bush, 2005). Both task-based and resting-state fMRI have been frequently applied in children with ADHD, and have demonstrated atypical functional activations in the frontal, temporal, parietal lobes, and cerebellar regions (Shaw et al., 2006; Cubillo et al., 2010, 2011; Rubia et al., 2010). The frontal cortex can be divided into five major functional sub-regions: the orbital, dorsolateral, mesial (all which make up the PFC), the premotor, and motor regions. Social inhibition and impulse control are associated with the OFC (Fischer et al., 1990). Abnormal functional activations in OFC have been suggested to influence behavioral inhibition in children with ADHD (Bush, 2010). The DLPFC, another most frequently reported region of functional impairment in ADHD, has been implicated in planning, working memory and attentional processes (Danielson et al., 2011). In addition, one fMRI study conducted in adults with childhood ADHD showed reduced activations in bilateral inferior prefrontal cortices (IFC), left parietal lobe, caudate and thalamus, and reduced inter-regional functional connectivity between right inferior fronto-frontal, fronto-striatal, and fronto-parietal neural networks during a stop and switching task, when compared to controls (Cubillo et al., 2010).

Structures of the cingulo-fronto-pariental (CFP) cognitive/attention network, including the fronto-striatal and fronto-parietal pathways, are thought to be the primary substrate for most attention and executive functions (Bush, 2011). The main regions that comprise the CFP network are the lateral frontal pole, dorsal anterior cingulate cortex (dACC), DLPFC, ventrolateral PFC (VLPFC), caudate, cerebellum, and the parietal cortex (Bush, 2010). This network controls goal-directed processes and provides the ability to respond to changing task demands (Castellanos, 2012). Significantly decreased activations have been reported in

DLPFC, VLPFC, IFC, and superior parietal cortex (SPC) in ADHD, during multiple cognitive performance tasks and in resting-state (Rubia et al., 2010; Bush, 2011; Castellanos, 2012).

The dACC is an important component of the fronto-striatal circuitry of the CFP network, which has been consistently reported to have abnormal activation in ADHD (Sun et al., 2012). The dACC has a critical role in attention, cognitive processing, target detection, novelty detection, response selection, response inhibition, error detection, and motivation (Bush, 2010). Hypotheses about its functions include reward-based decision-making, response selection, error detection, and predicting task difficulty, which have shown to be impaired in children and adults with ADHD (Seidman et al., 2005). An attention task-based fMRI study found hypo-activation of the dACC in adults with ADHD when compared to controls (Bush, 2011). Resting-state fMRI studies frequently reported disrupted functional connectivity between the dACC and PCC (Castellanos et al., 2008), and abnormal developmental pattern of the dACC–DMN interactions in ADHD subjects (Fair, 2010; Sun et al., 2012). The atypical connectivity in ADHD may relate to delayed or disrupted maturation. ADHD adults presented with abnormal dACC-PCC connectivity patterns when compared to age-matched TD adults. Connectivity patterns were similar between the ADHD group and the young TD subjects, indicating atypical brain maturation in the ADHD group (Sato, 2012). In addition, significantly increased functional connectivity between the dACC and the bilateral thalamus, bilateral cerebellum, and bilateral insula have been shown during resting-state in children with ADHD, compared to TDC (Tian, 2006).

The thalamus is a key subcortical structure of the cortico-striato-thalamo-cortical (CSTC) loops that serve attentional and cognitive processing. Significantly reduced regional activations in bilateral thalami (especially in the pulvinar nuclei), significantly decreased functional connectivity between bilateral pulvinar and right prefrontal regions, and significantly increased connectivity between the right pulvinar and bilateral occipital regions have been reported in children with ADHD, during a visual sustained attention task-based fMRI study (Li et al., 2012). Another study has found reduced functional connectivity between thalamus and basal ganglia areas (especially in putamen) in children with ADHD, during resting-state (Cao et al., 2009).

Altered topological features and inter-regional functional connectivity in large-scale brain networks encompassing cortical and subcortical regions have been increasingly reported, indicating systematic and more widespread brain alterations in ADHD. Resting-state fMRI has been used across laboratories to identify neural networks such as the DMN, dorsal, and ventral attentional networks, as well as motor, visual, and executive control systems (Fox et al., 2006; Buckner et al., 2008; Castellanos, 2012). The DMN is a distributed network of brain regions, which is more active during rest than during performance of sensory and cognitive demanding tasks. Studies have found significantly decreased functional connectivity among the brain regions of the DMN, and between those with putamen and thalamus (Cao et al., 2009; Qiu et al., 2011). Incremental deactivations of the regions in the DMN have been associated with increased task difficulty as well as during transition from rest-to-task states in ADHD (Konrad and Eickhoff, 2010; Liddle, 2011). Furthermore, by applying the graph theoretical approach (GTT), which has been used to characterize the topology of global and regional brain communications (Konrad and Eickhoff, 2010; Ahmadlou et al., 2012), a resting-state fMRI study found significantly increased local efficiency combined with a decreasing tendency in global efficiency of the DMN, and significantly decreased nodal efficiency in the medial prefrontal, temporal, occipital, and subcortical regions in children with ADHD, when compared to the control group (Wang, 2009). Castellanos (2012) have suggested that ADHD could be considered as a DMN disorder. In addition, a resting-state fMRI study, by running network based statistics (NBS) in 90 cortical and subcortical regions, demonstrated abnormal inter-regional connectivity of the frontal-amygdala-occipital network and frontal-temporal-occipital network in young adults with ADHD (Cocchi, 2012). Impaired inter-regional connectivity within reward-motivation regions and their decreased connectivity with regions from the DMN and dorsal attentional networks have also been reported, and suggest impaired interactions between control and reward pathways that might underlie attention and motivation deficits in ADHD (Tomasi and Volkow, 2012).

Altered topological features and inter-regional functional connectivity in large-scale brain networks in ADHD, which have been reviewed in the fMRI section, are convinced in EEG/ERP studies as well. A GTT-based study in resting-state EEG data reported abnormal cluster coefficients and path lengths of the nodes in the left hemisphere, which were recognizable in the delta band, in patients with ADHD when compared to controls (Ahmadlou et al., 2012). An NBS study in sustained attention task-based EEG data showed distinct frontal-central-parietal patterns in the theta and alpha frequency bands in adults with ADHD compared to controls, where ADHD subjects displayed a more robust homogeneous response pattern in the 120–260 ms time range that included the P1, N1, P2 component, with a majority of latency peaks characterized by alpha and theta activation in the fronto-central sites (Shahaf et al., 2012). Similar findings have been interpreted as revealing a compensatory mechanism activated by ADHD patients in early stages of stimulus processing, by which more attention was directed to the task (Prox et al., 2007).

DTI-BASED BRAIN NETWORKS IN ADHD

While functional brain imaging studies may reveal specific regions of dysfunction within the brain, it is important to know how the nodes within these networks are structurally connected. Micro-structural abnormalities in the WM may lead to disrupted functional communications between brain regions, ultimately resulting in disrupted behavioral functioning in ADHD (Nagel, 2011). DTI is an MRI method that provides *in vivo* information about the WM microstructure through water diffusion, which can reveal microscopic details about tissue architecture (Konrad and Eickhoff, 2010). Orientations of the WM tracts in the brain can be measured by the directions of diffusivity (Konrad and Eickhoff, 2010). The most common quantitative indices used to measure the WM integrity are mean diffusivity (MD) and fractional anisotropy (FA; Konrad and Eickhoff, 2010; Nagel, 2011).

Two primary analysis methods have been applied in DTI studies: voxel-based analysis (VBA) that allows for a complete overview of the WM integrity in the brain, and ROI-based analysis for more specific exploration of the WM abnormalities in certain brain regions. A recent meta-analysis reviewed the ROI-based studies assessing the WM integrity, and provided evidence of several disturbed WM regions in children with ADHD, including the inferior and superior longitudinal fasciculus, anterior corona radiate, cortico-spinal tract, cingulum, CC, internal capsule, caudate nucleus, and cerebellum (van Ewijk, 2012). Review of the VBA studies also confirmed WM changes in these regions, and found extensive differences across the four brain lobes, as well as areas within the basal ganglia, uncinate fasciculus, and forceps minor (van Ewijk, 2012).

Development of WM determinative and probabilistic tractography techniques has made it possible to estimate and visualize the structural connectivity of the WM pathways in human brain. Using tractography-based analyses, DTI studies have demonstrated increased FA in WM structures connecting parietal-occipital regions (Silk, 2009), and tracts connecting the temporal lobe and other distant cortical regions in children with ADHD compared to TDC, which were positively associated with symptom severity in the patient group (Peterson, 2011). Significantly reduced FA in the cortico-spinal tract (Carmona et al., 2005; Hamilton et al., 2008; Cubillo, 2010), the superior longitudinal fascicle that connects the prefrontal and parietal regions (Makris, 2008; Cubillo et al., 2010; Konrad, 2010), the cingulum bundle (Makris, 2008; Konrad, 2010), have also been reported in patients with ADHD. In addition, one study detected significantly increased MD in the frontal portion of the left fronto-occipital fasciculus in adults with ADHD when compared with controls (Konrad et al., 2006). DTI studies have also shown alterations within the cerebellar WM areas in children and adolescents with ADHD (Ashtari et al., 2005; Bechtel et al., 2009).

The neural pathways that are associated with the areas of abnormal WM reviewed above are the pathways connecting the cortical regions, cortical-striatum and cortical-cerebellum. The prevailing theory regarding the neurobiological basis of ADHD identified the fronto-striatal network as a probable substrate of cognitive and behavioral impairments seen in ADHD (Bush, 2005; van Ewijk, 2012). Studies found disturbed WM structural connectivity of the frontal-striatal network in both adults and children with ADHD, compared to group-matched controls (Konrad and Eickhoff, 2010; Tamm et al., 2012). Tract- specific analyses found reduced FA in bilateral fronto-striatal fiber tracts in children with ADHD, specifically in the orbitofrontal and ventrolateral tracts, associated with poor executive functioning performance (Shang, 2013). In addition, significant reductions of probabilistic WM connectivity between the thalamus and striatum has been reported in children with ADHD when compared to TDC (Xia et al., 2012).

The CC, the largest band of WM fibers in the brain that connects the left and right hemispheres, plays an important role in inter-hemispheric communication. Thus, abnormal microstructure of CC may affect cognitive functions that depend on bilateral collaboration (Vaidya, 2012). Across studies, children with ADHD showed reduced volume of the splenium, the posterior region of the CC that connects bilateral parieto–temporal cortices (Valera, 2007). Using both DTI and anatomical MRI, one study found microstructure abnormalities in the isthmus/splenium part of the CC, characterized by reduced FA values in adults with ADHD when compared to healthy controls (Dramsdahl, 2012). These results are in line with two earlier studies, which observed reduced FA in the isthmus in children with ADHD (Chao, 2009; Cao, 2010).

DISCUSSIONS

Attention-deficit/hyperactivity disorder is the most common neurodevelopmental disorder in childhood. Neuroimaging studies have attempted to identify the pathophysiology of the disorder by searching for abnormalities in brain regions and their connections that are involved in attention, executive function, motor control, response inhibition, working memory, and even during rest. We reviewed and summarized the important findings from the structural MRI, fMRI, EEG/ERP, and DTI studies, which have provided the abundant evidence of structural and functional alterations in widespread brain regions and their connections, in this severe and heritable brain disorder.

The majority of the existing neuroimaging studies, which have attempted to find the neurobiological underpinnings of ADHD, have focused on cortical regions and their connections, and has demonstrated global cortical maturation delay based on reduced cortical thickness and reduced GM and WM volumes, specifically in frontal lobe (Carmona et al., 2005), regional WM microstructural abnormalities in frontal, temporal and parietal lobes (Nagel, 2011; Dramsdahl, 2012; Shang, 2013), and aberrant neuronal activations, inter-regional functional connectivity and global network features over these cortical areas, during sensory and cognitive performance or even at rest (Wang, 2009; Ahmadlou et al., 2012; Castellanos, 2012; Cocchi, 2012; Shahaf et al., 2012). Furthermore, the existing studies also suggest that the structural and functional connectivity deficits and the ADHD symptoms might arise incidentally from a common etiologic mechanism, involving altered modulation of synaptic potentiating and pruning by dopamine and other factors during development, which result in altered patterns of cortico-cortical connectivity that might persist into adulthood (Liston et al., 2011).

Subcortical regions may also significantly contribute to the pathophysiology of ADHD. For example, the basal ganglia has been associated with the execution of appropriate goal-directed behaviors and may play a role in the behavioral impairments for response control seen in many children with ADHD (Qiu et al., 2009). Neuroimaging studies have demonstrated regional structural and functional deficits of the basal ganglia, especially in the striatum (Qiu et al., 2009; van Ewijk, 2012). Disturbed WM structural connectivity and atypical functional connectivity have been shown in the frontal-striatal network in both adults and children with ADHD (Konrad and Eickhoff, 2010; Tamm et al., 2012). It has been hypothesized that the impairments of the striatum and its brain connections are associated with the hyperactivity/impulsivity component in children with ADHD (van Ewijk, 2012).

However, the role of the thalamus and its mediating role in cortico-striatal and cortico-cortical pathways in ADHD have been relatively ignored. Very recently, investigation of high resolution structural MRI data revealed reduced bilateral thalamic volumes, as well as regional surface atrophy in the pulvinar nucleus of the left side thalamus in children with ADHD (Xia et al., 2012). In the same study, disturbed frontal-thalamo and thalamo-striatal WM connectivity have also been demonstrated in the children with ADHD. Furthermore, significantly reduced pulvinar activations and abnormal pulvinar-frontal and occipital-pulvinar functional connectivity have been shown in children with ADHD during a visual sustained attention task, which were also significantly correlated with their inattentiveness indices for clinical diagnoses (Li et al., 2012). This series of neuroimaging studies may drive the field forward by placing the pulvinar nuclei of the thalamus at the center of dysfunctional attentional networks in ADHD (Shaw, 2012).

As a summary, brain network associated dysfunctions have been found to be central in ADHD pathophysiology. It is important to gain a better understanding of how subcortical-cortical and cortical-cortical networks development is altered during the onset of the disorder. Thus, future studies should allocate greater resources on subcortical regions and relationships between subcortical and cortical regions in order to provide a better understanding of the etiology of the disorder.

ACKNOWLEDGMENTS

This work was partially supported by the Rose F. Kennedy Intellectual and Developmental Disabilities Research Center (RFK-IDDRC) through a program grant (HD071593) from the Eunice Kennedy Shriver National Institute of Child Health and Human Development (NICHD). It was also partially supported by the RFK-IDDRC Pilot and Feasibility Award to Dr. Xiaobo Li.

REFERENCES

Ahmadlou, M., Adeli, H., and Adeli, A. (2012). Graph theoretical analysis of organization of functional brain networks in ADHD. *Clin. EEG Neurosci.* 43, 5–13.

Akinbami, L. J., Liu, X., Pastor, P. N., and Reuben, C. A. (2011). Attention deficit hyperactivity disorder among children aged 5–17 years in the United States, 1998–2009. *NCHS Data Brief* 70, 1–8.

American Psychiatric Association (2000). *Diagnostic and statistical manual of mental disorders*, 4th Edn, (text revised Edn.) Washington: American Psychiatric Publishing.

Arnsten, A. F. T. (2006). Fundamentals of attention-deficit/hyperactivity disorder: circuits and pathways. *J. Clin. Psychiatry* 67(Suppl. 8), 7–12.

Ashtari, M., Kumra, S., Bhaskar, S. L., Clarke, T., Thaden, E., Cervellione, K. L., et al. (2005). Attention-deficit/hyperactivity disorder: a preliminary diffusion tensor imaging study. *Biol. Psychiatry* 57, 448–455.

Bartels, A., and Zeki, S. (2005). Brain dynamics during natural viewing conditions – a new guide for mapping connectivity in vivo. *Neuroimage* 24, 339–349.

Bechtel, N., Kobel, M., Penner, I. K., Klarhfer, M., Scheffler, K., Opwis, K., et al. (2009). Decreased fractional anisotropy in the middle cerebellar peduncle in children with epilepsy and/or attention deficit/hyperactivity disorder: a preliminary study. *Epilepsy Behav.* 15, 294–298.

Buckner, R. L., Andrews-Hanna, J. R., and Schacter, D. L. (2008). The brain's default network. *Ann. N. Y. Acad. Sci.* 1124, 1–38.

Bush, G. (2005). Functional neuroimaging of attention-deficit/hyperactivity disorder: a review and suggested future directions. *Biol. Psychiatry* 57, 1273–1284.

Bush, G. (2010). Attention-deficit/hyperactivity disorder and attention networks. *Neuropsychopharmacology* 35, 278–300.

Bush, G. (2011). Cingulate, frontal, and parietal cortical dysfunction in attention-deficit/hyperactivity disorder. *Biol. Psychiatry* 69, 1160–1167.

Cao, Q. (2010). The macrostructural and microstructural abnormalities of corpus callosum in children with attention deficit/hyperactivity disorder: a combined morphometric and diffusion tensor MRI study. *Brain Res.* 1310, 172–180.

Cao, X., Cao, Q., Long, X., Sun, L., Sui, M., Zhu, C., et al. (2009). Abnormal resting-state functional connectivity patterns of the putamen in medication-naïve children with attention deficit hyperactivity disorder. *Brain Res.* 1303, 195–206.

Carmona, S., Vilarroya, O., Bielsa, A., Tremols, V., Soliva, J. C., Rovira, M., et al. (2005). Global and regional gray matter reductions in ADHD: a voxel-based morphometric study. *Neurosci. Lett.* 389, 88–93.

Castellanos, F. X. (2002). Developmental trajectories of brain volume abnormalities in children and adolescents with attention-deficit/hyperactivity disorder. *JAMA* 288, 1740–1748.

Castellanos, F. X. (2012). Large-scale brain systems in ADHD: beyond the prefrontal-striatal model. *Trends Cogn. Sci.* 16, 17–26.

Castellanos, F. X., Margulies, D. S., Kelly, C., Uddin, L. Q., Ghaffari, M., Kirsch, A., et al. (2008). Cingulate-precuneus interactions: a new locus of dysfunction in adult attention-deficit/hyperactivity disorder. *Biol. Psychiatry* 63, 332–337.

Chao, T. C. (2009). Effects of interpolation methods in spatial normalization of diffusion tensor imaging data on group comparison of fractional anisotropy. *Magn. Reson. Imaging* 27, 681–690.

Cocchi, L. (2012). Altered functional brain connectivity in a non-clinical sample of young adults with attention-deficit/hyperactivity disorder. *J. Neurosci.* 32, 17753–17761.

Cubillo, A. (2010). Structural and functional brain imaging in adult attention-deficit/hyperactivity disorder. *Expert Rev. Neurother.* 10, 603–620.

Cubillo, A., Halari, R., Ecker, C., Giampietro, V., Taylor, E., and Rubia, K. (2010). Reduced activation and inter-regional functional connectivity of fronto-striatal networks in adults with childhood attention-deficit hyperactivity disorder (ADHD) and persisting symptoms during tasks of motor inhibition and cognitive switching. *J. Psychiatr. Res.* 44, 629–639.

Cubillo, A., Halari, R., Giampietro, V., Taylor, E., and Rubia, K. (2011). Fronto-striatal underactivation during interference inhibition and attention allocation in grown up children with attention deficit/hyperactivity disorder and persistent symptoms. *Psychiatry Res.* 193, 17–27.

Danielson, N. B., Guo, J. N., and Blumenfeld, H. (2011). The default mode network and altered consciousness in epilepsy. *Behav. Neurol.* 24, 55–65.

Dramsdahl, M. (2012). Adults with attention-deficit/hyperactivity disorder – a diffusion-tensor imaging study of the corpus callosum. *Psychiatry Res.* 201, 168–173.

Fair, D. A. (2010). Atypical default network connectivity in youth with attention-deficit/hyperactivity disorder. *Biol. Psychiatry* 68, 1084–1091.

Faraone, S. V. (2005). Molecular genetics of attention-deficit/hyperactivity disorder. *Biol. Psychiatry* 57, 1313–1323.

Fischer, M., Barkley, R. A., Edelbrock, C. S., and Smallish, L. (1990). The adolescent outcome of hyperactive children diagnosed by research criteria: II. Academic, attentional, and neuropsychological status. *J. Consult. Clin. Psychol.* 58, 580–588.

Fox, M. D., Corbetta, M., Snyder, A. Z., Vincent, J. L., and Raichle, M. E. (2006). Spontaneous neuronal activity distinguishes human dorsal and ventral attention systems. *Proc. Natl. Acad. Sci. U.S.A.* 103, 10046–10051.

Frodl, T., and Skokauskas, N. (2012). Meta-analysis of structural MRI studies in children and adults with attention deficit hyperactivity disorder indicates treatment effects. *Acta Psychiatr. Scand.* 125, 114–126.

Hamilton, L. S., Levitt, J. G., O'Neill, J., Alger, J. R., Luders, E., Phillips, O. R., et al. (2008). Reduced white matter integrity in attention-deficit hyperactivity disorder. *Neuroreport* 19, 1705–1708.

He, Y., and Evans, A. (2007). Graph theoretical modeling of brain connectivity. *Curr. Opin. Neurol.* 23, 341–350.

Konrad, A. (2010). Disturbed structural connectivity is related to inattention and impulsivity in adult attention deficit hyperactivity disorder. *Eur. J. Neurosci.* 31, 912–919.

Konrad, K., and Eickhoff, S. B. (2010). Is the ADHD brain wired differently? A review on structural and functional connectivity in attention deficit hyperactivity disorder. *Hum. Brain Mapp.* 31, 904–916.

Konrad, K., Neufang, S., Hanisch, C., Fink, G. R., and Herpertz-Dahlmann, B. (2006). Dysfunctional attentional networks in children with attention deficit/hyperactivity disorder: evidence from an event-related functional magnetic resonance imaging study. *Biol. Psychiatry* 59, 643–651.

Lahey, B. B., Pelham, W. E., Loney, J., Lee, S. S., and Willcutt, E. (2005). In stability of the DSM-IV subtypes of

ADHD from preschool through elementary school. *Arch. Gen. Psychiatry* 62, 896–902.

Lerch, J. P., Worsley, K., Shaw, W. P., Greenstein, D. K., Lenroot, R. K., Giedd, J., et al. (2006). Mapping anatomical correlations across cerebral cortex (MACACC) using cortical thickness from MRI. *Neuroimage* 31, 993–1003.

Li, X., Sroubek, A., Kelly, M. S., Lesser, I., Sussman, E., He, Y., et al. (2012). Atypical pulvinar-cortical pathways during sustained attention performance in children with attention-deficit/hyperactivity disorder. *J. Am. Acad. Child Adolesc. Psychiatry* 51, 1197–1207.

Liddle, E. B. (2011). Task-related default mode network modulation and inhibitory control in ADHD: effects of motivation and methylphenidate. *J. Child Psychol. Psychiatry* 52, 761–771.

Liston, C., Malter, C. M., Teslovich, T., Levenson, D., and Casey, B. J. (2011). Atypical prefrontal connectivity in attention-deficit/hyperactivity disorder: pathway to disease or pathological end point? *Biol. Psychiatry* 69, 1168–1177.

Makris, N. (2008). Attention and executive systems abnormalities in adults with childhood ADHD: a DT-MRI study of connections. *Cereb. Cortex* 18, 1210–1220.

Makris, N., Biederman, J., Valera, E. M., Bush, G., Kaiser, J., Kennedy, D. N., et al. (2007). Cortical thinning of the attention and executive function networks in adults with attention-deficit/hyperactivity disorder. *Cereb. Cortex* 17, 1364–1375.

Nagel, B. J. (2011). Altered white matter microstructure in children with attention-deficit/hyperactivity disorder. *J. Am. Acad. Child Adolesc. Psychiatry* 50, 283–292.

Peterson, D. J. (2011). Increased regional fractional anisotropy in highly screened attention-deficit hyperactivity disorder (ADHD). *J. Child Neurol.* 26, 1296–1302.

Proal, E, Reiss, P. T., Klein, R. G., Mannuzza, S., Gotimer, K., Ramos-Olazagasti, M. A., et al. (2011). Brain gray matter deficits at 33-year follow-up in adults with attention-deficit/hyperactivity disorder established in childhood. *Arch. Gen. Psychiatry* 68, 1122–1134.

Prox, V., Dietrich, D. E., Zhang, Y., Emrich, H. M., and Ohlmeier, M. D. (2007). Attentional processing in adults with ADHD as reflected by event-related potentials. *Neurosci. Lett.* 419, 236–241.

Qiu, A., Crocetti, D., Adler, M., Mahone, E. M., Denckla, M. B., Miller, M. I., et al. (2009). Basal ganglia volume and shape in children with attention deficit hyperactivity disorder. *Am. J. Psychiatry* 166, 74–82.

Qiu, M. G., Ye, Z., Li, Q. Y., Liu, G. J., Xie, B., and Wang, J. (2011). Changes of brain structure and function in ADHD children. *Brain Topogr.* 24, 243–252.

Rubia, K., Halari, R., Cubillo, A., Mohammad, A. M., Scott, S., and Brammer, M. (2010). Disorder-specific inferior prefrontal hypofunction in boys with pure attention-deficit/hyperactivity disorder compared to boys with pure conduct disorder during cognitive flexibility. *Hum. Brain Mapp.* 31, 1823–1833.

Sato, J. R. (2012). Abnormal brain connectivity patterns in adults with ADHD: a coherence study. *PLoS ONE* 7:e45671. doi: 10.1371/journal.pone.0045671

Seidman, L. J., Valera, E. M., and Makris, N. (2005). Structural brain imaging of attention-deficit/hyperactivity disorder. *Biol. Psychiatry* 57, 1263–1272.

Shahaf, G., Reches, A., Pinchuk, N., Fisher, T., Ben Bashat, G., Kanter, A., et al. (2012). Introducing a novel approach of network oriented analysis of ERPs, demonstrated on adult attention deficit hyperactivity disorder. *Clin. Neurophysiol.* 123, 1568–1580.

Shang, C. Y. (2013). Disturbed microstructural integrity of the frontostriatal fiber pathways and executive dysfunction in children with attention deficit hyperactivity disorder. *Psychol. Med.* 43, 1093–1107.

Shaw, P. (2011). Cortical development in typically developing children with symptoms of hyperactivity and impulsivity: support for a dimensional view of attention deficit hyperactivity disorder. *Am. J. Psychiatry* 168, 143–151.

Shaw, P. (2012). Attention-deficit/hyperactivity disorder and the battle for control of attention. *J. Am. Acad. Child Adolesc. Psychiatry* 51, 1116–1118.

Shaw, P., Eckstrand, K., Sharp, W., Blumenthal, J., Lerch, J. P., Greenstein, D., et al. (2007). Attention-deficit/hyperactivity disorder is characterized by a delay in cortical maturation. *Proc. Natl. Acad. Sci. U.S.A.* 104, 19649–19654.

Shaw, P., Lerch, J., Greenstein, D., Sharp, W., Clasen, L., Evans, A., et al. (2006). Longitudinal mapping of cortical thickness and clinical outcome in children and adolescents with attention-deficit/hyperactivity disorder. *Arch. Gen. Psychiatry* 63, 540–549.

Silk, T. J. (2009). White-matter abnormalities in attention deficit hyperactivity disorder: a diffusion tensor imaging study. *Hum. Brain Mapp.* 30, 2757–2765.

Sun, L., Cao, Q., Long, X., Sui, M., Cao, X., Zhu, C., et al. (2012). Abnormal functional connectivity between the anterior cingulate and the default mode network in drug-naïve boys with attention deficit hyperactivity disorder. *Psychiatry Res.* 201, 120–127.

Tamm, L., Barnea-Goraly, N., and Reiss, A. L. (2012). Diffusion tensor imaging reveals white matter abnormalities in attention-deficit/hyperactivity disorder. *Psychiatry Res.* 202, 150–154.

Tian, L. (2006). Altered resting-state functional connectivity patterns of anterior cingulate cortex in adolescents with attention deficit hyperactivity disorder. *Neurosci. Lett.* 400, 39–43.

Tomasi, D., and Volkow, N. D. (2012). Abnormal functional connectivity in children with attention-deficit/hyperactivity disorder. *Biol. Psychiatry* 71, 443–450.

Vaidya, C., (2012). "Neurodevelopmental abnormalities in ADHD," in *Behavioral Neuroscience of Attention Deficit Hyperactivity Disorder and Its Treatment*, 9th Eds, eds C. Stanford and R. Tannock (Berlin: Springer), 49–66.

Valera, E. M. (2007). Meta-analysis of structural imaging findings in attention-deficit/hyperactivity disorder. *Biol. Psychiatry* 61, 1361–1369.

van Ewijk, H. (2012). Diffusion tensor imaging in attention deficit/hyperactivity disorder: a systematic review and meta-analysis. *Neurosci. Biobehav. Rev.* 36, 1093–1106.

Wang, L. (2009). Altered small-world brain functional networks in children with attention-deficit/hyperactivity disorder. *Hum. Brain Mapp.* 30, 638–649.

Xia, S., Li, X., Kimball, A. E., Kelly, M. S., Lesser, I., and Branch, C. (2012). Thalamic shape and connectivity abnormalities in children with attention-deficit/hyperactivity disorder. *Psychiatry Res.* 204, 161–167.

Zielinski, B. A., Gennatas, E. D., Zhou, J., and Seeley, W. W. (2010). Network-level structural covariance in the developing brain. *Proc. Natl. Acad. Sci. U.S.A.* 107, 18191–18196.

5

Imaging structural and functional brain networks in temporal lobe epilepsy

Boris C. Bernhardt[1,2]*, SeokJun Hong[1], Andrea Bernasconi[1] and Neda Bernasconi[1]

[1] *Neuroimaging of Epilepsy Laboratory, Montreal Neurological Institute and Hospital, McGill University, Montreal, QC, Canada*
[2] *Department of Social Neuroscience, Max Planck Institute for Human Cognitive and Brain Sciences, Leipzig, Germany*

***Correspondence:**
Boris C. Bernhardt, Neuroimaging of Epilepsy Laboratory, Montreal Neurological Institute and Hospital, McGill University, 3801 University Street, H3A2B4, Montreal, QC, Canada
e-mail: boris@bic.mni.mcgill.ca

Early imaging studies in temporal lobe epilepsy (TLE) focused on the search for mesial temporal sclerosis, as its surgical removal results in clinically meaningful improvement in about 70% of patients. Nevertheless, a considerable subgroup of patients continues to suffer from post-operative seizures. Although the reasons for surgical failure are not fully understood, electrophysiological and imaging data suggest that anomalies extending beyond the temporal lobe may have negative impact on outcome. This hypothesis has revived the concept of human epilepsy as a disorder of distributed brain networks. Recent methodological advances in non-invasive neuroimaging have led to quantify structural and functional networks *in vivo*. While structural networks can be inferred from diffusion MRI tractography and inter-regional covariance patterns of structural measures such as cortical thickness, functional connectivity is generally computed based on statistical dependencies of neurophysiological time-series, measured through functional MRI or electroencephalographic techniques. This review considers the application of advanced analytical methods in structural and functional connectivity analyses in TLE. We will specifically highlight findings from graph-theoretical analysis that allow assessing the topological organization of brain networks. These studies have provided compelling evidence that TLE is a system disorder with profound alterations in local and distributed networks. In addition, there is emerging evidence for the utility of network properties as clinical diagnostic markers. Nowadays, a network perspective is considered to be essential to the understanding of the development, progression, and management of epilepsy.

Keywords: TLE, connectivity, MRI, graph-theory, connectome

INTRODUCTION

Epilepsy is one of the most prevalent neurological disorders, affecting ~1% of the general population. Of patients treated with antiepileptic drugs, about one third never achieve remission. Drug-resistance should be identified early and treated effectively, as uncontrolled epilepsy is harmful to the brain, has devastating socio-economic consequences, and is associated with increased mortality (Leonardi and Ustun, 2002; Pugliatti et al., 2007; Tellez-Zenteno et al., 2007; Cascino, 2009; Coan and Cendes, 2013). Epilepsy is broadly defined by a state of recurrent spontaneous seizures, which arise when balance between excitation and inhibition is disrupted (Scharfman, 2007; Engel et al., 2013). Compelling evidence from animal models, experimental paradigms, and clinical work in humans indicates that specific cortical and subcortical networks play a fundamental role in the genesis and expression of seizures (Avoli and Gloor, 1982; Bear et al., 1996; Bertram, 1997; Spencer, 2002).

Temporal lobe epilepsy (TLE) is the most common drug-resistant epilepsy in adults. TLE is traditionally associated with mesiotemporal sclerosis, defined by cell loss and gliosis in the hippocampus, entorhinal cortex, and amygdala. Surgical resection of this epileptogenic lesion is the current treatment of choice (Wiebe et al., 2001), and leads to freedom from seizures in the majority of cases. Nevertheless, even in carefully selected cases, ~30% of surgical candidates continue to have seizures (Mcintosh et al., 2004; Bernhardt et al., 2010). Although reasons for surgical failure are not fully understood, electrophysiological and imaging data suggest that anomalies extending beyond the temporal lobe may have negative impact on outcome. This hypothesis has revived the concept of human epilepsy as a disorder of distributed neural networks (Spencer, 2002; Bonilha et al., 2007b; Elsharkawy et al., 2009; Engel et al., 2013).

In the past decade, advances in imaging acquisition and postprocessing have permitted *in vivo* mapping of the regional distribution of network abnormalities in TLE patients. In particular, quantitative structural MRI studies based on volumetry, voxel-based morphometry, cortical thickness mapping, and structural covariance analysis have shown widespread, coordinated, and progressive cortical gray matter loss in temporal and extra-temporal regions, such as the thalamus, fronto-limbic, and fronto-central neocortices (Bernasconi et al., 2003b, 2004; Natsume et al., 2003; Bonilha et al., 2004; Lin et al., 2007; Bernhardt et al., 2008, 2009, 2010, 2012; Keller and Roberts, 2008; Mcdonald et al., 2008b,c). Findings of gray matter alterations have been complemented by diffusion MRI data of the white matter. These studies have shown disruptions in inter-regional fiber diffusivity both within and beyond mesiotemporal and temporo-limbic networks, suggestive of decreased fiber arrangement and altered myelin membranes (Concha et al., 2005; Rodrigo et al., 2007; Yogarajah and Duncan, 2008; Ahmadi et al., 2009). Furthermore, studies based on both electrophysiological techniques as well as functional MRI have provided evidence for region-specific shifts in intrinsic functional networks (Bettus et al., 2009; Voets et al., 2012). More recently, reports of disruptions of inter-regional structural and functional connections in TLE have been complemented by graph-theoretical approaches (Liao et al., 2010; Bernhardt et al., 2011; Bonilha et al., 2012). These techniques, derived from complex system analysis, lend tools to characterize topological aspects that relate to the specialization and integration of inter-connected brain networks (Watts and Strogatz, 1998; Sporns et al., 2004; Bullmore and Sporns, 2009; Guye et al., 2010). In TLE, such approaches provide a novel window to study connectivity, and have begun showing alterations in higher-order network configurations.

The aim of this review is to summarize the current state of imaging evidence for network abnormalities in TLE. We will first outline findings that have provided insights into the topographical extent of regional structural abnormalities in TLE. We will then discuss studies on low-level inter-regional abnormalities, using connectivity mapping techniques such as seed-based structural MRI covariance, functional MRI connectivity, and diffusion MRI tractography. Subsequently, we will discuss graph-theoretical analyses to address the topological organization of brain networks in TLE. We will conclude by commenting on the potential clinical relevance of current network-based MRI analysis in TLE.

REGIONAL PATTERNS OF STRUCTURAL PATHOLOGY

The hallmark lesion of TLE is hippocampal sclerosis. This lesion is characterized by various degrees of neuronal loss and gliosis within hippocampal subfields and the dentate gyrus (Sommer, 1880; Babb and Brown, 1987; Blumcke et al., 2002). In addition, up to 50% of TLE patients may show intense reorganization of neuronal networks, manifested by granule cell dispersion (Houser et al., 1992; Blumcke et al., 2002), selective loss of inhibitory neurons (De Lanerolle et al., 1989), as well as axonal sprouting (Babb et al., 1991). Histological reports of TLE patients and animal models of limbic epilepsy have consistently demonstrated that pathology is not limited to the hippocampus. Indeed, cell loss and gliosis may be found in proximal and even more distal temporo-limbic regions, including the amygdala (Yilmazer-Hanke et al., 2000), entorhinal cortex (Du et al., 1993, 1995), temporopolar (Choi et al., 1999; Meiners et al., 1999; Mitchell et al., 1999; Bothwell et al., 2001) and lateral temporal neocortices (Cavanagh and Meyer, 1956; Falconer et al., 1964; Turski et al., 1983; Clifford et al., 1987; Kuzniecky et al., 1987; Cavalheiro et al., 1991; Thom et al., 2009), as well as the thalamus (Turski et al., 1983; Clifford et al., 1987; Bertram et al., 2001; Sloan and Bertram, 2009). In animal models, tissue damage has been shown in extra-temporal neocortical regions, such as sensorimotor cortex, piriform, perirhinal, retrosplenial, and visual cortices. In humans, pathological data in regions remote from the temporal lobes in TLE is sparse. This is, in part, due to difficulties in obtaining immediate *postmortem* specimens and the surgical approach tailored to the temporal lobe. In their seminal postmortem study, Margerison and Corsellis described neuronal loss and gliosis in frontal and occipital cortices in about 20% of patients (Margerison and Corsellis, 1966). More recent autopsy reports have confirmed and further extended these observations by showing varying degrees of architectural abnormalities involving virtually all lobes (Eriksson et al., 2002; Blanc et al., 2011).

A large body of electro-clinical work suggests that the epileptogenic network in TLE is broad. Seizure activity may involve not only the hippocampus, but also several other subcortical and cortical structures, including the amygdala, entorhinal cortex, lateral temporal, inferior, as well as orbitofrontal cortices (Lieb et al., 1987, 1991) together with the medial thalamus (Cassidy and Gale, 1998; Rosenberg et al., 2006). The close spatial correspondence between histopathological alterations and electrophysiological anomalies in TLE has provided a strong motivation to study structural brain changes, which have been of a high clinical and scientific value in mapping causes and consequences of drug-resistant epilepsy. In particular, quantitative Magnetic Resonance Imaging (MRI) analysis has offered a unique perspective to study structural substrates of TLE *in vivo* and to gain further insights into their spatial patterns and clinical correlates (See **Figure 1**, for a schematic overview of structural MRI findings in TLE). Studies based on manual volumetric MRI analysis largely confirmed previous histological assessments, and provided a more comprehensive picture of the regional extent of structural abnormalities in TLE. Volumetric analysis demonstrated atrophy in multiple limbic structures, including the hippocampus, entorhinal cortex, amygdala (Cendes et al., 1993a,b; Bernasconi et al., 2001, 2003a,b), temporopolar, perirhinal, lateral temporal neocortices (Jutila et al., 2001; Moran et al., 2001; Sankar et al., 2008), and the thalamus (Dreifuss et al., 2001; Natsume et al., 2003; Bernhardt et al., 2012). In the hippocampus and thalamus, surface shape mapping has furthermore allowed localizing structural anomalies at a subregional level (Hogan et al., 2004; Kim et al., 2008; Bernhardt et al., 2012, in press). In the thalamus, for example, we found volume loss located primarily in mediodorsal segments (Bernhardt et al., 2012). Quantitative MRI postprocessing techniques, such as voxel-based morphometry (Bernasconi et al., 2004; Bonilha et al., 2004; Keller and Roberts, 2008) and analyses of cortical thickness have shown that TLE is associated with extensive regional neocortical abnormalities, encompassing not only mesiotemporal structures, but also prefrontal, fronto-central, cingulate, occipito-temporal, and lateral temporal neocortices (Lin et al., 2007; Bernhardt et al., 2008, 2009, 2010, 2012; Mcdonald et al., 2008c; Mueller et al., 2009b; Kemmotsu et al., 2011; Voets et al., 2011). Although the exact biological underpinnings of gray matter loss in different brain regions are not clear, they likely reflect a combination of neuronal loss and synaptic reorganization (Cascino et al., 1991; Sanabria et al., 2002; Blanc et al., 2011), possibly secondary to seizures (Sutula et al., 1988; Holmes, 2002; Cavazos et al., 2003). These findings have increased our understanding of whole-brain pathology associated with TLE. On the

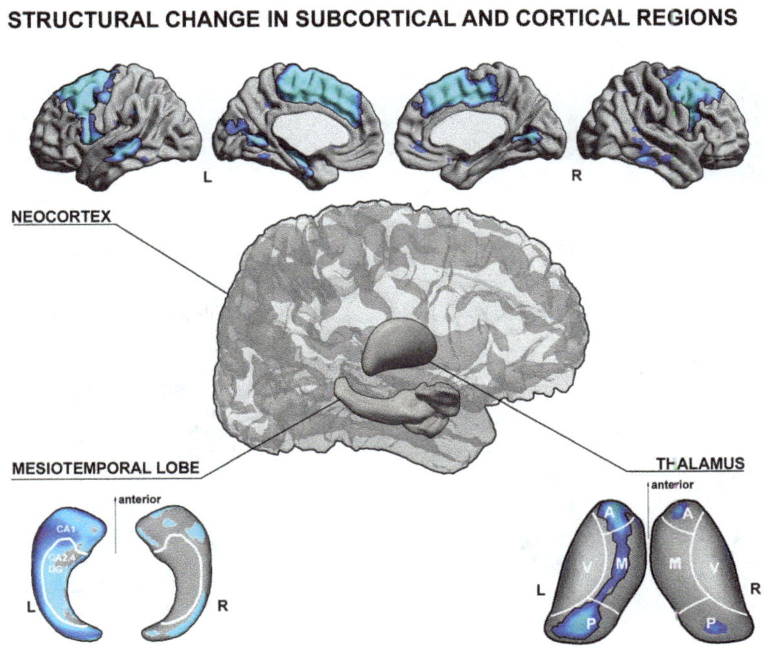

FIGURE 1 | Schematic illustration of gray matter structural anomalies in temporal lobe epilepsy. (top) Results from MRI-based cortical thickness analysis, showing cortical thinning in left temporal lobe epilepsy (TLE) patients with hippocampal atrophy relative to healthy controls in mesial and lateral temporal as well as fronto-central neocortices (Bernhardt et al., 2010). **(lower left)** Patterns of atrophy in TLE patients relative to controls in CA1 subregions of the ipsilateral hippocampus (Kim et al., 2008) and **(lower right)** mediodorsal segments of the thalamus (Bernhardt et al., 2012), both generated using spherical harmonic surface-shape modeling techniques of manual MRI segmentations. The shown analyses have been generated using the SurfStat toolbox for Matlab (Worsley et al., 2009). Further details on the statistical procedures can be found in the original publications.

other hand, new techniques such as hippocampal and thalamic surface-shape mapping (Kim et al., 2008; Bernhardt et al., 2012) have allowed searching for fine-grained, subregional structural anomalies within temporo-limbic seizure networks. Importantly, the MRI-derived knowledge of pathology is in overall agreement with data from animal models and *ex vivo* studies. These studies collectively support the concept of TLE as a disorder of distributed neural networks.

STRUCTURAL NETWORKS

Quantitative structural studies have provided a comprehensive mapping of structural pathology in TLE. Nevertheless, the commonly applied mass-univariate group comparisons provide only a snapshot of putative network abnormalities in TLE. Indeed, while such topographic maps may localize an ensemble of affected regions, they do not directly address how these regions inter-relate.

The term *structural connectivity* refers to anatomical associations between brain regions, defining the actual physical wiring (Stephan et al., 2000; Stone and Kotter, 2002; Sporns et al., 2005; Sporns, 2011). The gold standard to define such connections has been anterograde and retrograde tract-tracing techniques. Tracers show good accuracy and sensitivity, in particular for mapping long-range connections, and have resulted in a rich and detailed cartography of connectivity in several mammalian species (Felleman and Van Essen, 1991; Scannell et al., 1995; Modha and Singh, 2010). Their invasiveness however, limits their application to animal studies (Sporns, 2011).

In humans, two major indirect approaches have been employed to map structural networks: *diffusion MRI tractography* and *structural MRI covariance* (see **Figures 2A–D**). Structural networks derived from diffusion-weighted MRI data provide an approximation of the underlying white matter architecture (Le Bihan et al., 1986, 1996; Johansen-Berg and Behrens, 2006; Jbabdi and Johansen-Berg, 2011) by describing the directionality and magnitude of water diffusion at each imaging voxel. These data can be further processed by tractography algorithms (Mori et al., 1999; Behrens et al., 2003), which reconstruct fiber pathways running along plausible diffusion trajectories in voxel-space (**Figure 2A**). While somewhat challenged in regions where different fiber populations intersect (Behrens et al., 2003; Jones et al., 2012), such as the cortical gray matter, tractography can generate consistent results, particularly in deep white matter. Findings have shown overall a good correspondence with the animal tracing literature, and have been cross-validated by comparative sacrificial tracing studies in non-human primates (Mori et al., 1999; Parker et al., 2002; Dauguet et al., 2007). Moreover, it has been shown that factors such as fiber diameter and density, membrane permeability, myelination, as well as fiber packing (Beaulieu, 2002; Concha et al., 2010) can influence the directionality and magnitude of water displacement at a given voxel. Diffusion imaging may, thus, be used to assess microstructural and architectural integrity *in vivo*. The most widely used diffusion tensor parameters are fractional anisotropy (FA), an index of deviation of water diffusion from a random spherical displacement, and mean

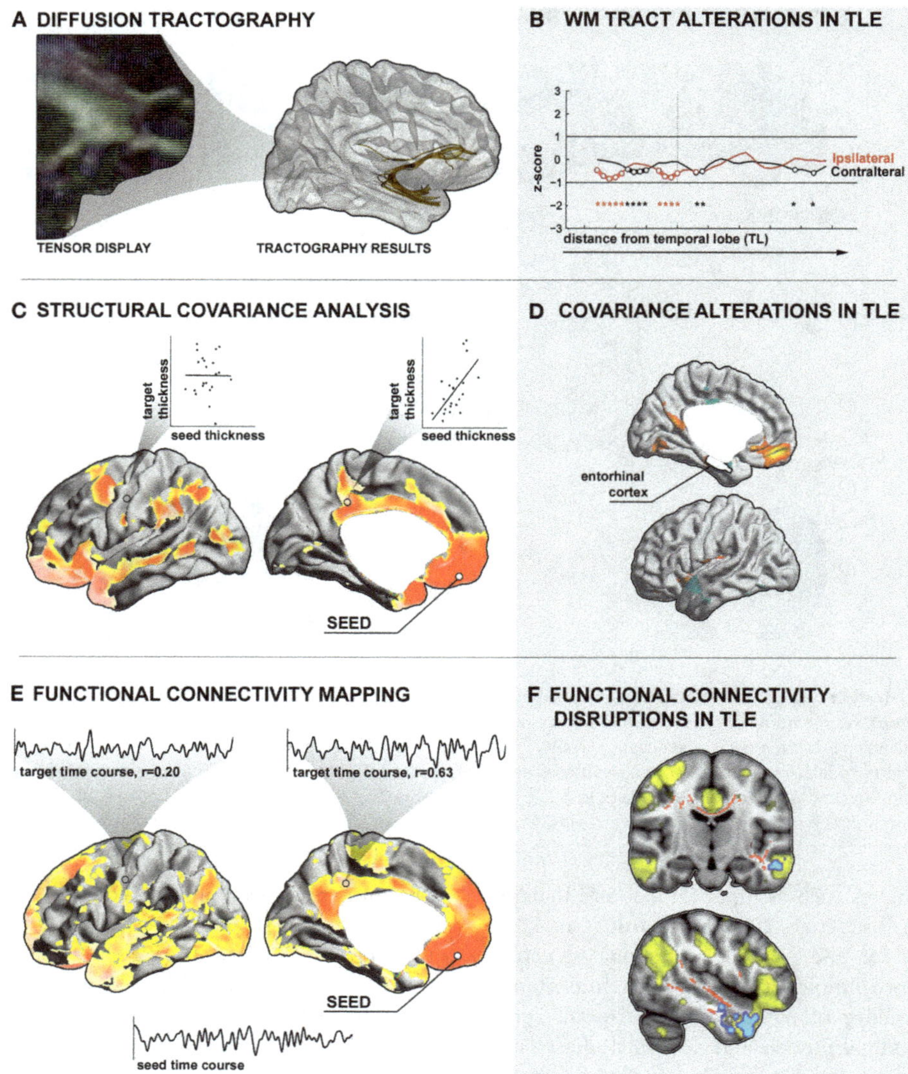

FIGURE 2 | Assessment of inter-regional connectivity. (A) Diffusion tractography. *Left:* Illustration of diffusion tensor directions superimposed on a fractional anisotropy map derived from diffusion MRI. *Right*: Seed-based deterministic tractography of the uncinate fasciculus. **(B)** Altered mean diffusivity along the uncinate fasciculus tract in a group of patients with temporal lobe epilepsy (TLE) relative to controls (Concha et al., 2012). Prior to analysis, the tract was subdivided into bins with respect to the anatomical distance to the temporal and frontal lobes. **(C)** Structural covariance analysis. Shown is the cortical thickness correlation map of the left medial orbital cortex seed with the remaining cortical mantle in a group of healthy controls. High positive correlations are interpreted as connections, low correlations as absence of connections. **(D)** Structural covariance alterations in TLE patients relative to controls between an entorhinal cortex seed and target regions in medial orbitofrontal cortices (Bernhardt et al., 2008). **(E)** Functional connectivity between a left medial orbitofrontal cortex seed and the rest of the cortical mantle in healthy controls. Insets show exemplary time courses of the seed region with selected cortical target regions with high and low correlations, respectively. **(F)** Voxel-wise functional connectivity abnormalities in TLE, highlighting target regions with altered time-series correlation to a spatial component that closely matches the "default mode" network (Voets et al., 2012).

diffusion (MD), a scalar marker of bulk diffusion at each voxel.

In TLE, previous diffusion MRI studies have consistently shown decreased FA in temporo-limbic tracts such as the fornix pathway (Concha et al., 2005; Ahmadi et al., 2009), parahippocampal fibers (Mcdonald et al., 2008a; Yogarajah and Duncan, 2008; Ahmadi et al., 2009), the uncinate fasciculus (Rodrigo et al., 2007; Diehl et al., 2008; Lin et al., 2008; Mcdonald et al., 2008a), and the cingulum bundle (Concha et al., 2008; Ahmadi et al., 2009), as well as in several frontal and posterior fiber tracts including the inferior and superior longitudinal fascicles (Focke et al., 2008; Lin et al., 2008; Mcdonald et al., 2008a; Ahmadi et al., 2009), the internal and external capsule (Arfanakis et al., 2002; Gross et al., 2006; Concha et al., 2008), and the corpus callosum (Arfanakis et al., 2002; Gross et al., 2006; Concha et al., 2008). Relative to the widespread pattern of FA changes, MD anomalies follow a more restricted distribution (Concha et al., 2005, 2008; Focke et al., 2008). In a recent study that assessed diffusion abnormalities along fiber tracts, our group could show that the effect size of MD alterations in TLE seems to decrease as a function of anatomical distance to the temporal lobe (**Figure 2B**), suggesting co-localization of these changes with the seizure focus (Concha et al., 2012).

The combined contribution of different microstructural and architectural properties to the diffusion signal precludes a straightforward, and universal biological interpretation of diffusion tensor indices and their alteration in disease (Jones et al., 2012). Diffusion MRI is, nevertheless, currently the only imaging method that can assess fiber architecture *in vivo* (Jones et al., 2012). Initial evidence from histopathological analysis of the fimbria-fornix pathways in operated TLE patients suggests that FA decreases may primarily reflect alterations in axonal membranes (Concha et al., 2010). MD changes, on the other hand, have been shown to vary with respect to the dynamics of seizure activity (Yu and Tan, 2008; Concha et al., 2012). Indeed, MD has been shown to decrease in the hyperacute phase after prolonged seizures or status epilepticus, likely due to intracellular cytotoxic edema. Conversely, few days following the subacute peri-ictal phase, MD may increase as a consequence of vasogenic edema (Scott et al., 2006). Neuronal loss and gliosis can lead to further MD increase as a consequence of the chronic expansion of the interstitial water content.

Structural networks may also be studied through covariance analysis of MRI-based morphological metrics, such as cortical thickness or gray matter volume (Bullmore et al., 1998; Mechelli et al., 2005; Lerch et al., 2006; Bernhardt et al., 2008, 2013). According to the framework of MRI covariance analysis, a high correlation in morphological markers between two regions across subjects can be interpreted as a network link, while a low correlation indicates no link (**Figure 2C**). Similar to diffusion tractography, this correlational framework does not infer direct anatomical connections between pairs of regions. Nonetheless, analyzing structural covariance may detect manifestations of persistent functional-trophic cross-talk, maturational inter-change, as well as common developmental and pathological influences (Lerch et al., 2006; Bullmore and Sporns, 2009; Zielinski et al., 2010; Bernhardt et al., 2011; Raznahan et al., 2011; Xia and He, 2011; Khundrakpam et al., 2012; Alexander-Bloch et al., 2013). One of the advantages of cortical thickness covariance analysis is the direct seeding from cortical gray matter regions in a high-resolution space that is in principle not limited by the imaging voxels of the underlying MR image, but by the sampling density of the points on the cortical mesh. Correlation analysis of structural features may furthermore represent a relatively pragmatic approach toward structural network mapping. In fact, the commonly used T1-weighted images, a standard component of every clinical imaging protocol, have a short acquisition time. Moreover, these images are generally unaffected by distortion and signal dropout artifacts in orbitofrontal and temporo-basal regions often occurring in echo-planar functional and diffusion MRI sequences.

In TLE, several recent covariance analyses have mapped abnormal structural correlations between mesiotemporal and neocortical regions (Bonilha et al., 2007a; Bernhardt et al., 2008; Mueller et al., 2009b), thalamic and neocortical regions (Mueller et al., 2009a; Bernhardt et al., 2012), and within cortico-cortical networks (Mueller et al., 2009a). Correlating the thickness of the entorhinal cortex to that of the neocortex, our group found decreased structural coordination between mesial temporal regions and lateral temporal neocortices, suggestive of a connectional breakdown within temporo-limbic circuits (**Figure 2D**; Bernhardt et al., 2008). Moreover, covariance analysis of thalamo-cortical circuits (Hetherington et al., 2007; Mueller et al., 2009a; Bernhardt et al., 2012) has shown coupled structural and metabolic change of the thalamus with neocortical (Bernhardt et al., 2012) and with mesiotemporal regions (Hetherington et al., 2007; Mueller et al., 2009a), emphasizing a key role of this structure in the pathological network of TLE.

Diffusion MRI and structural MRI covariance analysis tap into different facets of structural brain networks. While diffusion MRI analysis may be the method of choice to study white matter tracts, and their potential architectural disruptions, structural covariance analysis may sensitively assess alterations in the trophic-morphological coordination between gray matter regions. Both approaches have advanced our understanding of the fundamental architecture of inter-regional connections, and their disruptions in TLE.

FUNCTIONAL NETWORKS

The study of functional networks helps to elucidate *how* a structural architecture gives rise to alterations in neurophysiological dynamics. The term *functional connectivity* refers to the strength of statistical dependencies of neurophysiological signals between regions (**Figure 2E**).

Functional connectivity can be determined from time-series measured by functional MRI (Friston et al., 1993, 1996; Focke et al., 2008; Smith, 2012) or electrophysiological techniques, such as electroencephalography (EEG) (Lopes Da Silva et al., 1989; Tononi et al., 1994; Lachaux et al., 1999). Although functional MRI and EEG have complimentary temporal/spatial resolution tradeoffs, they can also be combined (Lemieux et al., 2011). In short, functional MRI does not directly measure neural activity, but only activity-dependent hemodynamic alterations, and has a relatively low temporal resolution in the range of 1–2 s [but see Feinberg et al. (2010); Smith et al. (2012), for a recent example of increasing the temporal resolution in functional MRI acquisitions]. Yet, this technique offers high spatial resolution in the millimeter range and allows imaging the entire brain (Lemieux et al., 2011). EEG, on the other hand, has a superior temporal resolution (in the order of milliseconds) but suffers from neurophysiological signals limited to the scalp.

One way to assess functional connectivity between different brain regions is through analysis of task-free (or, resting-state) paradigms, functional acquisitions during which the subject does not perform any task (Biswal et al., 1995, 2010; Greicius et al., 2003; Smith et al., 2009). Functional connectivity analysis of such task-free datasets has allowed the identification of brain networks that show strong coupling of intrinsic, spontaneous brain activity. Ample recent resting-state functional MRI assessments have revealed networks which are generally reproducible across subjects (Damoiseaux et al., 2006) that closely correspond to brain systems engaging in specific tasks (Biswal et al., 1995; Smith et al., 2009; Laird et al., 2011). Several studies have furthermore begun to explore the relationship between low-frequency resting-state networks derived from functional MRI and those measured from EEG (De Pasquale et al., 2010; Jann et al., 2010; Musso et al., 2010; Yuan et al., 2012). Moreover, several studies in primates have suggested a close correspondence between intrinsic functional MRI connections and known anatomical pathways (Mantini et al., 2011; Shen et al., 2012). In turn, other studies have demonstrated the utility of resting-state patterns to generate regional parcellations of specific anatomical areas (Margulies et al., 2007; Mars et al., 2011). Finally, analysis of resting-state connectivity patterns may be sensitive to detect disruptions of brain organization in disease conditions (Greicius, 2008; Fox and Greicius, 2010; Kelly et al., 2012).

Several EEG and combined EEG-fMRI studies have shown dynamic alterations in functional activations and connectivity patterns related to epileptic spikes (Gotman et al., 2006; Kobayashi et al., 2006; Laufs et al., 2007; Ponten et al., 2007; Bettus et al., 2011). Resting-state functional EEG and functional MRI connectivity analyses in TLE have also quantified chronic, inter-ictal changes in functional networks (Waites et al., 2006; Bettus et al., 2009). These studies have mainly focused on assessing associations of intrinsic signals between regions known to be involved in seizure activity, particularly among medial temporal lobe structures. Bettus and colleagues reported decreased functional connectivity in mesiotemporal regions proximal to the seizure focus; interestingly, ipsilateral decreases co-occurred with increased functional connectivity in contralateral regions (Bettus et al., 2009). Findings of contralateral connectivity increases are suggestive of compensatory network reorganization. Several studies have also suggested functional connectivity alterations in regions that comprise the "default mode" network (Raichle et al., 2001; Greicius et al., 2003; Voets et al., 2012), or between this network and other brain regions (Frings et al., 2009; Liao et al., 2010; Zhang et al., 2010). The default mode network includes a collection of medial frontal, midline parietal, and lateral parietal regions that show increased activation in the absence of a specific tasks, and whose function may closely relate to internal thought processes such as memory and mind-wandering (Buckner and Carroll, 2007; Christoff et al., 2009).

Changes in inter-regional functional coupling are thought to represent compensatory mechanisms secondary to structural pathology and seizure-related activity. Combining structural and functional image analysis, for example, our group recently showed disruptions in functional connectivity between mesiotemporal regions and neocortical target networks (**Figure 2F**) that may relate to abnormal gray matter density and altered diffusivity of inter-connecting fiber tracts (Voets et al., 2012) suggestive of a complex derangement in the structural-functional cross-links. There is also evidence for abnormal signal interactions in epileptic patients without a visible lesion on MRI (Vlooswijk et al., 2011). In addition, functional abnormalities have even been shown in regions unaffected by epileptic discharges (Bettus et al., 2011), suggestive of a widespread pathological process that alter the whole-brain intrinsic functional network architecture in TLE.

GRAPH THEORY—MODELING NETWORK TOPOLOGY

Conventional analysis approaches, mainly based on between-group comparisons have shown low-level regional and connectional alterations in TLE. These methods, however, are not tailored at capturing the complexity of whole-brain pathological interactions in TLE, which may affect higher-order, topological aspects of brain network organization.

Graph theory is a framework for the mathematical representation and analysis of complex systems. It has been applied to the analysis of artificial and biological networks (Watts and Strogatz, 1998). Graph theoretical analysis has recently attracted considerable attention in brain research because it provides a powerful formalism to quantitatively describe the topological organization of connectivity (Bullmore and Sporns, 2009; Guye et al., 2010; Bassett and Gazzaniga, 2011; Bullmore and Bassett, 2011; Alexander-Bloch et al., 2013). In graph theory terms, a network is a collection of nodes that are interconnected by edges. Nodes usually represent brain regions, while edges represent (structural or functional) connections. A pre-requisite to connectivity analysis is the proper designation of nodes as distinct gray matter regions. Various parcellation schemes have been proposed, including approximating Brodmann areas based on imaging-derived surrogates of myelination (Glasser and Van Essen, 2011; Bock et al., 2013), sulcation-based atlases (Van Essen, 2005; Desikan et al., 2006), high-resolution parcellations (Hagmann et al., 2008; Honey et al., 2009), as well as schemes that take the imaging voxels/vertices themselves as nodes (Lohmann et al., 2010; Tomasi and Volkow, 2011). In addition, several studies have also used data-driven techniques such as independent brain components to define network nodes (Yu et al., 2011b, 2013). Nodal definitions have shown to have a large influence on graph-theoretical parameters (Tohka et al., 2012), and the definition of reliable, biological meaningful parcellations schemes continues to be an active area of current research (Geyer et al., 2011; Glasser and Van Essen, 2011; Van Essen et al., 2012).

As described in previous sections, *in vivo* studies provide several definitions for network edges, both in the structural and functional domain (*see* **Figure 3**, for an example of functional and structural network generation). Accordingly, graph-theoretical analysis has been conducted across various modalities such as functional MRI (Salvador et al., 2005; He et al., 2009; Honey et al., 2009), electrophysiology (Stam, 2004; Bassett et al., 2006), diffusion-weighted MRI (Hagmann et al., 2007, 2008; Iturria-Medina et al., 2007; Gong et al., 2009), and structural covariance (He et al., 2007; Bassett et al., 2008; Chen et al., 2008; Bernhardt et al., 2011). Collectively, these studies have shown that the global topology of brain networks in healthy populations is neither random nor regular, but characteristic of a *small-world*. Small-world networks are defined by clusters of tightly inter-connected nodes, which are themselves linked to other clusters through few inter-connector links. This architecture results in overall short path

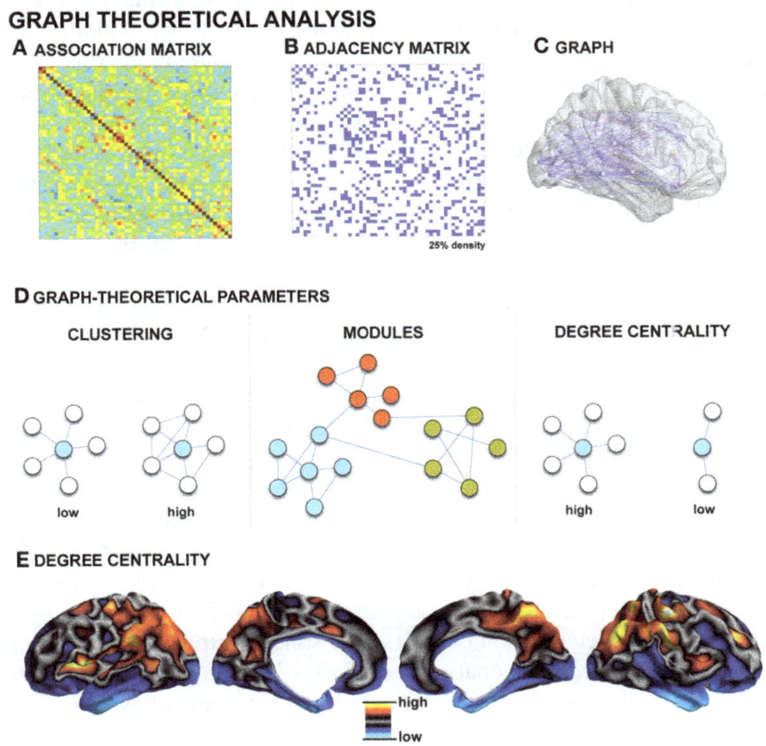

FIGURE 3 | Graph-theoretical analysis. **(A)** Association matrix quantifying the degree of connectivity (derived from techniques such as diffusion MRI tractography, structural covariance, or functional connectivity, see **Figure 2**). **(B)** Matrices commonly undergo a thresholding procedure to remove spurious edges. In this example, the highest 25% of associations are preserved, leading to a binary adjacency matrix. **(C)** Each binary matrix is equivalent to an undirected graph. **(D)** Topological parameters such as the clustering coefficient and path length can then be measured; networks can be partitioned in modules based on groupings of connectivity among nodes; hubs can be identified, for example, as nodes with high degree centrality (i.e., a high number of connections). **(E)** Cortical degree centrality map, based on resting-state functional connectivity data from a single healthy control subject.

lengths between individual nodes and an overall high degree of clustering (Watts and Strogatz, 1998), an architecture that enables both the specialization and integration of information transfer at relatively low wiring costs (Sporns et al., 2004). Graph-theoretical methods may be used to examine intermediary levels of organization. Communities (also called modules) are groups of nodes that are richly connected to one another within the larger framework of the entire network (Meunier et al., 2010; Bullmore and Bassett, 2011). Modularity is one of the most ubiquitous properties of complex, large-scale networks (Bullmore and Sporns, 2009), and modules may express some degree of hierarchical organization (Bassett et al., 2008; Meunier et al., 2010; Bullmore and Bassett, 2011). Theoretically, there are several advantages to a modular and hierarchical organization, including greater adaptability and robustness to changing environmental conditions (Meunier et al., 2010). Moreover, it has been suggested that the more modular and hierarchically organized a system is, the more diverse its functional activation patterns (Alexander-Bloch et al., 2010; Kaiser and Hilgetag, 2010). Modularity may be undermined by disease processes, as suggested by disrupted modularity in schizophrenia (Bassett et al., 2008; Alexander-Bloch et al., 2010; Yu et al., 2011a), and frontal lobe epilepsy (Vaessen et al., 2012a).

Besides the characterization of global and modular properties of large-scale networks, graph-theoretical techniques allow the localization of key regions within the network layout, so-called *hubs*, through centrality-based metrics (Bullmore and Sporns, 2009; Van Den Heuvel and Sporns, 2011; Zuo et al., 2012). According to formulations of centrality, hubs can be defined as regions with a high degree centrality, which means that they have a high number of connections to other nodes (Zuo et al., 2012); they can be identified on the basis of high betweeness centrality, which signifies they are located along pathways of efficient information flow (Zuo et al., 2012); finally, they can be identified through a high eigenvector centrality, which is a recursive formulation quantifying connections to other highly connected hubs (Lohmann et al., 2010; Zuo et al., 2012). Depending on their embedding in specific modules and connectivity profiles, hubs can be further classified as to whether they primarily mediate within- or between-module connectivity (Sporns et al., 2007). Assessing hubs promises to highlight critical key regions in structural and functional networks, and may thus provide a better understanding of their potential role in pathological processes (Bullmore and Sporns, 2012). In Alzheimer's disease, for example, functional hubs coincide with regions of high amyloid-beta deposition (Buckner et al., 2009). Central hubs may form a so-called *rich club*, a collection of mutually densely linked nodes with disproportionally high centrality (Van Den Heuvel and Sporns, 2011; Harriger et al., 2012). This architecture is thought to contribute to the robustness of the core constituents of the brain network. In humans, a rich club inferred from diffusion MRI has been shown to comprise lateral prefrontal, midline and lateral parietal, as well as the hippocampus, putamen, and thalamus (Van Den Heuvel and Sporns, 2011). In the macaque monkey, rich club regions have been shown to be preferentially located on short paths through the network, thereby contributing effectively to global communication (Harriger et al., 2012).

In focal epilepsy, relatively few studies have employed graph-theoretical analysis of brain networks derived from MRI (Liao et al., 2010; Bernhardt et al., 2011; Bonilha et al., 2012; Vaessen et al., 2012b). We previously showed that in drug-resistant TLE, structural networks derived from inter-regional MRI-based cortical thickness correlations are characterized by increased clustering and path length, a finding indicative of a more regular global topology (Bernhardt et al., 2011). These findings were complemented by the parallel observation of reduced network robustness, a measure of organizational stability (Bernhardt et al., 2011), and subtle alterations in the distribution of network hubs pointing toward a more paralimbic distribution in patients relative to controls. In a longitudinal study, we showed that structural network disruptions intensify over time. Furthermore, relating network parameters to postsurgical seizure outcome data indicated that patients who continued to have seizures after surgery had more marked network disruptions relative to those who became seizure-free (Bernhardt et al., 2011). These findings speak to the hypothesis that seizure recurrence after surgery may, in part, be related to an extended epileptogenic network (Ryvlin, 2003; Bernhardt et al., 2010). Our findings therefore suggest a possible clinical potential for network data in the presurgical workup.

Our finding of a more regularized topology of structural cortico-cortical networks in drug-resistant TLE closely resembled results from graph-theoretical analyses of intracerebral EEG recordings during focal seizures (Ponten et al., 2007; Kramer et al., 2008; Schindler et al., 2008) and scalp EEG data of generalized absence seizures (Ponten et al., 2009). Indeed, electrophysiological work has suggested that seizures may be associated with a sudden regularization of functional networks. It may, thus, be plausible that network synchronization during the ictal phase may influence mutual inter-cortical trophic exchanges, ultimately leading to progressive and long-lasting remodeling of inter-regional structural networks.

Few other studies assessed the topology of brain networks derived from MRI in TLE using graph-theoretical methods. A diffusion MRI tractography of structures belonging to the limbic network showed increased clustering and centrality in 12 patients with unilateral TLE (Bonilha et al., 2012). Analysis of whole-brain resting-state functional networks in patients with bilateral TLE has revealed both atypical low-level connectivity (i.e., increases in temporal and decreases in fronto-parietal connectivity) and topological disruptions, indicative of decreased clustering and path length (Liao et al., 2010). These studies have further demonstrated that TLE is associated with topological disruptions in large-scale structural and functional networks. Results have nevertheless been somewhat divergent, possibly as a result of heterogeneous patient populations and diverse network construction methods.

CONCLUSIONS AND FUTURE DIRECTIONS

Advances in brain network construction and graph theoretical modeling have permitted a characterization of topological aspects of healthy and abnormal brain connectivity. While an extensive literature has shown regional as well as low-level connectional disruptions in TLE, studies focusing on disruptions of network topology have been so far rather sparse. The unified and elegant framework of graph theoretical analysis promises to further consolidate our understanding of how functional networks interact with their structural substrate. Moreover, given initial observations of a relationship between the extent of network damage and post-surgical seizure outcome, establishing subject-specific profiles of network properties has great potential to assist in clinical decision-making.

REFERENCES

Ahmadi, M. E., Hagler, D. J. Jr., Mcdonald, C. R., Tecoma, E. S., Iragui, V. J., Dale, A.M., et al. (2009). Side matters: diffusion tensor imaging tractography in left and right temporal lobe epilepsy. *AJNR. Am. J. Neuroradiol.* 30, 1740–1747. doi: 10.3174/ajnr.A1650

Alexander-Bloch, A., Giedd, J. N., and Bullmore, E. (2013). Imaging structural co-variance between human brain regions. *Nat. Rev. Neurosci.* 14, 322–336. doi: 10.1038/nrn3465

Alexander-Bloch, A. F., Gogtay, N., Meunier, D., Birn, R., Clasen, L., Lalonde, F., et al. (2010). Disrupted modularity and local connectivity of brain functional networks in childhood-onset schizophrenia. *Front. Syst. Neurosci.* 4:147. doi: 10.3389/fnsys.2010.00147

Arfanakis, K., Hermann, B. P., Rogers, B. P., Carew, J. D., Seidenberg, M., and Meyerand, M. E. (2002). Diffusion tensor MRI in temporal lobe epilepsy. *Magn. Reson. Imaging* 20, 511–519. doi: 10.1016/S0730-725X(02)00509-X

Avoli, M., and Gloor, P. (1982). Interaction of cortex and thalamus in spike and wave discharges of feline generalized penicillin epilepsy. *Exp. Neurol.* 76, 196–217. doi: 10.1016/0014-4886(82)90112-1

Babb, T. L., and Brown, W. J. (1987). "Pathological findings in epilepsy," in *Surgical Treatment of the Epilepsies*, ed J. Engel Jr. (New York, NY: Raven), 511–540.

Babb, T. L., Kupfer, W. R., Pretorius, J. K., Crandall, P. H., and Levesque, M. F. (1991). Synaptic reorganization by mossy fibers in human epileptic fascia dentata. *Neuroscience* 42, 351–363. doi: 10.1016/0306-4522(91)90380-7

Bassett, D. S., Bullmore, E., Verchinski, B. A., Mattay, V. S., Weinberger, D. R., and Meyer-Lindenberg, A. (2008). Hierarchical organization of human cortical networks in health and schizophrenia. *J. Neurosci.* 28, 9239–9248. doi: 10.1523/JNEUROSCI.1929-08.2008

Bassett, D. S., and Gazzaniga, M. S. (2011). Understanding complexity in the human brain. *Trends Cogn. Sci.* 15, 200–209. doi: 10.1016/j.tics.2011.03.006

Bassett, D. S., Meyer-Lindenberg, A., Achard, S., Duke, T., and Bullmore, E. (2006). Adaptive reconfiguration of fractal small-world human brain functional networks. *Proc. Natl. Acad. Sci. U.S.A.* 103, 19518–19523. doi: 10.1073/pnas.0606005103

Bear, J., Fountain, N. B., and Lothman, E. W. (1996). Responses of the superficial entorhinal cortex *in vitro* in slices from naive and chronically epileptic rats. *J. Neurophysiol.* 76, 2928–2940.

Beaulieu, C. (2002). The basis of anisotropic water diffusion in the nervous system - a technical review. *NMR Biomed.* 15, 435–455. doi: 10.1002/nbm.782

Behrens, T. E., Johansen-Berg, H., Woolrich, M. W., Smith, S. M., Wheeler-Kingshott, C. A., Boulby, P. A., et al. (2003). Non-invasive mapping of connections between human thalamus and cortex using diffusion imaging. *Nat. Neurosci.* 6, 750–757. doi: 10.1038/nn1075

Bernasconi, N., Andermann, F., Arnold, D. L., and Bernasconi, A. (2003a). Entorhinal cortex MRI assessment in temporal, extratemporal, and idiopathic generalized epilepsy. *Epilepsia* 44, 1070–1074. doi: 10.1046/j.1528-1157.2003.64802.x

Bernasconi, N., Bernasconi, A., Caramanos, Z., Antel, S. B., Andermann, F., and Arnold, D. L. (2003b). Mesial temporal damage in temporal lobe epilepsy: a volumetric MRI study of the hippocampus, amygdala and parahippocampal region. *Brain* 126, 462–469. doi: 10.1093/brain/awg034

Bernasconi, N., Bernasconi, A., Caramanos, Z., Dubeau, F., Richardson, J., Andermann, F., et al. (2001). Entorhinal cortex atrophy in epilepsy patients exhibiting normal hippocampal volumes. *Neurology* 56, 1335–1339. doi: 10.1212/WNL.56.10.1335

Bernasconi, N., Duchesne, S., Janke, A., Lerch, J., Collins, D. L., and Bernasconi, A. (2004). Whole-brain voxel-based statistical analysis of gray matter and white matter in temporal lobe epilepsy. *Neuroimage* 23, 717–723. doi: 10.1016/j.neuroimage.2004.06.015

Bernhardt, B. C., Bernasconi, N., Concha, L., and Bernasconi, A. (2010). Cortical thickness analysis in temporal lobe epilepsy: reproducibility and relation to outcome. *Neurology* 74, 1776–1784. doi: 10.1212/WNL.0b013e3181e0f80a

Bernhardt, B. C., Bernasconi, N., Kim, H., and Bernasconi, A. (2012). Mapping thalamocortical network pathology in temporal lobe epilepsy. *Neurology* 78, 129–136. doi: 10.1212/WNL.0b013e31823efd0d

Bernhardt, B. C., Chen, Z., He, Y., Evans, A. C., and Bernasconi, N. (2011). Graph-theoretical analysis reveals disrupted small-world organization of cortical thickness correlation networks in temporal lobe epilepsy. *Cereb. Cortex* 21, 2147–2157. doi: 10.1093/cercor/bhq291

Bernhardt, B. C., Klimecki, O. M., Leiberg, S., and Singer, T. (2013). Structural covariance networks of dorsal anterior insula predict females' individual differences in empathic responding. *Cereb. Cortex* doi: 10.1093/cercor/bht072. [Epub ahead of print].

Bernhardt, B. C., Kim, H., and Bernasconi, N. (in press). Patterns of subregional disease progression in temporal lobe epilepsy. *Neurology*.

Bernhardt, B. C., Worsley, K. J., Besson, P., Concha, L., Lerch, J. P., Evans, A. C., et al. (2008). Mapping limbic network organization in temporal lobe epilepsy using morphometric correlations: insights on the relation between mesiotemporal connectivity and cortical atrophy. *Neuroimage* 42, 515–524. doi: 10.1016/j.neuroimage.2008.04.261

Bernhardt, B. C., Worsley, K. J., Kim, H., Evans, A. C., Bernasconi, A., and Bernasconi, N. (2009). Longitudinal and cross-sectional analysis of atrophy in pharmacoresistant temporal lobe epilepsy. *Neurology* 72, 1747–1754. doi: 10.1212/01.wnl.0000345969.57574.f5

Bertram, E. H. (1997). Functional anatomy of spontaneous seizures in a rat model of limbic epilepsy. *Epilepsia* 38, 95–105. doi: 10.1111/j.1528-1157.1997.tb01083.x

Bertram, E. H., Mangan, P. S., Zhang, D., Scott, C. A., and Williamson, J. M. (2001). The midline thalamus: alterations and a potential role in limbic epilepsy. *Epilepsia* 42, 967–978. doi: 10.1046/j.1528-1157.2001.042008967.x

Bettus, G., Guedj, E., Joyeux, F., Confort-Gouny, S., Soulier, E., Laguitton, V., et al. (2009). Decreased basal fMRI functional connectivity in epileptogenic networks and contralateral compensatory mechanisms. *Hum. Brain Mapp.* 30, 1580–1591. doi: 10.1002/hbm.20625

Bettus, G., Ranjeva, J. P., Wendling, F., Benar, C. G., Confort-Gouny, S., Regis, J., et al. (2011). Interictal functional connectivity of human epileptic networks assessed by intracerebral EEG and BOLD signal fluctuations. *PLoS ONE* 6:e20071. doi: 10.1371/journal.pone.0020071

Biswal, B., Yetkin, F. Z., Haughton, V. M., and Hyde, J. S. (1995). Functional connectivity in the motor cortex of resting human brain using echo-planar MRI. *Magn. Reson. Med.* 34, 537–541. doi: 10.1002/mrm.1910340409

Biswal, B. B., Mennes, M., Zuo, X. N., Gohel, S., Kelly, C., Smith, S. M., et al. (2010). Toward discovery science of human brain function. *Proc. Natl. Acad. Sci. U.S.A.* 107, 4734–4739. doi: 10.1073/pnas.0911855107

Blanc, F., Martinian, L., Liagkouras, I., Catarino, C., Sisodiya, S. M., and Thom, M. (2011). Investigation of widespread neocortical pathology associated with hippocampal sclerosis in epilepsy: a postmortem study. *Epilepsia* 52, 10–21. doi: 10.1111/j.1528-1167.2010.02773.x

Blumcke, I., Thom, M., and Wiestler, O. D. (2002). Ammon's horn sclerosis: a maldevelopmental disorder associated with temporal lobe epilepsy. *Brain Pathol.* 12, 199–211.

Bock, N. A., Hashim, E., Janik, R., Konyer, N. B., Weiss, M., Stanisz, G. J., et al. (2013). Optimizing T(1)-weighted imaging of cortical myelin content at 3.0T. *Neuroimage* 65, 1–12. doi: 10.1016/j.neuroimage.2012.09.051

Bonilha, L., Nesland, T., Martz, G. U., Joseph, J. E., Spampinato, M. V., Edwards, J. C., et al. (2012). Medial temporal lobe epilepsy is associated with neuronal fibre loss and paradoxical increase in structural connectivity of limbic structures. *J. Neurol. Neurosurg. Psychiatr.* 83, 903–909. doi: 10.1136/jnnp-2012-302476

Bonilha, L., Rorden, C., Castellano, G., Pereira, F., Rio, P. A., Cendes, F., et al. (2004). Voxel-based morphometry reveals gray matter network atrophy in refractory medial temporal lobe epilepsy. *Arch. Neurol.* 61, 1379–1384. doi: 10.1001/archneur.61.9.1379

Bonilha, L., Rorden, C., Halford, J. J., Eckert, M., Appenzeller, S., Cendes, F., et al. (2007a). Asymmetrical extra-hippocampal grey matter loss related to hippocampal atrophy in patients with medial temporal lobe epilepsy. *J. Neurol. Neurosurg. Psychiatr.* 78, 286–294. doi: 10.1136/jnnp.2006.103994

Bonilha, L., Yasuda, C. L., Rorden, C., Li, L. M., Tedeschi, H., De Oliveira, E., et al. (2007b). Does resection of the medial temporal lobe improve the outcome of temporal lobe epilepsy surgery? *Epilepsia* 48, 571–578. doi: 10.1111/j.1528-1167.2006.00958.x

Bothwell, S., Meredith, G. E., Phillips, J., Staunton, H., Doherty, C., Grigorenko, E., et al. (2001). Neuronal hypertrophy in the neocortex of patients with temporal lobe epilepsy. *J. Neurosci.* 21, 4789–4800.

Buckner, R. L., and Carroll, D. C. (2007). Self-projection and the brain. *Trends Cogn. Sci.* 11, 49–57. doi: 10.1016/j.tics.2006.11.004

Buckner, R. L., Sepulcre, J., Talukdar, T., Krienen, F. M., Liu, H., Hedden, T., et al. (2009). Cortical hubs revealed by intrinsic functional connectivity: mapping, assessment of stability, and relation to Alzheimer's disease. *J. Neurosci.* 29, 1860–1873. doi: 10.1523/JNEUROSCI.5062-08.2009

Bullmore, E., and Sporns, O. (2009). Complex brain networks: graph theoretical analysis of structural and functional systems. *Nat. Rev. Neurosci.* 10, 186–198. doi: 10.1038/nrn2575

Bullmore, E., and Sporns, O. (2012). The economy of brain network organization. *Nat. Rev. Neurosci.* 13, 336–349. doi: 10.1038/nrn3214

Bullmore, E. T., and Bassett, D. S. (2011). Brain graphs: graphical models of the human brain connectome. *Annu. Rev. Clin. Psychol.* 7, 113–140. doi: 10.1146/annurev-clinpsy-040510-143934

Bullmore, E. T., Woodruff, P. W., Wright, I. C., Rabe-Hesketh, S., Howard, R. J., Shuriquie, N., et al. (1998). Does dysplasia cause anatomical dysconnectivity in schizophrenia? *Schizophr. Res.* 30, 127–135. doi: 10.1016/S0920-9964(97)00141-2

Cascino, G. D. (2009). Temporal lobe epilepsy is a progressive neurologic disorder: time means neurons! *Neurology* 72, 1718–1719. doi: 10.1212/WNL.0b013e3181a4e465

Cascino, G. D., Jack, C. R. Jr., Parisi, J. E., Sharbrough, F. W., Hirschorn, K. A., Meyer, F. B., et al. (1991). Magnetic resonance imaging-based volume studies in temporal lobe epilepsy: pathological correlations. *Ann. Neurol.* 30, 31–36. doi: 10.1002/ana.410300107

Cassidy, R. M., and Gale, K. (1998). Mediodorsal thalamus plays a critical role in the development of limbic motor seizures. *J. Neurosci.* 18, 9002–9009.

Cavalheiro, E. A., Leite, J. P., Bortolotto, Z. A., Turski, W. A., Ikonomidou, C., and Turski, L. (1991). Long-term effects of pilocarpine in rats: structural damage of the brain triggers kindling and spontaneous recurrent seizures. *Epilepsia* 32, 778–782. doi: 10.1111/j.1528-1157.1991.tb05533.x

Cavanagh, J. B., and Meyer, A. (1956). Aetiological aspects of Ammon's horn sclerosis associated with temporal lobe epilepsy. *Br. Med. J.* 2, 1403–1407. doi: 10.1136/bmj.2.5006.1403

Cavazos, J. E., Zhang, P., Qazi, R., and Sutula, T. P. (2003). Ultrastructural features of sprouted mossy fiber synapses in kindled and kainic acid-treated rats. *J. Comp. Neurol.* 458, 272–292. doi: 10.1002/cne.10581

Cendes, F., Andermann, F., Gloor, P., Evans, A., Jones-Gotman, M., Watson, C., et al. (1993a). MRI volumetric measurement of amygdala and hippocampus in temporal lobe epilepsy. *Neurology* 43, 719–725. doi: 10.1212/WNL.43.4.719

Cendes, F., Andermann, F., Gloor, P., Lopes-Cendes, I., Andermann, E., Melanson, D., et al. (1993b). Atrophy of mesial structures in patients with temporal lobe epilepsy: cause or consequence of repeated seizures? *Ann. Neurol.* 34, 795–801. doi: 10.1002/ana.410340607

Chen, Z. J., He, Y., Rosa-Neto, P., Germann, J., and Evans, A. C. (2008). Revealing modular architecture of human brain structural networks by using cortical thickness from MRI. *Cereb. Cortex* 18, 2374–2381. doi: 10.1093/cercor/bhn003

Choi, D., Na, D. G., Byun, H. S., Suh, Y. L., Kim, S. E., Ro, D. W., et al. (1999). White-matter change in mesial temporal sclerosis: correlation of MRI with PET, pathology, and clinical features. *Epilepsia* 40, 1634–1641. doi: 10.1111/j.1528-1157.1999.tb02050.x

Christoff, K., Gordon, A. M., Smallwood, J., Smith, R., and Schooler, J. W. (2009). Experience sampling during fMRI reveals default network and executive system contributions to mind wandering. *Proc. Natl. Acad. Sci. U.S.A.* 106, 8719–8724. doi: 10.1073/pnas.0900234106

Clifford, D. B., Olney, J. W., Maniotis, A., Collins, R. C., and Zorumski, C. F. (1987). The functional anatomy and pathology of lithium-pilocarpine and high- dose pilocarpine seizures. *Neuroscience* 23, 953–968. doi: 10.1016/0306-4522(87)90171-0

Coan, A. C., and Cendes, F. (2013). Epilepsy as progressive disorders: what is the evidence that can guide our clinical decisions and how can neuroimaging help? *Epilepsy Behav.* 26, 313–321. doi: 10.1016/j.yebeh.2012.09.027

Concha, L., Beaulieu, C., Collins, D. L., and Gross, D. W. (2008). White matter diffusion abnormalities in temporal lobe epilepsy with and without mesial temporal sclerosis. *J. Neurol. Neurosurg. Psychiatr.* 80, 312–319. doi: 10.1136/jnnp.2007.139287

Concha, L., Beaulieu, C., and Gross, D. W. (2005). Bilateral limbic diffusion abnormalities in unilateral temporal lobe epilepsy. *Ann. Neurol.* 57, 188–196. doi: 10.1002/ana.20334

Concha, L., Kim, H., Bernasconi, A., Bernhardt, B. C., and Bernasconi, N. (2012). Spatial patterns of water diffusion along white matter tracts in temporal lobe epilepsy. *Neurology* 79, 455–462. doi: 10.1212/WNL.0b013e31826170b6

Concha, L., Livy, D. J., Beaulieu, C., Wheatley, B. M., and Gross, D. W. (2010). *In vivo* diffusion tensor imaging and histopathology of the fimbria-fornix in temporal lobe epilepsy. *J. Neurosci.* 30, 996–1002. doi: 10.1523/JNEUROSCI.1619-09.2010

Damoiseaux, J. S., Rombouts, S. A., Barkhof, F., Scheltens, P., Stam, C. J., Smith, S. M., et al. (2006). Consistent resting-state networks across healthy subjects. *Proc. Natl. Acad. Sci. U.S.A.* 103, 13848–13853. doi: 10.1073/pnas.0601417103

Dauguet, J., Peled, S., Berezovskii, V., Delzescaux, T., Warfield, S. K., Born, R., et al. (2007). Comparison of fiber tracts derived from *in-vivo* DTI tractography with 3D histological neural tract tracer reconstruction on a macaque brain. *Neuroimage* 37, 530–538. doi: 10.1016/j.neuroimage.2007.04.067

De Lanerolle, N. C., Kim, J. H., Robbins, R. J., and Spencer, D. D. (1989). Hippocampal interneuron loss and plasticity in human temporal lobe epilepsy. *Brain Res.* 495, 387–395. doi: 10.1016/0006-8993(89)90234-5

De Pasquale, F., Della Penna, S., Snyder, A. Z., Lewis, C., Mantini, D., Marzetti, L., et al. (2010). Temporal dynamics of spontaneous MEG activity in brain networks. *Proc. Natl. Acad. Sci. U.S.A.* 107, 6040–6045. doi: 10.1073/pnas.0913863107

Desikan, R. S., Segonne, F., Fischl, B., Quinn, B. T., Dickerson, B. C., Blacker, D., et al. (2006). An automated labeling system for subdividing the human cerebral cortex on MRI scans into gyral based regions of interest. *Neuroimage* 31, 968–980. doi: 10.1016/j.neuroimage.2006.01.021

Diehl, B., Busch, R. M., Duncan, J. S., Piao, Z., Tkach, J., and Luders, H. O. (2008). Abnormalities in diffusion tensor imaging of the uncinate fasciculus relate to reduced memory in temporal lobe epilepsy. *Epilepsia* 49, 1409–1418. doi: 10.1111/j.1528-1167.2008.01596.x

Dreifuss, S., Vingerhoets, F. J., Lazeyras, F., Andino, S. G., Spinelli, L., Delavelle, J., et al. (2001). Volumetric measurements of subcortical nuclei in patients with temporal lobe epilepsy. *Neurology* 57, 1636–1641. doi: 10.1212/WNL.57.9.1636

Du, F., Eid, T., Lothman, E. W., Köhler, C., and Schwarcz, R. (1995). Preferential neuronal loss in layer III of the medial entorhinal cortex in rat models of temporal lobe epilepsy. *J. Neurosci.* 15, 6301–6313.

Du, F., Whetsell, W. O., Abou-Khalil, B., and Blumenkopf, B. (1993). Preferential neuronal loss in layer III of the entorhinal cortex in patients with temporal lobe epilepsy. *Epilepsy Res.* 16, 223–233. doi: 10.1016/0920-1211(93)90083-J

Elsharkawy, A. E., Alabbasi, A. H., Pannek, H., Oppel, F., Schulz, R., Hoppe, M., et al. (2009). Long-term outcome after temporal lobe epilepsy surgery in 434 consecutive adult patients. *J. Neurosurg.* 110, 1135–1146. doi: 10.3171/2008.6.JNS17613

Engel, J. Jr., Thompson, P. M., Stern, J. M., Staba, R. J., Bragin, A., and Mody, I. (2013). Connectomics and epilepsy. *Curr. Opin. Neurol.* 26, 186–194. doi: 10.1097/WCO.0b013e32835ee5b8

Eriksson, S. H., Rydenhag, B., Uvebrant, P., Malmgren, K., and Nordborg, C. (2002). Widespread microdysgenesis in therapy-resistant epilepsy–a case report on post-mortem findings. *Acta Neuropathol. (Berl.)* 103, 74–77. doi: 10.1007/s004010100426

Falconer, M. A., Serafetinides, E. A., and Corsellis, J.A.N. (1964). Etiology and pathogenesis of temporal lobe epilepsy. *Arch. Neurol.* 10, 233–248. doi: 10.1001/archneur.1964.00460150003001

Feinberg, D. A., Moeller, S., Smith, S. M., Auerbach, E., Ramanna, S., Gunther, M., et al. (2010). Multiplexed echo planar imaging for sub-second whole brain FMRI and fast diffusion imaging. *PLoS ONE* 5:e15710. doi: 10.1371/journal.pone.0015710

Felleman, D. J., and Van Essen, D. C. (1991). Distributed hierarchical processing in the primate cerebral cortex. *Cereb. Cortex* 1, 1–47. doi: 10.1093/cercor/1.1.1

Focke, N. K., Yogarajah, M., Bonelli, S. B., Bartlett, P. A., Symms, M. R., and Duncan, J. S. (2008). Voxel-based diffusion tensor imaging in patients with mesial temporal lobe epilepsy and hippocampal sclerosis. *Neuroimage* 40, 728–737. doi: 10.1016/j.neuroimage.2007.12.031

Fox, M. D., and Greicius, M. (2010). Clinical applications of resting state functional connectivity. *Front. Syst. Neurosci.* 4:19. doi: 10.3389/fnsys.2010.00019

Frings, L., Schulze-Bonhage, A., Spreer, J., and Wagner, K. (2009). Remote effects of hippocampal damage on default network connectivity in the human brain. *J. Neurol.* 256, 2021–2029. doi: 10.1007/s00415-009-5233-0

Friston, K. J., Frith, C. D., Fletcher, P., Liddle, P. F., and Frackowiak, R. S. (1996). Functional topography: multidimensional scaling and functional connectivity in the brain. *Cereb. Cortex* 6, 156–164. doi: 10.1093/cercor/6.2.156

Friston, K. J., Frith, C. D., Liddle, P. F., and Frackowiak, R. S. (1993). Functional connectivity: the principal-component analysis of large (PET) data sets. *J. Cereb. Blood Flow Metab.* 13, 5–14. doi: 10.1038/jcbfm.1993.4

Geyer, S., Weiss, M., Reimann, K., Lohmann, G., and Turner, R. (2011). Microstructural parcellation of the human cerebral cortex - from Brodmann's post-mortem map to *in vivo* mapping with high-field magnetic resonance imaging. *Front. Hum. Neurosci.* 5:19. doi: 10.3389/fnhum.2011.00019

Glasser, M. F., and Van Essen, D. C. (2011). Mapping human cortical areas *in vivo* based on myelin content as revealed by T1- and T2-weighted MRI. *J. Neurosci.* 31, 11597–11616. doi: 10.1523/JNEUROSCI.2180-11.2011

Gong, G., He, Y., Concha, L., Lebel, C., Gross, D. W., Evans, A. C., et al. (2009). Mapping anatomical connectivity patterns of human cerebral cortex using *in vivo* diffusion tensor imaging tractography. *Cereb. Cortex* 19, 524–536. doi: 10.1093/cercor/bhn102

Gotman, J., Kobayashi, E., Bagshaw, A. P., Benar, C. G., and Dubeau, F. (2006). Combining EEG and fMRI: a multimodal tool for epilepsy research. *J. Magn. Reson. Imaging* 23, 906–920. doi: 10.1002/jmri.20577

Greicius, M. (2008). Resting-state functional connectivity in neuropsychiatric disorders. *Curr. Opin. Neurol.* 21, 424–430. doi: 10.1097/WCO.0b013e328306f2c5

Greicius, M. D., Krasnow, B., Reiss, A. L., and Menon, V. (2003). Functional connectivity in the resting brain: a network analysis of the default mode hypothesis. *Proc. Natl. Acad. Sci. U.S.A.* 100, 253–258. doi: 10.1073/pnas.0135058100

Gross, D. W., Concha, L., and Beaulieu, C. (2006). Extratemporal white matter abnormalities in mesial temporal lobe epilepsy demonstrated with diffusion tensor imaging. *Epilepsia* 47, 1360–1363. doi: 10.1111/j.1528-1167.2006.00603.x

Guye, M., Bettus, G., Bartolomei, F., and Cozzone, P. J. (2010). Graph theoretical analysis of structural and functional connectivity MRI in normal and pathological brain networks. *MAGMA* 23, 409–421. doi: 10.1007/s10334-010-0205-z

Hagmann, P., Cammoun, L., Gigandet, X., Meuli, R., Honey, C. J., Wedeen, V. J., et al. (2008). Mapping the structural core of human cerebral cortex. *PLoS Biol.* 6:e159. doi: 10.1371/journal.pbio.0060159

Hagmann, P., Kurant, M., Gigandet, X., Thiran, P., Wedeen, V. J., Meuli, R., et al. (2007). Mapping human whole-brain structural networks with diffusion MRI. *PLoS ONE* 2:e597. doi: 10.1371/journal.pone.0000597

Harriger, L., Van Den Heuvel, M. P., and Sporns, O. (2012). Rich club organization of macaque cerebral cortex and its role in network communication. *PLoS ONE* 7:e46497. doi: 10.1371/journal.pone.0046497

He, Y., Chen, Z. J., and Evans, A. C. (2007). Small-world anatomical networks in the human brain revealed by cortical thickness from MRI. *Cereb. Cortex* 17, 2407–2419. doi: 10.1093/cercor/bhl149

He, Y., Wang, J., Wang, L., Chen, Z. J., Yan, C., Yang, H., et al. (2009). Uncovering intrinsic modular organization of spontaneous brain activity in humans. *PLoS ONE* 4:e5226. doi: 10.1371/journal.pone.0005226

Hetherington, H. P., Kuzniecky, R. I., Vives, K., Devinsky, O., Pacia, S., Luciano, D., et al. (2007). A subcortical network of dysfunction in TLE measured by magnetic resonance spectroscopy. *Neurology* 69, 2256–2265. doi: 10.1212/01.wnl.0000286945.21270.6d

Hogan, R. E., Wang, L., Bertrand, M. E., Willmore, L. J., Bucholz, R. D., Nassif, A. S., et al. (2004). MRI-based high-dimensional hippocampal mapping in mesial temporal lobe epilepsy. *Brain* 127, 1731–1740. doi: 10.1093/brain/awh197

Holmes, G. L. (2002). Seizure-induced neuronal injury: animal data. *Neurology* 59, S3–S6. doi: 10.1212/WNL.59.9_suppl_5.S3

Honey, C. J., Sporns, O., Cammoun, L., Gigandet, X., Thiran, J. P., Meuli, R., et al. (2009). Predicting human resting-state functional connectivity from structural connectivity. *Proc. Natl. Acad. Sci. U.S.A.* 106, 2035–2040. doi: 10.1073/pnas.0811168106

Houser, C. R., Swartz, B. E., Walsh, G. O., and Delgado-Escueta, A. V. (1992). "Granule cell disorganization in the dentate gyrus: possible alterations of neuronal migration in human temporal lobe epilepsy," in *Molecular Neurobiology of Epilepsy*, eds J. Engel Jr., C. Wasterlain, E. A. Cavalheiro, U. Heinemann, and G. Avanzini (Amsterdam: Elsevier Science), 41–47.

Iturria-Medina, Y., Canales-Rodriguez, E. J., Melie-Garcia, L., Valdes-Hernandez, P. A., Martinez-Montes, E., Aleman-Gomez, Y., et al. (2007). Characterizing brain anatomical connections using diffusion weighted MRI and graph theory. *Neuroimage* 36, 645–660. doi: 10.1016/j.neuroimage.2007.02.012

Jann, K., Kottlow, M., Dierks, T., Boesch, C., and Koenig, T. (2010). Topographic electrophysiological signatures of FMRI Resting State Networks. *PLoS ONE* 5:e12945. doi: 10.1371/journal.pone.0012945

Jbabdi, S., and Johansen-Berg, H. (2011). Tractography: where do we go from here? *Brain Connect.* 1, 169–183. doi: 10.1089/brain.2011.0033

Johansen-Berg, H., and Behrens, T. E. (2006). Just pretty pictures? What diffusion tractography can add in clinical neuroscience. *Curr. Opin. Neurol.* 19, 379–385. doi: 10.1097/01.wco.0000236618.82086.01

Jones, D. K., Knosche, T. R., and Turner, R. (2012). White matter integrity, fiber count, and other fallacies: the do's and don'ts of diffusion MRI. *Neuroimage* 73, 239–254. doi: 10.1016/j.neuroimage.2012.06.081

Jutila, L., Ylinen, A., Partanen, K., Alafuzoff, I., Mervaala, E., Partanen, J., et al. (2001). MR volumetry of the entorhinal, perirhinal, and temporopolar cortices in drug-refractory temporal lobe epilepsy. *AJNR. Am. J. Neuroradiol.* 22, 1490–1501.

Kaiser, M., and Hilgetag, C. C. (2010). Optimal hierarchical modular topologies for producing limited sustained activation of neural networks. *Front. Neuroinform.* 4:8. doi: 10.3389/fninf.2010.00008

Keller, S. S., and Roberts, N. (2008). Voxel-based morphometry of temporal lobe epilepsy: an introduction and review of the literature. *Epilepsia* 49, 741–757. doi: 10.1111/j.1528-1167.2007.01485.x

Kelly, C., Biswal, B. B., Craddock, R. C., Castellanos, F. X., and Milham, M. P. (2012). Characterizing variation in the functional connectome: promise and pitfalls. *Trends Cogn. Sci.* 16, 181–188. doi: 10.1016/j.tics.2012.02.001

Kemmotsu, N., Girard, H. M., Bernhardt, B. C., Bonilha, L., Lin, J. J., Tecoma, E. S., et al. (2011). MRI analysis in temporal lobe epilepsy: cortical thinning and white matter disruptions are related to side of seizure onset. *Epilepsia* 52, 2257–2266. doi: 10.1111/j.1528-1167.2011.03278.x

Khundrakpam, B. S., Reid, A., Brauer, J., Carbonell, F., Lewis, J., Ameis, S., et al. (2012). Developmental changes in organization of structural brain networks. *Cereb. Cortex* 23, 2072–2085. doi: 10.1093/cercor/bhs187

Kim, H., Besson, P., Colliot, O., Bernasconi, A., and Bernasconi, N. (2008). Surface-based vector analysis using heat equation interpolation: a new approach to quantify local hippocampal volume changes. *Med. Image. Comput. Comput. Assist. Interv.* 11, 1008–1015. doi: 10.1007/978-3-540-85988-8_120

Kobayashi, E., Bagshaw, A. P., Benar, C. G., Aghakhani, Y., Andermann, F., Dubeau, F., et al. (2006). Temporal and extratemporal BOLD responses to temporal lobe interictal spikes. *Epilepsia* 47, 343–354. doi: 10.1111/j.1528-1167.2006.00427.x

Kramer, M. A., Kolaczyk, E. D. and Kirsch, H. E. (2008). Emergent network topology at seizure onset in humans. *Epilepsy Res.* 79, 173–186. doi: 10.1016/j.eplepsyres.2008.02.002

Kuzniecky, R. I., De La Sayette, V., Ethier, R., Melanson, D., Andermann, F., Berkovic, S. F., et al. (1987). Magnetic resonance imaging in temporal lobe epilepsy: pathological correlations. *Ann. Neurol.* 22, 341–347. doi: 10.1002/ana.410220310

Lachaux, J. P., Rodriguez, E., Martinerie, J., and Varela, F. J. (1999). Measuring phase synchrony in brain signals. *Hum. Brain Mapp.* 8, 194–208. doi: 10.1002/(SICI)1097-0193(1999)8:4<194::AID-HBM4>3.0.CO;2-C

Laird, A. R., Fox, P. M., Eickhoff, S. B., Turner, J. A., Ray, K. L., Mckay, D. R., et al. (2011). Behavioral interpretations of intrinsic connectivity networks. *J. Cogn. Neurosci.* 23, 4022–4037. doi: 10.1162/jocn_a_00077

Laufs, H., Hamandi, K., Salek-Haddadi, A., Kleinschmidt, A. K., Duncan, J. S., and Lemieux, L. (2007). Temporal lobe interictal epileptic discharges affect cerebral activity in "default mode" brain regions. *Hum. Brain Mapp.* 28, 1023–1032. doi: 10.1002/hbm.20323

Le Bihan, D., Breton, E., Lallemand, D., Grenier, P., Cabanis, E., and Laval-Jeantet, M. (1986). MR imaging of intravoxel incoherent motions: application to diffusion and perfusion in neurologic disorders. *Radiology* 161, 401–407.

Le Bihan, D., Turner, R., Douek, P., and Patronas, N. (1996). Diffusion MR imaging: clinical application. *AJNR Am. J. Neuroradiol.* 159, 591–599.

Lemieux, L., Daunizeau, J., and Walker, M. C. (2011). Concepts of connectivity and human epileptic activity. *Front. Syst. Neurosci.* 5:12. doi: 10.3389/fnsys.2011.00012

Leonardi, M., and Ustun, T. B. (2002). The global burden of epilepsy. *Epilepsia* 43(Suppl. 6), 21–25. doi: 10.1046/j.1528-1157.43.s.6.11.x

Lerch, J. P., Worsley, K., Shaw, W. P., Greenstein, D. K., Lenroot, R. K., Giedd, J., et al. (2006). Mapping anatomical correlations across cerebral cortex (MACACC) using cortical thickness from MRI. *Neuroimage* 31, 993–1003. doi: 10.1016/j.neuroimage.2006.01.042

Liao, W., Zhang, Z., Pan, Z., Mantini, D., Ding, J., Duan, X., et al. (2010). Altered functional connectivity and small-world in mesial temporal lobe epilepsy. *PLoS ONE* 5:e8525. doi: 10.1371/journal.pone.0008525

Lieb, J. P., Dasheiff, R. M., and Engel, J. Jr. (1991). Role of the frontal lobes in the propagation of mesial temporal lobe seizures. *Epilepsia* 32, 822–837. doi: 10.1111/j.1528-1157.1991.tb05539.x

Lieb, J. P., Hoque, K., Skomer, C. E., and Song, X. W. (1987). Inter-hemispheric propagation of human mesial temporal lobe seizures: a coherence/phase analysis. *Electroencephalogr. Clin. Neurophysiol.* 67, 101–119. doi: 10.1016/0013-4694(87)90033-2

Lin, J. J., Riley, J. D., Juranek, J., and Cramer, S. C. (2008). Vulnerability of the frontal-temporal connections in temporal lobe epilepsy. *Epilepsy Res.* 82, 162–170. doi: 10.1016/j.eplepsyres.2008.07.020

Lin, J. J., Salamon, N., Lee, A. D., Dutton, R. A., Geaga, J. A., Hayashi, K. M., et al. (2007). Reduced neocortical thickness and complexity mapped in mesial temporal lobe epilepsy with hippocampal sclerosis. *Cereb. Cortex* 17, 2007–2018. doi: 10.1093/cercor/bhl109

Lohmann, G., Margulies, D. S., Horstmann, A., Pleger, B., Lepsien, J., Goldhahn, D., et al. (2010). Eigenvector centrality mapping for analyzing connectivity patterns in fMRI data of the human brain. *PLoS ONE* 5:e10232. doi: 10.1371/journal.pone.0010232

Lopes Da Silva, F., Pijn, J. P., and Boeijinga, P. (1989). Interdependence of EEG signals: linear vs. nonlinear associations and the significance of time delays and phase shifts. *Brain Topogr.* 2, 9–18. doi: 10.1007/BF01128839

Mantini, D., Gerits, A., Nelissen, K., Durand, J. B., Joly, O., Simone, L., et al. (2011). Default mode of brain function in monkeys. *J. Neurosci.* 31, 12954–12962. doi: 10.1523/JNEUROSCI.2318-11.2011

Margerison, J. H., and Corsellis, J. A. (1966). Epilepsy and the temporal lobes. A clinical, electroencephalographic and neuropathological study of the brain in epilepsy, with particular reference to the temporal lobes. *Brain* 89, 499–530. doi: 10.1093/brain/89.3.499

Margulies, D. S., Kelly, A. M., Uddin, L. Q., Biswal, B. B., Castellanos, F. X., and Milham, M. P. (2007). Mapping the functional connectivity of anterior cingulate cortex. *Neuroimage* 37, 579–588. doi: 10.1016/j.neuroimage.2007.05.019

Mars, R. B., Jbabdi, S., Sallet, J., O'Reilly, J. X., Croxson, P. L., Olivier, E., et al. (2011). Diffusion-weighted imaging tractography-based parcellation of the human parietal cortex and comparison with human and macaque resting-state functional connectivity. *J. Neurosci.* 31, 4087–4100. doi: 10.1523/JNEUROSCI.5102-10.2011

Mcdonald, C. R., Ahmadi, M. E., Hagler, D. J., Tecoma, E. S., Iragui, V. J., Gharapetian, L., et al. (2008a). Diffusion tensor imaging correlates of memory and language impairments in temporal lobe epilepsy. *Neurology* 71, 1869–1876. doi: 10.1212/01.wnl.0000327824.05348.3b

Mcdonald, C. R., Hagler, D. J. Jr., Ahmadi, M. E., Tecoma, E., Iragui, V., Dale, A. M., et al. (2008b). Subcortical and cerebellar atrophy in mesial temporal lobe epilepsy revealed by automatic segmentation. *Epilepsy Res.* 79, 130–138. doi: 10.1016/j.eplepsyres.2008.01.006

Mcdonald, C. R., Hagler, D. J. Jr., Ahmadi, M. E., Tecoma, E., Iragui, V., Gharapetian, L., et al. (2008c). Regional neocortical thinning in mesial temporal lobe epilepsy. *Epilepsia* 49, 794–803. doi: 10.1111/j.1528-1167.2008.01539.x

Mcintosh, A. M., Kalnins, R. M., Mitchell, L. A., Fabinyi, G. C., Briellmann, R. S., and Berkovic, S. F. (2004). Temporal lobectomy: long-term seizure outcome, late recurrence and risks for seizure recurrence. *Brain* 127, 2018–2030. doi: 10.1093/brain/awh221

Mechelli, A., Friston, K. J., Frackowiak, R. S., and Price, C. J. (2005). Structural covariance in the human cortex. *J. Neurosci.* 25, 8303–8310. doi: 10.1523/JNEUROSCI.0357-05.2005

Meiners, L. C., Witkamp, T. D., De Kort, G. A., Van Huffelen, A. C., Van Der, G. Y., Jansen, G. H., et al. (1999). Relevance of temporal lobe white matter changes in hippocampal sclerosis. Magnetic resonance imaging and histology. *Invest. Radiol.* 34, 38–45. doi: 10.1097/00004424-199901000-00006

Meunier, D., Lambiotte, R., and Bullmore, E. T. (2010). Modular and hierarchically modular organization of brain networks. *Front. Neurosci.* 4:200. doi: 10.3389/fnins.2010.00200

Mitchell, L. A., Jackson, G. D., Kalnins, R. M., Saling, M. M., Fitt, G. J., Ashpole, R. D., et al. (1999). Anterior temporal abnormality in temporal lobe epilepsy: a quantitative MRI and histopathologic study. *Neurology* 52, 327–336. doi: 10.1212/WNL.52.2.327

Modha, D. S., and Singh, R. (2010). Network architecture of the long-distance pathways in the macaque brain. *Proc. Natl. Acad. Sci. U.S.A.* 107, 13485–13490. doi: 10.1073/pnas.1008054107

Moran, N. F., Lemieux, L., Kitchen, N. D., Fish, D. R., and Shorvon, S. D. (2001). Extrahippocampal temporal lobe atrophy in temporal lobe epilepsy and mesial temporal sclerosis. *Brain* 124, 167–175. doi: 10.1093/brain/124.1.167

Mori, S., Crain, B. J., Chacko, V. P., and Van Zijl, P. C. (1999). Three-dimensional tracking of axonal projections in the brain by magnetic resonance imaging. *Ann. Neurol.* 45, 265–269. doi: 10.1002/1531-8249(199902)45:2<265::AID-ANA21>3.0.CO;2-3

Mueller, S. G., Laxer, K. D., Barakos, J., Cheong, I., Finlay, D., Garcia, P., et al. (2009a). Involvement of the thalamocortical network in TLE with and without mesiotemporal sclerosis. *Epilepsia*. doi: 10.1111/j.1528-1167.2009.02413.x

Mueller, S. G., Laxer, K. D., Barakos, J., Ian, C., Garcia, P., and Weiner, M. W. (2009b). Widespread neocortical abnormalities in temporal lobe epilepsy with and without mesial sclerosis. *Neuroimage* 46, 353–359. doi: 10.1016/j.neuroimage.2009.02.020

Musso, F., Brinkmeyer, J., Mobascher, A., Warbrick, T., and Winterer, G. (2010). Spontaneous brain activity and EEG microstates. A novel EEG/fMRI analysis approach to explore resting-state networks. *Neuroimage* 52, 1149–1161. doi: 10.1016/j.neuroimage.2010.01.093

Natsume, J., Bernasconi, N., Andermann, F., and Bernasconi, A. (2003). MRI volumetry of the thalamus in temporal, extratemporal, and idiopathic generalized epilepsy. *Neurology* 60, 1296–1300. doi: 10.1212/01.WNL.0000058764.34968.C2

Parker, G. J., Stephan, K. E., Barker, G. J., Rowe, J. B., Macmanus, D. G., Wheeler-Kingshott, C. A., et al. (2002). Initial demonstration of *in vivo* tracing of axonal projections in the macaque brain and comparison with the human brain using diffusion tensor imaging and fast marching tractography. *Neuroimage* 15, 797–809. doi: 10.1006/nimg.2001.0994

Ponten, S. C., Bartolomei, F., and Stam, C. J. (2007). Small-world networks and epilepsy: graph theoretical analysis of intracerebrally recorded mesial temporal lobe seizures. *Clin. Neurophysiol.* 118, 918–927. doi: 10.1016/j.clinph.2006.12.002

Ponten, S. C., Douw, L., Bartolomei, F., Reijneveld, J. C., and Stam, C. J. (2009). Indications for network regularization during absence seizures: weighted and unweighted graph theoretical analyses. *Exp. Neurol.* 217, 197–204. doi: 10.1016/j.expneurol.2009.02.001

Pugliatti, M., Beghi, E., Forsgren, L., Ekman, M., and Sobocki, P. (2007). Estimating the cost of epilepsy in Europe: a review with economic modeling. *Epilepsia* 48, 2224–2233.

Raichle, M. E., Macleod, A. M., Snyder, A. Z., Powers, W. J., Gusnard, D. A., and Shulman, G. L. (2001). A default mode of brain function. *Proc. Natl. Acad. Sci. U.S.A.* 98, 676–682. doi: 10.1073/pnas.98.2.676

Raznahan, A., Lerch, J. P., Lee, N., Greenstein, D., Wallace, G. L., Stockman, M., et al. (2011). Patterns of coordinated anatomical change in human cortical development: a longitudinal neuroimaging study of maturational coupling. *Neuron* 72, 873–884. doi: 10.1016/j.neuron.2011.09.028

Rodrigo, S., Oppenheim, C., Chassoux, F., Golestani, N., Cointepas, Y., Poupon, C., et al. (2007). Uncinate fasciculus fiber tracking in mesial temporal lobe epilepsy. Initial findings. *Eur. Radiol.* 17, 1663–1668. doi: 10.1007/s00330-006-0558-x

Rosenberg, D. S., Mauguiere, F., Demarquay, G., Ryvlin, P., Isnard, J., Fischer, C., et al. (2006). Involvement of medial pulvinar thalamic nucleus in human temporal lobe seizures. *Epilepsia* 47, 98–107. doi: 10.1111/j.1528-1167.2006.00375.x

Ryvlin, P. (2003). Beyond pharmacotherapy: surgical management. *Epilepsia* 44(Suppl. 5), 23–28. doi: 10.1046/j.1528-1157.44.s.5.4.x

Salvador, R., Suckling, J., Schwarzbauer, C., and Bullmore, E. (2005). Undirected graphs of frequency-dependent functional connectivity in whole brain networks. *Philos. Trans. R. Soc. Lond. B Biol. Sci.* 360, 937–946. doi: 10.1098/rstb.2005.1645

Sanabria, E. R., Da Silva, A. V., Spreafico, R., and Cavalheiro, E. A. (2002). Damage, reorganization, and abnormal neocortical hyperexcitability in the pilocarpine model of temporal lobe epilepsy. *Epilepsia* 43(Suppl. 5), 96–106. doi: 10.1046/j.1528-1157.43.s.5.31.x

Sankar, T., Bernasconi, N., Kim, H., and Bernasconi, A. (2008). Temporal lobe epilepsy: differential pattern of damage in temporopolar cortex and white matter. *Hum. Brain Mapp.* 29, 931–944. doi: 10.1002/hbm.20437

Scannell, J. W., Blakemore, C., and Young, M. P. (1995). Analysis of connectivity in the cat cerebral cortex. *J. Neurosci.* 15, 1463–1483.

Scharfman, H. E. (2007). The neurobiology of epilepsy. *Curr. Neurol. Neurosci. Rep.* 7, 348–354. doi: 10.1007/s11910-007-0053-z

Schindler, K. A., Bialonski, S., Horstmann, M. T., Elger, C. E., and Lehnertz, K. (2008). Evolving functional network properties and synchronizability during human epileptic seizures. *Chaos* 18, 033119. doi: 10.1063/1.2966112

Scott, R. C., King, M. D., Gadian, D. G., Neville, B. G., and Connelly, A. (2006). Prolonged febrile seizures are associated with hippocampal vasogenic edema and developmental changes. *Epilepsia* 47, 1493–1498. doi: 10.1111/j.1528-1167.2006.00621.x

Shen, K., Bezgin, G., Hutchison, R. M., Gati, J. S., Menon, R. S., Everling, S., et al. (2012). Information processing architecture of functionally defined clusters in the macaque cortex. *J. Neurosci.* 32, 17465–17476. doi: 10.1523/JNEUROSCI.2709-12.2012

Sloan, D. M., and Bertram, E. H. 3rd. (2009). Changes in midline thalamic recruiting responses in the prefrontal cortex of the rat during the development of chronic limbic seizures. *Epilepsia* 50, 556–565. doi: 10.1111/j.1528-1167.2008.01790.x

Smith, S. M. (2012). The future of FMRI connectivity. *Neuroimage* 62, 1257–1266. doi: 10.1016/j.neuroimage.2012.01.022

Smith, S. M., Fox, P. T., Miller, K. L., Glahn, D. C., Fox, P. M., Mackay, C. E., et al. (2009). Correspondence of the brain's functional architecture during activation and rest. *Proc. Natl. Acad. Sci. U.S.A.* 106, 13040–13045. doi: 10.1073/pnas.0905267106

Smith, S. M., Miller, K. L., Moeller, S., Xu, J., Auerbach, E. J., Woolrich, M. W., et al. (2012). Temporally-independent functional modes of spontaneous brain activity. *Proc. Natl. Acad. Sci. U.S.A.* 109, 3131–3136. doi: 10.1073/pnas.1121329109

Sommer, W. (1880). Erkrankung des ammonshorns als aetiologisches moment der epilepsie. *Arch. Psychiatr. Nervenkr.* 10, 631–675. doi: 10.1007/BF02224538

Spencer, S. S. (2002). Neural networks in human epilepsy: evidence of and implications for treatment. *Epilepsia* 43, 219–227. doi: 10.1046/j.1528-1157.2002.26901.x

Sporns, O. (2011). The human connectome: a complex network. *Ann. N.Y. Acad. Sci.* 1224, 109–125. doi: 10.1111/j.1749-6632.2010.05888.x

Sporns, O., Chialvo, D. R., Kaiser, M., and Hilgetag, C. C. (2004). Organization, development and function of complex brain networks. *Trends Cogn. Sci.* 8, 418–425. doi: 10.1016/j.tics.2004.07.008

Sporns, O., Honey, C. J., and Kotter, R. (2007). Identification and classification of hubs in brain networks. *PLoS ONE* 2:e1049. doi: 10.1371/journal.pone.0001049

Sporns, O., Tononi, G., and Kotter, R. (2005). The human connectome: a structural description of the human brain. *PLoS Comput. Biol.* 1:e42. doi: 10.1371/journal.pcbi.0010042

Stam, C. J. (2004). Functional connectivity patterns of human magnetoencephalographic recordings: a 'small-world' network? *Neurosci. Lett.* 355, 25–28. doi: 10.1016/j.neulet.2003.10.063

Stephan, K. E., Hilgetag, C. C., Burns, G. A., O'neill, M. A., Young, M. P., and Kotter, R. (2000). Computational analysis of functional connectivity between areas of primate cerebral cortex. *Philos. Trans. R. Soc. Lond. B Biol. Sci.* 355, 111–126. doi: 10.1098/rstb.2000.0552

Stone, J. V., and Kotter, R. (2002). Making connections about brain connectivity. *Trends Cogn. Sci.* 6, 327–328. doi: 10.1016/S1364-6613(02)01943-5

Sutula, T., He, X. X., Cavazos, J., and Scott, G. (1988). Synaptic reorganization in the hippocampus induced by abnormal functional activity. *Science* 239, 1147–1150. doi: 10.1126/science.2449733

Tellez-Zenteno, J. F., Dhar, R., Hernandez-Ronquillo, L., and Wiebe, S. (2007). Long-term outcomes in epilepsy surgery: antiepileptic drugs, mortality, cognitive and psychosocial aspects. *Brain* 130, 334–345. doi: 10.1093/brain/awl316

Thom, M., Eriksson, S., Martinian, L., Caboclo, L. O., Mcevoy, A. W., Duncan, J. S., et al. (2009). Temporal lobe sclerosis associated with hippocampal sclerosis in temporal lobe epilepsy: neuropathological features. *J. Neuropathol. Exp. Neurol.* 68, 928–938. doi: 10.1097/NEN.0b013e3181b05d67

Tohka, J., He, Y., and Evans, A. C. (2012). The impact of sampling density upon cortical network analysis: regions or points. *Magn. Reson. Imaging* 30, 978–992. doi: 10.1016/j.mri.2012.02.029

Tomasi, D., and Volkow, N. D. (2011). Functional connectivity hubs in the human brain. *Neuroimage* 57, 908–917. doi: 10.1016/j.neuroimage.2011.05.024

Tononi, G., Sporns, O., and Edelman, G. M. (1994). A measure for brain complexity: relating functional segregation and integration in the nervous system. *Proc. Natl. Acad. Sci. U.S.A.* 91, 5033–5037. doi: 10.1073/pnas.91.11.5033

Turski, W. A., Cavalheiro, E. A., Schwarz, M., Czuczwar, S. J., Kleinrok, Z., and Turski, L. (1983). Limbic seizures produced by pilocarpine in rats: behavioural, electroencephalographic and neuropathological study. *Behav. Brain Res.* 9, 315–335. doi: 10.1016/0166-4328(83)90136-5

Vaessen, M. J., Braakman, H. M., Heerink, J. S., Jansen, J. F., Debeij-Van Hall, M. H., Hofman, P. A., et al. (2012a). Abnormal modular organization of functional networks in cognitively impaired children with frontal lobe epilepsy. *Cereb. Cortex* 23, 1997–2006. doi: 10.1093/cercor/bhs186

Vaessen, M. J., Jansen, J. F., Vlooswijk, M. C., Hofman, P. A., Majoie, H. J., Aldenkamp, A. P., et al. (2012b). White matter network abnormalities are associated with cognitive decline in chronic epilepsy. *Cereb. Cortex* 22, 2139–2147. doi: 10.1093/cercor/bhr298

Van Den Heuvel, M. P., and Sporns, O. (2011). Rich-club organization of the human connectome. *J. Neurosci.* 31, 15775–15786. doi: 10.1523/JNEUROSCI.3539-11.2011

Van Essen, D. C. (2005). A Population-Average, Landmark- and Surface-based (PALS) atlas of human cerebral cortex. *Neuroimage* 28, 635–662. doi: 10.1016/j.neuroimage.2005.06.058

Van Essen, D. C., Glasser, M. F., Dierker, D. L., and Harwell, J. (2012). Cortical parcellations of the macaque monkey analyzed on surface-based atlases. *Cereb. Cortex* 22, 2227–2240. doi: 10.1093/cercor/bhr290

Vlooswijk, M. C., Vaessen, M. J., Jansen, J. F., De Krom, M C., Majoie, H. J., Hofman, P. A., et al. (2011). Loss of network efficiency associated with cognitive decline in chronic epilepsy. *Neurology* 77, 938–944. doi: 10.1212/WNL.0b013e31822cfc2f

Voets, N. L., Beckmann, C. F., Cole, D. M., Hong, S., Bernasconi, A., and Bernasconi, N. (2012). Structural substrates for resting network disruption in temporal lobe epilepsy. *Brain.* doi: 10.1093/brain/aws137

Voets, N. L., Bernhardt, B. C., Kim, H., Yoon, U., and Bernasconi, N. (2011). Increased temporolimbic cortical folding complexity in temporal lobe epilepsy. *Neurology* 76, 138–144. doi: 10.1212/WNL.0b013e318205d521

Waites, A. B., Briellmann, R. S., Saling, M. M., Abbott, D. F., and Jackson, G. D. (2006). Functional connectivity networks are disrupted in left temporal lobe epilepsy. *Ann. Neurol.* 59, 335–343. doi: 10.1002/ana.20733

Watts, D. J., and Strogatz, S. H. (1998). Collective dynamics of 'small-world' networks. *Nature* 393, 440–442. doi: 10.1038/30918

Wiebe, S., Blume, W. T., Girvin, J. P., and Eliasziw, M. (2001). A randomized, controlled trial of surgery for temporal-lobe epilepsy. *N. Engl. J. Med.* 345, 311–318. doi: 10.1056/NEJM200108023450501

Worsley, K. J., Taylor, J. E., Carbonell, F., Chung, M. K., Duerden, E., Bernhardt, B., et al. (2009). SurfStat: a matlab toolbox for the statistical analysis of univariate and multivariate surface and volumetric data using linear mixed effects models and random field theory. *Neuroimage* 47, S102. doi: 10.1016/S1053-8119(09)70882-1

Xia, M., and He, Y. (2011). Magnetic resonance imaging and graph theoretical analysis of complex brain networks in neuropsychiatric disorders. *Brain Connect.* 1, 349–365. doi: 10.1089/brain.2011.0062

Yilmazer-Hanke, D. M., Wolf, H. K., Schramm, J., Elger, C. E., Wiestler, O. D., and Blumcke, I. (2000). Subregional pathology of the amygdala complex and entorhinal region in surgical specimens from patients with pharmacoresistant temporal lobe epilepsy. *J. Neuropathol. Exp. Neurol.* 59, 907–920.

Yogarajah, M., and Duncan, J. S. (2008). Diffusion-based magnetic resonance imaging and tractography in epilepsy. *Epilepsia* 49, 189–200. doi: 10.1111/j.1528-1167.2007.01378.x

Yu, J. T., and Tan, L. (2008). Diffusion-weighted magnetic resonance imaging demonstrates parenchymal pathophysiological changes in epilepsy. *Brain Res. Rev.* 59, 34–41. doi: 10.1016/j.brainresrev.2008.04.008

Yu, Q., Plis, S. M., Erhardt, E. B., Allen, E. A., Sui, J., Kiehl, K. A., et al. (2011a). Modular organization of functional network connectivity in healthy controls and patients with schizophrenia during the resting state. *Front. Syst. Neurosci.* 5:103. doi: 10.3389/fnsys.2011.00103

Yu, Q., Sui, J., Rachakonda, S., He, H., Gruner, W., Pearlson, G., et al. (2011b). Altered topological properties of functional network connectivity in schizophrenia during resting state: a small-world brain network study. *PLoS ONE* 6:e25423. doi: 10.1371/journal.pone.0025423

Yu, Q., Sui, J., Liu, J., Plis, S. M., Kiehl, K. A., Pearlson, G., et al. (2013). Disrupted correlation between low frequency power and connectivity strength of resting state brain networks in schizophrenia. *Schizophr. Res.* 143, 165–171. doi: 10.1016/j.schres.2012.11.001

Yuan, H., Zotev, V., Phillips, R., Drevets, W. C., and Bodurka, J. (2012). Spatiotemporal dynamics of the brain at rest–exploring EEG microstates as electrophysiological signatures of BOLD resting state networks.

Neuroimage 60, 2062–2072. doi: 10.1016/j.neuroimage.2012.02.031

Zhang, Z., Lu, G., Zhong, Y., Tan, Q., Liao, W., Wang, Z., et al. (2010). Altered spontaneous neuronal activity of the default-mode network in mesial temporal lobe epilepsy. *Brain Res.* 1323, 152–160. doi: 10.1016/j.brainres.2010.01.042

Zielinski, B. A., Gennatas, E. D., Zhou, J., and Seeley, W. W. (2010). Network-level structural covariance in the developing brain. *Proc. Natl. Acad. Sci. U.S.A.* 107, 18191–18196. doi: 10.1073/pnas.1003109107

Zuo, X. N., Ehmke, R., Mennes, M., Imperati, D., Castellanos, F. X., Sporns, O., et al. (2012). Network centrality in the human functional connectome. *Cereb. Cortex* 22, 1862–1875. doi: 10.1093/cercor/bhr269

6

Development of functional brain connectivity in the young brain

G. E. Anna-Jasmijn Hoff[1], M. P. Van den Heuvel[2]*, Manon J. N. L. Benders[1], Karina J. Kersbergen[1] and L. S. De Vries[1]

[1] Department of Neonatology, Wilhelmina Children's Hospital, University Medical Center Utrecht, Utrecht, Netherlands
[2] Department of Psychiatry, Brain Center Rudolf Magnus, University Medical Center Utrecht, Utrecht, Netherlands

Correspondence:
M. P. Van den Heuvel, Department of Psychiatry, Brain Center Rudolf Magnus, University Medical Center Utrecht, Universiteitsweg 100, 3584 CG Utrecht, Netherlands
e-mail: m.p.vandenheuvel@umcutrecht.nl

Our brain is a complex network of structurally and functionally interconnected regions, shaped to efficiently process and integrate information. The development from a brain equipped with basic functionalities to an efficient network facilitating complex behavior starts during gestation and continues into adulthood. Resting-state functional MRI (rs-fMRI) enables the examination of developmental aspects of functional connectivity (FC) and functional brain networks. This review will discuss changes observed in the developing brain on the level of network FC from a gestational age of 20 weeks onwards. We discuss findings of resting-state fMRI studies showing that functional network development starts during gestation, creating a foundation for each of the resting-state networks (RSNs) to be established. Visual and sensorimotor areas are reported to develop first, with other networks, at different rates, increasing both in network connectivity and size over time. Reaching childhood, marked fine-tuning and specialization takes place in the regions necessary for higher-order cognitive functions.

Keywords: resting-state functional MRI, functional connectivity, brain development

INTRODUCTION

The change from basic behavioral patterns during the first months after birth to being able to reason logically as an adult illustrates that development of the brain with age is very important. Although these cognitive manifestations of brain development are impressive, brain maturation may be even better appreciated by the macroscopic anatomical changes which the brain undergoes before birth. Considerable increases in both cortical folding and volume have been studied from 26 weeks gestational age (**Figure 1**) (Dubois et al., 2008; Ment et al., 2009). Even though this process continues also beyond the age of 2, important changes in cortical folding and volume are observed before 2 years of age. From the age of 2 onwards, both cognitive and behavioral development becomes more prominent, while the extent of macroscopic anatomical changes and myelination is fairly limited compared to changes before the age of 2 (Paus et al., 1999). Thus, development of these domains during late human development is more likely to rely on microstructural or functional changes (Yakovlev and Lecours, 1967; Paus et al., 1999).

For studying brain development, previous research has shed light on different aspects of the early developing brain, such as cerebral volume, cortical morphology, gray/white matter ratios, and brain metabolism (Chugani, 1998; Dubois et al., 2008; Hüppi, 2011). Studies have revealed several aspects of brain structure and function using techniques such as conventional MRI, diffusion-tensor imaging (DTI), positron emission tomography (PET), and electroencephalography (EEG) (Chugani, 1998; Smit et al., 2012; Vasung et al., 2013). An imaging technique to study the functional interactions between brain regions is resting-state functional MRI (rs-fMRI), which measures the level of correlation between endogenous brain signals. Evidence is emerging that this spontaneous activity is predominantly of a neuronal origin and can thus reflect functional connectivity (FC) within the brain (Fox and Raichle, 2007; Leopold and Maier, 2011). In case of a significant overlap of spontaneous activation patterns of two spatially distant brain regions, a level of FC is assumed and a so-called resting-state network (RSN) can be identified (Fox et al., 2005; Fox and Raichle, 2007). At least eight resting-state networks, among others motor, visual, attentional, and default-mode networks, have been described in adult humans (**Figure 2**) (Damoiseaux et al., 2006; Smith et al., 2009; Van den Heuvel and Hulshoff Pol, 2010). Also animal studies in rodents (Becerra et al., 2011; Jonckers et al., 2011) and monkeys (Hutchison et al., 2011; Mars et al., 2011) have shown analogous large-scale brain networks, validating concepts of functional network connectivity in humans.

This review will address some of the developmental changes that can be observed in the functional networks of the young brain using rs-fMRI. First, to illustrate how the early human brain develops qualitatively, connectivity patterns of preterm and full-term children up to the age of 2 will be discussed. After a concise description of late human brain development, i.e. from 2 years of age onwards, the focus will shift toward quantitative measurements of brain development. Lastly, a brief summary, a discussion of a number of technical limitations of rs-fMRI as well as future directions for research will be provided.

EARLY HUMAN DEVELOPMENT

In recent years, early brain maturation has been studied by examining the resting-state dynamics in both prenatal and postnatal life. Recently, two studies have conducted fetal rs-fMRI showing that it may be possible to map FC of healthy fetuses (Schöpf et al., 2012; Thomason et al., 2013). Almost half of all bilateral functional networks could be identified *in utero* from 24 weeks gestational age onwards, with increasing connectivity strength toward full-term age (Thomason et al., 2013). Similar maturation effects have been observed in prematurely born infants (Fransson et al., 2007; Doria et al., 2010; Smyser et al., 2010). Five functional networks were indentified in extremely preterm to early preterm infants at term-equivalent age, encompassing the primary visual cortex, bilateral sensorimotor area, bilateral auditory cortex, precuneus area, lateral parietal cortex, cerebellum, and the medial and dorsolateral prefrontal cortex (**Figure 3**) (Fransson et al., 2007). Additionally, default-mode and executive control RSNs have been reported in very preterm to late preterm infants as well (Doria et al., 2010). One network in the prematurely born infants (**Figure 3**, network **D**) could not be directly linked to a comparable network known in adults. Also, immaturity of the identified networks was characterized by less extension into the posterior-anterior direction compared to adult networks. Although contradicting results have been reported on lateralization of developing networks in which also unilateral networks have been described (Liu et al., 2008), more evidence seems to be present for bilateral FC patterns, already present at the neonatal stage (Fransson et al., 2007, 2009; Lin et al., 2008; Kelly et al., 2009; Gao et al., 2013). Based on the consistent findings of both fetal and neonatal rs-fMRI studies it can be hypothesized that the foundations of resting-state networks are already laid down before term age, with rapid neural growth in the last trimester of pregnancy (Doria et al., 2010).

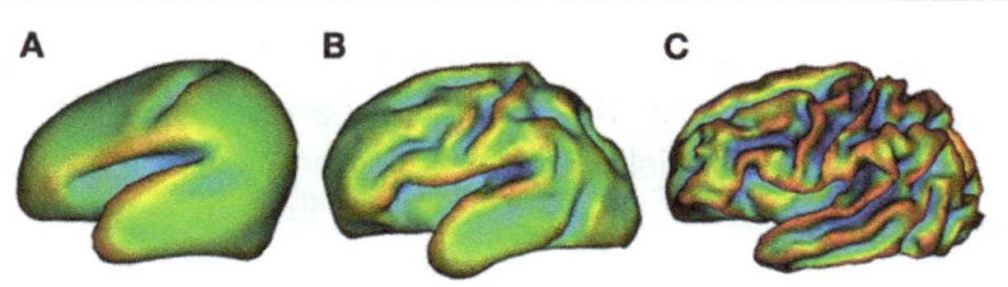

FIGURE 1 | Cortical folding at 26 weeks (A), 29 weeks (B), and 36 weeks gestational age (C). This illustrates considerable macroscopic changes of the developing preterm brain. Images are generated by brain surface rendering with a mathematical morphology approach. The different colors delineate surface curvature. Reproduced with permission from Elsevier (Ment et al., 2009).

The default-mode network (DMN) is a network that received considerable attention in FC studies in children. The adult DMN encompasses the posterior cingulate cortex (PCC), the precuneus, the medial prefrontal cortex (mPFC), the orbital frontal gyrus, the anterior cingulate cortex (ACC), the inferolateral temporal cortex, the parahippocampal gyrus as well as the bilateral parietal cortex (Raichle et al., 2001; Thomason et al., 2008; Van den Heuvel et al., 2009; Damaraju et al., 2010). Which exact collection of functions the network employs in humans has not yet been elucidated. However, the DMN is considered to be important for internally focused tasks, such as episodic memory, self-referential thought, and other social cognitive processes (Buckner et al., 2008; Uddin et al., 2010). Resting-state studies that could not detect a DMN in preterm infants have suggested the existence of a pre-DMN, or "proto-DMN" (Fransson et al., 2007, 2009, 2011; Doria et al., 2010; Power et al., 2010; Smyser et al., 2010). This network, composed of the bilateral parietal cortex and the precuneus/PCC, has been suggested to be a fragment of the posterior part of the adult DMN, forming the basics of the DMN at term age (Doria et al., 2010).

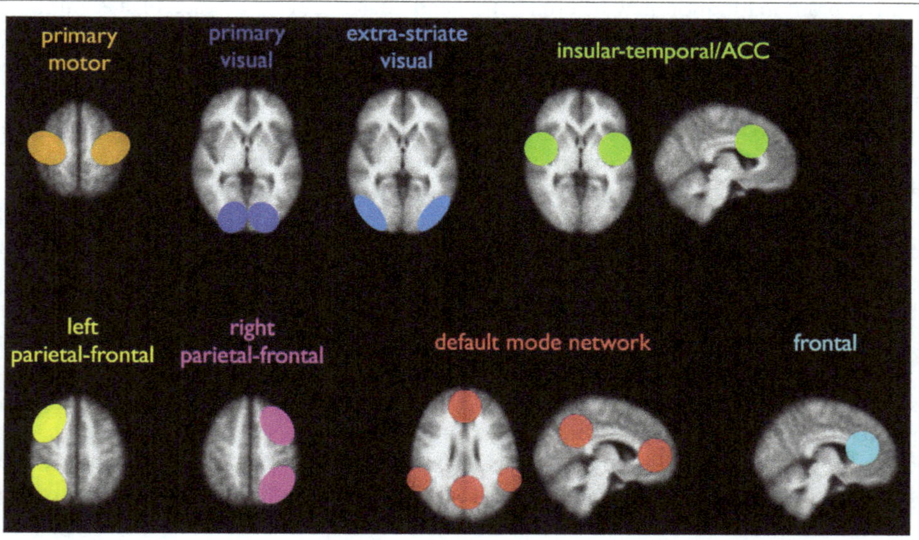

FIGURE 2 | Illustration of eight commonly reported resting-state networks (RSNs), consisting of distant areas that show functional coupling. Both unilateral and bilateral connectivity networks have been consistently reported in adults. Reproduced with permission from Elsevier (Van den Heuvel and Hulshoff Pol, 2010).

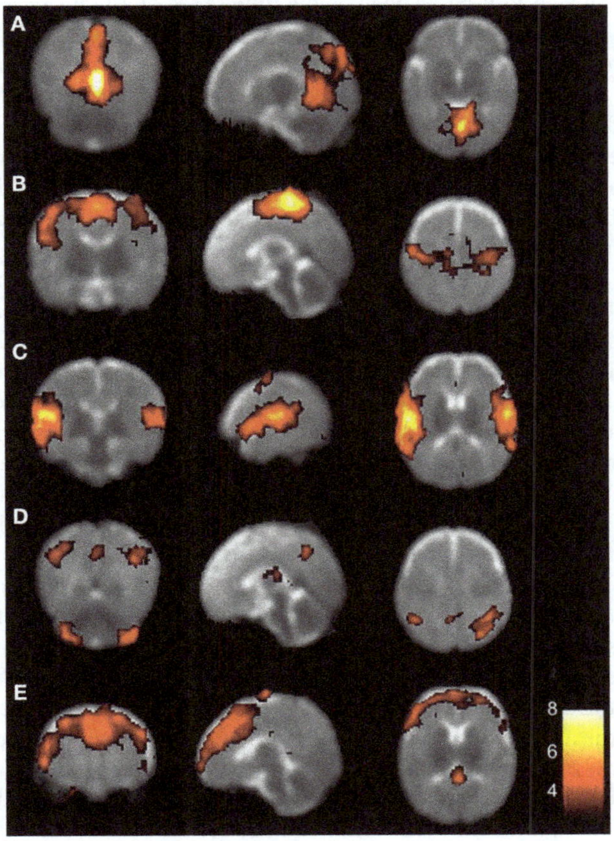

FIGURE 3 | The five resting-state networks consistently found in preterm infants. Each row depicts one resting-state network represented on an axial T2-weighted template, with on the left hand side the left hemisphere. Colors indicate correlation strength, with increasing correlation strength toward the yellow part of the spectrum. **(A)** primary visual areas; **(B)** bilateral somatosensory and motor cortices; **(C)** bilateral temporal/inferior parietal cortex encompassing the primary auditory cortex; **(D)** posterior lateral and midline parts of the parietal cortex and lateral aspects of the cerebellum; **(E)** medial and lateral sections of the anterior prefrontal cortex. With permission reproduced from (Fransson et al., 2007).

Even though the frameworks of the DMN and other RSNs can be recognized at term age, some networks appear to be more developed than others. For example, FC of the visual and auditory networks is relatively mature compared to other networks in preterm infants around 36 weeks of gestation (Lin et al., 2008; Doria et al., 2010). Medial regions develop through different connectivity patterns as compared to lateral regions (Smyser et al., 2010). In these medial regions, such as in the anterior cingulate, an increase in interhemispheric connectivity can already be detected as early as 26 weeks post-menstrual age (PMA) (Smyser et al., 2010; Thomason et al., 2013). Seeds in lateral brain regions, for instance in the sensorimotor cortex, have connections that extend over a relatively large distance to their homotopic counterparts. Interhemispheric connectivity between these laterally located areas still cannot be detected by 38 weeks PMA (Smyser et al., 2010). They appear to first intensify local connection strength before the connection toward the homotopic counterpart is established (Smyser et al., 2010). Increasingly coherent interhemispheric activity and high thalamic FC during the period of accelerated neural development demonstrates the critical importance of this last period of pregnancy for brain network maturation (Smyser et al., 2010, 2011; Uddin et al., 2010; Thomason et al., 2013).

THE FIRST YEARS OF LIFE

Next to different developmental rates of connectivity strength, development of network size appears to differ between networks as well. Changes in network size, represented by a percentage of brain volume, have been observed during the first years of life. Comparing infants of 2 weeks with infants at 2 years of age, several RSNs have shown to exhibit a significant increase in FC as well as cerebral volumes of cortical connectivity (Lin et al., 2008). However, the latter study showed that growth of network volume is not necessarily associated with a simultaneous increase in FC strength across all RSNs. Whereas FC strength of the sensorimotor RSNs is comparable to the visual RSNs, the sensorimotor network exhibits the most significant increase in volume between 2 weeks and 1 year, preceding the growth of the visual network, which occurs predominantly between 1 and 2 years of age (Lin et al., 2008). Lack of linear correlation between increases in connectivity strength and network size also applies to the DMN in the first 2 years (Gao et al., 2009). With a gradual increase in network size and a decrease in fragmentation during this period, it is possible that the more fragmented state of the DMN early in development could be a sign of immaturity, in which the network achieves adult-like properties around 1 year of age (Fair et al., 2008; Gao et al., 2009; de Bie et al., 2011). The dorsal attention network synchronizes in a similar way, although its configuration also seems to be influenced by network-network interactions with the DMN (Gao et al., 2013).

LATE HUMAN DEVELOPMENT

From the age of 2 years onwards, neurodevelopment is characterized by a gain in higher-order cognitive abilities, such as attention and memory. Networks supporting these abilities show differences between children and adults, which is assumed to reflect a process of maturation. For example, EEG in healthy 5–8-year-old children has demonstrated that RSNs associated with higher-order cognitive functions, such as the DMN, cingulo-opercular, ventral, and dorsal frontoparietal RSNs, still have a primitive architecture compared to adults (de Bie et al., 2011). Characteristics of such a primitive architecture are lower overall FC, weak within-network connectivity and presence of aberrant connections between distant brain areas as compared to adults. The sensorimotor area, which starts its development relatively early (de Bie et al., 2011), did not show these immature characteristics. Rather, FC of the sensorimotor area, which is similar to adults, may suggest mature-like characteristics of primary networks by the age of 7 (de Bie et al., 2011). As for the DMN, a more integrated network is found in teenagers and young adults (Fair et al., 2008, 2009). By the age of 10, each of the major regions of the DMN are present, with areas in the mPFC, the PCC, the left and right medial temporal lobe and the left and right angular gyrus (Supekar et al., 2010). Small spatial differences from adult patterns persist and FC of all RSNs, including the DMN, is still reduced. At 12 years of age, overall FC as well as network size is still decreased in comparison with adults (Jolles et al., 2011). However, areas associated with higher cognitive and emotional processing (for instance the executive control system, the dorsal attention system and the DMN) showed locally increased FC compared to the level of connectivity in these areas in adults. Hence, the basic configuration of RSNs may be subject to fine-tuning and specialization during the first years of adolescence, especially in the regions necessary for higher-order cognitive functions. Some studies have suggested that brain maturation may be reflected by a decrease in connectivity of short-range links and an increase of FC of long-range connections (Fair et al., 2007, 2008; Kelly et al., 2009; Supekar et al., 2009). Yet, caution is warranted regarding the interpretation of the results, as observed effects may at least be partly explained by effects of head motion, which has been shown to impose systemic effects on rs-fMRI measures (Power et al., 2012; Van Dijk et al., 2012).

QUANTITATIVE MEASUREMENTS OF BRAIN DEVELOPMENT: GRAPH THEORY

Graph theory describes and quantifies complex whole-brain networks (for a comprehensive review of graph theory, see Bullmore and Sporns, 2009), which allows interpretation of different quantitative measurements into qualitative aspects of whole-brain organization.

Initially, communication between networks seems to be mostly localized to areas in close anatomical proximity (Fair et al., 2007, 2009; Supekar et al., 2009; Gao et al., 2011). During development, large-scale brain networks transform from a locally oriented organization to a more integrated topology (Fair et al., 2007, 2009; Supekar et al., 2009; Gao et al., 2011). The presence of “functional hubs” is an example of how graph theoretical measures may provide insight into functional cerebral architecture. Functional hubs, which are brain areas with a high FC density, are thought to be important for efficient neural signaling and integration of information (Buckner et al., 2009; Tomasi and Volkow, 2011). Cortical hubs and their related cortical networks in healthy, full-term infants have been found to be bilaterally connected and mainly located in the homomodal primary sensorimotor, visual, and auditory brain regions (Fransson et al., 2011). As of the age of 2, the posterior cingulate cortex/retrosplenial (PCC/Rsp) connection exhibits considerable strength, which would make it suitable to function as a primary cortical hub within the developing DMN (Gao et al., 2009). With age, FC between hub and non-hub connections increases strongly, while connectivity between hubs remains relatively stable (Hwang et al., 2013).

METHODOLOGICAL CONSIDERATIONS

Currently, the approaches most commonly used for the analysis of the rs-fMRI data are seed-based or region-of-interest (ROI) analyses, independent component analysis (ICA) and graph theory. The latter approach is used for describing properties of the functional connections rather than establishing them; some applications of graph theory have been discussed in the previous section. In ROI-based analysis the time series of a brain region of interest are correlated to time series of other brain regions. The functional connections of this predefined area of the brain, or seed, can thus be determined. Its relative simplicity may be a disadvantage, as whole-brain connectivity patterns—without predefined brain regions to correlate to—cannot be evaluated. Also, it can be more difficult to detect novel links (Gao et al., 2009). Alternatively, this limitation does not apply to ICA, which enables formation of a whole-brain connectivity map. Although an a priori hypothesis is not necessary to run the statistics, the interpretation of the analysis is more difficult than the ROI-based analysis method (Fox and Raichle, 2007; de Bie et al., 2011). When further comparing seed-based analysis and ICA, the resting-state data results appear to correspond fairly well (Gao et al., 2011; Rosazza and Minati, 2011). Yet, the level of correspondence slightly decreases when more components are included in the analysis (Rosazza and Minati, 2011). The application of different preprocessing steps enhances the heterogeneity among rs-fMRI studies, further complicating comparison and uniform interpretation of rs-fMRI studies (Lee et al., 2013). In addition, rs-fMRI data may also be subject to other confounding effects possibly leading to misinterpretation. Potential and unknown effects of other neurophysiological processes or sedation on the rs-fMRI data (Nallasamy and Tsao, 2011; Birn, 2012), as well as the already mentioned sensitivity to effects of motion (Power et al., 2012; Van Dijk et al., 2012), with reported intra-individual differences (Honey et al., 2009) could impinge on reproducibility and question the neuronal nature of observed developmental effects.

EFFECTS OF PREMATURITY ON FC

Prematurity, especially in the context of a complicated postnatal course, may have adverse effects on gray matter volume, myelination, cerebral surface area, and overall cerebral volume (Hüppi et al., 1996; Inder et al., 2005; Kapellou et al., 2006). However, data on effects of prematurity on FC development are still limited. The networks identified in preterm infants have been reproduced in healthy full-term neonates, supporting at least similar RSN architecture (Fransson et al., 2009). In addition, despite small differences in the basal ganglia, the visual cortex and the cerebellum, no major differences have been reported between the anatomical locations of RSNs in preterm infants without serious postnatal complications and full-term controls (Damaraju et al., 2010; Doria et al., 2010; Smyser et al., 2010). The studies cited included prematurely born infants without acquired brain injury or early developmental problems and provided limited information on long-term neurodevelopmental outcome. Therefore, to what extent brain development of preterm infants may be different from full-term neonates warrants further exploration. Prematurely born infants with only minor cerebral abnormalities showed disruption in network architecture, especially in thalamo-cortical connections (Smyser et al., 2010). Compared to the networks of the full-term infant, preterm infants scanned at term-equivalent age had lower correlations and less connectivity between lateral seeds. Moreover, whereas infant born at term showed characteristics of a coherent network with possible DMN precursors, term-equivalent premature infants did not

(Smyser et al., 2010). Follow-up data of preterm infants at 36 months of age showed lower overall connectivity compared to full-term peers (Damaraju et al., 2010). Long-term effects of premature birth on FC have been observed in young adulthood, in which alternative functional circuits involved in language have been described (Constable et al., 2013).

Summarizing, a number of studies have looked at resting-state dynamics in premature populations, but only limited data is available on possible effects of prematurity on FC development. More studies in both preterm and healthy term infants with long-term follow-up are therefore required to improve insights into brain development.

DIRECTIONS FOR FUTURE RESEARCH

All of the aspects outlined in the previous section should be taken into consideration in the interpretation of developmental effects in rs-fMRI studies and also provide directions for further investigations. In addition, elucidating the structure-function relationship of networks by further combination of imaging techniques could improve insights into the mechanisms behind functional network development. Similar maturational effects can be observed with DTI measuring structural parameters (Vasung et al., 2013) and arterial spin labeling MRI to map perfusion (De Vis et al., 2013). Furthermore, the translational aspect of developmental connectivity patterns toward executive functions and behavior merits attention as well, which ultimately may improve prediction of neurodevelopmental outcome or disease progression by rs-fMRI techniques. Considering that the last trimester of pregnancy may be especially relevant for adequate FC development (Doria et al., 2010), studying effects of prematurity related to both brain maturation and neurocognitive outcome could be an important application. Full-term infants with neonatal encephalopathy, in whom prediction of cognitive outcome is often difficult, may also be a relevant study population. In addition, a possible effect of gender on RSN patterns has been suggested (Biswal et al., 2010; Weissman-Fogel et al., 2010; Zuo et al., 2010; Gong et al., 2011). Structural MRI studies have shown that in particular across puberty gradual sexual dimorphisms develop, with unknown relationships between gender, puberty and neural development (Blakemore, 2011). So far, only one study addressed gender differences in functional homotopy in children (Zuo et al., 2010). Therefore, to what extent gender effects might influence developmental patterns of FC in neonates, children or young adults remains unknown. Lastly, this review supports the notion that foundations of each of the RSNs are laid down before term age, after which fine-tuning and specialization of these networks take place. It has been suggested that a genetic substrate for functional networks may exist (e.g., Glahn et al., 2010). Twin-studies in children and adults indeed show significant effects of heritability, primarily on the level of whole-brain connectivity efficiency and functional organization (Fornito et al., 2011; Van den Heuvel et al., 2013). More research into the genetic control underlying functional network organization is needed, also toward possible identification of specific deficits in FC relevant for neuropsychiatric diseases, such as autism or schizophrenia.

CONCLUSION

This review described developmental changes observed in the functional networks of the brain from 20 weeks of gestation onwards using rs-fMRI. Even though the techniques used to acquire and analyze rs-fMRI data leave room for improvement, all of the efforts so far have led to significant insights into brain development. Even before term age, a network with foundations of each of the RSNs can be recognized (Doria et al., 2010; Fransson et al., 2011). RSNs differ in their growth trajectories, but fine-tuning and specialization of RSNs is generally characterized by increasing FC, network volume, and coherence. The next step in developmental fMRI research may be to explore the origins of inter-individual network variation as well as associations with cognitive functioning and behavior by combining structure and function at different ages, in both healthy and diseased states.

REFERENCES

Becerra, L., Pendse, G., Chang, P. C., Bishop, J., and Borsook, D. (2011). Robust reproducible resting state networks in the awake rodent brain. *PLoS ONE* 6:e25701. doi: 10.1371/journal.pone.0025701

Birn, R. M. (2012). The role of physiological noise in resting-state functional connectivity. *Neuroimage* 62, 864–870. doi: 10.1016/j.neuroimage.2012.01.016

Biswal, B. B., Mennes, M., Zuo, X. N., Gohel, S., Kelly, C., Smith, S. M., et al. (2010). Toward discovery science of human brain function. *Proc. Natl. Acad. Sci. U.S.A.* 107, 4734–4739. doi: 10.1073/pnas.0911855107

Blakemore, S. J. (2011). Imaging brain development: the adolescent brain. *Neuroimage* 61, 397–406. doi: 10.1016/j.neuroimage.2011.11.080

Buckner, R. L., Andrews-Hanna, J. R., and Schacter, D. L. (2008). The brain's default network: anatomy, function, and relevance to disease. *Ann. N.Y. Acad. Sci.* 1124, 1–38. doi: 10.1196/annals.1440.011

Buckner, R. L., Sepulcre, J., Talukdar, T., Krienen, F. M., Liu, H., Hedden, T., et al. (2009). Cortical hubs revealed by intrinsic functional connectivity: mapping, assessment of stability, and relation to Alzheimer's disease. *J. Neurosci.* 29, 1860–1873. doi: 10.1523/JNEUROSCI.5062-08.2009

Bullmore, E., and Sporns, O. (2009). Complex brain networks: graph theoretical analysis of structural and functional systems. *Nat. Rev. Neurosci.* 10, 186–198. doi: 10.1038/nrn2575

Chugani, H. T. (1998). A critical period of brain development: studies of cerebral glucose utilization with PET. *Prev. Med.* 27, 184–188. doi: 10.1006/pmed.1998.0274

Constable, B. R., Vohr, D., Scheinost, J. R., Benjamin, J. R., Fulbright, R. K., Lacadie, C., et al. (2013). A left cerebellar pathway mediates language in prematurely-born young adults. *Neuroimage* 64, 371–378. doi: 10.1016/j.neuroimage.2012.09 008

Damaraju, E., Phillips, J. R., Lowe, J. R., Ohls, R., Calhoun, V. D., and Caprihan, A. (2010). Resting-state functional connectivity differences in premature children. *Front. Syst. Neurosci.* 4:23. doi: 10.3389/fnsys.2010.00023

Damoiseaux, J. S., Rombouts, S. A., Barkhof, F., Scheltens, P., Stam, C. J., Smith, S. M., et al. (2006). Consistent resting-state networks across healthy subjects. *Proc. Natl. Acad. Sci. U.S.A.* 103, 13848–13853. doi: 10.1073/pnas.0601417103

de Bie, H. M., Boersma, M., Adriaanse, S., Veltman, D. J., Wink, A. M., Roosendaal, S. D., et al. (2011). Resting-state networks in awake five- to eight-year old children. *Hum. Brain Mapp.* 33, 1189–1201. doi: 10.1002/hbm.21280

De Vis, J. B., Petersen, E. T., de Vries, L. S., Groenendaal, F., Kersbergen, K. J., Alderliesten, T., et al. (2013). Regional changes in brain perfusion during brain maturation measured non-invasively with arterial spin labeling MRI in neonates. *Eur. J. Radiol.* 82, 538–543. doi: 10.1016/j.ejrad.2012.10.013

Doria, V., Beckmann, C. F., Arichi, T., Merchant, N., Groppo, M., Turkheimer, F. E., et al. (2010). Emergence of resting state networks in the preterm human brain. *Proc. Natl. Acad. Sci.*

U.S.A. 107, 20015–20020. doi: 10.1073/pnas.1007921107

Dubois, J., Benders, M., Cachia, A., Lazeyras, F., Ha-Vinh Leuchter, R., Sizonenko, S. V., et al. (2008). Mapping the early cortical folding process in the preterm newborn brain. *Cereb. Cortex* 18, 1444–1454. doi: 10.1093/cercor/bhm180

Fair, D. A., Cohen, A. L., Dosenbach, N. U. F., Church, J. A., Miezin, F. M., Barch, D. M., et al. (2008). The maturing architecture of the brain's default network. *Proc. Natl. Acad. Sci. U.S.A.* 105, 4028–4032. doi: 10.1073/pnas.0800376105

Fair, D. A., Cohen, A. L., Power, J. D., Dosenbach, N. U., Church, J. A., Miezin, F. M., et al. (2009). Functional brain networks develop from a "local to distributed" organization. *PLoS Comput. Biol.* 5:e1000381. doi: 10.1371/journal.pcbi.1000381

Fair, D. A., Dosenbach, N. U., Church, J. A., Cohen, A. L., Brahmbhatt, S., Miezin, F. M., et al. (2007). Development of distinct control networks through segregation and integration. *Proc. Natl. Acad. Sci. U.S.A.* 104, 13507–13512. doi: 10.1073/pnas.0705843104

Fornito, A., Zalesky, A., Bassett, D. S., Meunier, D., Ellison-Wright, I., Yucel, M., et al. (2011). Genetic influences on cost-efficient organization of human cortical functional networks. *J. Neurosci.* 31, 3261–3270. doi: 10.1523/JNEUROSCI.4858-10.2011

Fox, M. D., and Raichle, M. E. (2007). Spontaneous fluctuations in brain activity observed with functional magnetic resonance imaging. *Nat. Rev. Neurosci.* 8, 700–711. doi: 10.1038/nrn2201

Fox, M. D., Snyder, A. Z., Vincent, J. L., Corbetta, M., van Essen, D. C., and Raichle, M. E. (2005). The human brain is intrinsically organized into dynamic, anticorrelated functional networks. *Proc. Natl. Acad. Sci. U.S.A.* 102, 9673–9678. doi: 10.1073/pnas.0504136102

Fransson, P., Åden, U., Blennow, M., and Lagercrantz, H. (2011). The functional architecture of the infant brain as revealed by resting-state fMRI. *Cereb. Cortex* 21, 145–154. doi: 10.1093/cercor/bhq071

Fransson, P., Skiöld, B., Engström, M., Hallberg, B., Mosskin, M., Åden, U., et al. (2009). Spontaneous brain activity in the newborn brain during natural sleep–an fMRI study in infants born at full term. *Ped. Res.* 66, 301–305. doi: 10.1203/PDR.0b013e3181b1bd84

Fransson, P., Skiöld, B., Horsch, S., Nordell, A., Blennow, M., Lagercrantz, H., et al. (2007). Resting-state networks in the infant brain. *Proc. Natl. Acad. Sci. U.S.A.* 104, 15531–15536. doi: 10.1073/pnas.0704380104

Gao, W., Gilmore, J. H., Giovanello, K. S., Smith, J. K., Shen, D., Zhu, H., et al. (2011). Temporal and spatial evolution of brain network topology during the first years of life. *PLoS ONE* 6:e25278. doi: 10.1371/journal.pone.0025278

Gao, W., Gilmore, J. H., Maisog, J. M., Foss-Feig, J., Billington, M. E., Smith, J. K., et al. (2013). The synchronization within and interaction between the default and dorsal attention networks in early infancy. *Cereb. Cortex* 23, 594–603. doi: 10.1093/cercor/bhs043

Gao, W., Zhu, H., Giovanello, K. S., Smith, J. K., Shen, D., Gilmore, J. H., et al. (2009). Evidence on the emergence of the brain's default network from 2-week-old to 2-year-old healthy pediatric subjects. *Proc. Natl. Acad. Sci. U.S.A.* 106, 6790–6795. doi: 10.1073/pnas.0811221106

Glahn, D. C., Winkler, A. M., Kochunov, P., Almasy, L., Duggirala, R., Carless, M. A., et al. (2010). Genetic control over the resting brain. *Proc. Natl. Acad. Sci. U.S.A.* 107, 1223–1228. doi: 10.1073/pnas.0909969107

Gong, G., He, Y., and Evans, A. C. (2011). Brain connectivity: gender makes a difference. *Neuroscientist* 17, 575–591. doi: 10.1177/1073858410386492

Honey, C. J., Sporns, O., Cammoun, L., Gigandet, X., Thiran, J. P., Meuli, R., et al. (2009). Predicting human resting-state functional connectivity from structural connectivity. *Proc. Natl. Acad. Sci. U.S.A.* 106, 2035–2040. doi: 10.1073/pnas.0811168106

Hüppi, P. S. (2011). Cortical development in the fetus and the newborn: advanced MR techniques. *Top. Magn. Reson. Imaging* 22, 33–38. doi: 10.1097/RMR.0b013e3182416f78

Hüppi, P. S., Schuknecht, B., Boesch, C., Bossi, E., Felblinger, J., Fusch, C., et al. (1996). Structural and neurobehavioral delay in postnatal brain development of preterm infants. *Ped. Res.* 39, 895–901. doi: 10.1203/00006450-199605000-00026

Hutchison, R. M., Leung, L. S., Mirsattari, S. M., Gati, J. S., Menon, R. S., and Everling, S. (2011). Resting-state networks in the macaque at 7T. *Neuroimage* 56, 1546–1555. doi: 10.1016/j.neuroimage.2011.02.063

Hwang, K., Hallquist, M. N., and Luna, B. (2013). The development of hub architecture in the human functional brain network. *Cereb. Cortex* 23, 2380–2393. doi: 10.1093/cercor/bhs227

Inder, T. E., Warfield, S. K., Wang, H., Hüppi, P. S., and Volpe, J. J. (2005). Abnormal cerebral structure is present at term in premature infants. *Pediatrics* 115, 286–294. doi: 10.1542/peds.2004-0326

Jolles, D. D., van Buchem, M. A., Crone, E. A., and Rombouts, S. A. (2011). A comprehensive study of whole-brain functional connectivity in children and young adults. *Cereb. Cortex* 21, 385–391. doi: 10.1093/cercor/bhq104

Jonckers, E., van Audekerke, J., de Visscher, G., van der Linden, A., and Verhoye, M. (2011). Functional connectivity fMRI of the rodent brain: comparison of functional connectivity networks in rat and mouse. *PLoS ONE* 6:e18876. doi: 10.1371/journal.pone.0018876

Kapellou, O., Counsell, S. J., Kennea, N., Dyet, L., Saeed, N., Stark, J., et al. (2006). Abnormal cortical development after premature birth shown by altered allometric scaling of brain growth. *PLoS Med.* 3:e265. doi: 10.1371/journal.pmed.0030265

Kelly, A. M., Di Martino, A., Uddin, L. Q., Shehzad, Z., Gee, D. G., Reiss, P. T., et al. (2009). Development of anterior cingulate functional connectivity from late childhood to early adulthood. *Cereb. Cortex* 19, 640–657. doi: 10.1093/cercor/bhn117

Lee, M. H., Smyser, C. D., and Shimony, J. S. (2013). Resting-state fMRI: a review of methods and clinical applications. *AJNR Am. J. Neuroradiol.* doi: 10.3174/ajnr.A3263. [Epub ahead of print].

Leopold, D. A., and Maier, A. (2011). Ongoing physiological processes in the cerebral cortex. *Neuroimage* 62, 2190–2200. doi: 10.1016/j.neuroimage.2011.10.059

Lin, W., Zhu, Q., Gao, W., Chen, Y., Toh, C. H., Styner, M., et al. (2008). Functional connectivity MR imaging reveals cortical functional connectivity in the developing brain. *AJNR Am. J. Neuroradiol.* 29, 1883–1889. doi: 10.3174/ajnr.A1256

Liu, W. C., Flax, J. F., Guise, K. G., Sukul, V., and Benasich, A. A. (2008). Functional connectivity of the sensorimotor area in naturally sleeping infants. *Brain Res.* 1223, 42–49. doi: 10.1016/j.brainres.2008.05.054

Mars, R. B., Jbabdi, S., Sallet, J., O'Reilly, J. X., Croxson, P. L., Olivier, E., et al. (2011). Diffusion-weighted imaging tractography-based parcellation of the human parietal cortex and comparison with human and macaque resting-state functional connectivity. *J. Neurosci.* 31, 4087–4100. doi: 10.1523/JNEUROSCI.5102-10.2011

Ment, L. R., Hirtz, D., and Hüppi, P. S. (2009). Imaging biomarkers of outcome in the developing preterm brain. *Lancet Neurol.* 8, 1042–1055. doi: 10.1016/S1474-4422(09)70257-1

Nallasamy, N., and Tsao, D. Y. (2011). Functional connectivity in the brain: effects of anesthesia. *Neuroscientist* 17, 94–106. doi: 10.1177/1073858410374126

Paus, T., Zijdenbos, A., Worsley, K., Collins, D. L., Blumenthal, J., Giedd, J. N., et al. (1999). Structural maturation of neural pathways in children and adolescent: *in vivo* study. *Science* 283, 1908–1911. doi: 10.1126/science.283.5409.1908

Power, J. D., Barnes, K. A., Snyder, A. Z., Schlaggar, B. L., and Petersen, S. E. (2012). Spurious but systematic correlations in functional connectivity MRI networks arise from subject motion. *Neuroimage* 59, 2142–2154. doi: 10.1016/j.neuroimage.2011.10.018

Power, J. D., Fair, D. A., Schlaggar, B. L., and Petersen, S. E. (2010). The development of human functional brain networks. *Neuron* 67, 735–748. doi: 10.1016/j.neuron.2010.08.017

Raichle, M. E., MacLeod, A. M., Snyder, A. Z., Powers, W. J., Gusnard, D. A., and Shulman, G. L. (2001). A default mode of brain function. *Proc. Natl. Acad. Sci. U.S.A.* 98, 676–682. doi: 10.1073/pnas.98.2.676

Rosazza, C., and Minati, L. (2011). Resting-state brain networks: literature review and clinical applications. *Neurol. Sci.* 32, 773–785. doi: 10.1007/s10072-011-0636-y

Schöpf, V., Kasprian, G., Brugger, P. C., and Prayer, D. (2012). Watching the fetal brain at 'rest.' *Int. J. Dev. Neurosci.* 30, 11–17. doi: 10.1016/j.ijdevneu.2011.10.006

Smit, D. J. A., Boersma, M., Schnack, H. G., Micheloyannis, S., Boomsma, D. I., Hulshoff Pol, H. E., et al. (2012). The brain matures with stronger functional connectivity and decreased randomness of its network. *PLoS ONE* 7:e36896. doi: 10.1371/journal.pone.0036896

Smith, S. M., Fox, P. T., Miller, K. L., Glahn, D. C., Fox, P. M., Mackay, C. E., et al. (2009). Correspondence of the brain's functional architecture during activation and rest. *Proc. Natl. Acad. Sci. U.S.A* 106, 13040–13045. doi: 10.1073/pnas.0905267106

Smyser, C. D., Inder, T. E., Shimony, J. S., Hill, J. E., Degnan, A. J., Snyder, A. Z., et al. (2010). Longitudinal analysis of neural network development in preterm infants. *Cereb. Cortex* 20, 2852–2862. doi: 10.1093/cercor/bhq035

Smyser, C. D., Snyder, A. Z., and Neil, J. J. (2011). Functional connectivity MRI in infants: exploration of the functional organization of the developing brain. *Neuroimage* 56, 1437–1452. doi: 10.1016/j.neuroimage.2011.02.073

Supekar, K., Musen, M., and Menon, V. (2009). Development of large-scale functional brain networks in children. *PLoS Biol.* 7:e1000157. doi: 10.1371/journal.pbio.1000157

Supekar, K., Uddin, L. Q., Prater, K., Amin, H., Greicius, M. D., and Menon, V. (2010). Development of functional and structural connectivity within the default mode network in young children. *Neuroimage* 52, 290–301. doi: 10.1016/j.neuroimage.2010.04.009

Thomason, M. E., Chang, C. E., Glover, G. H., Gabrieli, J. D., Greicius, M. D., and Gotlib, I. H. (2008). Default-mode function and task-induced deactivation have overlapping brain substrates in children. *Neuroimage* 41, 1493–1503. doi: 10.1016/j.neuroimage.2008.03.029

Thomason, M. E., Dassanavake, M. T., Shen, S., Katkuri, Y., Alexis, M., Anderson, A. L., et al. (2013). Cross-hemispheric functional connectivity in the human fetal brain. *Sci. Transl. Med.* 5, 173ra24. doi: 10.1126/scitranslmed.3004978

Tomasi, D., and Volkow, N. D. (2011). Functional connectivity hubs in the human brain. *Neuroimage* 57, 908–917. doi: 10.1016/j.neuroimage.2011.05.024

Uddin, L. Q., Supekar, K., and Menon, V. (2010). Typical and atypical development of functional human brain networks: insights from resting-state fMRI. *Front. Syst. Neurosci.* 4:21. doi: 10.3389/fnsys.2010.00021

Van den Heuvel, M. P., and Hulshoff Pol, H. E. (2010). Exploring the brain network: a review on resting-state fMRI functional connectivity. *Eur. Neuropsychopharmacol.* 20, 519–534. doi: 10.1016/j.euroneuro.2010.03.008

Van den Heuvel, M. P., Mandl, R. C. W., Kahn, R. S., and Hulshoff Pol, H. E. (2009). Functionally linked resting-state networks reflect the underlying structural connectivity architecture of the human brain. *Hum. Brain Mapp.* 30, 3127–3141. doi: 10.1002/hbm.20737

Van den Heuvel, M. P., van Soelen, I. L. C., Stam, C. J., Kahn, R. S., Boomsma, D. I., and Hulshoff Pol, H. E. (2013). Genetic control of functional brain network efficiency in children. *Eur. Neuropsychopharmacol.* 23, 19–23. doi: 10.1016/j.euroneuro.2012.06.007

Van Dijk, K. R., Sabuncu, M. R., and Buckner, R. L. (2012). The influence of head motion on intrinsic functional connectivity MRI. *Neuroimage* 59, 431–438. doi: 10.1016/j.neuroimage.2011.07.044

Vasung, L., Fischi-Gomez, E., and Hüppi, P. S. (2013). Multimodality evaluation of the pediatric brain: DTI and its competitors. *Pediatr. Radiol.* 43, 60–68. doi: 10.1007/s00247-012-2515-y

Weissman-Fogel, I., Moayedi, M., Taylor, K. S., Pope, G., and Davis, K. D. (2010). Cognitive and default-mode resting state networks: do male and female brains "rest" differently? *Hum. Brain Mapp.* 31, 1713–1726.

Yakovlev, P. I., and Lecours, A. R. (1967). "The myelogenetic cycles of regional maturation of the brain," in *Regional Development of the Brain in Early Life*, ed A. Minkowski (Oxford: Blackwell), 3–70.

Zuo, X. N., Kelly, C., Di Martino, A., Mennes, M., Margulies, D. S., Bangaru, S., et al. (2010). Growing together and growing apart: regional and sex differences in the lifespan developmental trajectories of functional homotopy. *J. Neurosci.* 30, 15034–15043. doi: 10.1523/JNEUROSCI.2612-10.2010

7

Graph theoretical analysis of developmental patterns of the white matter network

Zhang Chen[1], Min Liu[1], Donald W. Gross[2] and Christian Beaulieu[1]*

[1] Department of Biomedical Engineering, Faculty of Medicine and Dentistry, University of Alberta, Edmonton, AB, Canada
[2] Division of Neurology, Department of Medicine, Faculty of Medicine and Dentistry, University of Alberta, Edmonton, AB, Canada

***Correspondence:**
Christian Beaulieu, Department of Biomedical Engineering, 1098 Research Transition Facility, University of Alberta, 8308-114 Street, Edmonton, AB T6G 2V2, Canada
e-mail: christian.beaulieu@ualberta.ca

Understanding the development of human brain organization is critical for gaining insight into how the enhancement of cognitive processes is related to the fine-tuning of the brain network. However, the developmental trajectory of the large-scale white matter (WM) network is not fully understood. Here, using graph theory, we examine developmental changes in the organization of WM networks in 180 typically-developing participants. WM networks were constructed using whole brain tractography and 78 cortical regions of interest were extracted from each participant. The subjects were first divided into 5 equal sample size ($n = 36$) groups (early childhood: 6.0–9.7 years; late childhood: 9.8–12.7 years; adolescence: 12.9–17.5 years; young adult: 17.6–21.8 years; adult: 21.9–29.6 years). Most prominent changes in the topological properties of developing brain networks occur at late childhood and adolescence. During late childhood period, the structural brain network showed significant increase in the global efficiency but decrease in modularity, suggesting a shift of topological organization toward a more randomized configuration. However, while preserving most topological features, there was a significant increase in the local efficiency at adolescence, suggesting the dynamic process of rewiring and rebalancing brain connections at different growth stages. In addition, several pivotal hubs were identified that are vital for the global coordination of information flow over the whole brain network across all age groups. Significant increases of nodal efficiency were present in several regions such as precuneus at late childhood. Finally, a stable and functionally/anatomically related modular organization was identified throughout the development of the WM network. This study used network analysis to elucidate the topological changes in brain maturation, paving the way for developing novel methods for analyzing disrupted brain connectivity in neurodevelopmental disorders.

Keywords: graph theory, neurodevelopment, anatomical connectivity, modular networks, small world network

INTRODUCTION

Neuroimaging studies have demonstrated widespread and regionally specific structural and functional brain changes during development from infancy to adulthood. Structural magnetic resonance imaging (MRI) studies have reported age-related changes in brain volumes (Giedd et al., 1999; Good et al., 2001), areas (Thompson et al., 2000), cortical thickness (Sowell et al., 2004; Shaw et al., 2008), and regional gray matter (GM) and white matter (WM) density (Paus et al., 1999; Gogtay et al., 2004). The developmental changes in GM and WM on gross scale MRI may reflect synaptic pruning and myelination occurring at the neuronal level (Gogtay et al., 2004). Functional neuroimaging studies have demonstrated increased connectivity among distant regions and decreased connectivity among neighboring regions in brain maturation which suggests a mechanism of segregation of local regions and integration of distant regions into disparate subnetworks for the developing brain (Fair et al., 2008, 2009; Vogel et al., 2010). Diffusion tensor imaging (DTI) studies of WM have shown age-related increases in fractional anisotropy (FA) and decrease in overall diffusion with development [many studies but some include (Snook et al., 2005; Lebel et al., 2008; Tamnes et al., 2010)], including into young adulthood (Giorgio et al., 2008; Lebel and Beaulieu, 2011).

The recent advent of modern network analysis based on graph theory (Strogatz, 2001), has enabled the investigation of the large-scale topological organization of various structural and functional brain networks such as the small-world property, network efficiency and modularity (He et al., 2007; Bullmore and Sporns, 2009; He and Evans, 2010). The network metrics have also proven useful in modeling the large-scale functional and structural organization of the developing brain. Several functional brain network studies have reported age-related increases in the small-worldness (Wu et al., 2013) and a progression from local to distributed organization (Fair et al., 2009) in brain development. The analysis of the structural brain network constructed from regional cortical thickness correlations has revealed a non-linear developmental pattern in network metrics and that most topological changes happen at the late childhood stage (Khundrakpam et al., 2013).

Recently, there has been an increasing interest in the study of how graph metrics of the anatomical brain network change during development. Using DTI, Yap et al. (2011) examined WM networks of 39 healthy pediatric subjects with longitudinal data collected at average ages of 2 weeks, 1 year, and 2 years and demonstrated that the small-world architecture exists at birth with efficiency that increases in later stages of development. Two recent brain connectivity studies of WM maturation pattern using diffusion MRI tractography demonstrated linear and non-linear patterns of increasing structural efficiency with age between ages 2 and 18 years in 30 patients scanned clinically and otherwise deemed normal post-MRI (Hagmann et al., 2010) and between ages 12 and 30 years in 439 healthy subjects (Dennis et al., 2013). However, those studies were limited by different constraints such as a binarized brain network, limited sample size, or restricted age range (early adolescence to early adulthood), thus the developmental trajectory of the WM network from early childhood to adulthood remains unclear.

Therefore, the main goal of this study was to map the developmental changes of the structural brain network based on WM connectivity in 180 typically-developing subjects from 6 to 30 years of age. We hypothesized (i) non-linear age-related developmental trajectories of network metrics as most changes would be expected to happen at late childhood and adolescent stages, and (ii) altered modular organization in different age groups that reflects a process of fine-tuning in structural brain development.

MATERIALS AND METHODS

SUBJECTS

This study included 180 healthy right-handed subjects aged from 6 to 30 years. Health was verified by asking participants a series of questions to ensure there was no history of neurological or psychiatric disease or brain injury. All subjects gave informed consent; child assent and parent/guardian consent was obtained for volunteers under 18 years. The subjects were divided into 5 age groups with equal numbers of subjects and demographics of all groups are shown in **Table 1**.

IMAGE ACQUISITION

All data were acquired on a 1.5-T Siemens Sonata MRI scanner. Standard DTI was acquired using a dual spin-echo, single shot echo-planar imaging sequence with the following parameters: 40 3-mm-thick slices with no inter-slice gap, $TR = 6400$ ms, $TE = 88$ ms, 6 non-collinear diffusion sensitizing gradient directions with $b = 1000\,\text{s/mm}^2$, 8 averages, field-of-view $220 \times 220\,\text{mm}^2$, matrix of 96×128 zero-filled to 256×256, and scan time of 6:06 min. T1-weighted images were also acquired using MPRAGE with $TE = 4.38$ ms, $TR = 1870$ ms, $TI = 1100$ ms, and scan time of 4:29 min.

Table 1 | Group demographics.

Group	Early childhood	Late childhood	Adolescence	Young adult	Adult
Number	36	36	36	36	36
Male/female	16/20	19/17	15/21	18/18	16/20
Mean age, *SD* (*y*)	8.1 (1.1)	11.3 (0.9)	15.4 (1.4)	19.4 (1.1)	25.7 (2.7)
Age range (*y*)	6.0–9.8	9.9–12.7	12.9–17.6	17.6–21.8	21.9–29.7

STRUCTURAL BRAIN NETWORK CONSTRUCTION

Image preprocessing steps including motion and eddy current corrections were performed using FSL 5.0 for all DTI images (http://fsl.fmrib.ox.ac.uk/fsl/fslwiki). The T_1-weighted (MPRAGE) image of each subject was first linearly coregistered (**Figures 1A,B**) to its corresponding b0 image. Each transformed T_1 image was then non-linearly registered to a pre-segmented and validated volumetric template, the automated anatomical labeling (AAL) atlas (Tzourio-Mazoyer et al., 2002) as shown in **Figures 1B,C**. This parcellation divided the cortical surface into 78 regions (39 per hemisphere). See **Table 2** for the name of the regions and their corresponding abbreviations. The resulting inverse deformation map (T^{-1}) for each subject was then applied to warp the AAL template to the DTI native space of each subject using nearest neighbor interpolation method (**Figures 1E,F**) as each AAL region was defined as a brain network node. Whole brain WM tractography was performed using a brute-force streamline-tracking method (Basser et al., 2000) with a FA threshold of 0.2 and primary eigenvector turning angle of 45 degrees (**Figures 1A,D**). To limit false positive connections, two cortical regions were deemed connected if at least 10 connecting fibers with two end points were located between them; the same threshold was also applied in a recent brain network study (van den Heuvel et al., 2012). The effects of different node-connecting fiber number (FN) thresholds ranging from 3 to 10 were determined for our network analysis. We quantified the weight of each valid connection between two cortical regions (i and j) as the product of the connecting FN and mean FA of the connecting fiber, normalized by dividing the average volume of the two connecting regions to counteract the bias where larger cortical regions inherently project/receive more "virtual" fibers ($w_{ij} = \text{FN*FA/Volume}$). Several diffusion brain network studies have applied this weighting function (Lo et al., 2010; Brown et al., 2011). As a result, the structural brain network of each participant was represented by a symmetric 78×78 matrix (**Figure 1G**).

To examine the small-worldness and modular organization of the WM networks for all different age groups, one weighted backbone network for each age group was generated to capture the underlying anatomical connectivity patterns using a previously published method by our group (Gong et al., 2009). In summary, to identify the highly consistent cortical connections, a non-parametric one-tailed sign test was applied. For each pair of cortical regions, the sign test was performed with the null hypothesis that there is no existing connection. The Bonferroni method was applied to correct for multiple comparisons at $P < 0.05$. The use of this conservative statistical criterion generated a symmetric weighted matrix as each edge weight was calculated as the mean of all existing edges in all subjects that captured underlying anatomical connectivity patterns in the human cerebral cortex (Gong et al., 2009).

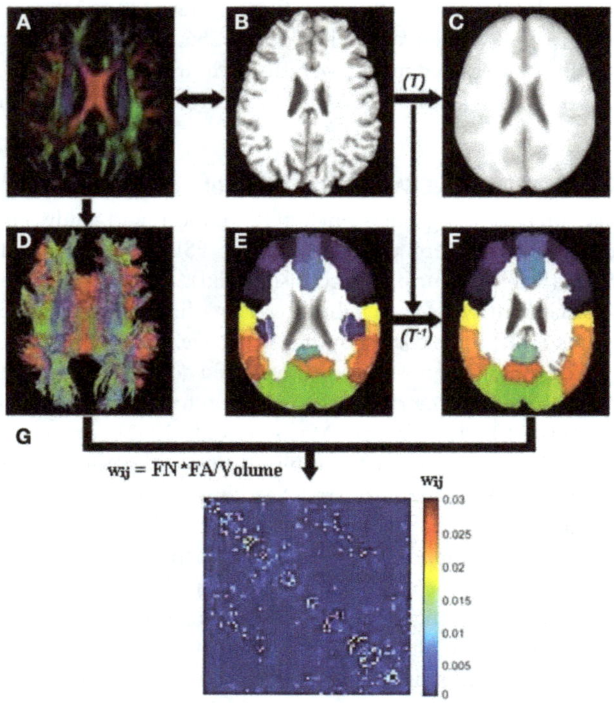

FIGURE 1 | Flowchart for the construction of the DTI white matter (WM) network for each subject. The T_1-weighted image of each subject **(B)** was first coregistered into DTI native space **(A)** using rigid transformation to the b0 image (not shown). The resultant T1 image was then non-linearly registered to the ICBM 152 template **(C)** in the MNI space to obtain transformation matrix *T*. The AAL template **(E)** was then inversely warped back to the individual DTI space **(F)** using the inverse transformation (T^{-1}). Whole brain white matter fibers were reconstructed using a deterministic tractography method in native DTI space **(D)**. The WM fibers connecting any pair of regions were located and the edge weight between the two regions was calculated from the FA, fiber number (FN) and average volume of the two cortical regions. **(G)** A sample white matter network for one subject.

NETWORK ANALYSIS

Several network topological properties were applied for the weighted anatomical brain network derived from each participant, including small-worldness, efficiency and modularity (Watts and Strogatz, 1998; Latora and Marchiori, 2001; Newman, 2006). The connection weights of all edges (w_{ij}) were normalized by the mean weight of the whole network to keep network cost at the same level for all subjects.

For a weighted network G with N nodes and K edges, the total strength S was defined as the mean of all edge weights in the network, $S(G) = \frac{1}{N} \sum_{i \neq j \in G}^{N_M} w_{ij}$ where i and j are two distinct nodes in graph G. The clustering coefficient (CC) of the weighted network G quantifies the likelihood whether the neighboring nodes of any network nodes are connected with each other (Onnela et al., 2005), which was defined as: $CC = \frac{1}{N} \sum_{j,k \in G} (w_{ij} w_{jk} w_{ik})^{1/3} / (k_i^*(k_i - 1)/2)$, where k_i is the number of connected neighbors of node i. The weighted characteristic path length L of a network is the average minimum connectional weights that link any two nodes of the network. To avoid the issue of disconnected nodes, L was measured here by using a "harmonic mean" distance between any pair of nodes such as the reciprocal of the average of the reciprocals (Newman, 2003). A real network would be considered small world if it meets the following criteria: $\gamma = C_p^{real}/C_p^{rand} > 1$ and $\lambda = L_p^{real}/L_p^{rand} \sim 1$ (Watts and Strogatz, 1998), where C_p^{rand} and L_p^{rand} are the mean CC and L of matched random networks that preserve the same number of nodes, edges and degree distribution as the real network (Maslov and Sneppen, 2002). In this study, we generated 1000 matched random networks for each group network.

The global efficiency E_{glob} of a weighted network G is defined as $E_{glob}(G) = \frac{1}{N(N-1)} \sum_{i \neq j \in G} \frac{1}{w_{ij}}$, where w_{ij} is the smallest connectional weight between node i and j and N is the number of nodes. It characterizes the efficiency of a system transporting information in parallel (Latora and Marchiori, 2003). The local efficiency E_{loc} of a weighted network G is defined as: $E_{loc}(G) = \frac{1}{N} \sum_{i \in G} E_{glob}(G_i)$, where G_i denotes the subgraph composed of the nearest neighbors of node i. The local efficiency represents the fault tolerance level of the network in response to the removal of a node (Latora and Marchiori, 2003).

The regional global efficiency E_{reg} of a given node i is defined as: $E_{nodal}(i) = \frac{1}{N-1} \sum_{i \neq j \in G} \frac{1}{w_{ij}}$, as it measures the average smallest path weight between given node i and all other nodes in the network. The node i was considered as a hub if its regional global efficiency was at least one standard deviation (SD) greater than the mean nodal efficiency of the whole network.

The modularity $Q(p)$ for a given partition p of a weighted brain structural network is defined as $Q(p) = \sum_{s=1}^{N_M} \left[\frac{w_s}{W} - \left(\frac{W_s}{2W} \right)^2 \right]$, where N_M is the number of modules, W is the total weight of the network, w_s is the sum of the connectional weights between all nodes in module s, and W_s is the sum of the nodal weights in module s. The modularity index quantifies the difference between the weight of intra-module links of the actual network and that of a random network in which connections are weighted at random (Newman, 2004). The aim of this module identification process is to find a specific partition p which yields the largest network modularity, $Q(p)$. Here a modified greedy optimization algorithm (Clauset et al., 2004; Danon et al., 2006) is used to find the modules of the network. The advantage of this modularity optimization method is that it takes into account the heterogeneity of module size observed in real networks (Danon et al., 2006).

We also determined the participation coefficient (PC) for each cortical region in terms of their inter-modular connection density (Guimera and Amaral, 2005; Guimera and Nunes Amaral, 2005; Sales-Pardo et al., 2007). The PC, P_i, measures the intermodular connectivity of node i, and is defined as: $P_i = 1 - \sum_{s=1}^{N_M} \left(\frac{w_{is}}{w_i} \right)^2$, where N_M is the number of modules and w_{is} is intermodular connectional weight between the node i and module s. w_i is the total weight of node i in the network. The PC of node i will be close to 0 if all weights are within its module.

Table 2 | Seventy eight cortical regions of interest defined in the study and their abbreviations (L: left hemisphere, R: right hemisphere).

Index (L, R)	Region	Abb.	Index (L, R)	Regions	Abb.
(1, 40)	Gyrus rectus	REC	(21, 60)	Precuneus	PCUN
(2, 41)	Olfactory cortex	OLF	(22, 61)	Superior occipital gyrus	SOG
(3, 42)	Superior frontal gyrus, orbital part	ORBsup	(23, 62)	Middle occipital gyrus	MOG
(4, 43)	Superior frontal gyrus, medial orbital	ORBsupmed	(24, 63)	Inferior occipital gyrus	IOG
(5, 44)	Middle frontal gyrus orbital part	ORBmid	(25, 64)	Calcarine fissure and surrounding cortex	CAL
(6, 45)	Inferior frontal gyrus, orbital part	ORBinf	(26, 65)	Cuneus	CUN
(7, 46)	Superior frontal gyrus, dorsolateral	SFGdor	(27, 66)	Lingual gyrus	LING
(8, 47)	Middle frontal gyrus	MFG	(28, 67)	Fusiform gyrus	FFG
(9, 48)	Inferior frontal gyrus, opercular part	IFGoperc	(29, 68)	Heschl gyrus	HES
(10, 49)	Inferior frontal gyrus, triangular part	IFGtriang	(30, 69)	Superior temporal gyrus	STG
(11, 50)	Superior frontal gyrus, medial	SFGmed	(31, 70)	Middle temporal gyrus	MTG
(12, 51)	Supplementary motor area	SMA	(32, 71)	Inferior temporal gyrus	ITG
(13, 52)	Paracentral lobule	PCL	(33, 72)	Temporal pole: superior temporal gyrus	TPOsup
(14, 53)	Precentral gyrus	PreCG	(34, 73)	Temporal pole: middle temporal gyrus	TPOmid
(15, 54)	Rolandic operculum	ROL	(35, 74)	Parahippocampal gyrus	PHG
(16, 55)	Postcentral gyrus	PoCG	(36, 75)	Anterior cingulate and paracingulate gyrus	ACG
(17, 56)	Superior parietal gyrus	SPG	(37, 76)	Median cingulate and paracingulate gyrus	DCG
(18, 57)	Inferior parietal, but supramarginal and angular gyri	IPL	(38, 77)	Posterior cingulate gyrus	PCG
(19, 58)	Supramarginal gyrus	SMG	(39, 78)	Insula	INS
(20, 59)	Angular gyrus	ANG			

The node i was considered as an inter-modular hub if its PC value was at least one SD greater than the mean PC of the whole network.

STATISTICAL ANALYSIS

Between-group differences analysis of all the global network metrics (S, CC, L, E_{glob}, E_{loc}, E_{reg}, Q) was performed between adjacent age groups using the General linear model (GLM) with age and gender included as covariates. The nodal properties (E_{reg}, z, P) were corrected by false discovery rate at $q = 0.05$ (Genovese et al., 2002; Zeisel et al., 2011).

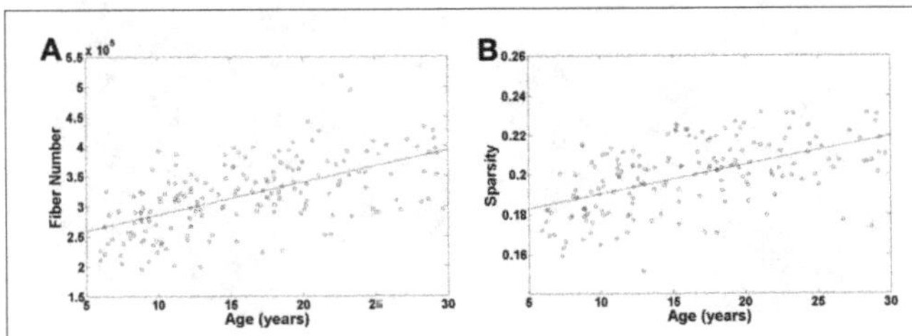

FIGURE 2 | Age-related changes in fiber number and sparsity of white matter network in all the individual subjects. Both fiber number and sparsity demonstrate increases with age.

RESULTS

AGE-RELATED CHANGES IN FIBER NUMBER AND NETWORK SPARSITY

To examine the age effect on the tractography results, we mapped age-related changes in the FN and sparsity of white matter network as shown in **Figures 2A,B**. We found that age has an incremental effect on both the FN and sparsity, where both increase by a factor of ~1.6 and ~1.2, respectively, from age 6 to 30 years. These increases are presumably due to the known elevations of FA in WM with age. Given the fact that our network edge weighting function depends on FN and FA, it is expected that the connectivity strength of the network would also increase with age.

SMALL-WORLD EFFICIENCY OF DEVELOPING WM NETWORKS

To examine the small-worldness of the WM networks for all different age groups, using a previously published method by our group (Gong et al., 2009), one weighted backbone network for each age group was generated to capture the underlying anatomical connectivity patterns as shown in **Figure 3**. Compared with their corresponding 1000 random networks, all five age groups showed strong small-worldness ($\sigma_{\text{early childhood}} = 3.54$, $\sigma_{\text{late childhood}} = 3.19$, $\sigma_{\text{adolescence}} = 3.25$, $\sigma_{\text{young adult}} = 3.12$, $\sigma_{\text{adult}} = 3.19$).

GLOBAL NETWORK PROPERTIES AND THEIR AGE-RELATED TRAJECTORIES

Over all subjects in each age group, the total network weight, CC, Lp, modularity (Q), E_{glob} and E_{loc} was calculated for the WM network and the age-related trajectories are shown in **Figure 4**. The total network weight displayed significant increases in three of the four developing stages, whereas the other metrics such as L_p, Q, E_{glob}, and E_{loc} demonstrated non-linear alteration patterns where most changes happened from young childhood to late childhood that then leveled off. Both L_p and Q decreased significantly from young childhood to late childhood but stabilized at older ages. Global network efficiency increased significantly from young childhood to late childhood but also stabilized

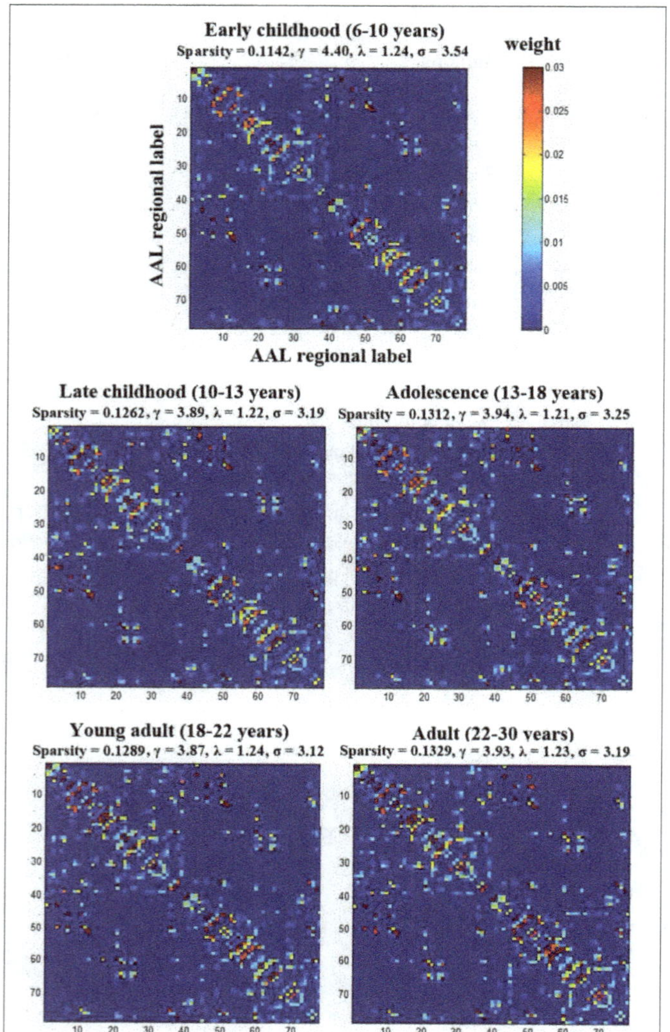

FIGURE 3 | The small-worldness of the WM networks for the five age groups. Each group was represented by one weighted backbone network to capture the underlying anatomical connectivity patterns. Compared with their corresponding random networks, all age groups showed strong small-worldness (i.e., σ >> 1). The numbers reflect the structural indices indicated in **Table 2**.

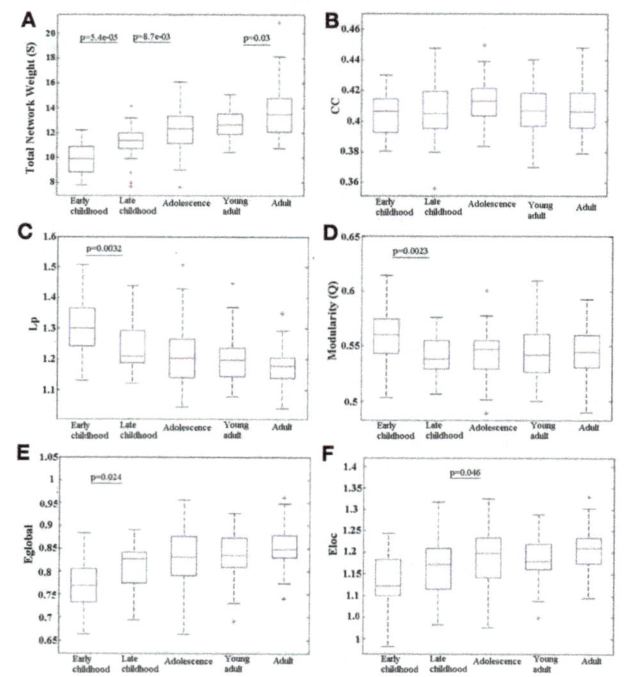

FIGURE 4 | Age-related changes in different network metrics for the developing WM network from early childhood to adult. (A) Total network strength (S), **(B)** Clustering coefficient (CC), **(C)** Shortest path length (L_p), **(D)** Modularity (Q), **(E)** Global efficiency (E_{glob}), and **(F)** Local efficiency (E_{loc}). Significant changes between any adjacent age groups are indicated by their *p* value. An increase with age is observed in S over the full age span. E_{glob} increases only between the two youngest age groups and E_{loc} only between late childhood and adolescence; in both cases, the efficiency values then stay elevated. Reductions are observed in L_p and Q from early to late childhood that is then maintained low. There is no change in CC between any adjacent age groups. The + signs indicate outliers.

later. Local network efficiency increased significantly from late childhood to adolescence and stabilized afterwards.

REGIONAL EFFICIENCY OF THE DEVELOPING WM NETWORKS

We found consistent hubs regions, measured here as the AAL areas with highest regional global efficiency, such as bilateral PCUN, SFGdor, and SFGmed, that are shared by all age groups as shown in **Figure 5**. Comparing the regional efficiency changes from group to group in these hubs, seven regions had increased nodal efficiency ($P < 0.05$, FDR corrected) from early childhood to late childhood and two regions from late childhood to adolescence (**Figure 6**). Most regional changes from early to late childhood are in the default-mode system, including bilateral PCUN and left DCG. Left STG and right INS were found to have increased efficiency from late childhood to adolescence.

MODULAR ORGANIZATION AND CONNECTOR HUBS OF THE DEVELOPING WM NETWORKS

The modular organization of the developing structural brain networks for the five different age groups is shown in **Table 3** and **Figure 7**. Six modules (1–6) were detected in all age groups indicating strong stability (Greicius et al., 2003) in the modularity of the developing brain network. Despite decreased modularity from early to late childhood, the modular structures of both groups were almost identical. Module 1 was mostly composed of bilateral orbitofrontal regions (ORBsup, ORBsupmed, ORBmid, REC) in early and late childhood that becomes more lateralized in adolescence. Right orbitofrontal regions become connected with right temporal and occipital regions that resembles the ventral visual system (Grill-Spector et al., 2008) and left orbitofrontal regions become part of lateral frontal system. Module 2 consists of mostly occipital regions (SOG, CAL, CUN) throughout the youngest age groups except at adulthood when the left occipital regions become part of left ventral visual system (Grill-Spector et al., 2008). Lateralized modules 3 (left hemisphere) and 4 (right hemisphere) consist of regions mostly across frontal, parietal and temporal lobes from each hemisphere from early to late childhood. However, module 4

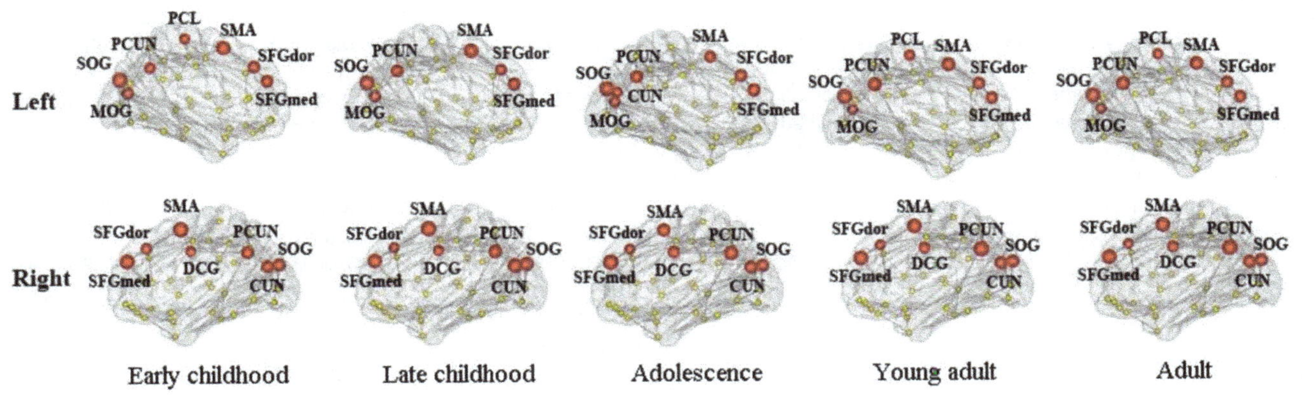

FIGURE 5 | Global hubs of the developing WM network defined by their nodal efficiency. Association hub regions such as bilateral PCUN, SFGdor, and SFGmed are consistent over all age groups. Note that all brain images are viewed from the medial side (also for **Figures 6, 7**).

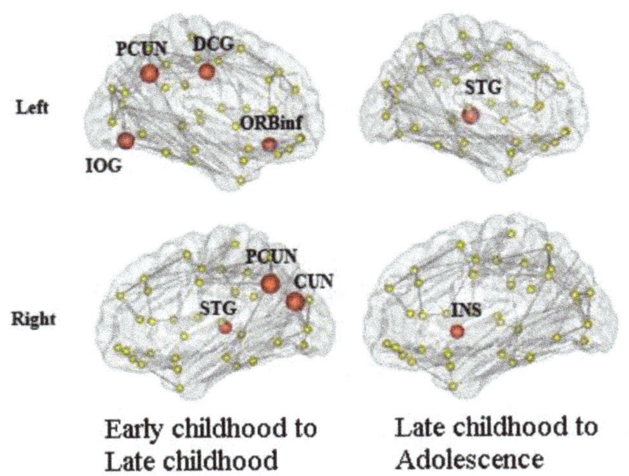

FIGURE 6 | Regions with significantly increased nodal efficiency from early childhood to late childhood and late childhood to adolescence. Seven regions had increased nodal efficiency ($P < 0.05$, FDR corrected) from early childhood to late childhood and two regions from late childhood to adolescence. Most regional changes from early to late childhood are in the default-mode system, including bilateral PCUN and left DCG. Left STG and right INS have increased efficiency from late childhood to adolescence.

is pruned to a mainly frontal-parietal system from adolescence onwards and module 3 doesn't reach a similar outcome until adulthood. Modules 5 and 6 are two of the most consistent modules during development and include mostly bilateral frontal (SFG, MFG) and posterior parietal (PCUN, DCG, SMA) regions, respectively.

The distribution of inter-modular hubs based on PC of each region for different age groups was very consistent (**Figure 8**). They were mostly located within posterior cortex, including bilateral PCUN, SPL, and MOG. Large frontal hubs such as bilateral SFGdor appeared in late childhood and remained significant afterwards.

To ensure the change of modular organization didn't result from the different sparsity of the five age groups, an additional analysis was performed where we normalized all group networks sparsity to the lowest sparsity at 0.1142 (early childhood) as weaker connections were removed from the other networks with higher sparsity (late childhood, 0.1262, adolescence, 0.1312, young adult, 0.1289, adult, 0.1329) and re-examined the modularity of the networks. We found extremely consistent modularity (0.56 previous vs. 0.56 with normalized sparsity in late childhood, 0.56 vs. 0.56 in adolescence, 0.55 vs. 0.56 in young adults, and 0.58 vs. 0.56 in adults) and modular organization compared with our original networks. Thus, we could presume that changes in the backbone network and its modular organization were not due to different matrix densities.

DISCUSSION

The present study utilized DTI tractography and network theory to characterize changes to the global structural WM network with age from early childhood to adulthood. Our main results are demonstrations of (1) a non-linear age effect on most network topological properties of brain WM network in development where most changes happen at late childhood stage (10–13 years), such as increased global network efficiency and decreased modularity, suggesting a shift of organization toward a more randomized configuration, (2) consistent hubs involving several major functional systems across all age groups and significant nodal changes only happening from early childhood to adolescence, (3) anatomically localized modules in the development of brain WM network, and (4) key connector hubs during development of the WM network.

First, using graph theoretical analysis, small-world network architecture was demonstrated in the WM networks of all age groups. During the last decade, graph theoretical analysis has been widely applied to both the functional (Stam, 2004; Bassett et al., 2006; Achard and Bullmore, 2007) and anatomical (He et al., 2007; Hagmann et al., 2008; Gong et al., 2009) brain networks and one common finding is the existence of "small-worldness" in all types of network, as defined by high CC and low characteristic path length. Recent structural brain network studies have also

Table 3 | Cortical regions in each module of developing white matter network.

Module	Early childhood	Late childhood	Adolescence	Young adult	Adult
1	ORBsupmed.L ORBsupmed.R ORBsup.L ORBmid.L ORBinf.L REC.L REC.R OLF.L OLF.R	ORBsupmed.L ORBsupmed.R REC.L REC.R OLF.L OLF.R	ORBsup.R ORBmid.R ORBinf.R TPOsup.R TPOmid.R REC.R OLF.R IOG.R FFG.R HES.R STG.R MTG.R ITG.R MOG.R PHG.R	ORBsupmed.L ORBsup.R ORBsupmed.R ORBmid.R ORBinf.R TPOsup.R TPOmid.R REC.L REC.R OLF.L OLF.R IOG.R FFG.R HES.R STG.R MTG.R ITG.R MOG.R	ORBsup.R ORBmid.R ORBinf.R TPOsup.R TPOmid.R MOG.R IOG.R FFG.R HES.R STG.R MTG.R ITG.R PHG.R REC.R OLF.R INS.R
2	SOG.L SOG.R CAL.L CAL.R CUN.L CUN.R LING.R	SOG.L SOG.R CAL.L CAL.R CUN.L CUN.R LING.R PHG.R	SOG.L CAL.L CUN.L PCG.L SOG.R CAL.R CUN.R LING.R PCG.R	SOG.L SOG.R CAL.L CAL.R CUN.L CUN.R LING.L LING.R PHG.L PHG.R	TPOmid.L SOG.L SOG.R MOG.L IOG.L CAL.L CAL.R CUN.L CUN.R LING.L LING.R FFG.L ITG.L PHG.L
3	IFGoperc.L IFGtriang.L TPOsup.L TPOmid.L PreCG.L ROL.L PoCG.L SPG.L IPL.L SMG.L ANG.L MOG.L IOG.L LING.L FFG.L HES.L STG.L MTG.L ITG.L PHG.L INS.L	ORBsup.L ORBmid.L ORBinf.L IFGoperc.L IFGtriang.L TPOsup.L TPOmid.L PreCG.L ROL.L PoCG.L SPG.L IPL.L SMG.L ANG.L MOG.L IOG.L LING.L FFG.L HES.L STG.L MTG.L ITG.L PHG.L INS.L	ORBmid.L ORBinf.L IFGoperc.L IFGtriang.L TPOsup.L TPOmid.L PreCG.L ROL.L PoCG.L SPG.L IPL.L SMG.L ANG.L MOG.L IOG.L LING.L FFG.L HES.L STG.L MTG.L ITG.L PHG.L INS.L	ORBsup.L ORBmid.L ORBinf.L IFGoperc.L TPOsup.L TPOmid.L INS.L PreCG.L ROL.L PoCG.L SPG.L IPL.L SMG.L ANG.L MOG.L IOG.L FFG.L HES.L STG.L MTG.L ITG.L	IFGoperc.L IFGtriang.L TPOsup.L PreCG.L ROL.L PoCG.L SPG.L IPL.L SMG.L ANG.L HES.L STG.L MTG.L INS.L
4	ORBsup.R ORBmid.R ORBinf.R IFGoperc.R IFGtriang.R TPOsup.R TPOmid.R PHG.R INS.R PreCG.R ROL.R PoCG.R SPG.R IPL.R SMG.R ANG.R MOG.R IOG.R FFG.R HES.R STG.R MTG.R ITG.R	ORBsup.R ORBmid.R ORBinf.R IFGoperc.R IFGtriang.R TPOsup.R TPOmid.R INS.R PreCG.R ROL.R PoCG.R SPG.R IPL.R SMG.R ANG.R MOG.R IOG.R FFG.R HES.R STG.R MTG.R ITG.R	IFGoperc.R IFGtriang.R PreCG.R PoCG.R ROL.R SPG.R IPL.R SMG.R ANG.R INS.R	SFGdor.R IFGoperc.R IFGtriang.R PreCG.R PoCG.R MFG.R ROL.R SPG.R IPL.R SMG.R ANG.R INS.R	SFGdor.R IFGoperc.R IFGtriang.R PreCG.R PoCG.R MFG.R ROL.R SPG.R IPL.R SMG.R ANG.R

(Continued)

Table 3 | Continued

Module	Early childhood	Late childhood	Adolescence	Young adult	Adult
5	SFGdor.L SFGdor.R SFGmed.L SFGmed.R ACG.L ACG.R MFG.L MFG.R	SFGdor.L SFGdor.R ORBsup.L ORBsupmed.L ORBsupmed.R SFGmed.L SFGmed.R REC.L OLF.L MFG.L MFG.R ACG.L ACG.R	SFGdor.L SFGmed.L SFGmed.R IFGtriang.L MFG.L ACG.L ACG.R	SFGdor.L SFGmed.L SFGmed.R MFG.L IFGtriang.L ACG.L ACG.R	SFGdor.L SFGmed.L SFGmed.R ORBsup.L ORBsupmed.R ORBsupmed.L ORBmid.L ORBinf.L MFG.L ACG.L ACG.R REC.L OLF.L
6	PCUN.L PCUN.R DCG.L DCG.R PCG.L PCG.R PCL.L PCL.R SMA.L SMA.R	PCUN.L PCUN.R DCG.L DCG.R PCG.L PCG.R PCL.L PCL.R SMA.L SMA.R	PCUN.L PCUN.R DCG.L DCG.R PCL.L PCL.R SMA.L SMA.R	PCL.L PCUN.L PCUN.R DCG.L DCG.R PCG.L PCG.R PCL.R SMA.L SMA.R	PCUN.L PCUN.R DCG.L DCG.R PCG.L PCG.R PCL.L PCL.R SMA.L

revealed that small-world topology and modular organization are established during early brain development (<2 years) to support rapid synchronization and information transfer with minimal rewiring cost (Fan et al., 2011; Yap et al., 2011). Thus, our results are in agreement with previous findings that the WM network maintains small-world efficiency at all stages of development.

Total network weight shows increases in three of the four developing stages, although the greatest change is between the two youngest groups pre-adolescence. Our finding is consistent with a previous WM network study that reported a significant increase in the average node strength in a group of subjects aged from 18 months to 18 years where it was suggested that increased network weight indicates increased nodal strength and greater physiological efficacy, particularly of long pathways (Hagmann et al., 2010). A functional network study has also reported increased functional integration due to a decrease of average path length during the same period and suggested it was related to increased axonal diameter and myelin thickness of long association fiber tracts (Supekar et al., 2009). We also found significant age-related decreases in the shortest path length and modularity and increase in the global efficiency of the developing WM network from early childhood to late childhood indicating greater integration among distant brain regions and a shift of topological organization to a more randomized configuration. Previous WM network (Hagmann et al., 2010) and cortical thickness network (Khundrakpam et al., 2013) studies of brain development also demonstrated a similar pattern of network metrics evolution between age 2 and 18 years and between 5 and 18 years, respectively. However, the WM network study had applied a linear fit for all the network metrics vs. age even though network metrics such as efficiency and clustering seemed to have leveled off after late childhood in their paper (Hagmann et al., 2010). Using a similar approach to ours, (Khundrakpam et al., 2013) demonstrated a leveling off of various cortical thickness network metrics after the early adolescence stage.

Consistent global hub regions, indicated by higher regional efficiency, are observed across all age groups. Hub regions are predominately association cortices that receive convergent inputs from multiple cortical regions. Regions such as SFG and PCUN have been constantly identified as the hub regions in both structural (He et al., 2007; Gong et al., 2009) and functional brain networks (Achard and Bullmore, 2007). A recent structural brain network study also identified them as the hub regions from age 2 years suggesting that they are established at a very early age (Hagmann et al., 2010). We also found that the regions with the most age-related increases in efficiency are in the default-mode system, including bilateral PCUN and left DCG. A functional brain network study has reported a less well-developed default mode network connectivity in early childhood compared with adults, especially within posterior regions such as PCUN (Fair et al., 2008). However, evidence from structural covariance network analysis has demonstrated significant pruning in the default mode system from early childhood to late childhood (Zielinski et al., 2010). Thus, we could speculate that nodal efficiency of default mode regions might plateau by late childhood.

In this study, a stable and functionally/anatomically related modular organization was demonstrated in the developing WM network. Six modules comprising regions with known functions or connections were identified in the developing WM network. Modules 1, 2, 5 and 6 were mostly composed of orbitofrontal, occipital, frontal, and posterior parietal regions that could correspond to sensory integration, visual, executive function, and default mode network, respectively, (Duncan and Owen, 2000; Raichle et al., 2001; Kringelbach, 2005). Modular network analysis has provided rich quantitative insights into the organization of complex brain networks. Studies in mammalian anatomical brain networks have revealed clusters that overlap with many known brain functions (Hilgetag et al., 2000;

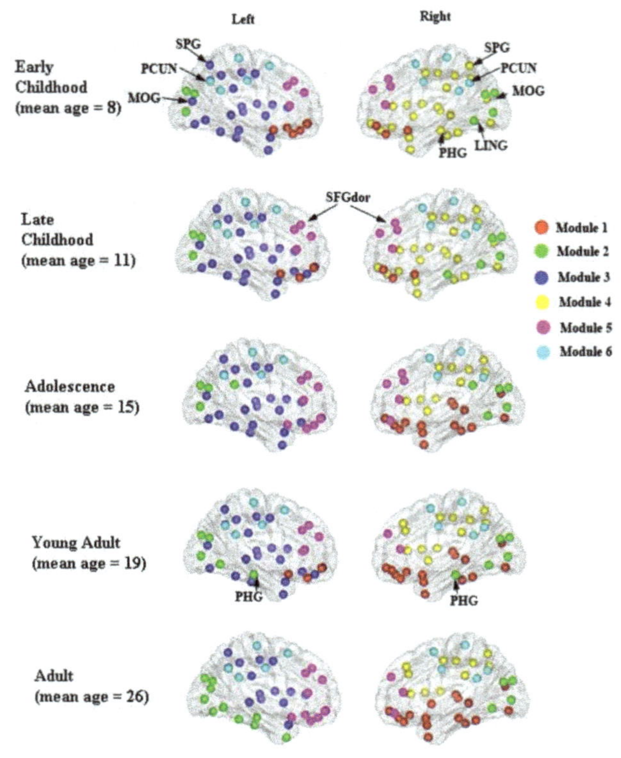

FIGURE 7 | Modular organization of the developing WM networks. Six **modules (1–6)** were detected in all age groups and are represented by red, green, purple, yellow, pink, and blue colors. See **Table 3** for a detailed list of modular regions. Module 1 was mostly composed of bilateral orbitofrontal regions (ORBsup, ORBsupmed, ORBmid, REC) in early and late childhood and becomes more lateralized from adolescence onwards. Module 2 consists of mostly occipital regions (SOG, CAL, CUN) bilaterally. Lateralized modules 3 (left hemisphere) and 4 (right hemisphere) consist of regions mostly across frontal, parietal and temporal lobes within each hemisphere. Modules 5 and 6 are two of the most consistent modules during development that include mostly bilateral frontal (SFG, MFG) and posterior parietal (PCUN, DCG, SMA) regions, respectively.

Zhou et al., 2006). Previous neuroimaging studies have also demonstrated anatomically- and functionally-related modules in the human brain structural network using diffusion spectrum imaging (Hagmann et al., 2008) and the functional network using resting-state functional MRI (Salvador et al., 2005; Ferrarini et al., 2009; He et al., 2009; Meunier et al., 2009; Valencia et al., 2009). Also, network modules identified by cortical thickness network analysis are comprised of brain regions known to subserve distinct brain functions such as executive function, vision, and default mode network (Chen et al., 2008, 2011). Two recent DTI studies also revealed non-random and dynamic modular organization of structural brain network in the first 2 years of brain development (Fan et al., 2011; Yap et al., 2011). Two lateralized modules (3 and 4) that correspond to the frontal-parietal network were also observed in the developing WM network. The adult human brain exhibits distinct hemispheric asymmetries in both structure and function. These asymmetries are thought to originate from evolutionary, developmental, hereditary, experiential, and pathological factors (Toga and Thompson, 2003). Thus, we could speculate that the lateralized network modules might result from the functional and structural hemispheric asymmetries.

Taken together, our results suggest an efficient modular organization in the WM network from early childhood and are consistent with modular behavior reported in previous structural and functional brain network studies and more importantly, a lateralized developmental pattern in some of the modules. The inter-modular hubs are the main connectors between modules and their existence in frontal and posterior cortex in the developing brain are consistent with previous WM network (Yap et al., 2011) and cortical thickness network (Khundrakpam et al., 2013) analysis. Resting state functional networks have also reported a high density of strong functional connections in posterior cortex (Achard et al., 2006). Thus, we could speculate that the inter-modular hubs uncovered in this study are well-established at childhood and are responsible for the connections between different functional systems of the developing brain.

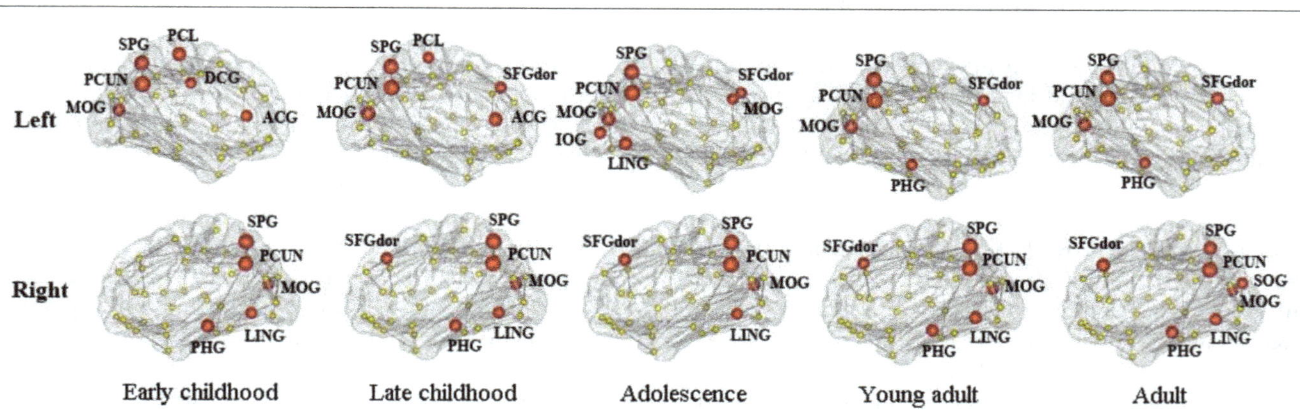

FIGURE 8 | The distribution of inter-modular hubs based on participation coefficient (PC) of each region for different age groups. They were mostly located within posterior cortex, including bilateral PCUN, SPL, and MOG. Large frontal hubs such as bilateral SFGdor appeared in late childhood and remained significant afterwards.

A few methodological issues need to be addressed. Two drawbacks of our study include the acquisition of DTI data with six diffusion directions at low *b* values of 1000 s/mm^2 and the use of deterministic tractography which will give errors in such an unsupervised tractography method given abrupt terminations at low FA crossing fiber regions or erroneous connections due to errors in the primary eigenvector direction. Multiple gradient directions can reduce the uncertainty of the primary eigenvector direction and limit potential bias as a function of tract orientation, both concerns for deterministic tractography of WM tracts (Landman et al., 2007). However, a recent study from our group has demonstrated six-direction data can also provide average diffusion measures like FA over a specific tract with comparable robustness to 30- or 60-direction data and yield appropriate parameter values for many major WM tracts (Lebel et al., 2012), which is encouraging as our edge weights were calculated based on the average FA of all voxels over the whole tract connecting two nodes. However, this does not overcome potential false positive connections or missed connections from the deterministic tractography algorithm. We attempted to minimize the former by invoking a minimum FN between regions but an incorrect connection that is consistent among the subjects within a group would still be included in the network analysis. DTI data with more than six directions also permit other advantages such as alternative analysis methods (e.g., probabilistic tractography) (Dennis et al., 2013). Higher *b* values than typically acquired are also advantageous for resolving crossing fibers and increasing the accuracy of tractography derived connections (Tournier et al., 2008). Another limitation of the study is that the age ranges of the groups covered a 3.1 to 4.7 year age range for the four youngest groups. In this study, a general linear model was applied to remove those age effects within all groups before performing the between-group comparison. In future study, smaller age ranges within groups may provide more specific indices of timing for the WM network maturation. Third, a FN threshold of 10 was applied to minimize the inclusion of random connections between two cortical regions. Currently, there are no standard approaches in determining the threshold value for the number of connecting fibers between regions as small thresholds such as 3 streamlines (Shu et al., 2011) produced networks with large sparsity with many spurious connections. Thus, our choice of higher threshold reduces, but does not eliminate, the risk of false-positive connections due to noise or the limitations in deterministic tractography. Recently, a threshold of 10 connecting streamlines or more was also applied in a brain network study (van den Heuvel et al., 2012) in which they considered that edges comprising fewer than 10 streamlines were potentially spurious and were deleted from the connection matrix. To examine the influence of the threshold, we tested a range of thresholds from 3 to 10 fibers and results including all network parameters are shown in **Table A1**. Although the network efficiency decreased as the sparsity decreased, the small worldness of the network remained intact. Most importantly, the group differences among adjacent age groups also remained consistent across all applied thresholds which indicates that the network comparison results are not sensitive to the threshold choices. Cortical regions in our study are defined by an a priori volumetric template (AAL) that was employed to automatically parcellate the entire cerebral cortex into different regions. Different templates used in various studies might cause discrepancy in the specific results, though the main trend of the network properties is expected to remain intact.

Various weighting functions for cortical-cortical connections have been applied in previous brain network analyses of brain development including 1/mean diffusivity (Hagmann et al., 2010) and proportional FN (Dennis et al., 2013), whereas we used the product of tract FA (known to increase exponentially with development over this age range but at unique rates per tract—Lebel et al., 2008) and AAL regional volume-normalized FN that has been used by others in studies of Alzheimer's Disease and aging (Lo et al., 2010; Brown et al., 2011). Other diffusion indices such as mean diffusivity (MD), axial diffusivity (AD) or radial diffusivity (RD) could have been examined instead of FA as a basis of "weighting" the network connections. However, to our best knowledge, while a few studies have applied MD as an edge weighting function (Hagmann et al., 2010; Li et al., 2012), none have used AD or RD. While changes in MD and FA for the WM typically occur together during maturation, with *MD* values decreasing and *FA* values increasing, the processes by which the two parameters change are theoretically different (Schmithorst et al., 2002; Huppi and Dubois, 2006) and they do not change at the same rate (Lebel et al., 2008). Axial and RD, under certain circumstances, may be more specific to underlying biological processes, such as myelin and axonal changes (Song et al., 2002). A recent study has demonstrated changes of FA in corticospinal tract and anterior corona radiata during development (2 to 40 years) that were attributed to the different rate changes in AD and RD (Faria et al., 2010). Thus, one would expect different WM network organization if using different weighting functions. Therefore, future studies could consider using multiple diffusion tensor measures such as FA, MD, AD and RD.

In conclusion, a graph theoretical approach was used to demonstrate age-related alterations in the large scale network properties of the developing WM network from early childhood (6 years) to adulthood (30 years). It was shown that increased network weight signifies a reshaping of the WM network from early childhood to late childhood with increased integration and decreased segregation. These findings are compatible with the notion that structural and functional brain networks become stable after late childhood. Our results also have implications for understanding how the modular organizational alterations in the large-scale structural brain networks underlie maturation of cognitive function in brain development. This study may pave the way for developing novel methods for analyzing disrupted brain connectivity in neurodevelopmental disorders.

ACKNOWLEDGMENTS

Operating funding from the Canadian Institutes of Health Research, and salary awards from the China Scholarship Council (Min Liu) and Alberta Innovates—Health Solutions (Christian Beaulieu).

REFERENCES

Achard, S., and Bullmore, E. (2007). Efficiency and cost of economical brain functional networks. *PLoS Comput. Biol.* 3:e17. doi: 10.1371/journal.pcbi.0030017

Achard, S., Salvador, R., Whitcher, B., Suckling, J., and Bullmore, E. (2006). A resilient, low-frequency, small-world human brain functional network with highly connected association cortical hubs. *J. Neurosci.* 26, 63–72. doi: 10.1523/JNEUROSCI.3874-05.2006

Basser, P. J., Pajevic, S., Pierpaoli, C., Duda, J., and Aldroubi, A. (2000). *In vivo* fiber tractography using DT-MRI data. *Magn. Reson. Med.* 44, 625–632. doi: 10.1002/1522-2594(200010)44:4<625::AID-MRM17>3.0.CO;2-O

Bassett, D. S., Meyer-Lindenberg, A., Achard, S., Duke, T., and Bullmore, E. (2006). Adaptive reconfiguration of fractal small-world human brain functional networks. *Proc. Natl. Acad. Sci. U.S.A.* 103, 19518–19523. doi: 10.1073/pnas.0606005103

Brown, J. A., Terashima, K. H., Burggren, A. C., Ercoli, L. M., Miller, K. J., Small, G. W., et al. (2011). Brain network local interconnectivity loss in aging APOE-4 allele carriers. *Proc. Natl. Acad. Sci. U.S.A.* 108, 20760–20765. doi: 10.1073/pnas.1109038108

Bullmore, E., and Sporns, O. (2009). Complex brain networks: graph theoretical analysis of structural and functional systems. *Nat. Rev.* 10, 186–198. doi: 10.1038/nrn2575

Chen, Z. J., He, Y., Rosa-Neto, P., Germann, J., and Evans, A. C. (2008). Revealing modular architecture of human brain structural networks by using cortical thickness from MRI. *Cereb. Cortex* 18, 2374–2381. doi: 10.1093/cercor/bhn003

Chen, Z. J., He, Y., Rosa-Neto, P., Gong, G., and Evans, A. C. (2011). Age-related alterations in the modular organization of structural cortical network by using cortical thickness from MRI. *Neuroimage* 56, 235–245. doi: 10.1016/j.neuroimage.2011.01.010

Clauset, A., Newman, M. E., and Moore, C. (2004). Finding community structure in very large networks. *Phys. Rev. E* 70, 066111. doi: 10.1103/PhysRevE.70.066111

Danon, L., Diaz-Guilera, A., and Arenas, A. (2006). The effect of size heterogeneity on community identification in complex networks. *J. Stat. Mech. Theory Exp.* P11010. doi: 10.1088/1742-5468/2006/11/P11010

Dennis, E. L., Jahanshad, N., McMahon, K. L., de Zubicaray, G. I., Martin, N. G., Hickie, I. B., et al. (2013). Development of brain structural connectivity between ages 12 and 30: a 4-Tesla diffusion imaging study in 439 adolescents and adults. *Neuroimage* 64, 671–684. doi: 10.1016/j.neuroimage.2012.09.004

Duncan, J., and Owen, A., M. (2000). Common regions of the human frontal lobe recruited by diverse cognitive demands. *Trends Neurosci.* 23, 475–483. doi: 10.1016/S0166-2236(00)01633-7

Fair, D. A., Cohen, A. L., Dosenbach, N. U., Church, J. A., Miezin, F. M., Barch, D. M., et al. (2008). The maturing architecture of the brain's default network. *Proc. Natl. Acad. Sci. U.S.A.* 105, 4028–4032. doi: 10.1073/pnas.0800376105

Fair, D. A., Cohen, A. L., Power, J. D., Dosenbach, N. U., Church, J. A., Miezin, F. M., et al. (2009). Functional brain networks develop from a "local to distributed" organization. *PLoS Comput. Biol.* 5:e1000381. doi: 10.1371/journal.pcbi.1000381

Fan, Y., Shi, F., Smith, J. K., Lin, W., Gilmore, J. H., and Shen, D. (2011). Brain anatomical networks in early human brain development. *Neuroimage* 54, 1862–1871. doi: 10.1016/j.neuroimage.2010.07.025

Faria, A. V., Zhang, J., Oishi, K., Li, X., Jiang, H., Akhter, K., et al. (2010). Atlas-based analysis of neurodevelopment from infancy to adulthood using diffusion tensor imaging and applications for automated abnormality detection. *Neuroimage* 52, 415–428. doi: 10.1016/j.neuroimage.2010.04.238

Ferrarini, L., Veer, I. M., Baerends, E., van Tol, M. J., Renken, R. J., van der Wee, N. J., et al. (2009). Hierarchical functional modularity in the resting-state human brain. *Hum. Brain Mapp.* 30, 2220–2231. doi: 10.1002/hbm.20663

Genovese, C. R., Lazar, N. A., and Nichols, T. (2002). Thresholding of statistical maps in functional neuroimaging using the false discovery rate. *Neuroimage* 15, 870–878. doi: 10.1006/nimg.2001.1037

Giedd, J. N., Blumenthal, J., Jeffries, N. O., Castellanos, F. X., Liu, H., Zijdenbos, A., et al. (1999). Brain development during childhood and adolescence: a longitudinal MRI study. *Nat. Neurosci.* 2, 861–863. doi: 10.1038/13158

Giorgio, A., Watkins, K. E., Douaud, G., James, A. C., James, S., De Stefano, N., et al. (2008). Changes in white matter microstructure during adolescence. *Neuroimage* 39, 52–61. doi: 10.1016/j.neuroimage.2007.07.043

Gogtay, N., Giedd, J. N., Lusk, L., Hayashi, K. M., Greenstein, D., Vaituzis, A. C., et al. (2004). Dynamic mapping of human cortical development during childhood through early adulthood. *Proc. Natl. Acad. Sci. U.S.A.* 101, 8174–8179. doi: 10.1073/pnas.0402680101

Gong, G., He, Y., Concha, L., Lebel, C., Gross, D. W., Evans, A. C., et al. (2009). Mapping anatomical connectivity patterns of human cerebral cortex using *in vivo* diffusion tensor imaging tractography. *Cereb. Cortex* 19, 524–536. doi: 10.1093/cercor/bhn102

Good, C. D., Johnsrude, I. S., Ashburner, J., Henson, R. N., Friston, K. J., and Frackowiak, R. S. (2001). A voxel-based morphometric study of ageing in 465 normal adult human brains. *Neuroimage* 14, 21–36. doi: 10.1006/nimg.2001.0786

Greicius, M. D., Krasnow, B., Reiss, A. L., and Menon, V. (2003). Functional connectivity in the resting brain: a network analysis of the default mode hypothesis. *Proc. Natl. Acad. Sci. U.S.A.* 100, 253–258. doi: 10.1073/pnas.0135058100

Grill-Spector, K., Golarai, G., and Gabrieli, J. (2008). Developmental neuroimaging of the human ventral visual cortex. *Trends Cogn. Sci.* 12, 152–162. doi: 10.1016/j.tics.2008.01.009

Guimera, R., and Amaral, L. A. (2005). Cartography of complex networks: modules and universal roles. *J. Stat. Mech.* 2005, nihpa35573. doi: 10.1088/1742-5468/2005/02/P02001

Guimera, R., and Nunes Amaral, L. A. (2005). Functional cartography of complex metabolic networks. *Nature* 433, 895–900. doi: 10.1038/nature03288

Hagmann, P., Cammoun, L., Gigandet, X., Meuli, R., Honey, C. J., Wedeen, V. J., et al. (2008). Mapping the structural core of human cerebral cortex. *PLoS Biol.* 6:e159. doi: 10.1371/journal.pbio.0060159

Hagmann, P., Sporns, O., Madan, N., Cammoun, L., Pienaar, R., Wedeen, V. J., et al. (2010). White matter maturation reshapes structural connectivity in the late developing human brain. *Proc. Natl. Acad. Sci. U.S.A.* 107, 19067–19072. doi: 10.1073/pnas.1009073107

He, Y., Chen, Z. J., and Evans, A. C. (2007). Small-world anatomical networks in the human brain revealed by cortical thickness from MRI. *Cereb. Cortex* 17, 2407–2419. doi: 10.1093/cercor/bhl149

He, Y., and Evans, A. (2010). Graph theoretical modeling of brain connectivity. *Curr. Opin. Neurol.* 23, 341–350. doi: 10.1097/WCO.0b013e32833aa567

He, Y., Wang, J., Wang, L., Chen, Z. J., Yan, C., Yang, H., et al. (2009). Uncovering intrinsic modular organization of spontaneous brain activity in humans. *PLoS ONE* 4:e5226. doi: 10.1371/journal.pone.0005226

Hilgetag, C. C., O'Neill, M. A., and Young, M. P. (2000). Hierarchical organization of macaque and cat cortical sensory systems explored with a novel network processor. *Philos. Trans. R. Soc. Lond. B* 355, 71–89. doi: 10.1098/rstb.2000.0550

Huppi, P. S., and Dubois, J. (2006). Diffusion tensor imaging of brain development. *Semin. Fetal Neonatal Med.* 11, 489–497. doi: 10.1016/j.siny.2006.07.006

Khundrakpam, B. S., Reid, A., Brauer, J., Carbonell, F., Lewis, J., Ameis, S., et al. (2013). Developmental changes in organization of structural brain networks. *Cereb. Cortex* 23, 2072–2085. doi: 10.1093/cercor/bhs187

Kringelbach, M. L. (2005). The human orbitofrontal cortex: linking reward to hedonic experience. *Nat. Rev.* 6, 691–702. doi: 10.1038/nrn1747

Landman, B. A., Farrell, J. A., Jones, C. K., Smith, S. A., Prince, J. L., and Mori, S. (2007). Effects of diffusion weighting schemes on the reproducibility of DTI-derived fractional anisotropy, mean diffusivity, and principal eigenvector measurements at 1.5T. *NeuroImage* 36, 1123–1138. doi: 10.1016/j.neuroimage.2007.02.056

Latora, V., and Marchiori, M. (2001). Efficient behavior of small-world networks. *Phys. Rev. Lett.* 87, 198701. doi: 10.1103/PhysRevLett.87.198701

Latora, V., and Marchiori, M. (2003). Economic small-world behavior in weighted networks. *Eur. Phys. J. B* 32, 249–263. doi: 10.1140/epjb/e2003-00095-5

Lebel, C., and Beaulieu, C. (2011). Longitudinal development of human brain wiring continues from childhood into adulthood. *J. Neurosci.* 31, 10937–10947. doi: 10.1523/JNEUROSCI.5302-10.2011

Lebel, C., Walker, L., Leemans, A., Phillips, L., and Beaulieu, C. (2008). Microstructural maturation of the human brain from childhood to adulthood. *Neuroimage* 40, 1044–1055. doi: 10.1016/j.neuroimage.2007.12.053

Lebel, C., Benner, T., and Beaulieu, C. (2012). Six is enough? Comparison of diffusion parameters measured using six or more diffusion-encoding gradient directions with deterministic tractography. *Magn Reson Med* 68, 474–483. doi: 10.1002/mrm.23254

Li, Y., Jewells, V., Kim, M., Chen, Y., Moon, A., Armao, D., et al. (2012). Diffusion tensor imaging based network analysis detects alterations of neuroconnectivity in patients with clinically early relapsing-remitting multiple sclerosis. *Hum. Brain Mapp.* doi: 10.1002/hbm.22158. [Epub ahead of print].

Lo, C. Y., Wang, P. N., Chou, K. H., Wang, J., He, Y., and Lin, C. P. (2010). Diffusion tensor tractography reveals abnormal topological organization in structural cortical networks in Alzheimer's disease. *J. Neurosci.* 30, 16876–16885. doi: 10.1523/JNEUROSCI.4136-10.2010

Maslov, S., and Sneppen, K. (2002). Specificity and stability in topology of protein networks. *Science* 296, 910–913. doi: 10.1126/science.1065103

Meunier, D., Achard, S., Morcom, A., and Bullmore, E. (2009). Age-related changes in modular organization of human brain functional networks. *Neuroimage* 44, 715–723. doi: 10.1016/j.neuroimage.2008.09.062

Newman, M. E. (2003). The structure and function of Complex Networks. *SIAM Rev.* 45, 167–256. doi: 10.1137/S0036 14450342480

Newman, M. E. (2004). Analysis of weighted networks. *Phys. Rev. E* 70, 056131. doi: 10.1103/PhysRevE.70.056131

Newman, M. E. (2006). Modularity and community structure in networks. *Proc. Natl. Acad. Sci. U.S.A.* 103, 8577–8582. doi: 10.1073/pnas.0601602103

Onnela, J. P., Saramaki, J., Kertesz, J., and Kaski, K. (2005). Intensity and coherence of motifs in weighted complex networks. *Phys. Rev.* 71, 065103. doi: 10.1103/PhysRevE.71.065103

Paus, T., Zijdenbos, A., Worsley, K., Collins, D. L., Blumenthal, J., Giedd, J. N., et al. (1999). Structural maturation of neural pathways in children and adolescents: *in vivo* study. *Science* 283, 1908–1911. doi: 10.1126/science.283.5409.1908

Raichle, M. E., MacLeod, A. M., Snyder, A. Z., Powers, W. J., Gusnard, D. A., and Shulman, G. L. (2001). A default mode of brain function. *Proc. Natl. Acad. Sci. U.S.A.* 98, 676–682. doi: 10.1073/pnas.98.2.676

Sales-Pardo, M., Guimera, R., Moreira, A. A., and Amaral, L. A. (2007). Extracting the hierarchical organization of complex systems. *Proc. Natl. Acad. Sci. U.S.A.* 104, 15224–15229. doi: 10.1073/pnas.0703740104

Salvador, R., Suckling, J., Coleman, M. R., Pickard, J. D., Menon, D., and Bullmore, E. (2005). Neurophysiological architecture of functional magnetic resonance images of human brain. *Cereb. Cortex* 15, 1332–1342. doi: 10.1093/cercor/bhi016

Schmithorst, V. J., Wilke, M., Dardzinski, B. J., and Holland, S. K. (2002). Correlation of white matter diffusivity and anisotropy with age during childhood and adolescence: a cross-sectional diffusion-tensor MR imaging study. *Radiology* 222, 212–218. doi: 10.1148/radiol.2221010626

Shaw, P., Kabani, N. J., Lerch, J. P., Eckstrand, K., Lenroot, R., Gogtay, N., et al. (2008). Neurodevelopmental trajectories of the human cerebral cortex. *J. Neurosci.* 28, 3586–3594. doi: 10.1523/JNEUROSCI.5309-07.2008

Shu, N., Liu, Y., Li, K., Duan, Y., Wang, J., Yu, C., et al. (2011). Diffusion tensor tractography reveals disrupted topological efficiency in white matter structural networks in multiple sclerosis. *Cereb. Cortex* 21, 2565–2577. doi: 10.1093/cercor/bhr039

Snook, L., Paulson, L. A., Roy, D., Phillips, L., and Beaulieu, C. (2005). Diffusion tensor imaging of neurodevelopment in children and young adults. *Neuroimage* 26, 1164–1173. doi: 10.1016/j.neuroimage.2005.03.016

Song, S. K., Sun, S. W., Ramsbottom, M. J., Chang, C., Russell, J., and Cross, A. H. (2002). Dysmyelination revealed through MRI as increased radial (but unchanged axial) diffusion of water. *Neuroimage* 17, 1429–1436. doi: 10.1006/nimg.2002.1267

Sowell, E. R., Thompson, P. M., Leonard, C. M., Welcome, S. E., Kan, E., and Toga, A. W. (2004). Longitudinal mapping of cortical thickness and brain growth in normal children. *J. Neurosci.* 24, 8223–8231. doi: 10.1523/JNEUROSCI.1798-04.2004

Stam, C. J. (2004). Functional connectivity patterns of human magnetoencephalographic recordings: a 'small-world' network. *Neurosci. Lett.* 355, 25–28. doi: 10.1016/j.neulet.2003.10.063

Strogatz, S. H. (2001). Exploring complex networks. *Nature* 410, 268–276. doi: 10.1038/35065725

Supekar, K., Musen, M., and Menon, V. (2009). Development of large-scale functional brain networks in children. *PLoS Biol.* 7:e100 0157. doi: 10.1371/journal.pbio.1000157

Tamnes, C. K., Ostby, Y., Fjell, A. M., Westlye, L. T., Due-Tonnessen, P., and Walhovd, K. B. (2010). Brain maturation in adolescence and young adulthood: regional age-related changes in cortical thickness and white matter volume and microstructure. *Cereb. Cortex* 20, 534–548. doi: 10.1093/cercor/bhp118

Thompson, P. M., Giedd, J. N., Woods, R. P., MacDonald, D., Evans, A. C., and Toga, A. W. (2000). Growth patterns in the developing brain detected by using continuum mechanical tensor maps. *Nature* 404, 190–193. doi: 10.1038/35004593

Toga, A. W., and Thompson, P. M. (2003). Mapping brain asymmetry. *Nat. Rev.* 4, 37–48. doi: 10.1038/nrn1009

Tournier, J. D., Yeh, C. H., Calamante, F., Cho, K. H., Connelly, A., and Lin, C. P. (2008). Resolving crossing fibres using constrained spherical deconvolution: validation using diffusion-weighted imaging phantom data. *Neuroimage* 42, 617–625. doi: 10.1016/j.neuro image.2008.05.002

Tzourio-Mazoyer, N., Landeau, B., Papathanassiou, D., Crivello, F., Etard, O., Delcroix, N., et al. (2002). Automated anatomical labeling of activations in SPM using a macroscopic anatomical parcellation of the MNI MRI single-subject brain. *Neuroimage* 15, 273–289. doi: 10.1006/nimg.2001.0978

Valencia, M., Pastor, M. A., Fernandez-Seara, M. A., Artieda, J., Martinerie, J., and Chavez, M. (2009). Complex modular structure of large-scale brain networks. *Chaos* 19, 023119. doi: 10.1063/1.3129783

van den Heuvel, M. P., Kahn, R. S., Goni, J., and Sporns, O. (2012). High-cost, high-capacity backbone for global brain communication. *Proc. Natl. Acad. Sci. U.S.A.* 109, 11372–11377. doi: 10.1073/pnas.1203593109

Vogel, A. C., Power, J. D., Petersen, S. E., and Schlaggar, B. L. (2010). Development of the brain's functional network architecture. *Neuropsychol. Rev.* 20, 362–375. doi: 10.1007/s11065-010-9145-7

Watts, D. J., Strogatz, S. H. (1998). Collective dynamics of 'small-world' networks. *Nature* 393, 440–442. doi: 10.1038/30918

Wu, K., Taki, Y., Sato, K., Hashizume, H., Sassa, Y., Takeuchi, H., et al. (2013). Topological organization of functional brain networks in healthy children: differences in relation to age, sex, and intelligence. *PLoS ONE* 8:e55347. doi: 10.1371/journal.pone.0055347

Yap, P. T., Fan, Y., Chen, Y., Gilmore, J. H., Lin, W., and Shen, D. (2011). Development trends of white matter connectivity in the first years of life. *PLoS ONE* 6:e24678. doi: 10.1371/journal.pone.0024678

Zeisel, A., Zuk, O., and Domany, E. (2011). Fdr control with adaptive procedures and fdr monotonicity. *Ann. Appl. Stat.* 5, 943–968. doi: 10.1214/10-AOAS399

Zhou, C., Zemanova, L., Zamora, G., Hilgetag, C. C., and Kurths, J. (2006). Hierarchical organization unveiled by functional connectivity in complex brain networks. *Phys. Rev. Lett.* 97, 238103. doi: 10.1103/PhysRevLett.97.238103

Zielinski, B. A., Gennatas, E. D., Zhou, J., and Seeley, W. W. (2010). Network-level structural covariance in the developing brain. *Proc. Natl. Acad. Sci. U.S.A.* 107, 18191–18196. doi: 10.1073/pnas.1003109107

APPENDIX

Table A1 | White matter network parameters derived from different fiber-number node-to-node connection thresholds in all age groups.

FN threshold	Groups	Eglob	Eloc	*Q*	σ
3	Early childhood	0.93 ± 0.07	1.32 ± 0.07	0.55 ± 0.03	3.15
	Late childhood	0.98 ± 0.07	1.35 ± 0.08	0.54 ± 0.02	3.02
	Adolescence	1.02 ± 0.09	1.38 ± 0.09	0.54 ± 0.02	2.92
	Young adult	1.02 ± 0.07	1.37 ± 0.06	0.54 ± 0.02	2.76
	Adult	1.03 ± 0.07	1.39 ± 0.06	0.54 ± 0.02	2.90
4	Early childhood	0.89 ± 0.07	1.27 ± 0.06	0.56 ± 0.02	3.22
	Late childhood	0.94 ± 0.07	1.30 ± 0.07	0.54 ± 0.02	3.02
	Adolescence	0.97 ± 0.08	1.33 ± 0.08	0.54 ± 0.02	2.95
	Young adult	0.97 ± 0.06	1.33 ± 0.06	0.54 ± 0.02	2.82
	Adult	0.99 ± 0.06	1.36 ± 0.06	0.54 ± 0.02	2.96
5	Early childhood	0.86 ± 0.07	1.25 ± 0.06	0.55 ± 0.02	3.29
	Late childhood	0.91 ± 0.07	1.27 ± 0.07	0.54 ± 0.02	3.09
	Adolescence	0.94 ± 0.08	1.30 ± 0.08	0.54 ± 0.02	3.06
	Young adult	0.94 ± 0.06	1.30 ± 0.05	0.54 ± 0.02	2.95
	Adult	0.96 ± 0.06	1.31 ± 0.06	0.54 ± 0.02	3.01
6	Early childhood	0.84 ± 0.07	1.22 ± 0.06	0.55 ± 0.03	3.33
	Late childhood	0.88 ± 0.06	1.24 ± 0.07	0.54 ± 0.02	3.08
	Adolescence	0.91 ± 0.08	1.27 ± 0.08	0.54 ± 0.02	3.10
	Young adult	0.91 ± 0.06	1.27 ± 0.05	0.54 ± 0.03	3.00
	Adult	0.93 ± 0.06	1.29 ± 0.05	0.54 ± 0.02	3.04
7	Early childhood	0.82 ± 0.07	1.19 ± 0.07	0.56 ± 0.03	3.37
	Late childhood	0.86 ± 0.06	1.22 ± 0.07	0.54 ± 0.02	3.01
	Adolescence	0.89 ± 0.08	1.25 ± 0.08	0.54 ± 0.02	3.18
	Young adult	0.89 ± 0.06	1.25 ± 0.05	0.54 ± 0.02	3.01
	Adult	0.90 ± 0.05	1.26 ± 0.05	0.54 ± 0.02	3.08
8	Early childhood	0.80 ± 0.06	1.17 ± 0.07	0.56 ± 0.03	3.40
	Late childhood	0.84 ± 0.06	1.20 ± 0.06	0.54 ± 0.02	3.14
	Adolescence	0.87 ± 0.07	1.23 ± 0.07	0.54 ± 0.02	3.23
	Young adult	0.87 ± 0.06	1.22 ± 0.05	0.54 ± 0.02	3.06
	Adult	0.89 ± 0.05	1.24 ± 0.05	0.54 ± 0.02	3.12
9	Early childhood	0.78 ± 0.06	1.15 ± 0.06	0.56 ± 0.02	3.48
	Late childhood	0.82 ± 0.05	1.18 ± 0.06	0.54 ± 0.02	3.21
	Adolescence	0.85 ± 0.07	1.21 ± 0.07	0.54 ± 0.02	3.25
	Young adult	0.85 ± 0.05	1.20 ± 0.05	0.54 ± 0.02	3.09
	Adult	0.87 ± 0.05	1.22 ± 0.05	0.54 ± 0.02	3.14
10	Early childhood	0.77 ± 0.06	1.13 ± 0.06	0.56 ± 0.03	3.54
	Late childhood	0.81 ± 0.05	1.16 ± 0.06	0.54 ± 0.02	3.12
	Adolescence	0.83 ± 0.07	1.19 ± 0.07	0.54 ± 0.02	3.25
	Young adult	0.84 ± 0.05	1.19 ± 0.05	0.54 ± 0.02	3.12
	Adult	0.85 ± 0.05	1.21 ± 0.05	0.54 ± 0.02	3.19

Adjacent groups show significant differences or trend in network properties are highlighted in shaded cells. FN: fiber number, Eglob: global efficiency, Eloc: local efficiency, Q: modularity, σ: small worldness.

8

A systematic investigation of the invariance of resting-state network patterns: Is resting-state fMRI ready for pre-surgical planning?

K. Kollndorfer[1], F. Ph. S. Fischmeister[2], G. Kasprian[1], D. Prayer[1] and V. Schöpf[1]*

[1] *Department of Radiology, Division of Neuro- and Musculoskeletal Radiology, Medical University of Vienna, Vienna, Austria*
[2] *Department of Neurology, Study Group Clinical fMRI, Medical University of Vienna, Vienna, Austria*

Correspondence:
V. Schöpf, Department of Radiology, Division of Neuro- and Musculoskeletal Radiology, Medical University of Vienna, Waehringer Guertel 18-20, 1090 Vienna, Austria.
e-mail: veronika.schoepf@meduniwien.ac.at

Objectives: Measurements of resting-state networks (RSNs) have been used to investigate a wide range of diseases, such as dementia or epilepsy. This raises the question whether this method could also serve as a pre-surgical planning tool. Generating reliable functional connectivity patterns is of crucial importance, particularly for pre-surgical planning, as these patterns may directly affect the outcome.

Methods: This study investigated the reproducibility of four commonly used resting-state conditions: fixation of a black crosshair on a white screen; fixation of the center of a black screen; eyes-closed and fixation of the words "Entspann dich!" (Engl., "relax"). Ten healthy, right-handed male subjects (mean age, 25 years; SD 2) participated in the experiment. The spatial overlap for different RSNs across the four conditions was calculated.

Results: The spatial overlap across all four conditions was calculated for each seed region on a single subject and at the group level. Activation maps at the single-subject and group levels were highly stable, especially for the reading network (RNW). The lowest consistency measures were found for the visual network (VIN). At the single-subject level spatial overlap values ranged from 0.31 (VIN) to 0.45 (RNW).

Conclusion: These findings suggest that RSN measurements are a reliable tool to assess language-related networks in clinical settings. Generally, resting-state conditions showed comparable activation patterns, therefore no specific conditions appears to be preferable.

Keywords: functional connectivity, resting-state network (RSN), resting-state, fMRI, default mode network, reproducibility

INTRODUCTION

The possibility of performing functional magnetic resonance imaging (fMRI) without stimulation, as an easy way to obtain insight into the spatiotemporal distribution of resting-state networks (RSNs), has revolutionized neuroscience research. It has been demonstrated that RSNs are organized as specific functional networks across the brain, demonstrating characteristic spatial and temporal changes independent of condition (sleep, task performance, rest, anesthesia) or age (fetuses, preterms, infants, adults) (see, e.g., Schöpf et al., 2012a,b). In particular, in patient groups that show a lack of task cooperation, as, for example, in patients with neurodegenerative or neuropsychiatric diseases (Auer, 2008), resting-state fMRI has become quite popular as a method by which to gain new insights into these diseases (Fox and Greicius, 2010). RSNs are typically characterized by spontaneous low-frequency fluctuations (<0.1 Hz) and are observed throughout the whole brain.

In several previous studies, state-dependent differences were observed in the functional connectivity of resting-state networks (fcRSN) (Fransson, 2006; Newton et al., 2007; Bianciardi et al., 2009; Yan et al., 2009; Van Dijk et al., 2010). Some of these studies (Yan et al., 2009; Van Dijk et al., 2010) compared the differences between frequently presented resting-state conditions: eyes-open with fixation; eyes-open without fixation; and eyes-closed. Independent of the resting-state condition, subjects or patients are usually instructed to relax, not to think of anything in particular, and not to fall asleep during the scanning session. These studies have shown that the eyes-open conditions evoked higher functional connectivity of the default mode network (DMN) than the eyes-closed condition. Apart from lower-vigilance states, such as mind wandering, day dreaming, or musing about the recent past (Mason et al., 2007; Buckner et al., 2008), the DMN is associated with monitoring the functions of sensory input (Gilbert et al., 2007; Hahn et al., 2007). Therefore, activities within the DMN seem to be attenuated when the eyes are closed. However, Fox et al. (2005) found no differences in the DMN between resting-state conditions for the eyes-closed condition, the eyes-open without fixation in low-level illumination condition, and the eyes-open condition with fixation of a crosshair.

A recently published study on the interpretation of deactivations in neuroimaging studies (Hayes and Huxtable, 2012) suggested resting-state fMRI measurements before and after task- or stimulus-related fMRI experiments would enable better interpretation of activity in the task itself. In this context, the stability of RSN patterns, independent of the resting-state condition, is of major importance.

The variations in the results of fcRSN measurements raise questions concerning the reproducibility, accuracy, and specificity of resting-state fMRI not only for basic neuroscience research. Resting-state connectivity measures are also proposed as a promising practical tool in a wide range of clinical applications, especially for pre-surgical planning (e.g., epilepsy) (see, e.g., Lui et al., 2008; Bettus et al., 2009). Hence, generating reliable functional connectivity measurements is of particular importance. The reproducibility of functional connectivity measurements within one subject and across subjects has been discussed critically. A recent study (Chou et al., 2012) obtained high reproducibility within one subject, but substantial variation in fcRSNs between subjects. However, other investigations found a high degree of reproducibility for functional connectivity in the DMN (Meindl et al., 2010) and in the motor network (Amann et al., 2009) across subjects, as well as a significant correspondence between different statistical methods (Rosazza et al., 2012). In most clinical resting-state studies, factors like differences in disease duration, incidence of precipitating factors, cognitive dysfunction, and surgical outcome, are considered, but the rest-task itself and how patients were instructed to perform in the resting-state has been given less attention.

In this study, we investigated the reproducibility of RSNs in a homogenous group of 10 healthy subjects, who underwent four different resting-state sessions, while factors that could potentially influence reproducibility were held constant. These four resting-state conditions have been commonly used in previous studies: (1) crosshair (rest_cross): participants had to fixate on a black crosshair on a white screen; (2) black screen (rest_black): subjects were instructed to focus on the center of a black screen; (3) eyes-closed (rest_eyes_closed): participants had to rest with their eyes-closed; and finally (4) subjects were asked to fixate on the presented words "Entspann dich!" (Engl., "relax") written in black letters on a white screen (rest_relax).

The prospective use of resting-state fMRI measures in a clinical set-up for the purpose of enabling pre-surgical planning, it is of crucial importance that the designs generate a stable and reliable signal. As fMRI reproducibility characteristics can be strongly dependent on the chosen paradigm designs (Bennett and Miller, 2010), it is important to formally examine reproducibility measures for specific conditions. Therefore, we analyzed differences in functional connectivity patterns induced by the four resting-state conditions (1–4) in distinct networks: the DMN; the visual network (VIN); the sensorimotor network (SMN); the reading network (RNW); and the auditory network (AUD).

MATERIALS AND METHODS

SUBJECTS

Ten healthy, right-handed male subjects (mean age, 25 years; SD 2) were included in the study. All participants had normal or corrected-to-normal vision. All subjects were informed about the aim of the study and gave their written, informed consent prior to inclusion. The study was approved by the Ethics Committee of the Medical University of Vienna. Measurements were performed at approximately the same time of the day, between 5:00 and 9:00 p.m.

IMAGING METHODS

Measurements were performed on a 3 Tesla TIM Trio system (Siemens Medical Solution, Erlangen, Germany) using single-shot gradient-recalled echo-planar imaging (EPI). Twenty slices (1 mm gap, 4 mm thickness) with an FOV of 210 × 210 mm and TE/TR 42/2000 ms were acquired. Slices were aligned with the connection line between the anterior and posterior commissure. Each subject underwent four resting-state conditions, each lasting for 5 min. The light in the scanning room was turned off throughout the whole measurement period.

RESTING-STATE CONDITIONS

Across all four conditions, participants were instructed not to think of anything in particular and not to fall asleep.

(1) Rest_cross: subjects were visually presented with a black crosshair on a white background image using an MR-compatible visual stimulation system (NordicNeuroLab, Bergen, NO) and were instructed to focus on the crosshair at all times.
(2) Rest_black: subjects were visually presented with a blank, black screen and instructed to focus on the center.
(3) Rest_closed: subjects were instructed to keep their eyes-closed during the whole run and visual presentation was turned off.
(4) Rest_relax: subjects were visually presented with the words "Entspann dich!" (Engl., "relax") in black letters centered on a white screen and instructed to focus on the words.

Eye movement and fixation of the target were monitored using an MR-compatible eye tracker (ViewPoint EyeTracker, Arrington Research, Scottsdale, AZ) at all times. The order of the runs was identical for all subjects.

DATA ANALYSIS

Image preprocessing for all four runs was performed separately with SPM8 (http://www.fil.ion.ucl.ac.uk/spm/), including slice-timing and motion correction, normalization to an MNI template, and smoothing. Correlation maps were generated by computing the cross-correlation coefficient on a single-voxel basis for different regions of interest (ROIs; see **Figure 1**). Seed regions were chosen according to previously published literature and specified on the standard brain using the WFU PickAtlas

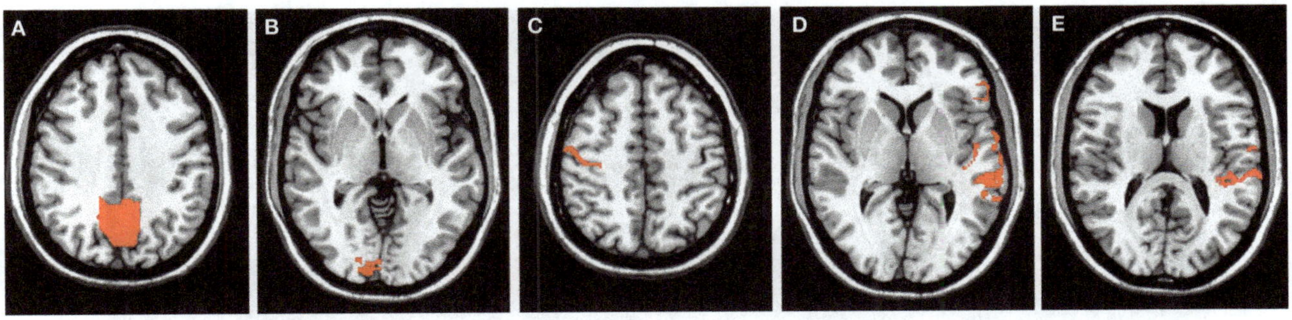

FIGURE 1 | Seed regions (red areas) for all investigated networks. (A) Precuneus (DMN); **(B)** primary visual cortex (BA17; VIN); **(C)** right primary motor cortex (BA 4; SMN); **(D)** left reading areas (RNW); and **(E)** left auditory cortex (BA 41, BA 42; AUD).

(Maldjian et al., 2003, 2004) and processed using MarsBaR v0.43 (Brett et al., 2002). Chosen seed regions comprised the precuneus (DMN see, e.g., Cole et al., 2010), the right primary visual cortex (BA17; VIN see, e.g., Bianciardi et al., 2009), the right primary motor cortex (BA 4; SMN see, e.g., Biswal et al., 1995), the left reading areas (BA 22, BA 44, BA 45; RNW see, e.g., Koyama et al., 2010), and the left auditory cortex (BA 41, BA 42; AUD see, e.g., Cordes et al., 2000). Correlation maps were converted to z-values using Fisher's r-to-z transformation, as implemented in Matlab (Matlab 7.8.0, Release 2009 Mathworks Inc., Sherborn, MA, USA) to enable parametric statistical comparison. Only positive correlations were mapped for this investigation. Single-subject analysis for all four conditions (rest_cross, rest_black, rest_eyes_closed, rest_relax) was conducted for all seed regions. A within-subject ANOVA factoring the four conditions was performed separately for all seed regions, followed by T-contrasts to compare all conditions in pairs. All resulting statistical parametric maps were thresholded at $p < 0.001$ (uncorrected) using a cluster extent threshold of 10 contiguous voxels.

As a measure of consistency of the spatial patterns, an overlap of activation maps for all four conditions was calculated at the single-subject level and group level [see Equation (1)]. For comparison of consistency across all four conditions and across all possible combinations of three conditions, an overlap was calculated at the single-subject and at the group level.

The spatial overlap for each condition and each seed voxel (Rombouts et al., 1997, 1998) was calculated by

$$R_{\mathrm{OVERLAP}}(i) = n \times \frac{A_{\mathrm{OVERLAP}}(i)}{\sum_j A_{j(i)}} \qquad (1)$$

where i represents the different seed regions, j the different resting-state conditions, n the number of conditions, $A_{j(i)}$ the quantity of activated voxels for seed region i in condition j, and $A_{\mathrm{OVERLAP}}(i)$ the quantity of identical supra-threshold voxels for all conditions for seed region i. A_{OVERLAP} is a measure to describe the quantity of voxels that are activated across all conditions. R_{OVERLAP} ranges from 0 (no spatial overlap) to 1 (exact overlap) and can be expressed as a percentage. This measure represents the consistency of the spatial extent of the functional connectivity, independent from the way, resting-state was induced. The application of this whole brain consistency measure was motivated by the fact that we did not want to restrict our measurements to a predefined ROI (e.g., Raemaekers et al., 2007; Caceres et al., 2009).

RESULTS

After successfully completing all four fMRI runs, subjects were asked which of the four resting-state conditions created the greatest state of relaxation. The majority of subjects (6/10) rated rest_relax, the last condition, to be the easiest condition in which to stay relaxed during the scan. Three subjects declared the rest_eyes_closed condition, and one subject the rest_cross condition, to induce the greatest state of relaxation.

A complete description and visualization of all contrasts, conditions, and seed regions can be found in **Figure A1** and **Table A1** (both in Appendix). Results of the calculated linear T-contrast uncovered significant differences within network-specific areas for most comparisons across all resting-state conditions and all networks analyzed.

SINGLE-SUBJECT ANALYSIS

Results revealed a high consistency for all investigated RSN across the four conditions within one subject, but considerable differences between subjects (see **Figure 2**). Spatial overlaps of any two conditions within one subject ranged from 0.58 to 0.66 (exemplarily calculated for subject 3 for the DMN; for visualization see **Figure 2**), whereas overlaps of one condition between two subjects ranged from 0.39 to 0.57 (exemplarily calculated for subject 2 and 3 for the DMN; for visualization see **Figure 2**). The highest overlap across all conditions was found for the RNW (0.45), and the lowest overlap was seen in the VIN (0.31; see **Table 1** and **Figure 3**). Results further revealed that all overlaps calculated for any combination of three conditions led to comparable spatial overlap.

GROUP ANALYSIS

Although group activation maps showed high consistency across all four conditions, significant variations were found in all investigated networks. For the DMN, these differences involved the precuneus, the medial temporal and frontal gyrus, the pre- and postcentral gyrus, the inferior parietal gyrus, and the

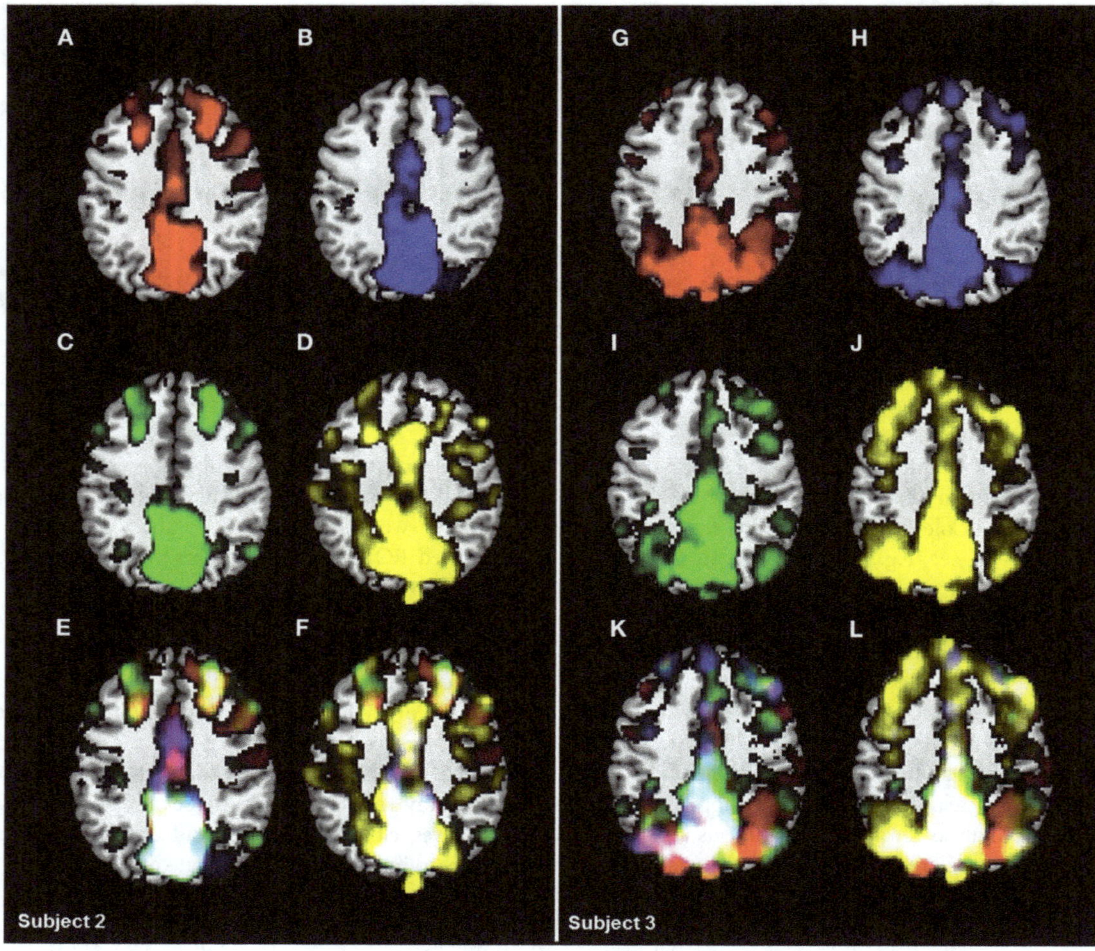

FIGURE 2 | Comparison of the DMN based on two single-subject activation maps for all four conditions. (A/G): black screen (rest_black), **(B/H):** fixation of a crosshair (rest_cross), **(C/I):** fixation of the words "Entspann dich!" (Engl. "relax") and **(D/J):** eyes-closed (rest_eyes_closed). Results revealed a substantial consistency across all four conditions **(F/L)** in one subject (spatial overlaps of any two conditions ranging from 0.58 to 0.66 in subject 3), but considerable differences of activation maps between two subjects for the same condition (spatial overlaps ranging from 0.39 to 0.57). However, a significant increase of overlap was found excluding the eyes-closed condition **(E/K)**.

Table 1 | Mean overlap at the single-subject level for all four conditions compared to the overlap of any possible combination of three conditions.

Overlap	DMN Mean (SD)	VIN Mean (SD)	AUD Mean (SD)	SMN Mean (SD)	RNW Mean (SD)
All four conditions	0.39 (0.10)	0.31 (0.09)	0.37 (0.07)	0.40 (0.11)	0.45 (0.11)
Without rest_cross	0.48 (0.07)	0.37 (0.10)	0.48 (0.09)	0.50 (0.10)	0.54 (0.10)
Without rest_black	0.48 (0.12)	0.38 (0.11)	0.46 (0.11)	0.48 (0.11)	0.56 (0.10)
Without rest_eyes_closed	0.46 (0.09)	0.40 (0.09)	0.44 (0.08)	0.45 (0.10)	0.51 (0.10)
Without rest_relax	0.47 (0.10)	0.40 (0.09)	0.44 (0.10)	0.46 (0.13)	0.54 (0.13)

paracentral lobule. Significant changes in the network-specific areas were obtained in the calcarine gyrus, the fusiform gyrus, the lingual gyrus, and the superior and medial occipital cortex. The rest_cross condition resulted in the highest functional connectivity in the right precuneus, whereas, in the resting-state condition, rest_relax functional connectivity in the precuneus was found on left side. The least precuneus functional connectivity was induced by the rest_black condition.

Significant differences in the VIN have been found across the four resting-state conditions in the calcarine gyrus, the fusiform gyrus, the lingual gyrus, and the superior occipital cortex. All of these brain areas are associated with the

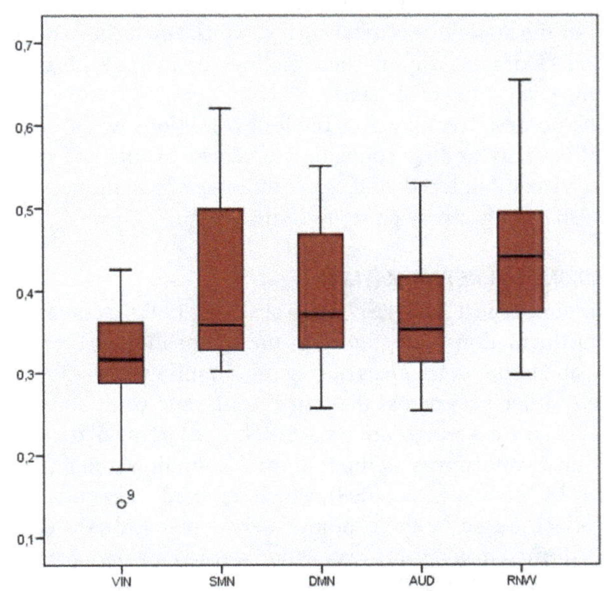

FIGURE 3 | Boxplot of overlap across all four conditions at the single-subject level.

Table 2 | Overlap at the group level for all four conditions compared to the overlap of any possible combination of three conditions.

Overlap	DMN	VIN	AUD	SMN	RNW
All four conditions	0.71	0.41	0.55	0.70	0.82
Without rest_cross	0.75	0.51	0.68	0.72	0.84
Without rest_black	0.79	0.43	0.70	0.77	0.84
Without rest_eyes_closed	0.76	0.41	0.54	0.75	0.87
Without rest_relax	0.74	0.62	0.54	0.73	0.86

VIN. The rest_cross condition, compared to all other conditions (rest_black, rest_eyes_closed, rest_relax), induced the highest functional connectivity in the left lingual gyrus and the right fusiform gyrus. The rest_eyes_closed condition evoked less functional connectivity in the superior occipital cortex. Significant differences within the SMN involved areas such as the precentral gyrus, the supplementary motor area (SMA), and the postcentral gyrus. A decreased functional connectivity in the left postcentral gyrus was found in the rest_black condition. For the RNW, differences were found in the left medial temporal gyrus and the left superior temporal gyrus. Results revealed significant differences in the AUD for the superior temporal gyrus, the insular cortex, the postcentral gyrus, and the supramarginal gyrus.

The spatial consistency analysis of the group maps across resting-state conditions revealed substantial overlap in supra-threshold voxels ($p < 0.001$, FWE corrected) for all ROIs (see **Table 2**).

The spatial overlap of any possible combination of three conditions was calculated for detecting one specific condition that induces most variability. The results show that all overlaps of three conditions revealed comparable overlaps, leading to the conclusion that no specific conditions appears to be preferable at group level. Therefore, no specific conditions appears to induce more variance in general.

DISCUSSION

fMRI is a validated and frequently used tool in pre-surgical planning for the mapping of language or motor areas (Roessler et al., 2005). Difficulties with this method may arise when patients have restricted motor or language abilities, as active participation is necessary in most fMRI paradigms. In contrast, resting-state fMRI is a method that does not require active task performance. Therefore, it is a promising tool to overcome the challenge of active participation in clinical practice. RSN measurements have experimentally been used in pre-surgical planning (Böttger et al., 2011). To date, initial experience has been gained by comparing fcRSN with functional connectivity patterns generated by a finger tapping paradigm (Zhang et al., 2009). The results of that study revealed high consistency of fcRSN patterns compared to task-based mapping of functional connectivity patterns. Less attention has been given to the impact of the resting-state condition.

In this study, we were able to demonstrate stable networks across different resting-state conditions. An analysis of the robustness of the group-mean response was performed for all resting-state conditions. Differences across the four conditions occurred in all networks investigated. However, we found that the group-level activation maps were highly stable across conditions. As previous studies have shown considerable between-subject variations (Chou et al., 2012), the analysis of consistency across the conditions was also calculated on a single-subject level. We were able to replicate these findings as single-subject overlaps for all four conditions differed across subjects within a range from 0.14 to 0.65. According to Gorgolewski et al. (2013), a reliable task may be characterized by a significantly higher within- than between-subject overlap. Results of our study revealed higher overlaps across different conditions within one subject (overlaps of any two conditions ranging from 0.58 to 0.66) than overlaps for two different subjects for the same conditions (overlaps ranging from 0.39 to 0.57).

Motion related artifacts are one of the most challenging problems in fMRI used for pre-surgical planning (Bullmore et al., 1999; Seto et al., 2001) and at very high field, as parallel imaging reconstruction artifacts, eddy currents and B0 changes due to motion increase (Beisteiner et al., 2011; Robinson et al., in revision). Known problems are head motion in slice selecting direction during one TR causing spin history effects and between image volumes causing signal changes near the ventricles and at the edge of the brain (Friston et al., 1996). Head motion artifacts are particularly severe in patient studies. Gorgolewski et al. (2013) reported stimulus related motion to be the confounding factor in explaining reliability between sessions. Therefore, resting-state fMRI could serve as a supplementary technique in pre-surgical planning not presenting with stimulus correlated motion artifacts.

In addition to the DMN, we extended our analysis to other networks, such as the VIN, the SMN, the AUD, and the RNW.

These networks are of increasing importance in clinical and pre-surgical mapping studies. Thus, our results may be highly relevant for the planning and task specification of future clinical RSN trials.

The results of our single-subject analysis revealed a stable reproducibility for all investigated networks on a single-subject level, but considerable differences between subjects. These findings are in line with the results of Chou et al. (2012), who obtained high reliability of the DMN within one subject, but substantial variations across different subjects by calculating intraclass correlation coefficients (ICC) and coefficients of variance (COV). The highest overlap across all four conditions was found in the RNW (0.45), and the lowest overlap in the VIN (0.31). The poorer overlap in the VIN might have been the result of different visual input. Therefore, a spatial overlap was calculated for any possible combination of three conditions to evaluate if any condition significantly decreases variability. Exclusion of any condition led to a significant increase in spatial overlap, but no difference between any combinations of three conditions could be found. Therefore, no specific resting-state condition appears to be preferable.

A detailed discussion of our data in relation to the published literature is only possible on the topic of the DMN, as the other networks were not part of extensive investigations concerning differences across resting-state conditions. In the following paragraphs, all investigated networks will be discussed in detail.

DEFAULT MODE NETWORK (DMN)

The DMN includes parts of the medial temporal lobe, the medial prefrontal cortex, the posterior cingulated cortex, the precuneus, and the medial, lateral, and inferior parietal cortex (Buckner et al., 2008).

In this study, we found that all four resting-state conditions induced differences in functional connectivity networks within areas that are typically part of the DMN. Yan et al. (Yan et al., 2009) found differences among the three resting-state conditions of eyes-closed, eyes-open, and eyes-open with fixation. The eyes-closed condition evoked less functional connectivity, assuming that more evaluation of sensory information is needed with opened eyes, and therefore, an increased functional connectivity was found for the DMN. However, in our study, we even found differences between the three resting-state conditions with opened eyes. This variability in fcRSN activation patterns might be explained by distinctive eye movements across the four resting-state conditions (Morisita and Yagi, 2001).

For the DMN, we found a stable overlap of $R_{\mathrm{OVERLAP}} = 0.71$ across all conditions at a group level, representing a consistent spatial extent of functional connectivity independent of resting-state condition.

VISUAL NETWORK (VIN)

The VIN can be characterized by areas typically involved in processing visual stimuli, such as the mesial visual areas (e.g., striate cortex, lingual gyrus) and lateral visual areas, such as the occipital pole and the occipito-temporal regions (Rosazza and Minati, 2011). The eyes_closed condition induced less functional connectivity in the superior occipital cortex, which might be explained by the lack of visual input. These findings are in line with a study by Yang et al. (Yang et al., 2007).

The poorest overlap across the four conditions was found for the VIN. This finding could be elucidated by the use of different visually induced fcRSN conditions, which influence the functional connectivity patterns of the VIN.

SENSORIMOTOR NETWORK (SMN)

In the first report of a RSN (Biswal et al., 1995), spontaneous BOLD fluctuations were found in the sensorimotor cortex, the SMA, and in premotor areas during rest. In this investigation, significant differences across the four resting-state conditions were found in all areas representing the SMN. The finding of decreased functional connectivity in the rest_black condition is in line with a study by McAvoy et al. (2008), which reported a dissimilarity in networks induced by the conditions eyes-open and eyes-closed, where the first may reflect greater neuronal activity than the latter.

With an overlap of 70% across all four conditions, the SMN was found to be very robust. This high spatial reproducibility makes the SMN an interesting candidate for pre-surgical planning, e.g., to evaluate motor-related areas in patients with restricted motor abilities.

READING NETWORK (RNW)

Language-related areas are commonly examined for pre-surgical planning, using fMRI activation patterns during verb generation tasks, see for example (Holland et al., 2001; Eaton et al., 2008; Szaflarski et al., 2008; Tillema et al., 2008; Karunanayaka et al., 2010). Individual definition of language- and motor-related areas is of high importance, as it is widely accepted that there are no typical language or motor "centers." These functions are rather spread across wide cortical and subcortical networks. As patients with brain tumors or epilepsy often show restricted functioning, resting-state fMRI may act as an outstanding method for pre-surgical planning.

The highest consistency across all four resting-state conditions was obtained for the RNW. With an overlap of 0.82 at the group level, the spontaneous fluctuations across all conditions was extremely stable, hence fcRSN measurements seem to be an appropriate tool for the assessment of a language network in group studies. For any 3-fold combination a minimal spatial overlap of 0.84 was found ranging from 0.84 (excluding the condition rest_cross) to 0.87 (excluding the condition rest_eyes_closed). Thus, all four resting-state conditions examined in this study appear to show robust and reliable functional connectivity in the RNW and are thus appropriate for investigations of the RNW.

AUDITORY NETWORK (AUD)

The AUD involves the superior temporal gyrus, Heschl's gyrus, the insula, and the postcentral gyrus. The primary auditory cortex is known to interact with the angular gyrus, the supramarginal gyrus, Broca's area, and Wernicke's area.

Our results indicate that, among all conditions, rest_eyes_closed and rest_relax evoked the most differences concerning functional connectivity networks compared to the other conditions. With an overlap of $R_{OVERLAP} = 0.54$ in the AUD, the four resting-state conditions induced larger variability compared to the other networks, except the VIN. Yet, the underlying source of this moderate overlap remains unclear.

RATING OF RELAXATION

The majority of subjects rated the condition, rest_relax, as most relaxing. In this rest-task, however, less precuneus activation was found in the DMN. DMN activity is generally characterized by the absence of an active task. Without focusing attention on a task, thoughts tend to wander, participants imagine future events, or think about the recent past. In fact, participants perform an active task in the resting-state condition, rest_relax, by focusing their attention on relaxation. Subjects felt more relaxed, but mind wandering and daydreaming tendencies decreased, as the functional connectivity of the DMN is decreased compared to rest_cross or rest_black.

APPLICATION TO CLINICAL PRACTICE

Resting-state measurements are not only of interest for basic neuroscience research. These measurements have recently been shown to allow promising insights in the epileptic brain in clinical practice (e.g., Lui et al., 2008; Negishi et al., 2011; Morgan et al., 2012).

The results of a study by Lui et al. (2008) revealed a difference in the interictal activity of the precuneus in epilepsy patients with generalized rather than partial seizures, suggesting that the lack of precuneus activation in patients with generalized seizures may contribute to the more severe interictal deficits in cognitive functions. Morgan et al. (2012) also identified resting-state fMRI as a supporting tool for pre-surgical assessment.

According to Negishi et al. (2011), RSN measurements are also an appropriate technique to predict surgical outcome in epilepsy patients. A common treatment method for intractable epilepsy is surgery, which can considerably improve epileptic symptoms. However, surgical therapy is not risk-free, and postsurgical complications can lead to cognitive dysfunction. Therefore, it is necessary to assess the possible benefit of surgical treatment. A recently published investigation by Negishi et al. (2011) showed that preoperative measurements of RSNs may serve as a predictor of surgical outcome, as patients with recurrent seizures after surgery differed in their functional connectivity compared to seizure-free patients.

Seed-based resting-state fMRI must be discussed critically in clinical practice, as mapping of a seed region may cause complications. In pathologically altered brains, an activated region may be located differently, therefore additional variance, based on different locations of the seed regions, must be recognized. Moreover, the performance of seed-based resting-state fMRI is impossible if the seed region is occupied by a tumor or a lesion.

Alterations of RSN connectivity, especially in the DMN, have been shown in neurological and neurodegenerative disorders, such as Alzheimer's disease (Auer, 2008). Initial changes can be observed even in the preclinical stages. For a reliable interpretation of the results, especially in a clinical setting, the stability of generated networks is of crucial importance, and the way the resting-state is induced should be considered. Generally, resting-state conditions with eyes-opened are preferable, as they usually evoke higher functional connectivity. According to our findings, patients who undergo fMRI for investigation of speech- and reading-related areas may also be investigated with eyes-closed conditions, considering patient comfort due to disease-related impairments. For examination of the DMN, resting-state conditions in which subjects or patients are instructed to relax by visual presentation of a word or a sentence (e.g., "relax") should be avoided because of the lowered activity levels in the precuneus. Study protocols for fMRI resting-state measurements should be clearly defined for reliability of functional connectivity patterns and to complete information in reports. In pre-surgical planning, motion artifacts may cause considerable difficulties, as head motion artifacts are particularly severe in patients. Gorgolewski et al. (2013) identified motion as the main confounding factor in task-based fMRI. Therefore, resting-state fMRI may be a useful tool to overcome stimulus correlated motion-artifacts in pre-surgical planning.

LIMITATIONS

A possible limitation of this study is the identical sequence of resting-state conditions, i.e., there was no randomization of the different conditions across subjects. However, it is known from several studies using the Stroop test that reading is an automatic process (see, e.g., MacLeod, 1991), which does not require the subjects' focused attention. Therefore, to prevent possible influence and carry-over effects induced by the rest_relax condition on the resting-state conditions, the run order was kept identical for all subjects.

Another limitation is eye movements, which have been suggested to possibly influence activity patterns according to Ramot et al. (2011). However, an eye-tracking device in this study was used only to verify that the subject obeyed the instructions and had his/her eyes-opened or closed. Thus, we did not record eye movements or blinking during the scanning session. Such data should be collected in further investigations to determine the exact influence of eye movements on RSNs.

CONCLUSION

We were able to show that the degree of network pattern modulation induced by resting-state conditions varied across the investigated networks. The most consistent results were obtained for the RNW. Our results indicate that RSN patterns were not affected by the resting-state conditions within one subject but a considerable difference of overlap across subjects was obtained. Furthermore, we were able to show that fcRSN were highly stable at the group level, especially for the language-related network. As the overlap is comparable in any combination of three conditions, no specific condition seems to be preferable at single-subject or at group level.

ACKNOWLEDGMENTS

The authors thank the reviewers for their helpful comments on the manuscript, the subjects for their participation, and D. Prayer, AC, and GT for their special support. V. Schöpf and K. Kollndorfer are supported by the FWF (P23205-B09).

REFERENCES

Amann, M., Hirsch, J. G., and Gass, A. (2009). A serial functional connectivity MRI study in healthy individuals assessing the variability of connectivity measures: reduced interhemispheric connectivity in the motor network during continuous performance. *Magn. Reson. Imaging* 27, 1347–1359.

Auer, D. P. (2008). Spontaneous low-frequency blood oxygenation level-dependent fluctuations and functional connectivity analysis of the "resting" brain. *Magn. Reson. Imaging* 26, 1055–1064.

Beisteiner, R., Robinson, S., Wurnig, M., Hilbert, M., Merksa, K., Rath, J., et al. (2011). Clinical fMRI: Evidence for a 7 T benefit over 3 T. *Neuroimage* 57, 1015–1021.

Bennett, C. M., and Miller, M. B. (2010). How reliable are the results from functional magnetic resonance imaging? *Ann. N.Y. Acad. Sci.* 1191, 133–155.

Bettus, G., Guedj, E., Joyeux, F., Confort-Gouny, S., Soulier, E., Laguitton, V., et al. (2009). Decreased basal fMRI functional connectivity in epileptogenic networks and contralateral compensatory mechanisms. *Hum. Brain Mapp.* 30, 1580–1591.

Bianciardi, M., Fukunaga, M., Van Gelderen, P., Horovitz, S. G., De Zwart, J. A., and Duyn, J. H. (2009). Modulation of spontaneous fMRI activity in human visual cortex by behavioral state. *Neuroimage* 45, 160–168.

Biswal, B., Yetkin, F. Z., Haughton, V. M., and Hyde, J. S. (1995). Functional connectivity in the motor cortex of resting human brain using echo-planar MRI. *Magn. Reson. Med.* 34, 537–541.

Böttger, J., Margulies, D. S., Horn, P., Thomale, U. W., Podlipsky, I., Shapira-Lichter, I., et al. (2011). A software tool for interactive exploration of intrinsic functional connectivity opens new perspectives for brain surgery. *Acta Neurochir.* 153, 1561–1572.

Brett, M., Anton, J.-L., Valabregue, R., and Poline, J. P. (2002). "Region of interest analysis using an SPM toolbox," in *Presented at the 8th International Conference on Functional Mapping of the Human Brain*, Sendai, Available on CD-ROM in Neuroimage, 16.

Buckner, R. L., Andrews-Hanna, J. R., and Schacter, D. L. (2008). The brain's default network: anatomy, function, and relevance to disease. *Ann. N.Y. Acad. Sci.* 1124, 1–38.

Bullmore, E. T., Brammer, M. J., Rabe-Hesketh, S., Curtis, V. A., Morris, R. G., Williams, S. C., et al. (1999). Methods for diagnosis and treatment of stimulus-correlated motion in generic brain activation studies using fMRI. *Hum. Brain Mapp.* 7, 38–48.

Caceres, A., Hall, D. L., Zelaya, F. O., Williams, S. C. R., and Mehta, M. A. (2009). Measuring fMRI reliability with the intra-class correlation coefficient. *Neuroimage* 45, 758–768.

Chou, Y., Panych, L. P., Dickey, C. C., Petrella, J. R., and Chen, N. (2012). Investigation of long-term reproducibility of intrinsic connectivity network mapping: a resting-state fMRI study. *AJNR. Am. J. Neuroradiol.* 33, 833–838.

Cole, D. M., Smith, S. M., and Beckmann, C. F. (2010). Advances and pitfalls in the analysis and interpretation of resting-state FMRI data. *Front. Syst. Neurosci.* 4:8. doi: 10.3389/fnsys.2010.00008

Cordes, D., Haughton, V. M., Arfanakis, K., Wendt, G. J., Turski, P. A., Moritz, C. H., et al. (2000). Mapping functionally related regions of brain with functional connectivity MR imaging. *AJNR. Am. J. Neuroradiol.* 21, 1636–1644.

Eaton, K. P., Szaflarski, J. P., Altaye, M., Ball, A. L., Kissela, B. M., Banks, C., et al. (2008). Reliability of fMRI for studies of language in post-stroke aphasia subjects. *Neuroimage* 41, 311–322.

Fox, M. D., and Greicius, M. (2010). Clinical applications of resting state functional connectivity. *Front. Syst. Neurosci.* 4:19. doi: 10.3389/fnsys.2010.00019

Fox, M. D., Snyder, A. Z., Vincent, J. L., Corbetta, M., Van Essen, D. C., and Raichle, M. E. (2005). The human brain is intrinsically organized into dynamic, anticorrelated functional networks. *Proc. Natl. Acad. Sci. U.S.A.* 102, 9673–9678.

Fransson, P. (2006). How default is the default mode of brain function? Further evidence from intrinsic BOLD signal fluctuations. *Neuropsychologia* 44, 2836–2845.

Friston, K. J., Williams, S., Howard, R., Frackowiak, R. S., and Turner, R. (1996). Movement-related effects in fMRI time-series. *Magn. Reson. Med.* 35, 346–355.

Gilbert, S. J., Dumontheil, I., Simons, J. S., Frith, C. D., and Burgess, P. W. (2007). Comment on "Wandering minds: the default network and stimulus-independent thought." *Science* 317, 43; author reply 43.

Gorgolewski, K. J., Storkey, A. J., Bastin, M. E., Whittle, M. E., and Pernet, C. (2013). Single subject fMRI test-retest reliability metrics and confounding factors. *Neuroimage* 69, 231–243.

Hahn, B., Ross, T. J., and Stein, E. A. (2007). Cingulate activation increases dynamically with response speed under stimulus unpredictability. *Cereb. Cortex* 17, 1664–1671.

Hayes, D. J., and Huxtable, A. G. (2012). Interpreting deactivations in neuroimaging. *Front. Psychol.* 3:27. doi: 10.3389/fpsyg.2012.00027

Holland, S. K., Plante, E., Weber Byars, A., Strawsburg, R. H., Schmithorst, V. J., and Ball, W. S. (2001). Normal fMRI brain activation patterns in children performing a verb generation task. *Neuroimage* 14, 837–843.

Karunanayaka, P., Schmithorst, V. J., Vannest, J., Szaflarski, J. P., Plante, E., and Holland, S. K. (2010). A group independent component analysis of covert verb generation in children: a functional magnetic resonance imaging study. *Neuroimage* 51, 472–487.

Koyama, M. S., Kelly, C., Shehzad, Z., Penesetti, D., Castellanos, F. X., and Milham, M. P. (2010). Reading networks at rest. *Cereb. Cortex* 20, 2549–2559.

Lui, S., Ouyang, L., Chen, Q., Huang, X., Tang, H., Chen, H., et al. (2008). Differential interictal activity of the precuneus/posterior cingulate cortex revealed by resting state functional MRI at 3T in generalized vs. partial seizure. *J. Magn. Reson. Imaging* 27, 1214–1220.

MacLeod, C. M. (1991). Half a century of research on the Stroop effect: an integrative review. *Psychol. Bull.* 109, 163–203.

Maldjian, J. A., Laurienti, P. J., and Burdette, J. H. (2004). Precentral gyrus discrepancy in electronic versions of the Talairach atlas. *Neuroimage* 21, 450–455.

Maldjian, J. A., Laurienti, P. J., Kraft, R. A., and Burdette, J. H. (2003). An automated method for neuroanatomic and cytoarchitectonic atlas-based interrogation of fMRI data sets. *Neuroimage* 19, 1233–1239.

Mason, M. F., Norton, M. I., Van Horn, J. D., Wegner, D. M., Grafton, S. T., and Macrae, C. N. (2007). Wandering minds: the default network and stimulus-independent thought. *Science* 315, 393–395.

McAvoy, M., Larson-prior, L., Nolan, T. S., Vaishnavi, S. N., Raichle, E., Avossa, G., et al. (2008). Resting states affect spontaneous BOLD oscillations in sensory and paralimbic cortex. *J. Neurophysiol.* 100, 922–931.

Meindl, T., Teipel, S., Elmouden, R., Mueller, S., Koch, W., Dietrich, O., et al. (2010). Test-retest reproducibility of the default-mode network in healthy individuals. *Hum. Brain Mapp.* 31, 237–246.

Morgan, V. L., Sonmezturk, H. H., Gore, J. C., and Abou-Khalil, B. (2012). Lateralization of temporal lobe epilepsy using resting functional magnetic resonance imaging connectivity of hippocampal networks. *Epilepsia* 53, 1628–1635.

Morisita, M., and Yagi, T. (2001). The stability of human eye orientation during visual fixation and imagined fixation in three dimensions. *Auris Nasus Larynx* 28, 301–304.

Negishi, M., Martuzzi, R., Novotny, E. J., Spencer, D. D., and Constable, R. T. (2011). Functional MRI connectivity as a predictor of the surgical outcome of epilepsy. *Epilepsia* 52, 1733–1740.

Newton, A. T., Morgan, V. L., and Gore, J. C. (2007). Task demand modulation of steady-state functional connectivity to primary motor cortex. *Hum. Brain Mapp.* 28, 663–672.

Raemaekers, M., Vink, M., Zandbelt, B., Van Wezel, R. J. A., Kahn, R. S., and Ramsey, N. F. (2007). Test-retest reliability of fMRI activation during prosaccades and antisaccades. *Neuroimage* 36, 532–542.

Ramot, M., Wilf, M., Goldberg, H., Weiss, T., Deouell, L. Y., and Malach, R. (2011). Coupling between spontaneous (resting state) fMRI fluctuations and human oculo-motor activity. *Neuroimage* 58, 213–225.

Roessler, K., Donat, M., Lanzenberger, R., Novak, K., Geissler, A., Gartus, A., et al. (2005). Evaluation of preoperative high magnetic field motor functional MRI (3 Tesla) in glioma patients by navigated electrocortical stimulation and postoperative outcome. *J. Neurol. Neurosurg. Psychiatry* 76, 1152–1157.

Rombouts, S. A., Barkhof, F., Hoogenraad, F. G., Sprenger, M., and Scheltens, P. (1998). Within-subject reproducibility of visual activation patterns with functional magnetic resonance imaging using multislice echo planar imaging. *Magn. Reson. Imaging* 16, 105–113.

Rombouts, S. A., Barkhof, F., Hoogenraad, F. G., Sprenger, M., Valk, J., and Scheltens, P. (1997). Test-retest analysis with functional MR of the activated area in the human visual cortex. *AJNR. Am. J. Neuroradiol.* 18, 1317–1322.

Rosazza, C., and Minati, L. (2011). Resting-state brain networks: literature review and clinical applications. *Neurol. Sci.* 32, 773–785.

Rosazza, C., Minati, L., Ghielmetti, F., Mandelli, M. L., and Bruzzone, M. G. (2012). Functional connectivity during resting-state functional mr imaging: study of the correspondence between independent component analysis and region-of-interest-based methods. *Am. J. Neuroradiol.* 33, 180–187.

Schöpf, V., Kasprian, G., Brugger, P., and Prayer, D. (2012a). Watching the fetal brain at "rest". *Int. J. Dev. Neurosci.* 30, 11–17.

Schöpf, V., Kasprian, G., Schwindt, J., Kollndorfer, K., and Prayer, D. (2012b). Visualization of resting-state networks *in utero*. *Ultrasound Obstet. Gynecol.* 39, 487–488.

Seto, E., Sela, G., McIlroy, W. E., Black, S. E., Staines, W. R., Bronskill, M. J., et al. (2001). Quantifying head motion associated with motor tasks used in fMRI. *Neuroimage* 14, 284–297.

Szaflarski, J. P., Holland, S. K., Jacola, L. M., Lindsell, C., Privitera, M. D., and Szaflarski, M. (2008). Comprehensive presurgical functional MRI language evaluation in adult patients with epilepsy. *Epilepsy Behav.* 12, 74–83.

Tillema, J.-M., Byars, A. W., Jacola, L. M., Schapiro, M. B., Schmithorst, V. J., Szaflarski, J. P., et al. (2008). Cortical reorganization of language functioning following perinatal left MCA stroke. *Brain Lang.* 105, 99–111.

Tzourio-Mazoyer, N., Landeau, B., Papathansassiou, D., Crivello, F., Etard, O., Delcroix, N., et al. (2002). Automated anatomical labeling of activations in SPM using a macroscopic anatomical parcellation of the MNI MRI single-subject brain. *Neuroimage* 15, 273–289.

Van Dijk, K. R. A, Hedden, T., Venkataraman, A., Evans, K. C., Lazar, S. W., and Buckner, R. L. (2010). Intrinsic functional connectivity as a tool for human connectomics: theory, properties, and optimization. *J. Neurophysiol.* 103, 297–321.

Yan, C., Liu, D., He, Y., Zou, Q., Zhu, C., Zuo, X., et al. (2009). Spontaneous brain activity in the default mode network is sensitive to different resting-state conditions with limited cognitive load. *PLoS ONE* 4:e5743. doi: 10.1371/journal.pone.0005743

Yang, H., Long, X.-Y., Yang, Y., Yan, H., Zhu, C.-Z., Zhou, X.-P., et al. (2007). Amplitude of low frequency fluctuation within visual areas revealed by resting-state functional MRI. *Neuroimage* 36, 144–152.

Zhang, D., Johnston, J. M., Fox, M. D., Leuthardt, E. C., Grubb, R. L., Chicoine, M. R., et al. (2009). Preoperative sensorimotor mapping in brain tumor patients using spontaneous fluctuations in neuronal activity imaged with functional magnetic resonance imaging: initial experience. *Neurosurgery* 65, 226–236.

APPENDIX

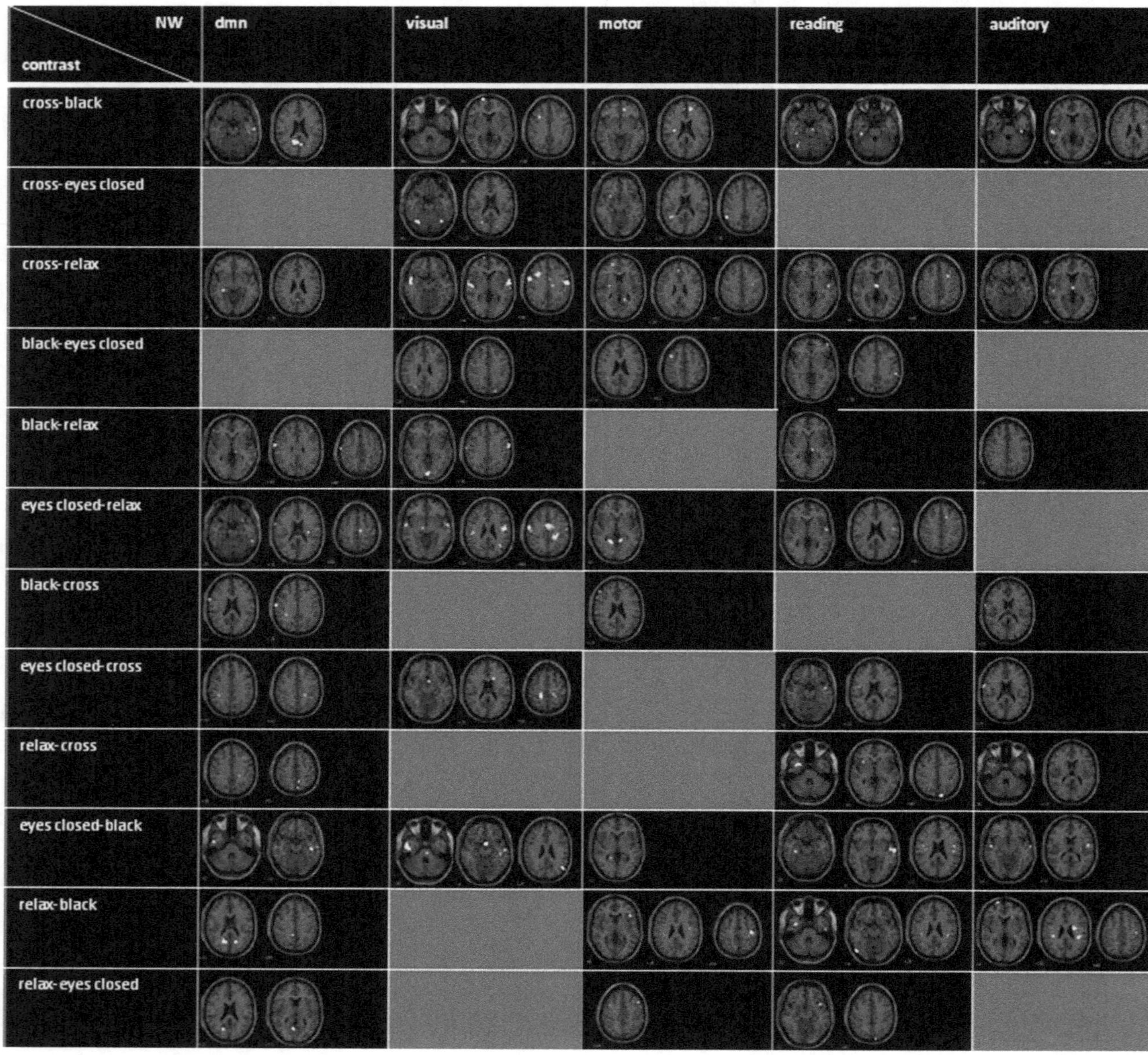

FIGURE A1 | Axial mean anatomical images overlaid by brain activation resulting from contrasts for all conditions and networks ($p < 0.001$ uncorrected for whole-brain volume analysis).

Table A1 | Detailed listing of all condition contrasts analyzed for all networks.

Contrast \ NW	DMN	Visual	Motor	Reading	Auditory
Cross-black	r precuneus (446; 4.89) r med temp g (47; 3.66) r med temp g (21; 3.41)	r sup front g (100; 4.10) r med front g (64; 4.01) r calcarine g (21; 3.85) r med temp g (25; 3.85) l med front g (31; 3.44) r fusiform g (28; 3.42) r sup temp g (32; 3.42) l precentral g (10; 3.40) r lingual g (10; 3.35)	l ant cingulum (68; 4.37) r parahippocampal g (21; 4.02) l precentral g (26; 3.82) r ant cingulum (20; 3.75) l sup med front g (69; 3.71) r insula (26; 3.66) r calcarine g (11; 3.64) r cerebellum (VI) (40; 3.63) l SMA (13; 3.51) l postcentral g (19; 3.50) r ant cingulum (13; 3.31)	r fusiform g (41; 3.93) r med temp g (30; 3.70) r fusiform g (48; 3.70) l parahippocampal g (15; 3.40)	l fusiform g (32; 4.22) r sup temp g (59; 3.65) r med temp g (14; 3.56) l insula (12; 3.40)
Cross-eyes closed		r fusiform g (106; 3.77) r sup occ c (39; 3.56) l lingual g (15; 3.53) l cerebellum (43; 3.42)	r ant cingulum (18; 3.67) r med temp g (70; 3.63) r inf parietal g (53; 3.50) l thalamus (35; 3.49) r insula (26; 3.48) r sup frontal g (31; 3.39) r med cingulum (15; 3.39) l ant cingulum (14; 3.37) l sup med frontal g (12; 3.33)		
Cross-relax	r hippocampus (35; 4.03) l paracentral l (33; 3.62) r precuneus (18; 3.28)	r precentral g (2237; 3.61) r med front g (200; 4.59) l sup temp g (401; 4.56) r sup temp g (644; 4.42) r precentral g (315; 4.25) r paracentral l (465; 4.23) r postcentral g (55; 408) r fusiform g (28; 3.83) l inf front g (tri) (82; 3.75) l insula (97; 3.70) l precentral g (17; 3.67) l cingulum (post) (41; 3.65) l insula (31; 3.58) r medial front g (65; 3.54) l medial front g (19; 3.53) r sup front g (27; 3.52) l sup temp g (17; 3.48) l sup parietal c (17; 3.82) l lingual g (13; 3.37) r sup temp g (48; 3.34)	r lingual g (20; 3.70) l precuneus (70; 3.64) l med cingulum (17; 3.61) r sup frontal g (59; 3.49) r ant cingulum (15; 3.48) l calcarine g (13; 3.46) r putamen (46; 3.34) l SMA (10; 3.26)	l thalamus (65; 3.57) l sup temp g (36; 3.51) l med frontal g (42; 3.46)	r sup temp g (18; 3.45) r thalamus (26; 3.34) l inf front g (orb) (10; 3.26)

(Continued)

Table A1 | Continued

Contrast \ NW	DMN	Visual	Motor	Reading	Auditory
Black-eyes closed		l sup occ c (25; 3.57) r sup occ c (11; 3.27)	r angular g (33; 3.58) r med front g (39; 3.41) r angular g (22; 3.40)	r sup temp g (13; 3.69) l supramargninal g (35; 3.69) l med front g (orb) (22; 3.45) l supramarginal g (12; 3.42) l inf parietal g (21; 3.81) r supramarginal g (11; 3.33)	
Black-relax	r precentral g (204; 4.83) l caudate (64; 3.69) l inf temp g (26; 3.67) l paracentral l (148; 3.66) r postcentral g (41; 3.55) l postcentral g (33; 3.43) l precuneus (10; 3.34)	r calcarine g (101; 4.22) r precentral c (46; 3.82) l postcentral g (158; 3.68) r precentral g (10; 3.35)		l thalamus (16; 3.78)	l precentral g (29; 3.43)
Eyes closed-relax	l med front g (11; 389) l cereb (17; 3.87) r precentral g (14; 3.66) r thalamus (21; 3.65) l insula c (16; 3.61) r paracentral l (35; 3.58) r thalamus (16; 3.49) l med temp g (16; 3.49) l inf temp g (31; 3.39)	r SMA (4981; 5.18) l precentral g (963; 485) l insula (229; 460) r heschl g (902; 4.39) r thalamus (902; 4.39) r fusiform g (80; 4.01) l sup temp g (37; 4.00) l precuneus (230; 3.94) l angular g (63; 3.79) l sup front g (97; 3.71) l thalamus (14; 3.65) l med front g (20; 3.61) l precentral g (66; 3.56) l putamen (42; 3.55) r med front g (27; 3.53) r inf temp g (21; 3.50) r sup tem g (41; 3.49) l calcarine g (14; 3.44) r med temp g (12; 3.41) l thalamus (32; 3.41) l inf temp g (13; 3.33) vermis (IV, V) (14; 3.28) r rolandic op (13; 3.25) r lingual g (11; 3.20)	r lingual g (149; 4.02) l lingual g (52; 3.83)	g sup temp g (68; 4.09) l sup front g (13; 3.60) r precentral g (25; 3.53)	

(Continued)

Table A1 | Continued

Contrast \ NW	DMN	Visual	Motor	Reading	Auditory
Black-cross	r precentral g (37; 4.19) l occ med g (22; 3.76) l thalamus (44; 3.72) r postcentral g (56; 3.68) r inf parietal g (25; 3.57)		r inf front g (tri) (58; 3.86) r inf front g (tri) (11; 3.56)		r postcentral g (59; 4.19)
Eyes closed-cross	l med cingulum (23; 3.82) r supramarginal g (12; 3.52)	l postcentral g (224; 4.15) l caudate n (46; 3.91) r paracentral l (152; 3.74) r med cingulum (10; 3.60) l sup temp pole (27; 3.59) l med temp g (17; 3.53) l thalamus (10; 3.53) l angular g (21; 3.34) l caudate n (14; 3.31)		r insula (16; 3.57) l med temp g (17; 3.39) r rolandic oper (10; 3.19)	r postcentral g (49; 3.49)
Relax-cross	l precuneus (28; 3.47) l precuneus (16; 3.39)			l sup occ g (60; 4.52) r med temp pole (132; 4.35) l hippocampus (14; 3.54) r caudate n (23; 3.54) l supramarginal g (13; 3.47) r lingual g (13; 3.47) r insula (23; 3.46)	l postcentral g (15; 3.95)
Eyes closed-black	l med temp g (56; 4.38) l med temp g (60; 3.95) r inf temp g (53; 3.83)	l rolandic oper (14; 3.60) r med temp g (135; 358) r med sup temp g (11; 3.35) r paracentral l (10; 3.26) l insula (10; 3.26)	r lingual g (20, 3.61)	l med temp g (193; 4.69) l insula (23; 4.01) l precentral g (44; 3.92) r rolandic oper (39; 3.81) l rolandic oper (23; 3.68) l cerebellum (crus I) (12; 3.66) r fusiform g (64; 3.61) l sup med front g (12; 3.53)	r sup temp g (33; 4.03) l postcentral g (63; 3.93) r med front g (10; 3.74) r rolandic oper (23; 3.67) r supramarginal g (31; 3.65) r inf occ g (14; 3.58) r precentral g (32; 3.58) l putamen (31; 3.54) l med temp (10; 3.46)

(Continued)

Table A1 | Continued

Contrast / NW	DMN	Visual	Motor	Reading	Auditory
Relax-black	r cuneus (213; 4.27) r precuneus (30; 3.74) l calcarine g (97; 3.61) l precuneus (11; 3.51) r sup front g (10; 3.30)		l postcentral g (126; 3.97) l insula (10; 3.81) l inf front g (tri) (47; 3.59) l sup med front g (15; 3.48)	l sup occ g (21; 4.38) r inf temp g (25; 3.96) r inf temp g (87; 3.87) l rolandic oper (24; 3.87) l precentral g (10; 3.84) l cerebellum (crus I) (33; 3.73) r sup front (orb) (22; 3.73) l inf temp g (11; 3.47) r precentral g (15; 3.30)	l supramarginal g (121; 4.50) r med cingulum (39; 4.07) l caudate n (134; 3.85) r supramarginal g (41; 3.80) r sup frontal g (32; 3.76) l inf front g (tri) (17; 3.70) r sup front g (orb) (23; 3.69) l hippocampus (20; 3.64) l fusiform g (10; 3.60) r inf occ g (12; 3.55) l post cingulum (11; 3.47) l caudate n (20; 3.38) r putamen (14; 3.35)
Relax-eyes closed	r cuneus (185; 3.99) l precuneus (15; 3.76)		l med front g (85; 3.67) r precentral g (34; 3.56) l med front g (14; 3.50)	l insula (29; 3.87)	

$p < 0.001$ uncorrected for whole brain volume analysis. Reported are significantly activated clusters with 10 or more voxels. Clusters were automatically labeled using the AAL toolbox (Tzourio-Mazoyer et al., 2002). Numbers in brackets refer to number of significantly activated voxels and the corresponding peak Z-value.

9

Task vs. rest—different network configurations between the coactivation and the resting-state brain networks

Xin Di, Suril Gohel, Eun H. Kim and Bharat B. Biswal*

Department of Biomedical Engineering, New Jersey Institute of Technology, Newark, NJ, USA

Correspondence:
Bharat B. Biswal, Department of Biomedical Engineering, New Jersey Institute of Technology, 607 Fenster Hall, University Heights, Newark, NJ 07102, USA
e-mail: bbiswal@yahoo.com

There is a growing interest in studies of human brain networks using resting-state functional magnetic resonance imaging (fMRI). However, it is unclear whether and how brain networks measured during the resting-state exhibit comparable properties to brain networks during task performance. In the present study, we investigated meta-analytic coactivation patterns among brain regions based upon published neuroimaging studies, and compared the coactivation network configurations with those in the resting-state network. The strength of resting-state functional connectivity between two regions were strongly correlated with the coactivation strength. However, the coactivation network showed greater global efficiency, smaller mean clustering coefficient, and lower modularity compared with the resting-state network, which suggest a more efficient global information transmission and between system integrations during task performing. Hub shifts were also observed within the thalamus and the left inferior temporal cortex. The thalamus and the left inferior temporal cortex exhibited higher and lower degrees, respectively in the coactivation network compared with the resting-state network. These results shed light regarding the reconfiguration of the brain networks between task and resting-state conditions, and highlight the role of the thalamus in change of network configurations in task vs. rest.

Keywords: brain network, coactivation, hub shift, meta-analysis, modularity, resting-state, small world, thalamus

INTRODUCTION

The human brain exhibits organized spontaneous fluctuations in the resting-state (Biswal et al., 1995), enabling researchers to study large-scale brain segregations and integrations (Bullmore and Sporns, 2009, 2012; Menon and Uddin, 2010). The spontaneous fluctuations reveal high synchronization between brain regions in the same brain system (Cordes et al., 2000; Greicius et al., 2003), and are relatively independent between different brain systems (Beckmann et al., 2005; Biswal et al., 2010). The whole brain segregation and integration can also be studied using graph theory based analysis (Bullmore and Sporns, 2009; Wang et al., 2010). For example, the brain network in the resting-state revealed modular structures, small world and scale free properties (Salvador et al., 2005; Achard et al., 2006; Achard and Bullmore, 2007; Nakamura et al., 2009; Yan and He, 2011).

Despite the growing popularity of resting-state fMRI to study brain functions, studies have yet to address a fundamental question regarding whether the brain at resting-state is comparable to the brain during task performing. Given that the evoked cerebral blood flow by different tasks account for less than 5% of the resting-state cerebral blood flow (Raichle, 2010), the resting-state brain already represents a large proportion of hemodynamic information which may reflect brain maintenance. Studies have also shown that task-related coactivation patterns correspond well with the brain systems that are measured during the resting-state (Toro et al., 2008; Smith et al., 2009). However, based on the economic theory of brain network organization, the brain network should be in an energy saving mode during the resting-state, while exhibiting dynamic network reconfiguration in the presence of a task demand to facilitate global and between systems information transmissions (Bullmore and Sporns, 2012). We predict that even though the connectivity in task conditions and the resting-state may be similar, substantial differences of network configurations may take place to support different task demands.

Changes in connectivity modulated by task are important to understand brain integration (Friston, 2011). Specific connections have been shown to be modulated by specific tasks (McLntosh and Gonzalez-Lima, 1994; McIntosh et al., 1994; Büchel and Friston, 1997; Rao et al., 2008). However, the modulations of connectivity are task specific, and it is difficult to modulate the whole brain network using a specific task. Thus, we adopted the same approach as Toro et al., and Smith et al. to examine task activations or group differences and their corresponding coactivation pattern across the whole brain (Toro et al., 2008; Smith et al., 2009). Specifically, we constructed brain networks comprised of 140 regions of interest (ROIs) from the whole brain based on both meta-analytic coactivation patterns (Yarkoni et al., 2011) and resting-state correlations of fMRI signals (Biswal et al., 2010). The online database Neurosynth (http://old.neurosynth.org/) was used to extract coactivation information, which contained 47,493 activations from 4393 studies (Yarkoni et al., 2011). We first asked whether the strength of coactivation between a pair of ROIs was correlated with their resting-state correlations. We then compared different network properties based on graph theory between the two brain networks (Bullmore and Sporns, 2009), including the small-worldness (Watts and

Strogatz, 1998), modularity (Newman, 2006), and hub distributions. We hypothesized that the brain when performing tasks will be more integrated and thus exhibit higher global efficiency and reduced modularity compared with the resting-state brain. In addition, we hypothesized that the brain hubs may shift from the default mode network (DMN) (Raichle et al., 2001; Greicius et al., 2003) regions to other brain regions that are critical during task executions.

METHODS

REGIONS OF INTEREST

One hundred and sixty functionally defined ROIs from Dosenbach et al. were adopted in the present analysis (Dosenbach et al., 2010). Twenty-four ROIs were removed because they were outside the Neurosynth mask. We included four more ROIs that were not represented within the 136 ROIs (Sabatinelli et al., 2011): the right amygdala (Montreal Neurological Institute, MNI, coordinates: 20, −4, −15), the left amygdala (−20, −6, −15), the right parahippocampus (14, −33, −7), and the left parahippocampus (−20, −33, −4). A total of 140 ROIs were used in the present study to construct brain networks (supplementary Table S1).

COACTIVATION NETWORK

The online database, Neurosynth, was used to construct the coactivation network (Yarkoni et al., 2011). The database search was conducted in November, 2012 when the database had 4393 studies and 47,493 activations. For each of the 140 ROIs, Neurosynth identified all the papers in the database that reported coordinates within 10 mm from the ROI center, and exported a whole brain z-score map representing the likelihood that a voxel coactivated with the given ROI (Yarkoni et al., 2011). The images were thresholded using a false discovery rate (FDR) criterion of $p < 0.05$. Thus, the Neurosynth search of all the ROIs resulted in 140 coactivation maps.

One hundred and forty spherical ROIs were defined using radii of 10 mm. The coactivation values of 140 ROIs were extracted from 140 coactivation maps, which resulted in a 140×140 matrix. Each row of the matrix represented the coactivation values of a given ROI with the other ROIs. Because the number of papers that was returned by each ROI inquiry was different, the coactivation values from different ROI inquiry may be biased. Therefore, we normalized each row by dividing the value from the ROI corresponding to that row, so that the diagonal values of the matrix were equaled to one. In addition, since the distribution of the coactivation values are skewed, all the values of the matrix were added by one, and were logarithmically transformed to facilitate a normal distribution. Finally, because the coactivation likelihood of region A with region B and the coactivation likelihood of region B with region A are generally similar but have slightly different values, the matrix was transposed, and averaged with the original matrix to create a symmetrical coactivation matrix.

RESTING-STATE NETWORK

We analyzed a resting-state fMRI data set to construct a resting-state network to compare with the coactivation network. The Oulu dataset from the 1000 Functional Connectomes Project was used (Biswal et al., 2010). This dataset originally contains 103 subjects. One subject's data was discarded because of large head motion (greater than 3 mm). Thus 102 subjects' data were included in the current analysis (36M/66F). The mean age was 21.5 years (range from 20 to 23 years). Two hundred and forty-five resting-state functional images were acquired for each subject ($TR = 1.8$ s, 28 slices). High resolution anatomical image was also acquired for each subject using MPRAGE sequence (Magnetization Prepared Rapid Acquisition Gradient Echo). More information for the data can be found at http://fcon_1000.projects.nitrc.org/fcpClassic/FcpTable.html. To rule out the possibility that the current results are due to sample bias of the resting-state dataset, we have conducted a separate analysis using another resting-state dataset, i.e., the Nathan Kline Institute (NKI) / Rockland Sample (http://fcon_1000.projects.nitrc.org/indi/pro/nki.html). Data analyses were identical to the Oulu dataset. Detailed methods and results of NKI dataset are reported in the supplementary material section.

Functional MRI images were processed using the SPM8 toolbox (http://www.fil.ion.ucl.ac.uk/spm/) under the MATLAB7.7 environment (www.mathworks.com). First, the MPRAGE anatomical image for each subject was segmented into gray matter (GM), white matter (WM), and cerebrospinal fluid (CSF) using the new segment routine in SPM8. The deformation field maps were also obtained in this step to later normalize the functional images. For each subject, the first five images of the fMRI images were discarded, resulting in 240 images per subject. The functional images were then motion corrected using the realign function. One subject's data were discarded after this step because the head motion was greater than 3 mm, resulting in 102 subjects in total. Next, the functional images were coregistered to the subjects' own anatomical images. Then, the deformation field map obtained from new segmentation step was applied to the functional images to normalize them into the standard MNI space.

One hundred and forty times series from the corresponding ROIs were extracted for each of the subjects. Six head motion parameters and their first order derivatives, first five eigenvectors from signals within WM masks, and first five eigenvectors from signals within CSF masks were regressed out using linear regression (Chai et al., 2012). No global signal regression was applied. Next, the time series were temporally filtered using a band-pass filter of 0.01–0.1 Hz. For each subject, a 140×140 correlation matrix was calculated using Kendall's rank correlation to minimize spurs correlations due to noises. The correlation matrices were transformed into Fisher's z, and averaged across subjects. Finally, the mean Fishers' z matrix was transformed back to correlation matrix using Fisher's inverse transform.

NETWORK ANALYSIS

Because the values in the coactivation matrix and the resting-state correlation matrix are essentially different, network sparsity thresholds were used to keep the number of edges of the two networks the same when comparing the two networks. The sparsity range was set between 6 and 40% with an increment of 1%. This range was used because typical sparsity of human neuron network is between this range, and the large scale brain networks revealed small world properties within this range (Achard and Bullmore,

2007; He et al., 2008). After thresholding, all the networks were binary (unweighted) undirected networks.

We first compared the two networks in terms of small world properties (global efficiency and mean clustering coefficient) and modularity. The global efficiency characterizes how efficient the whole brain network integrates information, and the mean clustering coefficient characterizes how efficient the information flows around local nodes (Watts and Strogatz, 1998). Modularity, also known as Newman's Q, characterizes the extent the whole brain network can be divided into sub-communities (Newman, 2006). The global efficiency, mean clustering coefficient, and modularity were calculated for the two networks at each sparsity level using the brain connectivity toolbox (Rubinov and Sporns, 2010). As a reference, random networks were generated 1000 times at each sparsity level. The three parameters were also calculated for the random networks, and were averaged across the 1000 random networks.

To determine the statistical significance, we created a null distribution of network differences by randomly shuffling the two networks 1000 times and calculating their differences of network properties for 1000 random networks. Specifically, at each sparsity level, we first identified edges that were different between the two networks. Next, we randomly assigned 50% of these different edges from the coactivation network to the resting-state network, and vice versa, resulting in two new mixed networks. We then calculated the three network parameters, i.e., the global efficiency, mean clustering coefficient and modularity, for the two mixed networks and obtained their differences between the two networks. The randomizations were performed 1000 times for each sparsity level to obtain a difference distribution. The difference of the three parameters between the coactivation network and the resting-state network were then compared with the randomized distribution to determine statistical significances. A critical threshold of $p < 0.001$ was used.

To demonstrate modular structures of the coactivation and the resting-state network, we thresholded the two networks at a sparsity level of 20%, and entered the two unweighted undirected networks into Gephi (https://gephi.org/) to determine their modular structures using the algorithm by Blondel et al. (2008). The two networks and their modular structures were rendered into a 2D surface using the Fruchterman–Reingold Algorithm (Fruchterman and Reingold, 1991).

We then examined whether the two networks displayed similar hub distribution (Achard et al., 2006). In the present study, we simply defined the importance of each node by calculating the number of edges connected to this node (also known as degree). We calculated the degrees for each node for the two networks at each sparsity level. Next, at each sparsity level, correlations of node degrees between the coactivation network and the resting-state network were calculated at the sparsity range of 6–40%. The correlations reflected the similarity of hub distributions of the two networks. There were only small correlations of degrees between the two networks (see Results below), i.e., a high degree node in the resting-state network was not necessarily a high degree node in the coactivation network. Hence, we subtracted the degrees between the two networks for each node at the sparsity level of 10, 20, and 30%. At each of the three sparsity levels, we sorted the degree differences. The two networks were also randomized using the method mentioned above, and the sorted degree differences were calculated. The randomization was conducted 1000 times, and the distribution of the sorted degree differences was obtained. Then, the original sorted degree differences between the coactivation network and resting-state network was compared with the distribution. Next, at each sparsity level, five nodes that had the largest degree differences and five nodes that had the least degree differences between the coactivation network and the resting-state network were identified. These nodes were rendered on a brain surface model using the BrainNet Viewer (http://www.nitrc.org/projects/bnv/).

RESULTS

COACTIVATION AND RESTING-STATE NETWORKS

The pattern of the coactivation and the resting-state correlation matrix were comparable (**Figures 1A,B**). Because the ROIs were arranged according to their network affiliations as reported by Dosenbach et al. (2010), square like structures along the diagonal were observed in both networks (see supplementary Table S1 for the network affiliations of the ROIs). In addition, the coactivation strengths and the resting-state correlation strengths among the 9730 (140 × 139/2) pairs of ROIs showed a strong linear relationship (**Figure 1C**), i.e., if two regions had higher correlation in the resting-state, they also had higher coactivation strength, and vice versa. The Pearson correlation between the coactivation strengths and connectivity strengths was 0.72 ($r^2 = 0.51$).

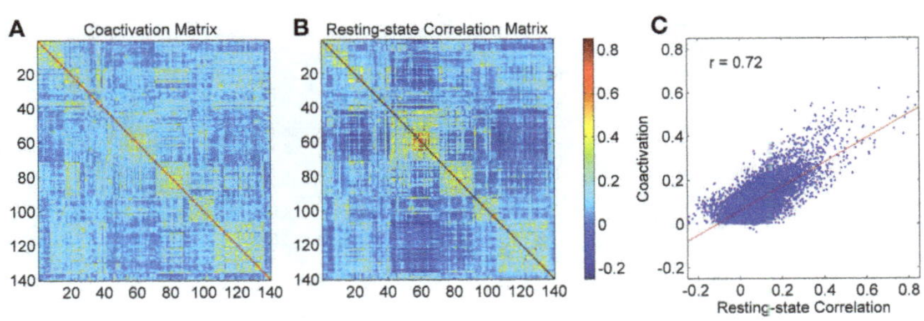

FIGURE 1 | Coactivation matrix (A), resting-state correlation matrix (B), and the relationship between coactivation strengths and resting-state correlations (C). Each dot in the scatter plot represents one pair of ROIs. The red line in panel **(C)** represents the linear fit.

SMALL WORLD AND MODULARITY

Both the coactivation network and the resting-state network revealed smaller global efficiency and larger clustering coefficient compared with the reference random networks, which characterizes the small world network properties (**Figure 2**). Direct comparison between the coactivation network and the resting-state network revealed greater global efficiency and smaller mean clustering coefficient for the coactivation network compared with the resting-state network at selected sparsity levels (highlighted by shading in **Figure 2**). Thresholding at a significance level of $p < 0.001$, greater global efficiency for the coactivation network were present at almost all the sparsity levels that were tested between 6 and 40% (except for 23%), while smaller mean clustering coefficient for the coactivation network were only present at the sparsity level between 28 and 40%.

Both the coactivation network and the resting-state network revealed higher modularity compared with the random networks (**Figure 3A**). The coactivation network generally revealed lower modularity than the resting-state network at sparsity level between 17 and 40% at the significance level of $p < 0.001$. **Figures 3B,C** demonstrated the modular structures of the coactivation network and the resting-state network at sparsity level of 20%. For the resting-state network, four modules were clearly visible with a large number of within module connections and a small number of between modules connections. In contrast, five modules for the coactivation network were difficult to distinguish since there were large numbers of between module connections.

HUB SHIFTS

At all sparsity levels between 6 and 40%, the correlations between node degrees of the coactivation network and the resting-state network were small (range from 0.17 to 0.38) (**Figure 4A**). We then plotted the node degrees of the coactivation network against the node degrees of the resting-state network at 10, 20, and 30% sparsity levels (**Figures 4B–D**). We observed that there were several nodes in the upper right corner or lower right corner of the scatter plots, which indicates that these nodes had higher degrees in one network but not in the other network.

Additional analysis showed that the distribution of degree differences between the coactivation network and the resting-state network were outside the distribution of sorted degree differences

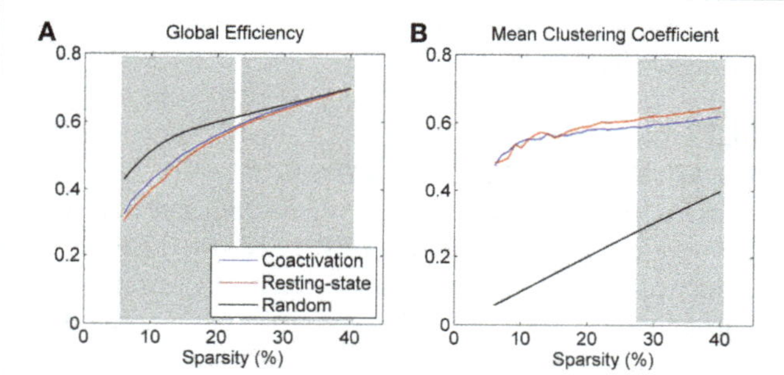

FIGURE 2 | Global efficiency (A) and mean clustering coefficient (B) for the coactivation, resting-state, and random networks as a function of connectivity sparsity. The shading areas represent significant differences between the coactivation and resting-state networks at $p < 0.001$ based on 1000 permutations.

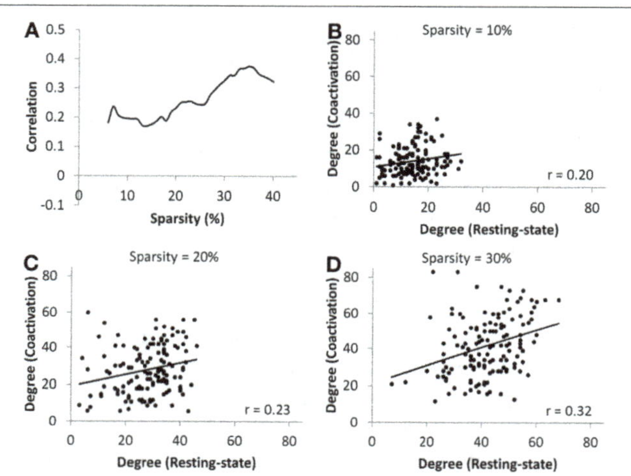

FIGURE 4 | (A) Correlations between nodes' degree of the coactivation network and the resting-state network as a function of connectivity sparsity. Panels **(B–D)** show the scatter plots of node degrees between the two networks at sparsity level of 10% **(B)**, 20% **(C)**, and 30% **(D)**, respectively. The lines in the scatter plots represent the linear fit.

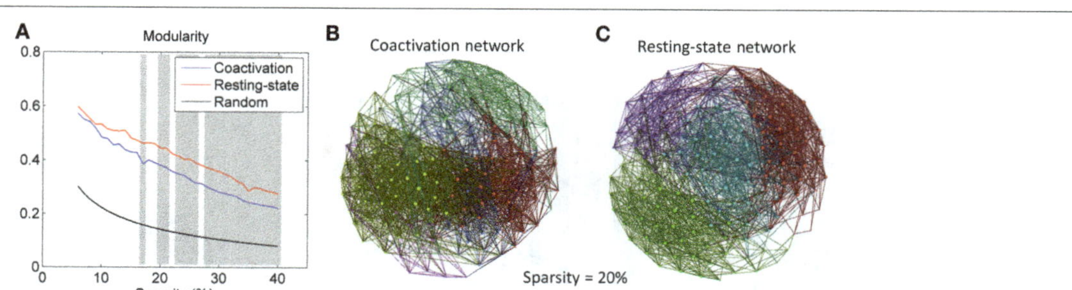

FIGURE 3 | (A) Modularity for the coactivation, resting-state, and random networks as a function of connectivity sparsity. The shading areas represent significant differences between the coactivation and resting-state networks at $p < 0.001$ based on 1000 permutations. Panels **(B,C)** demonstrate the modular structures for the coactivation network and the resting-state network at sparsity level 20%. The node colors in panels B and C encode different modules.

of randomized 1000 permutations (**Figures 5A–C**), indicating that the degree differences between the two networks are not likely due to random noises. We then subtracted the degrees in the activation network by the degrees in the resting-state network for all 140 nodes at sparsity levels of 10, 20, and 30%, respectively. The top five nodes that had the greatest degree differences between the two networks are illustrated in **Figures 5D–F** and **Table 1**. Across the three sparsity levels, the bilateral thalamus demonstrated higher degrees in the coactivation network compared with the resting-state network. Other regions, including the basal ganglia, inferior parietal lobule (IPL), posterior parietal cortex, medial frontal cortex (mFC), and anterior insula, also showed higher degrees in the coactivation network at various sparsity levels. In contrast, a node in the inferior temporal cortex revealed consistently higher degree in the resting-state network compared with the coactivation network. Other regions, including the precuneus, angular gyrus, inferior parietal sulcus (IPS), temporoparietal junction (TPJ), superior frontal cortex, parahippocampal gyrus, and inferior cerebellum, also showed higher degrees in the resting-state network at various sparsity levels. The connectivity of the thalamus and the left inferior cortex for the two networks at sparsity level of 20% are illustrated in **Figure 6**.

DISCUSSION

The current study compared the whole brain network configurations between the coactivation network and the resting-state network. We first observed a high correlation between the coactivation strength and the resting-state correlation across all pairs of ROIs. In other words, if a pair of brain regions has greater functional connectivity in the resting-state, they are more likely to have greater coactivation, and vice versa. This is in line with previous findings that the coactivation patterns correspond well with the resting-state connectivity and networks (Toro et al., 2008; Smith et al., 2009). However, further analysis revealed substantial differences in network configuration between the two networks. Specifically, the coactivation network revealed higher global efficiency, lower mean clustering coefficient, and lower modularity as compared with the resting-state network. Shifts in hub regions were also observed where the thalamus had greater degrees in the coactivation network than in the resting-state network, and a region in the left inferior temporal cortex had greater degrees in the resting-state network than in the coactivation network. These results were similar when using NKI-dataset (see supplementary materials).

The brain network exhibits a so-called "small-world" property (Watts and Strogatz, 1998) that the network has greater mean local efficiency but smaller global efficiency than random network. Small world properties have been initially shown in non-human primates (Sporns, 2000; Stephan et al., 2000) and later in human brain network using both the resting-state fMRI (Salvador et al., 2005; van den Heuvel et al., 2009) and diffusion weighted imaging (Hagmann et al., 2007; Gong et al., 2009). The current results revealed greater global efficiency and smaller mean local efficiency for the coactivation network as compared with the resting-state network, suggesting that the whole brain is connected more efficiently to support global information flow during task performing. These results are in line with the findings that the brain exhibits higher global efficiency as task difficulty increases (Kitzbichler et al., 2011), and in the awake state compared with the stage 1 sleep (Uehara et al., 2013).

The current study also revealed smaller modularity in the coactivation network as compared with the resting-state network. These results suggest that the whole brain is less segregated as independent modules when performing tasks as compared with the resting-state. In other words, there are more between module connections and less within module connections when performing tasks, while more within module connections and less between module connections exist in the resting-state. These results are in line with the economy theory of brain network that long range between system connections are more costly, so that dynamic connectivity between brain systems is only present upon task demands (Bullmore and Sporns, 2012). Consistent with this notion, brain network modularity reduces when the task demand

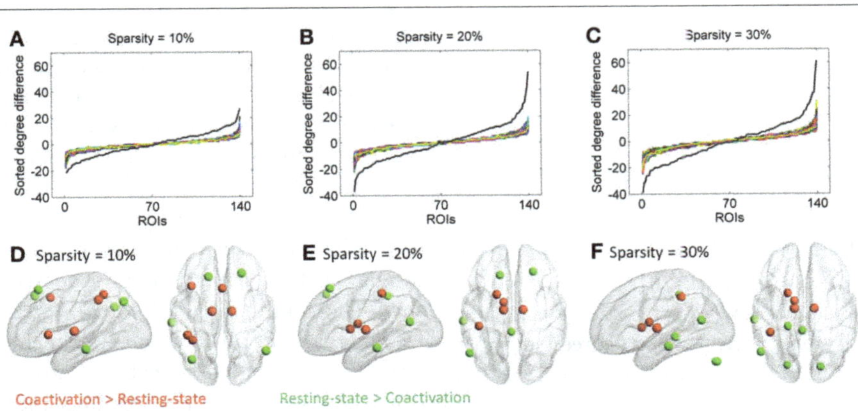

FIGURE 5 | Top row, sorted degree differences of 140 ROIs between the coactivation network and the resting-state network at sparsity of 10% (A), 20% (B), and 30%(C), respectively. The chromatic lines represent sorted degree differences of scrambled networks for 1000 permutations. Bottom row, five regions that have largest and least degree differences between the coactivation network and the resting-state network at sparsity of 10% **(D)**, 20% **(E)**, and 30% **(F)**, respectively.

Table 1 | Top five regions that have greater or smaller degree in the coactivation network as compared with in the resting-state network for the sparsity of 10, 20, and 30%, respectively.

MNI coordinates			Label	Degree differences Coactivation > correlation
x	*y*	*z*		
SPARSITY = 10%				
−12	**−12**	**6**	**Thalamus**	**27**
11	**−12**	**6**	**Thalamus**	**24**
−41	−40	42	IPL	21
−35	−46	48	Post-parietal	18
0	15	45	mFC	16
−36	18	2	Ant insula	16
−16	29	54	Sup frontal	−18
−36	−69	40	IPS	−18
23	33	47	Sup frontal	−19
−59	**−25**	**−15**	**Inf temporal**	**−21**
51	−59	34	Angular gyrus	−21
SPARSITY = 20%				
−12	**−12**	**6**	**Thalamus**	**54**
11	**−12**	**6**	**Thalamus**	**42**
−20	6	7	Basal ganglia	36
−12	−3	13	Thalamus	30
−41	−31	48	Post-parietal	30
23	33	47	Sup frontal	−23
−3	−38	45	Precuneus	−24
−52	−63	15	TPJ	−26
−16	29	54	Sup frontal	−28
−59	**−25**	**−15**	**Inf temporal**	**−37**
SPARSITY = 30%				
−12	**−12**	**6**	**Thalamus**	**61**
11	**−12**	**6**	**Thalamus**	**52**
−12	−3	13	Thalamus	37
−41	−40	42	IPL	37
−20	6	7	Basal ganglia	34
18	−81	−33	Inf cerebellum	−26
−3	−38	45	Precuneus	−26
−21	−79	−33	Inf cerebellum	−26
−52	−63	15	TPJ	−31
−20	−33	−4	Parahippocampal	−31
−59	**−25**	**−15**	**Inf temporal**	**−39**

Regions highlighted in bold represent the regions show consistent differences between the two networks across the three sparsity levels.

increases (Kitzbichler et al., 2011), and in awake state than during non-rapid eye movement sleep (Boly et al., 2012).

In addition to the whole brain network properties, the current study also identified hub regions by calculating degrees (number of connections) for each ROI. In contrast to the high correlation of network strengths between the coactivation network and the resting-state network, the correlations of node degrees between the two networks are small (around 0.3). This suggests a hub shift between task performance and resting-state (Fransson et al., 2011; Achard et al., 2012), which may reflect the adaptive brain reorganization that support the execution of tasks. However, the low correlations of degrees are inconsistent with a previous study showing a high correlation of degrees between a passive fixation condition and a continuous semantic classification task condition (Buckner et al., 2009). The differences may be due to the methodological differences used by Buckner et al. (voxel-wise analysis); the voxel-wise degree distributions are likely to be affected by the underlying brain anatomy, and the high correlation between the two degree maps may partially reflect the anatomical information. In addition, the differences may also be explained by the task adopted by Buckner et al., which is different from the current coactivation approach. Further studies are needed to investigate shifts in hubs elicited by different tasks.

The thalamus regions showed consistently higher degrees (the number of connections with other regions) in the coactivation network as compared with the resting-state network. The thalamus relays visual and auditory information gathered from the eyes and ears to the cerebral cortex (Hotta and Kameda, 1963). Different parts of the thalamus have intensive connections to wide spread cortical regions (Zhang et al., 2008; Eckert et al., 2012). In addition, the thalamus as a relay is important for corticocortical communication, and thus is suggested to be a potential hub for the brain function (Guillery, 1995). Previous resting-state fMRI studies occasionally identified the thalamus as a hub region (van den Heuvel et al., 2008), however, most of studies did not support this view (Achard et al., 2006; Buckner et al., 2009; Yan and He, 2011; Zuo et al., 2012). This may be because the centrality (as measured by degree or eigenvector centrality) of the thalamus is context specific (Lohmann et al., 2010; Gili et al., 2013). This is in line with the present result, and suggests that the thalamus mediates corticocortical communication during task, but this mediation is weakened in the resting-state.

In contrast, the left inferior temporal cortex region revealed higher degree in the resting-state network as compared with the coactivation network. This region is part of the DMN (Raichle et al., 2001; Buckner et al., 2008), which is generally deactivated during tasks (Shulman et al., 1997). Regions that are connected with the left inferior temporal cortex mostly constitute the DMN (**Figure 6D**). Consistent with previous studies of brain centrality (Achard et al., 2006; Buckner et al., 2009), the left inferior temporal cortex showed high centrality in resting-state. But, the current analysis also revealed that the degree is significantly less in the coactivation network. This may reflect the less involvement of this region during tasks as compared with the resting-state (Shulman et al., 1997).

By comparing network configurations of the coactivation network with the resting-state network, the current analysis provides insight on the different brain modes during task and resting-state. The brain during task exhibits greater small-worldness that facilitates global information transmission, and smaller modularity that facilitate information transmission between different systems. These results motivate future studies to investigate brain network configurations in different task conditions. In addition, the current analysis identified the thalamus as a hub region only in the coactivation network but not the resting-state network, suggesting that the role of thalamus in the brain network may be overlooked when studying the resting-state brain network.

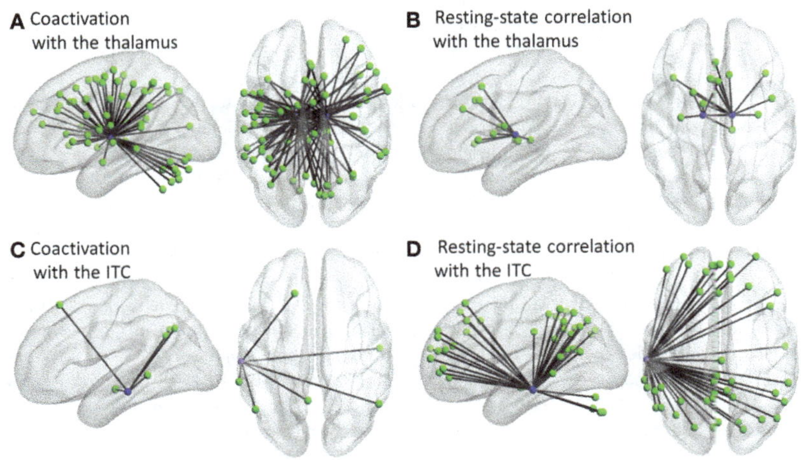

FIGURE 6 | Connectivity of the thalamus (A,B) and left inferior temporal cortex (ITC) (C,D) for the coactivation (A,C) and resting-state correlation (B,D) networks at sparsity of 20%.

A difficulty of studying thalamus connectivity is that the thalamus is spatially heterogeneous, so that different substructures connect to different brain regions (Zhang et al., 2008; Eckert et al., 2012). Future studies may need to use fine spatial scales to investigate the thalamus and its effect on network configurations (Wang et al., 2009; Hayasaka and Laurienti, 2010).

Recently, several efforts have been made to study brain networks using inter-individual covariance from different imaging modalities, for example brain structures (Mechelli et al., 2005; Chen et al., 2008), brain metabolisms (Horwitz et al., 1984; Di et al., 2012), and resting-state brain parameters (Zhang et al., 2011; Taylor et al., 2012). Although these studies provide information on brain integration, the lack of theoretical basis causes difficulty in combining results from different imaging modalities. The current study may provide a theoretical framework to relate the different levels of brain network (e.g., anatomical, metabolic, and hemodynamic) in terms of local/global efficiencies and modular integrations. Future work on systematically comparing different levels of brain network configuration will facilitate in testing theories of brain organization such as the economic theory (Bullmore and Sporns, 2012).

ACKNOWLEDGMENTS

This study was supported by a National Institute of Health grant 5R01AG032088.

REFERENCES

Achard, S., and Bullmore, E. (2007). Efficiency and cost of economical brain functional networks. *PLoS Comput. Biol.* 3:e17. doi: 10.1371/journal.pcbi.0030017

Achard, S., Delon-Martin, C., Vértes, P. E., Renard, F., Schenck, M., Schneider, F., et al. (2012). Hubs of brain functional networks are radically reorganized in comatose patients. *Proc. Natl. Acad. Sci. U.S.A.* 109, 20608–20613. doi: 10.1073/pnas.1208933109

Achard, S., Salvador, R., Whitcher, B., Suckling, J., and Bullmore, E. (2006). A resilient, low-frequency, small-world human brain functional network with highly connected association cortical hubs. *J. Neurosci.* 26, 63–72. doi: 10.1523/JNEUROSCI.3874-05.2006

Beckmann, C. F., DeLuca, M., Devlin, J. T., and Smith, S. M. (2005). Investigations into resting-state connectivity using independent component analysis. *Philos. Trans. R. Soc. Lond. B Biol. Sci.* 360, 1001–1013. doi: 10.1098/rstb.2005.1634

Biswal, B., Yetkin, F. Z., Haughton, V. M., and Hyde, J. S. (1995). Functional connectivity in the motor cortex of resting human brain using echo-planar MRI. *Magn. Reson. Med.* 34, 537–541. doi: 10.1002/mrm.1910340409

Biswal, B. B., Mennes, M., Zuo, X.-N., Gohel, S., Kelly, C., Smith, S. M., et al. (2010). Toward discovery science of human brain function. *Proc. Natl. Acad. Sci. U.S.A.* 107, 4734–4739. doi: 10.1073/pnas.0911855107

Blondel, V. D., Guillaume, J.-L., Lambiotte, R., and Lefebvre, E. (2008). Fast unfolding of communities in large networks. *J. Statis. Mech. Theory Exp.* 2008:P10008. doi: 10.1088/1742-5468/2008/10/P10008

Boly, M., Perlbarg, V., Marrelec, G., Schabus, M., Laureys, S., Doyon, J., et al. (2012). Hierarchical clustering of brain activity during human nonrapid eye movement sleep. *Proc. Natl. Acad. Sci. U.S.A.* 109, 5856–5861. doi: 10.1073/pnas.1111133109

Büchel, C., and Friston, K. J. (1997). Modulation of connectivity in visual pathways by attention: cortical interactions evaluated with structural equation modelling and fMRI. *Cereb. Cortex* 7, 768–778. doi: 10.1093/cercor/7.8.768

Buckner, R. L., Andrews-Hanna, J. R., and Schacter, D. L. (2008). The brain's default network: anatomy, function, and relevance to disease. *Ann. N.Y. Acad. Sci.* 1124, 1–38. doi: 10.1196/annals.1440.011

Buckner, R. L., Sepulcre, J., Talukdar, T., Krienen, F. M., Liu, H., Hedden, T., et al. (2009). Cortical hubs revealed by intrinsic functional connectivity: mapping, assessment of stability, and relation to Alzheimer's disease. *J. Neurosci.* 29, 1860–1873. doi: 10.1523/JNEUROSCI.5062-08.2009

Bullmore, E., and Sporns, O. (2009). Complex brain networks: graph theoretical analysis of structural and functional systems. *Nat. Rev. Neurosci.* 10, 186–198. doi: 10.1038/nrn2575

Bullmore, E., and Sporns, O. (2012). The economy of brain network organization. *Nat. Rev. Neurosci.* 13, 336–349. doi: 10.1038/nrn3214

Chai, X. J., Castañón, A. N., Ongür, D., and Whitfield-Gabrieli, S. (2012). Anticorrelations in resting state networks without global signal regression. *Neuroimage* 59, 1420–1428. doi: 10.1016/j.neuroimage.2011.08.048

Chen, Z. J., He, Y., Rosa-Neto, P., Germann, J., and Evans, A. C. (2008). Revealing modular architecture of human brain structural networks by using cortical thickness from MRI. *Cereb. Cortex* 18, 2374–2381. doi: 10.1093/cercor/bhn003

Cordes, D., Haughton, V. M., Arfanakis, K., Wendt, G. J., Turski, P. A., Moritz, C. H., et al. (2000). Mapping functionally related regions of brain with functional connectivity MR imaging. *Am. J. Neuroradiol.* 21, 1636–1644.

Di, X., Biswal, B. B., and Alzheimer's Disease Neuroimaging Initiative. (2012). Metabolic brain covariant networks as revealed by FDG-PET with reference to resting-state fMRI networks. *Brain Connect.* 2, 275–283. doi: 10.1089/brain.2012.0086

Dosenbach, N. U. F., Nardos, B., Cohen, A. L., Fair, D. A., Power, J. D., Church, J. A., et al. (2010). Prediction of individual brain maturity using fMRI. *Science* 329, 1358–1361. doi: 10.1126/science.1194144

Eckert, U., Metzger, C. D., Buchmann, J. E., Kaufmann, J., Osoba, A., Li, M., et al. (2012). Preferential networks of the mediodorsal nucleus and centromedian-parafascicular complex of the thalamus–a DTI tractography study. *Hum. Brain Mapp.* 33, 2627–2637. doi: 10.1002/hbm.21389

Fransson, P., Aden, U., Blennow, M., and Lagercrantz, H. (2011). The functional architecture of the infant brain as revealed by resting-state fMRI. *Cereb. Cortex* 21, 145–154. doi: 10.1093/cercor/bhq071

Friston, K. J. (2011). Functional and effective connectivity: a review. *Brain Connect.* 1, 13–36. doi: 10.1089/brain.2011.0008

Fruchterman, T. M. J., and Reingold, E. M. (1991). Graph drawing by force-directed placement. *Softw. Pract. Exp.* 21, 1129–1164. doi: 10.1002/spe.4380211102

Gili, T., Saxena, N., Diukova, A., Murphy, K., Hall, J. E., and Wise, R. G. (2013). The thalamus and brainstem act as key hubs in alterations of human brain network connectivity induced by mild propofol sedation. *J. Neurosci.* 33, 4024–4031. doi: 10.1523/JNEUROSCI.3480-12.2013

Gong, G., He, Y., Concha, L., Lebel, C., Gross, D. W., Evans, A. C., et al. (2009). Mapping anatomical connectivity patterns of human cerebral cortex using *in vivo* diffusion tensor imaging tractography. *Cereb. Cortex* 19, 524–536. doi: 10.1093/cercor/bhn102

Greicius, M. D., Krasnow, B., Reiss, A. L., and Menon, V. (2003). Functional connectivity in the resting brain: a network analysis of the default mode hypothesis. *Proc. Natl. Acad. Sci. U.S.A.* 100, 253–258. doi: 10.1073/pnas.0135058100

Guillery, R. W. (1995). Anatomical evidence concerning the role of the thalamus in corticocortical communication: a brief review. *J. Anat.* 187(Pt 3), 583–592.

Hagmann, P., Kurant, M., Gigandet, X., Thiran, P., Wedeen, V. J., Meuli, R., et al. (2007). Mapping human whole-brain structural networks with diffusion MRI. *PLoS ONE* 2:e597. doi: 10.1371/journal.pone.0000597

Hayasaka, S., and Laurienti, P. J. (2010). Comparison of characteristics between region-and voxel-based network analyses in resting-state fMRI data. *Neuroimage* 50, 499–508. doi: 10.1016/j.neuroimage.2009.12.051

He, Y., Chen, Z., and Evans, A. (2008). Structural insights into aberrant topological patterns of large-scale cortical networks in Alzheimer's disease. *J. Neurosci.* 28, 4756–4766. doi: 10.1523/JNEUROSCI.0141-08.2008

Horwitz, B., Duara, R., and Rapoport, S. I. (1984). Intercorrelations of glucose metabolic rates between brain regions: application to healthy males in a state of reduced sensory input. *J. Cereb. Blood Flow Metab.* 4, 484–499. doi: 10.1038/jcbfm.1984.73

Hotta, T., and Kameda, K. (1963). Interactions between somatic and visual or auditory responses in the thalamus of the cat. *Exp. Neurol.* 8, 1–13. doi: 10.1016/0014-4886(63)90003-7

Kitzbichler, M. G., Henson, R. N. A., Smith, M. L., Nathan, P. J., and Bullmore, E. T. (2011). Cognitive effort drives workspace configuration of human brain functional networks. *J. Neurosci.* 31, 8259–8270. doi: 10.1523/JNEUROSCI.0440-11.2011

Lohmann, G., Margulies, D. S., Horstmann, A., Pleger, B., Lepsien, J., Goldhahn, D., et al. (2010). Eigenvector centrality mapping for analyzing connectivity patterns in fMRI data of the human brain. *PLoS ONE* 5:e10232. doi: 10.1371/journal.pone.0010232

McIntosh, A., Grady, C., Ungerleider, L., Haxby, J., Rapoport, S., and Horwitz, B. (1994). Network analysis of cortical visual pathways mapped with PET. *J. Neurosci.* 14, 655–666.

McLntosh, A. R., and Gonzalez-Lima, F. (1994). Structural equation modeling and its application to network analysis in functional brain imaging. *Hum. Brain Mapp.* 2, 2–22. doi: 10.1002/hbm.460020104

Mechelli, A., Friston, K. J., Frackowiak, R. S., and Price, C. J. (2005). Structural covariance in the human cortex. *J. Neurosci.* 25, 8303–8310. doi: 10.1523/JNEUROSCI.0357-05.2005

Menon, V., and Uddin, L. Q. (2010). Saliency, switching, attention and control: a network model of insula function. *Brain Struct. Funct.* 214, 655–667. doi: 10.1007/s00429-010-0262-0

Nakamura, T., Hillary, F. G., and Biswal, B. B. (2009). Resting network plasticity following brain injury. *PLoS ONE* 4:e8220. doi: 10.1371/journal.pone.0008220

Newman, M. E. J. (2006). Modularity and community structure in networks. *Proc. Natl. Acad. Sci. U.S.A.* 103, 8577–8582. doi: 10.1073/pnas.0601602103

Raichle, M. E. (2010). Two views of brain function. *Trends Cogn. Sci.* 14, 180–190. doi: 10.1016/j.tics.2010.01.008

Raichle, M. E., MacLeod, A. M., Snyder, A. Z., Powers, W. J., Gusnard, D. A., and Shulman, G. L. (2001). A default mode of brain function. *Proc. Natl. Acad. Sci. U.S.A.* 98, 676–682. doi: 10.1073/pnas.98.2.676

Rao, H., Di, X., Chan, R. C. K., Ding, Y., Ye, B., and Gao, D. (2008). A regulation role of the prefrontal cortex in the fist-edge-palm task: evidence from functional connectivity analysis. *Neuroimage* 41, 1345–1351. doi: 10.1016/j.neuroimage.2008.04.026

Rubinov, M., and Sporns, O. (2010). Complex network measures of brain connectivity: uses and interpretations. *Neuroimage* 52, 1059–1069. doi: 10.1016/j.neuroimage.2009.10.003

Sabatinelli, D., Fortune, E. E., Li, Q., Siddiqui, A., Krafft, C., Oliver, W. T., et al. (2011). Emotional perception: meta-analyses of face and natural scene processing. *Neuroimage* 54, 2524–2533. doi: 10.1016/j.neuroimage.2010.10.011

Salvador, R., Suckling, J., Coleman, M. R., Pickard, J. D., Menon, D., and Bullmore, E. (2005). Neurophysiological architecture of functional magnetic resonance images of human brain. *Cereb. Cortex* 15, 1332–1342. doi: 10.1093/cercor/bhi016

Shulman, G. L., Fiez, J. A., Corbetta, M., Buckner, R. L., Miezin, F. M., Raichle, M. E., et al. (1997). Common blood flow changes across visual tasks: II. decreases in cerebral cortex. *J. Cogn. Neurosci.* 9, 648–663. doi: 10.1162/jocn.1997.9.5.648

Smith, S. M., Fox, P. T., Miller, K. L., Glahn, D. C., Fox, P. M., Mackay, C. E., et al. (2009). Correspondence of the brain's functional architecture during activation and rest. *Proc. Natl. Acad. Sci. U.S.A.* 106, 13040–13045. doi: 10.1073/pnas.0905267106

Sporns, O. (2000). Theoretical neuroanatomy: relating anatomical and functional connectivity in graphs and cortical connection matrices. *Cereb. Cortex* 10, 127–141. doi: 10.1093/cercor/10.2.127

Stephan, K. E., Hilgetag, C. C., Burns, G. A., O'Neill, M. A., Young, M. P., and Kötter, R. (2000). Computational analysis of functional connectivity between areas of primate cerebral cortex. *Philos. Trans. R. Soc. Lond. B Biol. Sci.* 355, 111–126.

Taylor, P. A., Gohel, S., Di, X., Walter, M., and Biswal, B. B. (2012). Functional covariance networks: obtaining resting-state networks from intersubject variability. *Brain Connect.* 2, 203–217. doi: 10.1089/brain.2012.0095

Toro, R., Fox, P. T., and Paus, T. (2008). Functional coactivation map of the human brain. *Cereb. Cortex* 18, 2553–2559. doi: 10.1093/cercor/bhn014

Uehara, T., Yamasaki, T., Okamoto, T., Koike, T., Kan, S., Miyauchi, S., et al. (2013). Efficiency of a "small-world" brain network depends on consciousness level: a resting-state fmri study. *Cereb. Cortex.* doi: 10.1093/cercor/bht004. [Epub ahead of print].

van den Heuvel, M. P., Stam, C. J., Boersma, M., and Hulshoff Pol, H. E. (2008). Small-world and scale-free organization of voxel-based resting-state functional connectivity in the human brain. *Neuroimage* 43, 528–539. doi: 10.1016/j.neuroimage.2008.08.010

van den Heuvel, M. P., Stam, C. J., Kahn, R. S., and Hulshoff Pol, H. E. (2009). Efficiency of functional brain networks and intellectual performance. *J. Neurosci.* 29, 7619–7624. doi: 10.1523/JNEUROSCI.1443-09.2009

Wang, J., Wang, L., Zang, Y., Yang, H., Tang, H., Gong, Q., et al. (2009). Parcellation-dependent small-world brain functional networks: a resting-state fMRI study. *Hum. Brain Mapp.* 30, 1511–1523. doi: 10.1002/hbm.20623

Wang, J., Zuo, X., and He, Y. (2010). Graph-based network analysis of resting-state functional MRI. *Front. Syst. Neurosci.* 4:16. doi: 10.3389/fnsys.2010.00016

Watts, D. J., and Strogatz, S. H. (1998). Collective dynamics of "small-world" networks. *Nature* 393, 440–442. doi: 10.1038/30918

Yan, C., and He, Y. (2011). Driving and driven architectures of directed small-world human brain functional networks. *PLoS ONE* 6:e23460. doi: 10.1371/journal.pone.0023460

Yarkoni, T., Poldrack, R. A., Nichols, T. E., Van Essen, D. C., and Wager, T. D. (2011). Large-scale automated synthesis of human functional neuroimaging data. *Nat. Methods* 8, 665–670. doi: 10.1038/nmeth.1635

Zhang, D., Snyder, A. Z., Fox, M. D., Sansbury, M. W., Shimony, J. S., and Raichle, M. E. (2008). Intrinsic functional relations between human cerebral cortex and thalamus. *J. Neurophysiol.* 100, 1740–1748. doi: 10.1152/jn.90463.2008

Zhang, Z., Liao, W., Zuo, X.-N., Wang, Z., Yuan, C., Jiao, Q., et al. (2011). Resting-state brain organization revealed by functional covariance networks. *PLoS ONE* 6:e28817. doi: 10.1371/journal.pone.0028817

Zuo, X.-N., Ehmke, R., Mennes, M., Imperati, D., Castellanos, F. X., Sporns, O., et al. (2012). Network centrality in the human functional connectome. *Cereb. Cortex* 22, 1862–1875. doi: 10.1093/cercor/bhr269

10

Parcellation of the cingulate cortex at rest and during tasks: A meta-analytic clustering and experimental study

Diana M. E. Torta[1,2]*, Tommaso Costa[1,2], Sergio Duca[2], Peter T. Fox[3] and Franco Cauda[1,2]

[1] *Department of Psychology, Università di Torino, Torino, Italy*
[2] *CCS fMRI-Brain Connectivity and Complex Systems Unit, Koelliker Hospital, Torino, Italy*
[3] *Research Imaging Institute, University of Texas Health Science Center at San Antonio, San Antonio, TX, USA*

Correspondence:
Diana M. E. Torta, Department of Psychology, Università di Torino, Via Po 14, 10123 Turin, Italy
e-mail: diana.torta@unito.it

Anatomical, morphological, and histological data have consistently shown that the cingulate cortex can be divided into four main regions. However, less is known about parcellations of the cingulate cortex when involved in active tasks. Here, we aimed at comparing how the pattern of clusterization of the cingulate cortex changes across different levels of task complexity. We parcellated the cingulate cortex using the results of a meta-analytic study and of three experimental studies. The experimental studies, which included two active tasks and a resting state protocol, were used to control the results obtained with the meta-analytic parcellation. We explored the meta-analytic parcellation by applying a meta-analytic clustering (MaC) to papers retrieved from the BrainMap database. The MaC is a meta-analytic connectivity driven parcellation technique recently developed by our group which allowed us to parcellate the cingulate cortex on the basis of its pattern of co-activations during active tasks. The MaC results indicated that the cingulate cortex can be parcellated into three clusters. These clusters covered different percentages of the cingulate parenchyma and had a different density of foci, with the first cluster being more densely connected. The control experiments showed different clusterization results, suggesting that the co-activations of the cingulate cortex are highly dependent on the task that is tested. Our results highlight the importance of the cingulate cortex as a hub, which modifies its pattern of co-activations depending on the task requests and on the level of task complexity. The neurobiological meaning of these results is discussed.

Keywords: meta-analytic clustering, voxel-based meta-analysis, meta-analytic connectivity modeling, activation likelihood estimation, data driven parcellation, k-means clustering, hierarchical clustering, voronoi parcellation

INTRODUCTION

The cingulate cortex is the thick part of the cerebral cortex surrounding the corpus callosum and is currently thought to be made up of four subregions (the four-region neurobiological model): The anterior cingulate cortex, which includes the perigenual cingulate cortex, the midcingulate cortex, the posterior cingulate cortex and the restrosplenial cingulate cortex (Vogt, 2009). Such four major subdivisions were built mainly on structural observations (Vogt and Pandya, 1987; Vogt et al., 1987, 1992, 2001, 2003; Vogt and Derbyshire, 2002; Vogt and Vogt, 2003; Vogt and Laureys, 2005; Fan et al., 2008; Palomero-Gallagher et al., 2008, 2009; Vogt, 2009) and were proposed to subserve specific functions, with the anterior cingulate cortex involved in affective evaluation (Allman et al., 2001), conflict monitoring (Carter et al., 1998, 1999; Botvinick et al., 2004), error monitoring and detection (Holroyd et al., 1998; Gehring and Knight, 2000; Gehring and Fencsik, 2001), response selection (Paus et al., 1993; Awh and Gehring, 1999) and attention control (Posner and Dehaene, 1994; Crottaz-Herbette and Menon, 2006); the midcingulate cortex involved in cognitive tasks such as attention for action (Pardo et al., 1990; Badgaiyan and Posner, 1998), response selection (Corbetta et al., 1991; Paus et al., 1993), error detection and competition monitoring (Carter et al., 1998), anticipation (Murtha et al., 1996), and working memory (Petit et al., 1998); the posterior cingulate cortex in tasks related to visuospatial orientation and navigation of the body in environmental space (Vogt and Laureys, 2005), self-reflection and autobiographical memory (Spreng et al., 2009); and finally, the retrosplenial cingulate cortex in memory and visuospatial functions (Vogt and Pandya, 1987; Vogt et al., 1987; Parker and Gaffan, 1997; Burgess et al., 2001; Vogt, 2005; Iaria et al., 2007; Keene and Bucci, 2008; Vann et al., 2009). Until recently this "segregationist model," for which each portion of the cingulate cortex subserves specific functions, has been adopted.

Recent studies have used magnetic resonance imaging (MRI) or functional MRI (fMRI) to investigate the connectivity based parcellation of the cingulate cortex. Beckmann and colleagues (2009) used probabilistic diffusion tractography (a measure of anatomical connectivity), to characterize the cingulate probabilistic connectivity. By applying a connectivity-based parcellation, they found nine distinct clusters in the cingulate cortex

Abbreviations: MaC, Meta-analytic clustering; fMRI, Functional magnetic resonance imaging; ROI, Region of interest; MACM, Meta-analytic connectivity modeling; ALE, Activation likelihood estimation.

(Beckmann et al., 2009). Yu and colleagues investigated the functional connectivity of each of the subregions proposed in the four-region model and showed that each subregion was characterized by a specific pattern of functional connectivity (Yu et al., 2011). This finding led the authors to conclude that the anatomical segregation is confirmed by functional segregation (Margulies et al., 2007; Yu et al., 2011). While the functional connectivity of some specific subregions of the cingulate cortex during rest has been progressively disclosed (Koski and Paus, 2000; Margulies et al., 2007; Yu et al., 2011), to date far less is known about the functional profile and the parcellation of the cingulate cortex during tasks.

The advent of databases such as BrainMap (Fox et al., 2005; Laird et al., 2005a,b, 2009a,b), which stores thousands of fMRI experiments together with their results, has allowed performing the so-called voxel-based meta-analyses. Using these databases, many different studies can be pooled together to investigate the functional properties of specific brain regions when involved in active tasks. As a result of this approach, recent views have proposed that the same subregions of the cingulate cortex are involved in different functions ("integrationist model"). For example, Shackman and colleagues (2011) observed that in the rostral anterior cingulate cortex, pain, affect, and cognition overlap. Similarly, Torta and Cauda (2011) have reported that the midcingulate cortex is recruited in a variety of tasks ranging from pain to affect to attention and motor tasks.

Altogether these findings suggest that fMRI parcellations of the cingulate cortex lead to different results depending on the methodological approach. In addition, it has been shown that high-dimensional parcellations support the view of a hierarchical nested structure within the hub regions of the brain (Leech et al., 2011). Here, we aimed at comparing how the pattern of clusterization of the cingulate cortex changes across different levels of task complexity (i.e., tasks and non-tasks such as resting state). We performed a meta-analytic study using a meta-analytic tool recently developed by our group: the meta-analytic clustering (MaC) (Cauda et al., 2012). This method permits a voxel-wise data-driven clusterization of the patterns of co-activation of the cingulate cortex during the widest number of active tasks (Cauda et al., 2012). This technique starts from the meta-analytic data and produces a meta-analytic connectivity-based parcellation in a data-driven fashion (Torta and Cauda, 2011). We verified the results of the MaC study by performing three additional fMRI experiments on healthy volunteers. In this way we could observe possible modifications of the parcellation of the cingulate cortex during the widest number of active tasks, during specific tasks and during resting state.

For the control fMRI experiments, we scanned participants during resting state (experiment 2), during the presentation of emotional faces (experiment 3) and during the administration of painful stimuli (experiment 4). These latter two tasks were chosen as known to activate the cingulate cortex (Apkarian et al., 2005; Friebel et al., 2011). Subsequently we parcellated the cingulate cortex on the basis of the results of the two experiments and compared such findings to those obtained with the meta-analytic parcellation.

MATERIALS AND METHODS

META-ANALYTIC STUDY

Database search

We queried the BrainMap database (Fox et al., 2005; Laird et al., 2005a,b, 2009a,b) for studies on healthy volunteers that recorded activations in the cingulate cortex. We did not select studies on the basis of the task performed as we were interested in investigating activations of the cingulate cortex in a broad range of cognitive tasks. Such a choice allowed us to characterize the parcellation of the cingulate cortex in a "working mode" irrespective of the task. The results of this search were saved in a series of files containing locations, papers and behavioral domains. For the meta-analysis, boundaries of the cingulate cortex were already coded in BrainMap, indeed we queried the database for all the papers that showed at least one focus in the cingulate cortex (http://www.brainmap.org/sleuth/). For subsequent analyses on in-house acquired fMRI data, the volume of interest (VOI) around the cingulate cortex was drawn by one of the authors (Franco Cauda), expert in neuroanatomical clustering, on the Colin 27 template (http://neuro.debian.net/pkgs/mni-colin27nifti.html) at the group level. The MNI cingulate coordinates were then converted to Talairach coordinates using the icbm2Tal transform (http://brainmap.org/icbm2tal/).

META-ANALYTIC CLUSTERING (MaC)

Data preparation

Here, we employed a methodology called MaC, delineated in a recent paper (Cauda et al., 2012). MaC works on meta-analytic connectivity modeling data (MACM; Robinson et al., 2010). Thus, as a first step, we performed a MACM. The MACM method is based on co-occurrences that are evaluated using the ALE approach. With a too small number of co-occurrences (i.e., foci) the ALE results are too dependent on the contribution of single foci (i.e., single studies) and are spatially very variable. As a consequence of this variability the parcellation results are unstable. Indeed the ALE method needs a minimum number of foci to produce a valid estimate (Laird et al., 2005a, 2009a; Eickhoff et al., 2009). To accomplish this need we created, in a completely unsupervised data-driven way, "blocks" of voxels each containing 50 foci.

The choice of 50 foci was supported by a simulation to evaluate the stability of the parcellation results using 10–100 foci in steps of 10. We parcellated the cingulate surface using blocks of different dimensions (namely with a different number of foci). For each dimension we repeated the entire process 100 times. We then checked the reliability of the results for each step evaluating if the results were stable for a given number of foci. The results were stable with blocks of $n > 40$ foci (see also Cauda et al., 2012) so we decided to opt for a minimum number of 50 foci as to further improve the stability obtained with 40 foci. We created blocks of voxels by employing the quad tree algorithm (Ballard and Brown, 1982). The quad tree is an algorithm that subdivides the two-dimensional space by decomposing the region into four equal quadrants and subsequently into four further subquadrants until each of the subquadrants contains the pre-defined number of foci (50 in our case). Thus, when the blocks meet the criterion, they are not subdivided further. In contrast, if more than 50 foci are found in a block, the algorithm further subdivides the block until the criterion of homogeneity is reached. As a result, we obtained 37 blocks containing 50 foci each but having different sizes. The quad tree decomposition returns a structure consisting of the y and z Talairach coordinates of each block and the corresponding papers in which Talairach coordinates of the foci appear. All parcellations were performed on a 3D mesh. To build the 3D mesh, a constant gray matter (GM) thickness was assumed, to allow subsequent methods to operate in 2D. Indeed, the 3D data from the database were projected to a plane passing through the coordinates $X = 0$ and then analyzed. For visualization purposes these data were back projected to a renderized brain surface on the basis of each voxel's original coordinate. All foci were projected within $+1$ and -5 mm from the GM plane to this surface. All these clustering analyses were performed using custom developed MATLAB scripts (Mathworks, Natick, MA, USA).

We calculated the MACM using the ALE algorithm (Laird et al., 2005a; Eickhoff et al., 2009) to pool the active foci of each quad tree. Each coordinate (focus) was modeled by a 3-D Gaussian distribution, defined by a full-width half-maximum (FWHM) of 10 mm (Turkeltaub et al., 2002). The ALE statistic was computed at every voxel in the brain. We made a valid assessment of the significance of the result by testing the values from the ALE images against null distributions. A threshold was applied, while controlling the false discovery rate (FDR) (Genovese et al., 2002) at a significance level of $p < 0.05$. Importantly, the ALE algorithm has been formulated to limit the inter-subject and inter-laboratory variability typical of neuroimaging studies. This algorithm estimates the spatial uncertainty of each focus and takes into account the possible differences among studies, as to avoid that single studies may drive the results.

We subdivided the cingulate cortex into areas with homogeneous co-activations by employing two kinds of cluster analysis (Cauda et al., 2010; Frades and Matthiesen, 2010): Hierarchical and k-means clustering and using as input the results of ALE analysis (MACM). Hierarchical clustering groups data over a variety of scales by creating a cluster tree; trees represent multilevel hierarchies where clusters at one level are joined as clusters at the next level. Importantly, hierarchical clustering does not require a priori impositions on the number of clusters and by creating the dendrogram it allows the visualization of the hierarchy within the data. The advantage of the hierarchical clustering is that it can handle different forms of similarity or distance. A distance matrix is the only requirement for hierarchical clustering. Furthermore, hierarchical clustering allows an embedded flexibility regarding the level of granularity; that is, the extent to which an entity is divided in smaller parts. We used the hierarchical clustering as we were interested in visualizing the hierarchical structure of the data. To verify the goodness of the hierarchical clustering we used the cophenetic distance. This measure describes how well the cluster tree reflects the data for different distance measures and allows to verify the consistency of each link. This method, together with the visual inspection of the dendrogram and the reordered distance matrix, represents a way to find the optimal number of clusters of the data (Ward, 1963). The matrix was composed of rows, representing the blocks formed by the quad tree algorithm, and columns representing the probability of activation obtained by the ALE analysis of each voxel in the brain. The data matrix was used to create the distance matrix. There are different criteria to evaluate the distances between clusters in the hierarchical clustering literature. In this case, we employed the Ward method that uses an analysis of variance approach (Ward, 1963). Subsequently, we employed the k-mean clustering to assess the results using as input the number of clusters obtained from the techniques described above.

Unlike hierarchical clustering, k-means operates on actual observations and creates a single level of clusters. K-means is a partition method in which objects are classified as belonging to one or k groups with k chosen a priori. The cluster membership is determined by calculating the centroid for each group and assigning each object to the group with the closest centroid. This approach minimizes the overall dispersion within cluster by operating an iterative reallocation of cluster members. Advantages of this methods are its time and space complexity and its order-independent properties. Order independency means that k-means generates the same partition of the data irrespective of the order in which patterns are presented.

The results of the k-means clustering were further verified using the average silhouette values (Rousseeuw, 1987). To calculate the hemisphere prevalence, for each cluster we overimposed the clusterization results of the left and the right cingulate cortex. Areas pertaining to the left cingulate cortex were colored in green, areas pertaining to the right cingulate cortex were colored in orange. Areas of overlap of the clusterization results of both sides were colored in red.

DENSITY ANALYSIS

We observed that voxels in the cingulate cortex were unequally activated by tasks. That is, the activation of some voxels was more frequent and some regions of the cingulate cortex were found to be characterized by a wider number of active voxels. In order to substantiate this observation, we performed a density analysis of the active foci in the cingulate cortex. This was done in order to obtain a deterministic method to calculate the density of foci. We decided not to use ALE for this aim because it modifies the probability kernel including information such as the number of subjects. In this way results are not exactly a measure of density of foci. For density, we intended the number of foci per unit of area. In order to analytically calculate the number of foci per unit per area, we used the Voronoi tessellation algorithm (Klein, 1989). A Voronoi tessellation is a decomposition of metric space by distances between sets of points. The Voronoi algorithm tessellates a surface into polygons in such a way that the area of each polygon is inversely proportional to the density of points (foci) in that area.

NETWORK ANALYSIS

It has been suggested that some portions of the cingulate cortex may act as hubs interconnecting different networks (Leech et al., 2011). Graph analysis techniques allow the investigation of how complex brain networks relate to each other (Bullmore and Sporns, 2009), therefore resulting particularly suitable for inspecting the presence of hub areas. Graph and network analyses build graphs of elements in such a way that the position of an element in the graph reflects its relationship with neighboring elements.

We reordered the distance matrix so as to place more edges closer to the diagonal. Reordering was performed using a routine of the Brain Connectivity Toolbox that minimizes the cost function of the matrix (Rubinov and Sporns, 2010). Then, using the data in the reordered distance matrix, we constructed a network and we optimally represented the results employing a force-directed algorithm: the Fruchterman-Reingold method (Fruchterman and Reingold, 1991). In this algorithm, the nodes are represented by steel rings and the edges are springs between them. The attractive force is analogous to the spring force and the repulsive force is analogous to the electrical force. The basic idea is to minimize the energy of the system by moving the nodes and changing the forces between them. A threshold was applied to the resulting image so that only the circles (blocks) with highest network connectivity (first quartile) were represented as color-filled.

EXPERIMENTS 2–4

We also performed three additional experiments on healthy volunteers.

PARTICIPANTS

We scanned two groups of healthy volunteers. The first group was composed of 10 right-handed adults (five females) (mean age = 22 ± 1.4) who participated in the resting state experiment (experiment 2) and in the experiment in which emotional faces were shown (experiment 3). The second group was composed of 17 healthy right-handed volunteers (eight females, mean age 28 ± 4.2) who participated in the experiment in which painful stimuli were applied to the hands (experiment 3). All of the participants were free of neurological or psychiatric disorders, not taking medications known to alter brain activity, and with no history of drug or alcohol abuse. We obtained the written informed consent of each subject, in accordance with the Declaration of Helsinki. The studies were approved by the institutional committee on ethical use of human subjects at the University of Turin.

TASKS AND ACQUISITION

Experiment 2—Resting state

The first group performed a 6-minute resting state task. During the resting state scan, participants were asked to relax, to not fall asleep and to not think of anything in particular while they were being scanned.

Experiment 3—Faces expressing emotions

The same 10 participants took part in an experiment in which faces expressing different emotions were shown to them while lying in the scanner. The stimuli consisted of faces showing anger, disgust, fear, happiness, sadness, and neutral expressions. The faces were taken from Biehl et al. (1997). A total of four Caucasian actors (two males and two females) showing both emotional and neutral expressions were used for a total of 24 images (six conditions × four actors). The task scans consisted of four runs of a slow event-related design. Each run consisted of 24 stimuli, four for each emotional and neutral condition, presented in random order. The subjects were instructed to look passively at the faces.

Experiment 4—Painful stimuli

The second group participated in a task in which painful mechanical stimuli were delivered to the hands. Painful mechanical stimuli were delivered with a 256 mN pinprick probe which activates the high-threshold mechanoreceptors (Baumgartner et al., 2010). During the four runs of this slow event-related design, the participants received a total of 48 stimuli on the left and right hand (no more than three consecutive stimuli on the same hand). They were instructed to relax, pay attention to the stimuli and report a subjective rating of intensity at the end of each block.

Data acquisition

Data acquisition was performed on a 1.5 Tesla INTERA™ scanner (Philips Medical Systems) with a SENSE high-field, high resolution (MRIDC) head coil that was optimized for functional imaging. The functional T2*-weighted images were acquired using echoplanar (EPI) sequences, with a repetition time (TR) of 2000 ms, an echo time (TE) of 50 ms, and a 90° flip angle. The acquisition matrix was 64 × 64, and the field of view (FoV) 200 mm. A total of 200 volumes were acquired; each volume consisted of 19 axial slices, parallel to the anterior-posterior (AC-PC) commissure line and covering the whole brain; slice thickness was 4.5 mm with a 0.5 mm gap. Two scans were added at the beginning of the functional scanning and the data were discarded to reach a steady-state magnetization before acquiring the experimental data.

In the same session, a set of three-dimensional high-resolution T_1-weighted structural images was acquired for each participant. This data-set was acquired using a Fast Field Echo (FFE) sequence, with a TR of 25 ms, ultra-short TE, and a 30° flip angle. The acquisition matrix was 256 × 256, and the field of view (FoV) 256 mm. The set consisted of 160 contiguous sagittal images covering the whole brain. In-plane resolution was 1 × 1 mm and slice thickness 1 mm (1 × 1 × 1 mm voxels).

ANALYSIS

The data were pre-processed using slice scan time correction, 3D motion correction, spatial smoothing (4 mm FWHM) and temporal filters (linear trend removal and band pass filter of 0.008–0.08 Hz).

After pre-processing, voxels belonging to the cingulate cortex were submitted to a voxel-wise unsupervised fuzzy c-mean clustering technique (Cauda et al., 2010, 2013). This data-driven method decomposes the original fMRI time series into a predefined number of spatiotemporal modes, which include a spatial map and an associated cluster centroid time course. The extent to which a voxel belongs to a cluster is defined by the similarity (as measured, e.g., by correlation) of its time course to the cluster centroid. We used this clusterization approach as it has been previously optimized for resting state and MACM (Cauda et al., 2010, 2011b).

We used two clustering approaches to compare the complexity of clustering of the MaC data to that of the experimental tasks.

First, we imposed the same number of clusters obtained for the MaC to the in-house acquired datasets. Second, we calculated the number of clusters of the experimental data without imposing the results of the MaC.

VALIDATION OF CLUSTERING PROCEDURES

We used the upper tail rule developed by Mojena to validate the number of clusters (Mojena, 1977). Statistical stopping rules for clustering methods allow selecting the "best" number of clusters in the data. Stopping rules define explicitly what is meant by a significant change in the clustering criterion. That is, these rules help define when a further partition is not necessary. The method developed by Mojena (1977) uses the relative sizes of the fusion level in the hierarchy. The algorithm selects the partition associated to the first level in the cluster number sequence which satisfies the following condition:

$$Zj + 1 > m + ksz$$

where m is the mean of the fusion level of the previous fusion level, sz is the standard deviation of those values, and k is the standard deviate. The knee of the curve of the cluster sequence is an indicator of the right number of clusters. In simple words, this method takes the distance matrix and calculates the types of aggregation by calculating mean and standard deviation of the number of nodes as a function of the imposed clusters. Then the knee is calculated as a second derivative of the curve. The peak that is obtained represents the "optimal" number of clusters according to the stopping criterion.

RESULTS

DATABASE SEARCH

The BrainMap query retrieved 1240 papers involving 24,540 subjects and a total of 1851 foci (see Table S1).

MACM CLUSTERING

The results of the dendrogram obtained from the hierarchical clustering suggested that the cingulate cortex can be optimally parcellated into three clusters (see **Figures 1**, **2**). The same result was confirmed by the silhouette plot. The silhouette plot is a measure of how close each point in one cluster is to points in the neighboring clusters. This method allows to understand of how well-separated the resulting clusters are.

We used the k-means method to cluster the MACM blocks into the three clusters as previously identified. To minimize the risk of inconsistent results obtained for the initial random placement of starting points, the k-means was computed 256 times (Nanetti et al., 2009). The same three clusters were identified all 256 times.

The results of the MaC evidenced that Cluster 1 covers 7% of the cingulate surface and is located in the dorsal anterior cingulate cortex (dACC). Cluster 2 covers 30% of the total cingulate surface, being predominantly located in the intermediate part of the cingulate cortex but also presenting two small locations in the anterior and posterior cingulate cortex. Cluster 3 covers 63% of the cingulate surface, encompassing the posterior but also the anterior parts of the cingulate cortex, and also presenting a small location in the midcingulate area (**Figures 2**, **3**).

Figure 4 shows the mean MACM connectivity of the three clusters. Our results indicate that cluster 1 is functionally connected to the parietal cortices (the inferior parietal lobe BA 40, the superior parietal lobe BA 7), frontal cortices (superior and middle frontal gyri BA 9, 10) and to some sensory (primary somatosensory cortices BA 2, 3) and motor (primary and premotor areas BA 4 and 6) areas. In addition, this cluster shows connections to the temporal lobe (superior and middle temporal gyri BA 21, 22, 39) and is slightly left lateralized in the anterior cingulate cortex and slightly right lateralized in the posterior cingulate cortex. Cluster 2 is co-active with the inferior, middle and superior frontal gyri (BA 45, 9, and 10), the parietal cortex (BA 7, 40, 43), and the temporal lobe (BA 37, 39). Moreover this cluster presents a strong co-activation with subcortical structures such as the thalamus, the red nucleus, and the caudate. This cluster is also characterized by a right-prevalence of activations in the posterior cingulate cortex. Cluster 3 is characterized by a more frontal and limbic functional connectivity which includes the superior and middle frontal gyri (BA 9 and 10) and hippocampal and parahippocampal structures. All three clusters are extensively co-active with other portions of the cingulate cortex and with the insula (see **Figure 4** and Tables S2–S4).

The probabilistic map (**Figure 5**) shows that the highest overlap between all the block-related MACM maps is in the anterior insula, dorsal cingulate cortex, dorsolateral prefrontal cortices, sensorimotor, precuneal, and posterior parietal cortices.

The lower part of **Figure 1** represents the network derived from the distance between blocks of the cingulate cortex. The points represent blocks and are coded with a color indicating the cluster to which they belong. In this image the distance between points represents the Euclidean distance between the MACM maps of each block. The network representation is optimized using multidimensional scaling. Points belonging to cluster 1 are centrally located and surrounded by points belonging to clusters 2 and 3. This method rearranges multidimensional entities in a 2D space such that the distance represents the similarity. In this way, similar entities are closer in space whereas dissimilar entities are placed apart.

The same finding was confirmed by the results presented in **Figure 6**, which shows the network representation of the Euclidean distances between blocks. Here the graphical network representation is optimized with the Fruchterman–Reingold method. The color-filled circles display blocks with the highest degree of connectivity. This analysis supports the idea that blocks in cluster 1 are hub areas.

A representation of which behavioral classes activate each cluster can be found in Figure S1.

DENSITY OF FOCI

Figure 7 displays the results of the Voronoi tessellation. The dACC showed the highest density of foci. Notably, this area was found to partially overlap with the location of cluster 1. Other

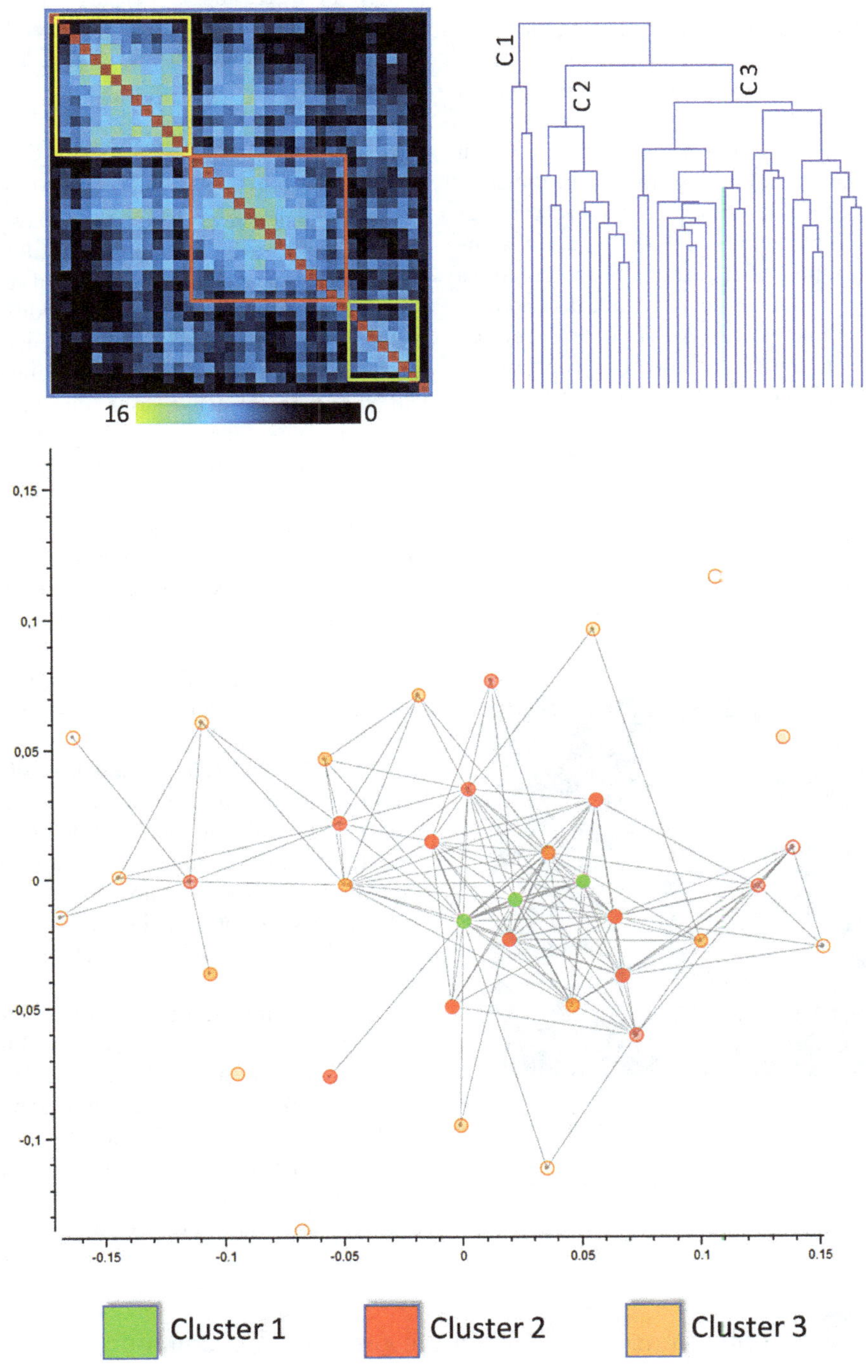

FIGURE 1 | Results of the clusterization of the cingulate cortex: distance matrix and multidimensional scaling (see also Figure 6 for network analysis). The upper left panel shows the results of the distance matrix. The upper right panel shows the dendrogram of the hierarchical clusterization, one of the algorithms used. The lower panel shows the Multidimensional scaling of the network derived from the distance between blocks of the cingulate cortex. The points represent blocks and are coded with a color indicating the cluster to which they belong. In this image the distance between points represents the Euclidean distance between the MACM maps of each block.

portions in the anterior cingulate cortex and in the cingulate motor zone showed a high density of foci. The two blocks showing the highest number of functional connections (see **Figure 6**) were found to be part of cluster 1 and were located in the dorsal cingulate cortex in the area with the highest density of foci. Together, these results indicate that such area exerts a pivotal role as a hub.

Figure S2 describes the behavioral related density of foci.

EXPERIMENTS 2–4

Images of the task-evoked activations and of the resting state protocol are shown in the supplementary material (Figures S3–S5).

The resting state parcellation shows a tripartite subdivision of the cingulate cortex with an anterior, a mid and a posterior cluster. In contrast, the parcellations based on the functional connectivity of the cingulate cortex when involved in the elaboration of emotional faces are less sharp and more complex (**Figure 8**). The parcellation based on responses to painful stimuli goes further in the direction of the results of the emotions paradigm: The clusters were found to be intermixed in a complex and blurred pattern of connectivity. Areas clearly connected with one network in the resting state showed, in contrast, an intermixed pattern of connectivity during tasks. That is, areas previously found to be characterized by homogeneous functional connectivity (e.g., cluster containing only voxels belonging to that cluster) are found to contain voxels also belonging to other clusters.

The results of the parcellation of the cingulate cortex based on the activations elicited by experimental tasks and obtained without imposing a priori the number of clusters, revealed a pattern of increasing complexity from the resting state data (2 clusters) to the emotion (3 clusters) and pain (5 clusters) paradigms (See **Figure 9** and Figure S6 for the results of the stopping criterion).

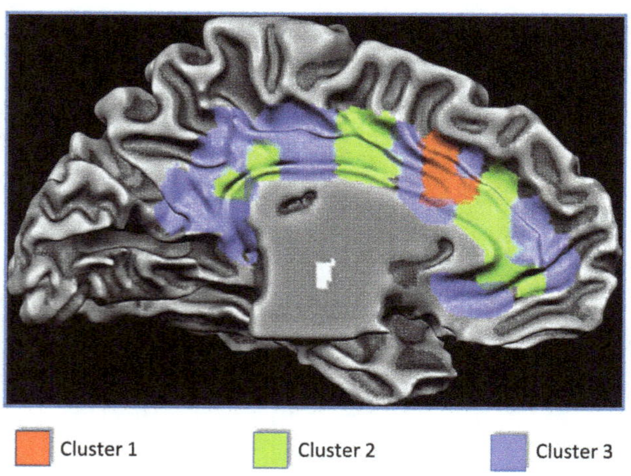

FIGURE 2 | Results of the clusterization of the cingulate cortex and anatomical location of the clusters.

DISCUSSION

This study was designed to investigate the pattern of clusterization of the cingulate cortex during the broadest range of tasks possible. We performed a meta-analytic study using a meta-analytic tool recently developed by our group: the MaC (Cauda et al., 2012). We further performed three additional fMRI experiments on healthy volunteers. In this way we could observe possible modifications of the parcellation of the cingulate cortex during the widest number of active tasks, during specific tasks and during resting state. Our main finding was that the cingulate cortex changes its pattern of co-activations depending on the level of task complexity. Indeed, the complexity of the pattern of parcellation increased and changed from the resting state experiment, to the two task-based experiments and the meta-analytic study. Importantly, we considered the task complexity not as reflecting a greater cognitive challenge, but rather as reflecting the kind of task (resting state-no task vs. active tasks) and the number of tasks (e.g., responses to painful stimulation vs. a general active mode, that is whenever a task is performed-meta-analytic study).

MaC CLUSTERING: CLUSTERING MACM RESULTS

Voxel-based meta-analyses have provided a fundamental contribution to the building of new insights into brain functions. In a previous study, we found that an ROI based parcellation of the cingulate cortex produced three clusters (Torta and Cauda, 2011). Such results were confirmed by those of the present study which indicate that using MaC, the cingulate cortex can be efficiently divided into three clusters (see **Figure 1**). These three clusters have different dimensions and cover a different percentage of the cingulate parenchyma. Although each cluster is characterized by specific co-activations (Corbetta et al., 1991, 2008; Corbetta and Shulman, 2002; Seeley et al., 2007; Beckmann et al., 2009; Menon and Uddin, 2010; Alexander and Brown, 2011), all three have extensive co-activations within the cingulate cortex and the insula (Cauda et al., 2011b, 2012) and share an "attentional" pattern of co-activation (Craig, 2003, 2009; Medford and Critchley, 2010;

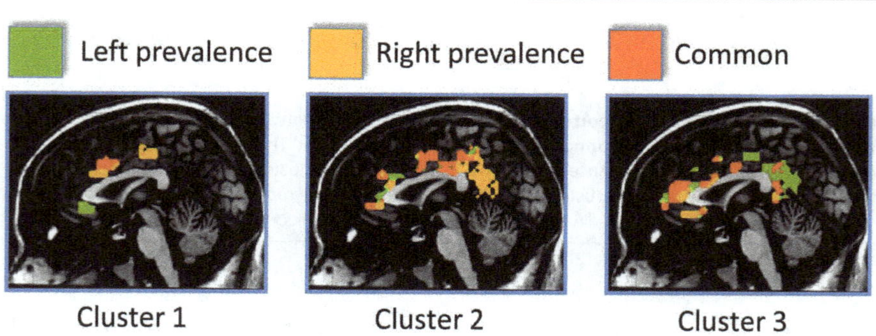

FIGURE 3 | The side differences for each cluster are shown here. Areas showing a left prevalence are coded in green, areas showing a right prevalence are coded in orange, areas equally lateralized are coded in red.

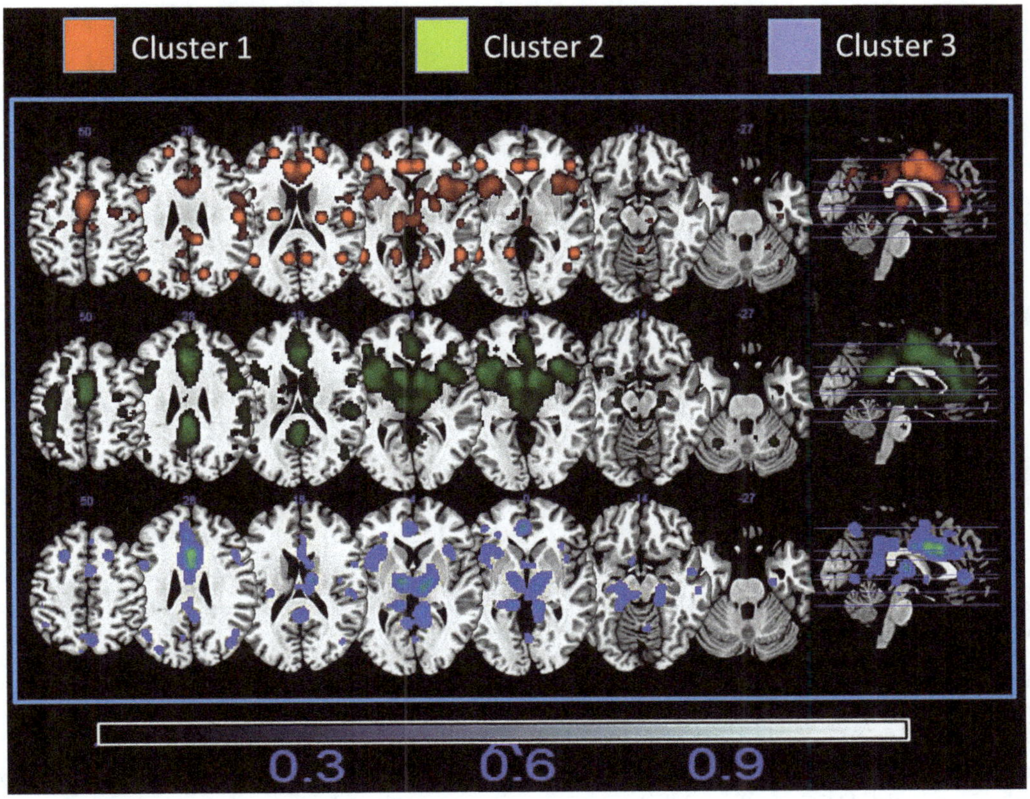

FIGURE 4 | Mean Meta-analytic connectivity of the three networks. ALE maps were computed at an FDR-corrected threshold of $p < 0.05$; minimum cluster dimension $k > 100\,\text{mm}^3$ and visualized using MRIcron (http://www.cabiatl.com/mricro/mricron/index.html).

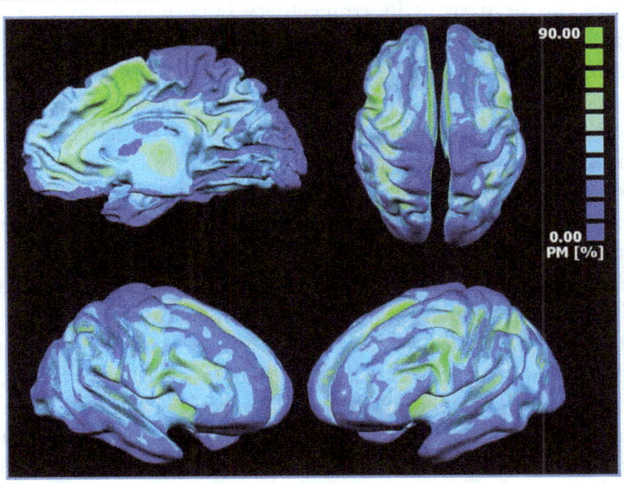

FIGURE 5 | Probabilistic map showing the superposition of the MACM of all blocks. The probabilistic map shows the probability of overlap between each block-related MACM map. The probability map is calculated by summing the voxel value of each block-related MACM map and dividing this value by the number of blocks. Single network maps before the creation of the probability maps were thresholded at $p < 0.05$, minimum cluster size $k > 100\,\text{mm}^3$. Regions in blue are characterized by a low probability of overlap, whereas green regions present a high probability of overlap.

Cauda et al., 2011b; Torta and Cauda, 2011). This overlap of common co-activations is maximal in the dACC and in the insula, as evidenced by the results of the probabilistic map (**Figure 5**). These findings support the view that the cingulate cortex and the insula form a saliency network devoted to the integration of information coming from the internal (e.g., homeostasis) and the external (e.g., sensory) environments (e.g., sensory inputs) (Vincent et al., 2008). In addition, this insular-cingulate system is thought to be in charge providing a stable "set maintenance" over the execution of tasks (Dosenbach et al., 2006). Moreover, we found that all clusters are strongly locally interconnected as evidenced by the presence of activity of the dACC and of the insula in the MACM profiles of the three clusters.

One possible criticism to our approach is that it may be considered not completely data driven. However, to obtain a voxel-wise analysis we first needed to aggregate a certain number of voxels to reach a minimum amount of foci. In this sense, our clustering cannot be entirely considered as voxelwise. Our method does not rely on pre-determined regions of interest but operates a local reduction of the resolution in a inverse relation to the density of foci. Other alternative solutions have been proposed (Bzdok et al., 2012). For instance, Bzdok and colleagues (2012) have obtained a partial voxel-wise clusterization by searching foci in the adjacency of a voxel, spreading the search to reach a minimum number of foci and then projecting the connectivity profile of these foci to the voxel.

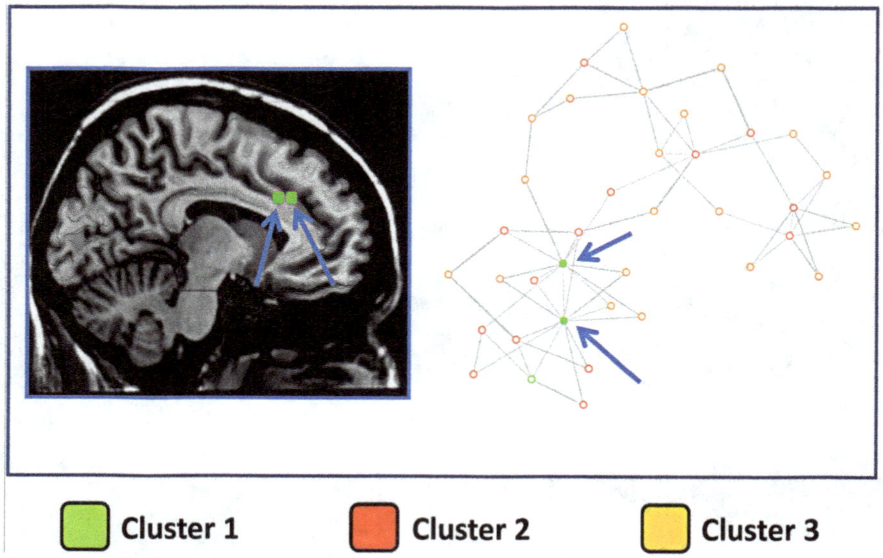

FIGURE 6 | Network derived from the distance between blocks of the cingulate cortex. Right panel: The points represent blocks and are coded with a color indicating the cluster to which they belong. In this image the distance between points represents the Euclidean distance between the MACM maps of each block. The network representation is optimized using a force-directed layout algorithm (Fruchterman–Reingold). Arrows indicate the two blocks with the highest number of connections. **Left panel**: the two blocks with the highest number of connections are graphically represented over a sliced standard brain surface.

HUBS OF THE CINGULATE CORTEX

The overlap of activations in the dACC, insula and thalamus (see **Figure 5**) suggests that such brain regions act as hubs through which homeostatic and sensory information is conveyed. This interpretation is also supported by the results of the Voronoi tessellation that pointed to the dACC as the area with the greatest density of foci. Indeed, it is highly likely that those areas having the greatest density of foci also have a greater number of connections. Further confirmation of the interpretation of the dACC as a hub area comes from the results of the distance matrix analysis (**Figure 1**, lower panel) and of the network analysis. Indeed, the findings of the graph analysis show that, in multidimensional scaling of MACM-based profiles, blocks of cluster 1 are close to each other and placed in a central position. These results indicated that such blocks have a similar and homogenous connectivity pattern. Moreover, they also suggest that cluster 1 may exert a pivotal role in regulating the activity of the other two clusters. A pivotal role of the cingulo-insular network in the regulation of the activity of other networks was suggested by Sridharan and colleagues (2008). These authors proposed that the cingulo-insular network plays a major role in switching between brain networks such as the central-executive network and the default-mode network (Sridharan et al., 2008). Interestingly, hypo-functionality of the dACC has been related to reduced awareness of the self. This would suggest that damage to hub areas may result in a failure to integrate stimuli coming from the external world into a coherent representation of the self (Amanzio et al., 2011).

PARCELLATION OF THE CINGULATE CORTEX WHEN AT REST AND WHEN INVOLVED IN ACTIVE TASKS

Whether the cingulate cortex has a segregated functional organization or not remains a matter of debate. Devinsky et al. (1995) and Bush et al. (2000) have reviewed evidence from neuroimaging, neurophysiological and anatomical data supporting the view that each part of the cingulate cortex is specialized in a family of cognitive operations, with the anterior cingulate more devoted to affective elaboration and the midcingulate to cognitive tasks. Previous studies, investigating the parcellation of the cingulate cortex on the basis of its connectivity (anatomical, Beckmann et al., 2009 or functional Yu et al., 2011) have upheld this view. A partial support for these results came also from a previous study performed by our group (Torta and Cauda, 2011). However, our present findings open up the possibility of a substantial divergence between the parcellation of the cingulate cortex when at rest and when involved in active tasks. Differences were also found depending on the kind and on the number of active tasks under exam. This result suggests that, when involved in active tasks, the cingulate cortex reconfigures its patterns of co-activation. In this view, the cingulate cortex may modify its connectivity from a resting state to a "working state": We, propose that such a modification may be related to the kind of task executed and consequently to how subpopulations of neurons modify their own specific time courses to begin to cooperate with different neuronal groups (see also Leech et al., 2011). This implies that such subdivisions are probably related to the kind of task and that, depending on the kind of task that is included in the analysis, they may change. In this sense, it may be argued that not even the MACM results allow a generalization of a "functional clustering" of the cingulate cortex, as also in BrainMap some tasks are more represented than others. The results of the experiments seem to support this view. However, two elements should be considered. First, these observations do not hamper the main results of our study, namely that the cingulate cortex reconfigures to a more complex parcellation when involved in active tasks. Second,

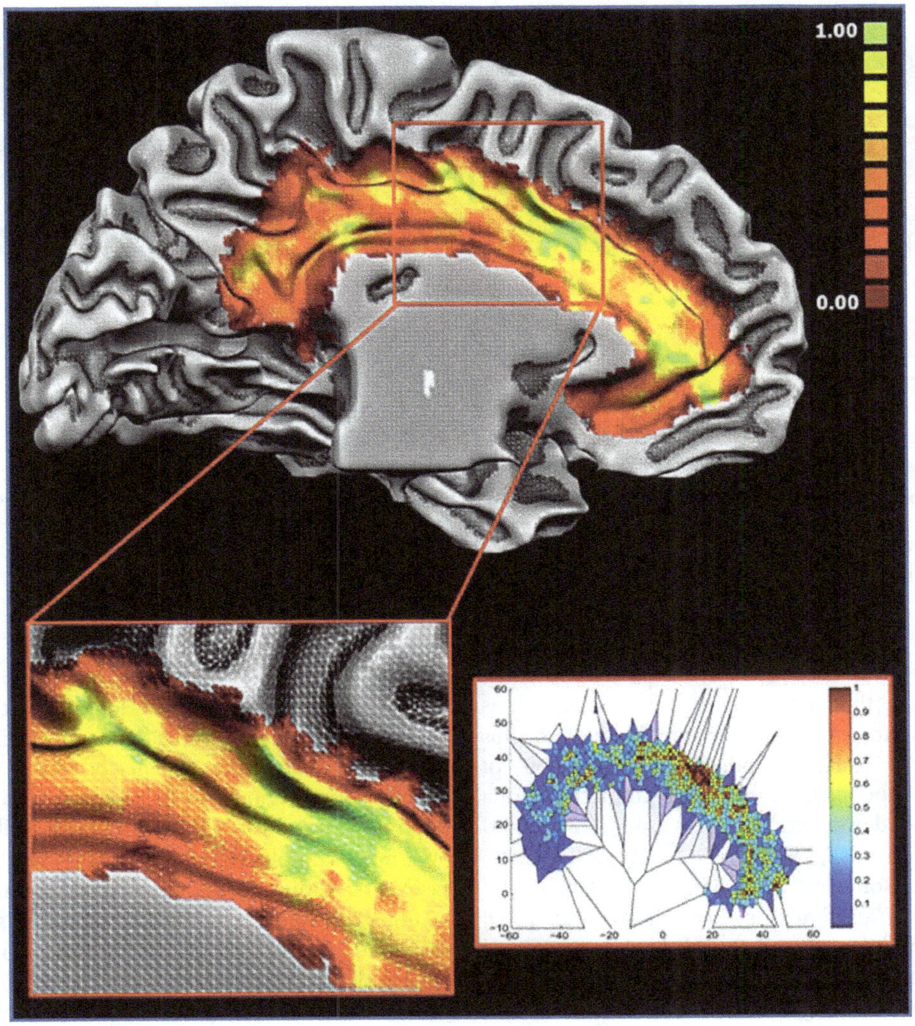

FIGURE 7 | Density of foci. Upper panel: colors from red to green represent increased foci density. **Lower right panel**: Voronoi tessellation of the cingulate cortex; colors from blue to red are inversely proportional to the Voronoi polygon area (i.e., Proportional to the density). All values are normalized.

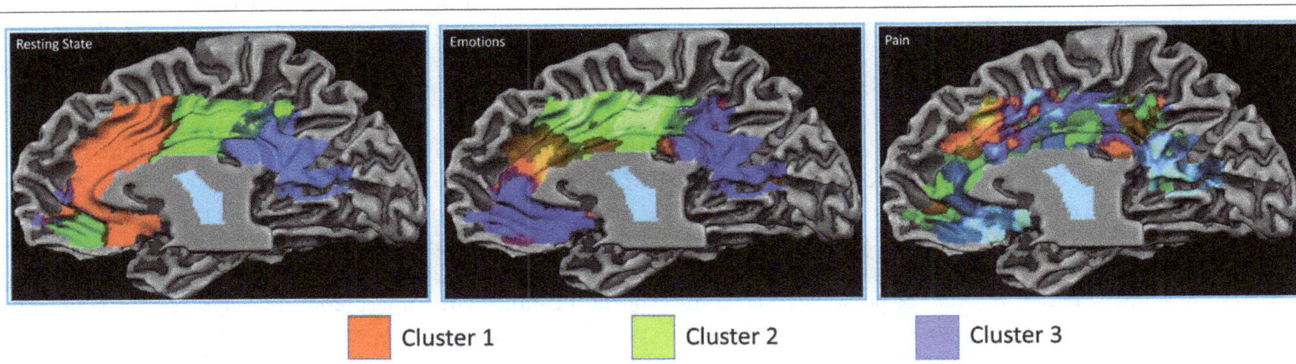

FIGURE 8 | Control experiments. Connectivity-based parcellation of the cingulate cortex in the three datasets. Probabilistic maps for functional connectivity defined clusters. The color scheme represents the probability of overlapping brain areas in each voxel across all the subjects. Maps are projected on an inflated 3D brain surface with the BrainVoyager QX surface tooL This parcellation was obtained by imposing the same number ɔf clusters obtained for the parcellation of the MaC data.

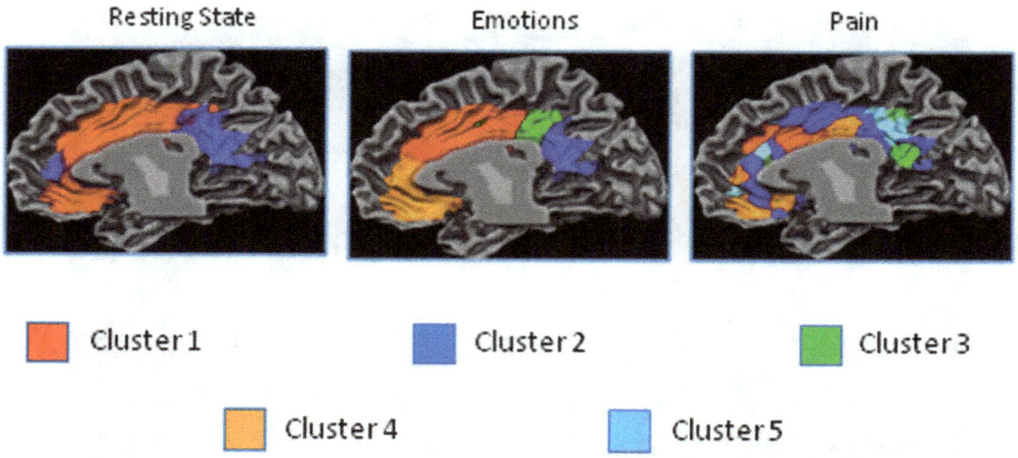

FIGURE 9 | Control experiments. Connectivity-based parcellation of the cingulate cortex in the three datasets. Probabilistic maps for functional connectivity defined clusters. The color scheme represents the probability of overlapping brain areas in each voxel across all the subjects. Maps are projected on an inflated 3D brain surface with the BrainVoyager QX surface tool. This parcellation was obtained by parcellating the data without imposing an a priori partition.

although some tasks are indeed more represented than others in BrainMap, it is also true that some cognitive functions such as attention are common across a great variety of tasks and thus more likely to be always recruited. Indeed, a growing body of literature indicates that the intrinsic functional connectivity of a brain region is modulated in function of a task, both during and after task execution (Liu et al., 1999; Friston and Buchel, 2000; Lowe et al., 2000; Hampson et al., 2002; Jiang et al., 2004; Peltier et al., 2005; Waites et al., 2005; Fransson, 2006; Hasson et al., 2009; Lewis et al., 2009; Tambini et al., 2010) and that the functional connectivity varies adaptively with a local efficiency that is higher locally and lower globally (Wang et al., 2012). Here, we did not directly measure functional connectivity, but used MACM, which is meant to assess the consistency of co-activations. However, it has been shown that MACM and resting state functional connectivity may lead to similar results (Cauda et al., 2011a). It is difficult to explain how such co-activations of brain areas across different paradigms and studies may emerge in absence of any functional connectivity between these areas [for a discussion see Koski and Paus (2000), Postuma and Dagher (2006), Laird et al. (2009b), Smith et al. (2009)]. Functional co-activations may be thus interpreted as forms of functional connectivity (Koski and Paus, 2000; Postuma and Dagher, 2006; Laird et al., 2009b; Smith et al., 2009). Furthermore, the mapping of functional connectivity via coordinate-based meta-analysis has been validated by comparing the results of MACM to resting-state connectivity (Smith et al., 2009). Both approaches produced very consistent results.

Another important question regards the possibility that complex "interdigitated" results may be related to under or over-decompositions in the clustering step. This issue specifically applies to clusterization in the control experiments. We used two different approaches to investigate if the cingulate cortex reconfigures its pattern of connectivity from resting state to "working state." First, we kept the number of clusters of the in-house acquired datasets equal to the number of clusters calculated for the meta-analytic data in order to have a one-by-one comparison between clusters. The logic behind this choice was to compare how the pattern changes across different levels of task complexity. Indeed, the evidence of greater functional complexity of a given region can be reflected either by an increase in the number of clusters (some of which probably very small) or by a more complex and interdigitated clusterization (as in our case). In addition, it should be considered that, as evidenced by Figure S2, single behavioral categories of stimuli do not activate contiguous cingulate areas but wide regions of interdigitated (sparse) blobs. This further supports the view that "sparseness" predominates in brain connectivity (Daubechies et al., 2009). However, as a second approach, in order to validate the results obtained with the first, we performed a parcellation of the resting state and task results, without imposing to the experimental datasets the same number of clusters as in the MaC. The results of this second analysis confirmed what we proposed with the previous approach, namely that from resting state to experimental tasks, there is an increase in the number of identified clusters (from 2 of the resting state to 5 of the pain task).

LIMITATIONS OF THE STUDY; NEUROBIOLOGICAL MEANING OF THE RESULTS AND CONTROVERSIES

Our results seem at odds with previous neurobiological evidence showing many additional partitions in the cingulate cortex (Bush et al., 2000; Vogt, 2009). However, some elements should be borne in mind when interpreting our findings. First, different parcellation schemes may co-exist in associative areas such as the insula (Cauda and Vercelli, 2012; Kelly et al., 2012). This could be explained by the intrinsically hierarchical nature of brain networks, as disclosed by neuroimaging studies (Doucet et al., 2011; Power et al., 2011; Yeo et al., 2011). Second, functional properties of these regions do not necessarily correspond to the anatomical subdivisions. For instance, it has been proposed that

different tasks and stimuli may activate the very same region of the cingulate cortex as this area may be devoted to elaborate some common characteristics of the tasks (Vogt, 2005). Third, the aim of our paper was not to provide compelling evidence to the parcellation of the cingulate cortex when during tasks. This is difficult, as in meta-analytic studies, many papers on different behavioral domains are pooled together. Thus, it may well be that different behavioral domains lead to different co-activations and thus to different parcellations. This is what we show with the control experiments. In addition, it has been demonstrated that clusterization of brain networks likely produces sparse rather than segregated results (Daubechies et al., 2009). All these elements may explain why it is possible to obtain a clusterization of the cingulate cortex that is different from previously suggested ones. In addition, it has been shown that individual anatomical differences may produce slightly diverging results when parcellating the cingulate cortex (Beckmann et al., 2009). We could not control for these factors in the meta-analytic study, thus our results might have been affected also by this. Importantly, the main objective of our study was to show that when the cingulate cortex is studied during tasks, the co-activations of its subparts diverge in a way that, when clustered together, is different from what we have known on the cingulate cortex so far. Finally, previous studies using meta-analytic procedures have already shown that our understanding of the cingulate cortex during tasks remains behind its anatomical understanding. Our clustering is based mainly on co-activations (MACM procedure), thus in this sense it is possible that a part of the cingulate cortex, as for example the anterior cingulate cortex, is connected with others as they are functionally linked at a network level, although the two components remain anatomically segregated.

In conclusion, we have shown that the cingulate cortex changes its pattern of co-activations depending on the level of task complexity. In addition, clusters resulting from a parcellation of the cingulate cortex during tasks, rather than being strongly functionally segregated, are likely to reflect the activity of hub areas densely interconnected with local and whole-brain networks. This opens up the possibility that areas that appear to be active for a wide range of active tasks are differentially recruited by each of them and echo the activity of other networks in the brain (Leech et al., 2011).

REFERENCES

Alexander, W. H., and Brown, J. W. (2011). Medial prefrontal cortex as an action-outcome predictor. *Nat. Neurosci.* 14, 1338–1344. doi: 10.1038/nn.2921

Allman, J. M., Hakeem, A., Erwin, J. M., Nimchinsky, E., and Hof, P. (2001). The anterior cingulate cortex. The evolution of an interface between emotion and cognition. *Ann. N.Y. Acad. Sci.* 935, 107–117. doi: 10.1111/j.1749-6632.2001.tb03476.x

Amanzio, M., Torta, D. M., Sacco, K., Cauda, F., D'Agata, F., Duca, S., et al. (2011). Unawareness of deficits in Alzheimer's disease: role of the cingulate cortex. *Brain* 134, 1061–1076. doi: 10.1093/brain/awr020

Apkarian, A. V., Bushnell, M. C., Treede, R. D., and Zubieta, J. K. (2005). Human brain mechanisms of pain perception and regulation in health and disease. *Eur. J. Pain* 9, 463–484. doi: 10.1016/j.ejpain.2004.11.001

Awh, E., and Gehring, W. J. (1999). The anterior cingulate cortex lends a hand in response selection. *Nat. Neurosci.* 2, 853–854. doi: 10.1038/13145

Badgaiyan, R. D., and Posner, M. I. (1998). Mapping the cingulate cortex in response selection and monitoring. *Neuroimage* 7, 255–260. doi: 10.1006/nimg.1998.0326

Ballard, D. H., and Brown, C. M. (1982). *Computer Vision.* Englewood Cliffs, NJ: Practise Hall.

Baumgartner, U., Iannetti, G. D., Zambreanu, L., Stoeter, P., Treede, R. D., and Tracey, I. (2010). Multiple somatotopic representations of heat and mechanical pain in the operculo-insular cortex: a high-resolution fMRI study. *J. Neurophysiol.* 104, 2863–2872. doi: 10.1152/jn.00253.2010

Beckmann, M., Johansen-Berg, H., and Rushworth, M. F. (2009). Connectivity-based parcellation of human cingulate cortex and its relation to functional specialization. *J. Neurosci.* 29, 1175–1190. doi: 10.1523/JNEUROSCI.3328-08.2009

Biehl, M., Matsumoto, D., Ekman, P., Hearn, V., Heider, K., Kudoh, T., et al. (1997). Matsumoto and Ekman's Japanese and Caucasian facial expressions of emotion (JACFEE): reliability data and cross-national differences. *J. Nonverbal Behav.* 21, 3–21. doi: 10.1023/A:1024902500935

Botvinick, M. M., Cohen, J. D., and Carter, C. S. (2004). Conflict monitoring and anterior cingulate cortex: an update. *Trends Cogn. Sci.* 8, 539–546. doi: 10.1016/j.tics.2004.10.003

Bullmore, E., and Sporns, O. (2009). Complex brain networks: graph theoretical analysis of structural and functional systems. *Nat. Rev. Neurosci.* 10, 186–198. doi: 10.1038/nrn2575

Burgess, N., Maguire, E. A., Spiers, H. J., and O'Keefe, J. (2001). A temporoparietal and prefrontal network for retrieving the spatial context of lifelike events. *Neuroimage* 14, 439–453. doi: 10.1006/nimg.2001.0806

Bush, G., Luu, P., and Posner, M. I. (2000). Cognitive and emotional influences in anterior cingulate cortex. *Trends Cogn. Sci.* 4, 215–222. doi: 10.1016/S1364-6613(00)01483-2

Bzdok, D., Laird, A. R., Zilles, K., Fox, P. T., and Eickhoff, S. B. (2012). An investigation of the structural, connectional, and functional subspecialization in the human amygdala. *Hum. Brain Mapp.* doi: 10.1002/hbm.22138. [Epub ahead of print].

Carter, C. S., Botvinick, M. M., and Cohen, J. D. (1999). The contribution of the anterior cingulate cortex to executive processes in cognition. *Rev. Neurosci.* 10, 49–57. doi: 10.1515/REVNEURO.1999.10.1.49

Carter, C. S., Braver, T. S., Barch, D. M., Botvinick, M. M., Noll, D., and Cohen, J. D. (1998). Anterior cingulate cortex, error detection, and the online monitoring of performance. *Science* 280, 747–749. doi: 10.1126/science.280.5364.747

Cauda, F., Cavanna, A., D'Agata, F., Sacco, K., Duca, S., and Geminiani, G. (2011a). Functional connectivity and coactivation of the nucleus accumbens: a combined resting state fMRI and structure-based meta analysis study. *J. Cogn. Neurosci.* 23, 2864–2877. doi: 10.1162/jocn.2011.21624

Cauda, F., D'Agata, F., Sacco, K., Duca, S., Geminiani, G., and Vercelli, A. (2011b). Functional connectivity of the insula in the resting brain. *Neuroimage* 55, 8–23. doi: 10.1016/j.neuroimage.2010.11.049

Cauda, F., Costa, T., Torta, D. M., Sacco, K., D'Agata, F., Duca, S., et al. (2012). Meta-analytic clustering of the insular cortex: characterizing the meta-analytic connectivity of the insula when involved in active tasks. *Neuroimage* 62, 343–355. doi: 10.1016/j.neuroimage.2012.04.012

Cauda, F., Torta, D. M., Sacco, K., D'Agata, F., Geda, E., Duca, S., et al. (2013). Functional anatomy of cortical areas characterized by Von Economo neurons. *Brain Struct. Funct.* 218, 1–20. doi: 10.1007/s00429-012-0382-9

Cauda, F., Geminiani, G., D'Agata, F., Sacco, K., Duca, S., Bagshaw, A. P., et al. (2010). Functional connectivity of the posteromedial cortex. *PLoS ONE* 5:e13107. doi: 10.1371/journal.pone.0013107

Cauda, F., and Vercelli, A. (2012). How many clusters in the insular cortex? *Cereb Cortex.* doi: 10.1093/cercor/bhs249. [Epub ahead of print].

Corbetta, M., Miezin, F. M., Dobmeyer, S., Shulman, G. L., and Petersen, S. E. (1991). Selective and divided attention during visual discriminations of shape, color, and speed: functional anatomy by positron emission tomography. *J. Neurosci.* 11, 2383–2402.

Corbetta, M., Patel, G., and Shulman, G. L. (2008). The reorienting system of the human brain: from environment to theory of mind. *Neuron* 58, 306–324. doi: 10.1016/j.neuron.2008.04.017

Corbetta, M., and Shulman, G. L. (2002). Control of goal-directed and stimulus-driven attention in the brain. *Nat. Rev. Neurosci.* 3, 201–215. doi: 10.1038/nrn755

Craig, A. D. (2003). Interoception: the sense of the physiological condition of the body. *Curr. Opin. Neurobiol.* 13, 500–505. doi: 10.1016/S0959-4388(03)00090-4

Craig, A. D. (2009). How do you feel–now? The anterior insula and human awareness. *Nat. Rev. Neurosci.* 10, 59–70. doi: 10.1038/nrn2555

Crottaz-Herbette, S., and Menon, V. (2006). Where and when the anterior cingulate cortex modulates attentional response: combined fMRI and ERP evidence. *J. Cogn. Neurosci.* 18, 766–780. doi: 10.1162/jocn.2006.18.5.766

Daubechies, I., Roussos, E., Takerkart, S., Benharrosh, M., Golden, C., D'Ardenne, K., et al. (2009). Independent component analysis for brain fMRI does not select for independence. *Proc. Natl. Acad. Sci. U.S.A.* 106, 10415–10422. doi: 10.1073/pnas.0903525106

Devinsky, O., Morrell, M. J., and Vogt, B. A. (1995). Contributions of anterior cingulate cortex to behaviour. *Brain* 118, 279–306. doi: 10.1093/brain/118.1.279

Dosenbach, N. U., Visscher, K. M., Palmer, E. D., Miezin, F. M., Wenger, K. K., Kang, H. C., et al. (2006). A core system for the implementation of task sets. *Neuron* 50, 799–812. doi: 10.1016/j.neuron.2006.04.031

Doucet, G., Naveau, M., Petit, L., Delcroix, N., Zago, L., Crivello, F., et al. (2011). Brain activity at rest: a multiscale hierarchical functional organization. *J. Neurophysiol.* 105, 2753–2763. doi: 10.1152/jn.00895.2010

Eickhoff, S. B., Laird, A. R., Grefkes, C., Wang, L. E., Zilles, K., and Fox, P. T. (2009). Coordinate-based activation likelihood estimation meta-analysis of neuroimaging data: a random-effects approach based on empirical estimates of spatial uncertainty. *Hum. Brain Mapp.* 30, 2907–2926. doi: 10.1002/hbm.20718

Fan, J., Hof, P. R., Guise, K. G., Fossella, J. A., and Posner, M. I. (2008). The functional integration of the anterior cingulate cortex during conflict processing. *Cereb. Cortex* 18, 796–805. doi: 10.1093/cercor/bhm125

Fox, P. T., Laird, A. R., Fox, S. P., Fox, P. M., Uecker, A. M., Crank, M., et al. (2005). BrainMap taxonomy of experimental design: description and evaluation. *Hum. Brain Mapp.* 25, 185–198. doi: 10.1002/hbm.20141

Frades, I., and Matthiesen, R. (2010). Overview on techniques in cluster analysis. *Methods Mol. Biol.* 593, 81–107. doi: 10.1007/978-1-60327-194-3_5

Fransson, P. (2006). How default is the default mode of brain function? Further evidence from intrinsic BOLD signal fluctuations. *Neuropsychologia* 44, 2836–2845. doi: 10.1016/j.neuropsychologia.2006.06.017

Friebel, U., Eickhoff, S. B., and Lotze, M. (2011). Coordinate-based meta-analysis of experimentally induced and chronic persistent neuropathic pain. *Neuroimage* 58, 1070–1080. doi: 10.1016/j.neuroimage.2011.07.022

Friston, K. J., and Buchel, C. (2000). Attentional modulation of effective connectivity from V2 to V5/MT in humans. *Proc. Natl. Acad. Sci. U.S.A.* 97, 7591–7596. doi: 10.1073/pnas.97.13.7591

Fruchterman, T. M. J., and Reingold, E. M. (1991). Graph drawing by force-directed placement. *Softw. Pract. Exper.* 21, 1129–1164. doi: 10.1002/spe.4380211102

Gehring, W. J., and Fencsik, D. E. (2001). Functions of the medial frontal cortex in the processing of conflict and errors. *J. Neurosci.* 21, 9430–9437.

Gehring, W. J., and Knight, R. T. (2000). Prefrontal-cingulate interactions in action monitoring. *Nat. Neurosci.* 3, 516–520. doi: 10.1038/74899

Genovese, C. R., Lazar, N. A., and Nichols, T. (2002). Thresholding of statistical maps in functional neuroimaging using the false discovery rate. *Neuroimage* 15, 870–878. doi: 10.1006/nimg.2001.1037

Hampson, M., Peterson, B. S., Skudlarski, P., Gatenby, J. C., and Gore, J. C. (2002). Detection of functional connectivity using temporal correlations in MR images. *Hum. Brain Mapp.* 15, 247–262. doi: 10.1002/hbm.10022

Hasson, U., Nusbaum, H. C., and Small, S. L. (2009). Task-dependent organization of brain regions active during rest. *Proc. Natl. Acad. Sci. U.S.A.* 106, 10841–10846. doi: 10.1073/pnas.0903253106

Holroyd, C. B., Dien, J., and Coles, M. G. (1998). Error-related scalp potentials elicited by hand and foot movements: evidence for an output-independent error-processing system in humans. *Neurosci. Lett.* 242, 65–68. doi: 10.1016/S0304-3940(98)00035-4

Iaria, G., Chen, J. K., Guariglia, C., Ptito, A., and Petrides, M. (2007). Retrosplenial and hippocampal brain regions in human navigation: complementary functional contributions to the formation and use of cognitive maps. *Eur. J. Neurosci.* 25, 890–899. doi: 10.1111/j.1460-9568.2007.05371.x

Jiang, T., He, Y., Zang, Y., and Weng, X. (2004). Modulation of functional connectivity during the resting state and the motor task. *Hum. Brain Mapp.* 22, 63–71. doi: 10.1111/j.1460-9568.2007.05371.x

Keene, C. S., and Bucci, D. J. (2008). Neurotoxic lesions of retrosplenial cortex disrupt signaled and unsignaled contextual fear conditioning. *Behav. Neurosci.* 122, 1070–1077. doi: 10.1037/a0012895

Kelly, C., Toro, R., Di Martino, A., Cox, C. L., Bellec, P., Castellanos, F. X., et al. (2012). A convergent functional architecture of the insula emerges across imaging modalities. *Neuroimage* 61, 1129–1142. doi: 10.1016/j.neuroimage.2012.03.021

Klein, R. (1989). *Concrete and Abstract Voronoi Diagrams.* Berlin, Heidelberg: Springer Verlag.

Koski, L., and Paus, T. (2000). Functional connectivity of the anterior cingulate cortex within the human frontal lobe: a brain-mapping meta-analysis. *Exp. Brain Res.* 133, 55–65.

Laird, A. R., Eickhoff, S. B., Kurth, F., Fox, P. M., Uecker, A. M., Turner, J. A., et al. (2009a). ALE meta-analysis workflows via the brainmap database: progress towards a probabilistic functional brain atlas. *Front. Neuroinform.* 3:23. doi: 10.3389/neuro.11.023.2009

Laird, A. R., Lancaster, J. L., and Fox, P. T. (2009b). Lost in localization? The focus is meta-analysis. *Neuroimage* 48, 18–20. doi: 10.1016/j.neuroimage.2009.06.047

Laird, A. R., Fox, P. M., Price, C. J., Glahn, D. C., Uecker, A. M., Lancaster, J. L., et al. (2005a). ALE meta-analysis: controlling the false discovery rate and performing statistical contrasts. *Hum. Brain Mapp.* 25, 155–164. doi: 10.1002/hbm.20136

Laird, A. R., Lancaster, J. L., and Fox, P. T. (2005b). BrainMap: the social evolution of a human brain mapping database. *Neuroinformatics* 3, 65–78.

Leech, R., Braga, R., and Sharp, D. J. (2011). Echoes of the brain within the posterior cingulate cortex. *J. Neurosci.* 32, 215–222. doi: 10.1523/JNEUROSCI.3689-11.2012

Lewis, C. M., Baldassarre, A., Committeri, G., Romani, G. L., and Corbetta, M. (2009). Learning sculpts the spontaneous activity of the resting human brain. *Proc. Natl. Acad. Sci. U.S.A.* 106, 17558–17563. doi: 10.1073/pnas.0902455106

Liu, Y., Gao, J. H., Liotti, M., Pu, Y., and Fox, P. T. (1999). Temporal dissociation of parallel processing in the human subcortical outputs. *Nature* 400, 364–366. doi: 10.1038/22547

Lowe, M. J., Dzemidzic, M., Lurito, J. T., Mathews, V. P., and Phillips, M. D. (2000). Correlations in low-frequency BOLD fluctuations reflect cortico-cortical connections. *Neuroimage* 12, 582–587. doi: 10.1006/nimg.2000.0654

Margulies, D. S., Kelly, A. M., Uddin, L. Q., Biswal, B. B., Castellanos, F. X., and Milham, M. P. (2007). Mapping the functional connectivity of anterior cingulate cortex. *Neuroimage* 37, 579–588. doi: 10.1016/j.neuroimage.2007.05.019

Medford, N., and Critchley, H. D. (2010). Conjoint activity of anterior insular and anterior cingulate cortex: awareness and response. *Brain Struct. Funct.* 214, 535–549. doi: 10.1007/s00429-010-0265-x

Menon, V., and Uddin, L. Q. (2010). Saliency, switching, attention and control: a network model of insula function. *Brain Struct. Funct.* 214, 655–667. doi: 10.1007/s00429-010-0262-0

Mojena, R. (1977). Hierarchical grouping methods and stopping rules: an evaluation. *Comput. J.* 20, 359–363. doi: 10.1093/comjnl/20.4.359

Murtha, S., Chertkow, H., Beauregard, M., Dixon, R., and Evans, A. (1996). Anticipation causes increased blood flow to the anterior cingulate cortex. *Hum. Brain Mapp.* 4, 103–112. doi: 10.1002/(SICI)1097-0193(1996)4:2<103::AID-HBM2>3.0.CO;2-7

Nanetti, L., Cerliani, L., Gazzola, V., Renken, R., and Keysers, C. (2009). Group analyses of connectivity-based cortical parcellation using repeated k-means clustering. *Neuroimage* 47, 1666–1677. doi: 10.1016/j.neuroimage.2009.06.014

Palomero-Gallagher, N., Mohlberg, H., Zilles, K., and Vogt, B. (2008). Cytology and receptor architecture of human anterior cingulate cortex. *J. Comp. Neurol.* 508, 906–926. doi: 10.1002/cne.21684

Palomero-Gallagher, N., Vogt, B. A., Schleicher, A., Mayberg, H. S., and Zilles, K. (2009). Receptor architecture of human cingulate cortex: evaluation of the four-region neurobiological model. *Hum. Brain Mapp.* 30, 2336–2355. doi: 10.1002/hbm.20667

Pardo, J. V., Pardo, P. J., Janer, K. W., and Raichle, M. E. (1990). The anterior cingulate cortex mediates processing selection in the Stroop attentional conflict paradigm. *Proc. Natl. Acad. Sci. U.S.A.* 87, 256–259. doi: 10.1073/pnas.87.1.256

Parker, A., and Gaffan, D. (1997). The effect of anterior thalamic and cingulate cortex lesions on object-in-place memory in monkeys. *Neuropsychologia* 35, 1093–1102. doi: 10.1016/S0028-3932(97)00042-0

Paus, T., Petrides, M., Evans, A. C., and Meyer, E. (1993). Role of the human anterior cingulate cortex in the control of oculomotor, manual, and speech responses: a positron emission tomography study. *J. Neurophysiol.* 70, 453–469.

Peltier, S. J., Laconte, S. M., Niyazov, D. M., Liu, J. Z., Sahgal, V., Yue, G. H., et al. (2005). Reductions in interhemispheric motor cortex functional connectivity after muscle fatigue. *Brain Res.* 1057, 10–16. doi: 10.1016/j.brainres.2005.06.078

Petit, L., Courtney, S. M., Ungerleider, L. G., and Haxby, J. V. (1998). Sustained activity in the medial wall during working memory delays. *J. Neurosci.* 18, 9429–9437.

Posner, M. I., and Dehaene, S. (1994). Attentional networks. *Trends Neurosci.* 17, 75–79.

Postuma, R. B., and Dagher, A. (2006). Basal ganglia functional connectivity based on a meta-analysis of 126 positron emission tomography and functional magnetic resonance imaging publications. *Cereb. Cortex* 16, 1508–1521. doi: 10.1093/cercor/bhj088

Power, J. D., Cohen, A. L., Nelson, S. M., Wig, G. S., Barnes, K. A., Church, J. A., et al. (2011). Functional network organization of the human brain. *Neuron* 72, 665–678. doi: 10.1016/j.neuron.2011.09.006

Robinson, J. L., Laird, A. R., Glahn, D. C., Lovallo, W. R., and Fox, P. T. (2010). Metaanalytic connectivity modeling: delineating the functional connectivity of the human amygdala. *Hum. Brain Mapp.* 31, 173–184. doi: 10.1002/hbm.20854

Rousseeuw, P. J. (1987). Silhouettes: a graphical aid to the interpretation and validation of cluster analysis. *J. Comp. Appl. Math.* 20, 53–65. doi: 10.1016/0377-0427(87)90125-7

Rubinov, M., and Sporns, O. (2010). Complex network measures of brain connectivity: uses and interpretations. *Neuroimage* 52, 1059–1069. doi: 10.1016/j.neuroimage.2009.10.003

Seeley, W. W., Menon, V., Schatzberg, A. F., Keller, J., Glover, G. H., Kenna, H., et al. (2007). Dissociable intrinsic connectivity networks for salience processing and executive control. *J. Neurosci.* 27, 2349–2356. doi: 10.1523/JNEUROSCI.5587-06.2007

Shackman, A. J., Salomons, T. V., Slagter, H. A., Fox, A. S., Winter, J. J., and Davidson, R. J. (2011). The integration of negative affect, pain and cognitive control in the cingulate cortex. *Nat. Rev. Neurosci.* 12, 154–167. doi: 10.1038/nrn2994

Smith, S. M., Fox, P. T., Miller, K. L., Glahn, D. C., Fox, P. M., MaCkay, C. E., et al. (2009). Correspondence of the brain's functional architecture during activation and rest. *Proc. Natl. Acad. Sci. U.S.A.* 106, 13040–13045. doi: 10.1073/pnas.0905267106

Spreng, R. N., Mar, R. A., and Kim, A. S. (2009). The common neural basis of autobiographical memory, prospection, navigation, theory of mind, and the default mode: a quantitative meta-analysis. *J. Cogn. Neurosci.* 21, 489–510. doi: 10.1162/jocn.2008.21029

Sridharan, D., Levitin, D. J., and Menon, V. (2008). A critical role for the right fronto-insular cortex in switching between central-executive and default-mode networks. *Proc. Natl. Acad. Sci. U.S.A.* 105, 12569–12574. doi: 10.1073/pnas.0800005105

Tambini, A., Ketz, N., and Davachi, L. (2010). Enhanced brain correlations during rest are related to memory for recent experiences. *Neuron* 65, 280–290. doi: 10.1016/j.neuron.2010.01.001

Torta, D. M., and Cauda, F. (2011). Different functions in the cingulate cortex, a meta-analytic connectivity modeling study. *Neuroimage* 56, 2157–2172. doi: 10.1016/j.neuroimage.2011.03.066

Turkeltaub, P. E., Eden, G. F., Jones, K. M., and Zeffiro, T. A. (2002). Meta-analysis of the functional neuroanatomy of single-word reading: method and validation. *Neuroimage* 16, 765–780. doi: 10.1006/nimg.2002.1131

Vann, S. D., Aggleton, J. P., and Maguire, E. A. (2009). What does the retrosplenial cortex do? *Nat. Rev. Neurosci.* 10, 792–802. doi: 10.1038/nrn2733

Vincent, J. L., Kahn, I., Snyder, A. Z., Raichle, M. E., and Buckner, R. L. (2008). Evidence for a frontoparietal control system revealed by intrinsic functional connectivity. *J. Neurophysiol.* 100, 3328–3342. doi: 10.1152/jn.90355.2008

Vogt, B. (2009). *Cingulate Neurobiology and Disease.* New York, NY: Oxford University Press.

Vogt, B., and Derbyshire, S. (2002). *Roles of the Human Anterior and Posterior Midcingulate Cortex in Pain Processing,* 10. Seattle, WA: IASP Press.

Vogt, B. A. (2005). Pain and emotion interactions in subregions of the cingulate gyrus. *Nat. Rev. Neurosci.* 6, 533–544. doi: 10.1038/nrn1704

Vogt, B. A., Berger, G. R., and Derbyshire, S. W. (2003). Structural and functional dichotomy of human midcingulate cortex. *Eur. J. Neurosci.* 18, 3134–3144. doi: 10.1111/j.1460-9568.2003.03034.x

Vogt, B. A., Finch, D. M., and Olson, C. R. (1992). Functional heterogeneity in cingulate cortex: the anterior executive and posterior evaluative regions. *Cereb. Cortex* 2, 435–443. doi: 10.1093/cercor/2.6.435-a

Vogt, B. A., and Laureys, S. (2005). Posterior cingulate, precuneal and retrosplenial cortices: cytology and components of the neural network correlates of consciousness. *Prog. Brain Res.* 150, 205–217. doi: 10.1016/S0079-6123(05)50015-3

Vogt, B. A., and Pandya, D. N. (1987). Cingulate cortex of the rhesus monkey: II. Cortical afferents. *J. Comp. Neurol.* 262, 271–289. doi: 10.1002/cne.902620208

Vogt, B. A., Pandya, D. N., and Rosene, D. L. (1987). Cingulate cortex of the rhesus monkey: I. Cytoarchitecture and thalamic afferents. *J. Comp. Neurol.* 262, 256–270. doi: 10.1002/cne.902620207

Vogt, B. A., and Vogt, L. (2003). Cytology of human dorsal midcingulate and supplementary motor cortices. *J. Chem. Neuroanat.* 26, 301–309. doi: 10.1016/j.jchemneu.2003.09.004

Vogt, B. A., Vogt, L. J., Perl, D. P., and Hof, P. R. (2001). Cytology of human caudomedial cingulate, retrosplenial, and caudal parahippocampal cortices. *J. Comp. Neurol.* 438, 353–376. doi: 10.1002/cne.1320

Waites, A. B., Stanislavsky, A., Abbott, D. F., and Jackson, G. D. (2005). Effect of prior cognitive state on resting state networks measured with functional connectivity. *Hum. Brain Mapp.* 24, 59–68. doi: 10.1002/hbm.20069

Wang, Z., Liu, J., Zhong, N., Qin, Y., Zhou, H., and Li, K. (2012). Changes in the brain intrinsic organization in both on-task state and post-task resting state. *Neuroimage* 62, 394–407. doi: 10.1016/j.neuroimage.2012.04.051

Ward, J. H. (1963). Hierarchical grouping to optimize an objective function. *J. Am. Statist. Assoc.* 58, 236–244. doi: 10.1080/01621459.1963.10500845

Yeo, B. T., Krienen, F. M., Sepulcre, J., Sabuncu, M. R., Lashkari, D., Hollinshead, M., et al. (2011). The organization of the human cerebral cortex estimated by intrinsic functional connectivity. *J. Neurophysiol.* 106, 1125–1165. doi: 10.1152/jn.00338.2011

Yu, C., Zhou, Y., Liu, Y., Jiang, T., Dong, H., Zhang, Y., et al. (2011). Functional segregation of the human cingulate cortex is confirmed by functional connectivity based neuroanatomical parcellation. *Neuroimage* 54, 2571–2581. doi: 10.1016/j.neuroimage.2010.11.018

11

Extraversion and neuroticism relate to topological properties of resting-state brain networks

Qing Gao[1]*, Qiang Xu[2], Xujun Duan[2], Wei Liao[2], Jurong Ding[2], Zhiqiang Zhang[3], Yuan Li[4], Guangming Lu[3] and Huafu Chen[2]*

[1] School of Mathematical Sciences, University of Electronic Science and Technology of China, Chengdu, China
[2] Key Laboratory for Neuroinformation of Ministry of Education, School of Life Science and Technology, University of Electronic Science and Technology of China, Chengdu, China
[3] Department of Medical Imaging, Jinling Hospital, Clinical School, Medical College, Nanjing University, Nanjing, Jiangsu, China
[4] School of Politics and Public Managements, University of Electronic Science and Technology of China, Chengdu, China

***Correspondence:**
Qing Gao, School of Mathematical Sciences, University of Electronic Science and Technology of China, No. 4, Section 2, N. Jianshe Rd., Chengdu 610054, China
e-mail: qingqing.gao@gmail.com;
Huafu Chen, Key Laboratory for Neuroinformation of Ministry of Education, School of Life Science and Technology, University of Electronic Science and Technology of China, No. 4, Section 2, N. Jianshe Rd., Chengdu 610054, China
e-mail: chenhf@uestc.edu.cn

With the advent and development of modern neuroimaging techniques, there is an increasing interest in linking extraversion and neuroticism to anatomical and functional brain markers. Here, we aimed to test the theoretically derived biological personality model as proposed by Eysenck using graph theoretical analyses. Specifically, the association between the topological organization of whole-brain functional networks and extraversion/neuroticism was explored. To construct functional brain networks, functional connectivity among 90 brain regions was measured by temporal correlation using resting-state functional magnetic resonance imaging (fMRI) data of 71 healthy subjects. Graph theoretical analysis revealed a positive association of extraversion scores and normalized clustering coefficient values. These results suggested a more clustered configuration in brain networks of individuals high in extraversion, which could imply a higher arousal threshold and higher levels of arousal tolerance in the cortex of extraverts. On a local network level, we observed that a specific nodal measure, i.e., betweenness centrality (BC), was positively associated with neuroticism scores in the right precentral gyrus (PreCG), right caudate nucleus, right olfactory cortex, and bilateral amygdala. For individuals high in neuroticism, these results suggested a more frequent participation of these specific regions in information transition within the brain network and, in turn, may partly explain greater regional activation levels and lower arousal thresholds in these regions. In contrast, extraversion scores were positively correlated with BC in the right insula, while negatively correlated with BC in the bilateral middle temporal gyrus (MTG), indicating that the relationship between extraversion and regional arousal is not as simple as proposed by Eysenck.

Keywords: resting-state, functional magnetic resonance imaging, graph topological properties, extraversion, neuroticism

INTRODUCTION

In Eysenck's personality theory, he proposed three fundamental dimensions of personality: extraversion, neuroticism, and psychoticism (Eysenck, 1967; Eysenck and Eysenck, 1985). It is now acknowledged that extraversion and neuroticism have their biological bases (Matthews and Gilliland, 1999), while the neuropsychology of the third dimension, psychoticism, has not been worked out in detail. The arousal theory of Eysenck (1967) related extraversion to arousability of the reticulo-cortical circuit and proposed a higher arousal threshold in cortex and higher levels of arousal tolerance in extraverts (Eysenck, 1967; Eysenck and Eysenck, 1985; Fischer et al., 1998). Neuroticism, on the other hand, is associated with arousability of the limbic circuit, such that individuals with higher neuroticism scores have greater activation levels and lower thresholds within subcortical structures (Eysenck, 1990; Wei et al., 2012).

With the advent and development of modern neuroimaging techniques, there is increasing interest in exploring neuroanatomical or neurofunctional correlates of extraversion and neuroticism, to test the theoretically proposed biological explanation of the two fundamental dimensions. Neuroanatomical studies have found extraversion was associated with structural/anatomic variations in the middle and inferior frontal regions, fusiform gyrus, and insula (INS), whereas neuroticism was associated with variations in the orbitofrontal cortex, precentral gyrus (PreCG), and amygdala (AMYG) (Rauch et al., 2005; Omura et al., 2005b; Wright et al., 2006, 2007; Sollberger et al., 2009; DeYoung, 2010). In neurofunctional studies, functional magnetic resonance imaging (fMRI) experiments have also demonstrated that specific brain regions that are engaged during cognitive-affective tasks were associated with specific personality dimensions. For example, activations in the prefrontal cortex, parietal cortex, anterior cingulated cortex (ACC), and middle temporal gyrus

(MTG) were correlated with extraversion (Canli et al., 2001; Eisenberger et al., 2005; Hutcherson et al., 2008; Tamura et al., 2012), while activations in the frontal cortex, dorsomedial prefrontal cortex, and AMYG were related to neuroticism (Canli et al., 2001; Haas et al., 2007; Hooker et al., 2008; Harenski et al., 2009). In addition, a positron emission tomography (PET) study assessing resting regional cerebral blood flow (rCBF) found that regions in ACC and temporal lobes were correlated with extraversion (Johnson et al., 1999). Extraversion was associated with regional cerebral glucose metabolism (rCMRglu) assessed by PET in right putamen, while neuroticism was associated with rCMRglu in the medial prefrontal cortex (MPFC) (Kim et al., 2008). These studies indicated specialized, spatially distributed regions were associated with personality dimensions of extraversion and neuroticism, respectively, and provided neurobiological evidence for the hypothesized biological model of Eysenck's personality.

Instead of detection activation paradigms by task-based fMRI, resting-state fMRI studies observe intrinsic spontaneous fluctuations in the blood oxygen level-dependent (BOLD) fMRI signal while avoiding the constraints of task-based approaches (Raichle et al., 2001; Fox and Raichle, 2007; Raichle and Snyder, 2007; Adelstein et al., 2011). There is accumulating evidence for local characteristics of resting brain functions associated with personality dimensions using resting-state fMRI (Kunisato et al., 2011; Wei et al., 2011, 2012; Hahn et al., 2012). Using regional homogeneity (ReHo) approach, our prior study found ReHo was correlated negatively with extraversion in the MPFC, and correlated positively in INS, cerebellum, and cingulate gyrus; whereas neuroticism had negative correlation with ReHo in left middle frontal gyrus (Wei et al., 2011). In addition, by using other local characteristics, i.e., the fractional amplitude of low-frequency fluctuations (fALFF), our previous study found positive correlations between LFF amplitude at Slow-5 and extraversion in MPFC and PCU, and between LFF amplitude at Slow-5 and neuroticism in right PreCG; LFF amplitude at Slow-4 was negatively associated with extraversion and neuroticism in left hippocampus (HIP) and bilateral superior temporal cortex (STC), respectively (Wei et al., 2012). **Table 1** summarizes the main results on the characteristics of resting brain functions associated with extraversion and neuroticism in recent resting-state fMRI studies.

From a functional integration perspective in the human brain, the multiple spatially distinct brain regions are functionally connected with coherent temporal dynamics (Friston et al., 1997; Sporns et al., 2000; Van Den Heuvel et al., 2009), making up complex and reciprocal brain networks even when we are at rest (Greicius et al., 2003; Damoiseaux et al., 2006; Van Den Heuvel et al., 2009). Such networks are thought to provide the physiological basis for information processing and mental representation (Canli, 2004; Bullmore and Sporns, 2009). Furthermore, evidence for small-world attributes of brain networks has been reported in the relative studies (Sporns et al., 2004; Stam, 2004; Eguiluz et al., 2005; Achard et al., 2006; Van Den Heuvel et al., 2009), indicating that small-world architectures in brain networks deviating from randomness reflect their specific functionality (Watts and Strogatz, 1998; Latora and Marchiori, 2001; Stam and Reijneveld, 2007; Bullmore and Sporns, 2009; Van Den Heuvel et al., 2009; He and Evans, 2010). Since personality factors may well be related to the networks in the brain (Canli, 2004; Wilt and Revelle, 2009), the analysis of task-independent, resting-state functional connectivity may reveal the intrinsically organized functional brain networks (Biswal et al., 1995), and allow for a better understanding of the neurobiological bases of extraversion and neuroticism. The recent study by Adelstein et al. (2011) found that extraversion and neuroticism were encoded within resting-state functional connectivity between seed regions and the lateral paralimbic regions and dorsomedial prefrontal cortex, respectively (Adelstein et al., 2011). However, the study was seed-based and lacked a network perspective on brain dynamics. In the present study, we hypothesized that the topological organization of the whole-brain functional networks would be associated with inter-individual variations in extraversion and neuroticism, and would link to Eysenck's cortical arousal theory of the two dimensions. To test our hypothesis, an exploratory analysis based on graph theory was thereby performed on the resting-state fMRI data of 71 healthy subjects, to detect the intrinsic resting-state

Table 1 | The main results on the characteristics of resting brain functions associated with extraversion and neuroticism in recent resting-state fMRI studies.

Method	fALFF (Kunisato et al., 2011)	Seed-based (ACC and PCU) FC (Adelstein et al., 2011)	ReHo (Wei et al., 2011)	fALFF (Slow-5 and Slow-4 bands) (Wei et al., 2012)
Extraversion	Striatum PCU SFG	FC between seed regions and lateral paralimbic regions	INS MCG MPFC MTG Cerebellum	MPFC and PCU at Slow-5 HIP at Slow-4
Neuroticism	MFG PCU	FC between seed regions and the dorsomedial prefrontal cortex	MFG	PreCG at Slow-5 STC at Slow-4

ACC, anterior cingulate cortex; fALFF, fractional amplitude of low-frequency fluctuations; FC, functional connectivity; HIP, hippocampus; INS, insula; MCG, middle cingulate gyrus; MFG, middle frontal gyrus; MPFC, medial prefrontal cortex; MTG, middle temporal gyrus; PCU, precuneus; PreCG, precentral gyrus; ReHo, regional homogeneity; SFG, superior frontal gyrus; STC, superior temporal cortex.

functional connectivity mechanisms underlying the two personality dimensions.

MATERIALS AND METHODS

PARTICIPANTS

We conducted the analysis with the same dataset in our previous study (Wei et al., 2011). Eighty-seven healthy right-handed subjects (48 males; age range: 17–36 yrs, mean age: 23.5 yrs) with no history of neurological or psychiatric disorders participated in the study. The present study was approved by the local Medical Ethics Committee at Jinling Hospital, Nanjing University School of Medicine, and the informed written consents were obtained from all participants.

PERSONALITY QUESTIONNAIRES

The revised Eysenck personality questionnaire short scale for Chinese (EPQ-RSC) (Eysenck, 1991; Qian et al., 2000) was used to assess personality dimensions of extraversion, neuroticism, and psychoticism of each subject before MRI scanning. Raw scores of the three dimensions were then converted into T-scores using the formula (Qian et al., 2000), respectively:

$$T = 50 + 10 \times \frac{\text{raw score} - \text{mean}}{\text{SD}},$$

where *mean* represents the mean value of the personality scores over all the subjects; *SD* is the standard deviation of the personality scores. We focused our analyses on extraversion and neuroticism whose resultant T-scores were used for calculating correlations with the brain network metrics.

IMAGE ACQUISITION

Resting-state fMRI images were acquired using a single-shot, gradient-recalled echo planar imaging (EPI) sequence on a 3.0-T Siemens Trio scanner (Jinling Hospital, Nanjing, China). The acquisition parameters were: $TR = 2000$ ms, $TE = 30$ ms, field of view (FOV) = 240 mm, image matrix size = 64×64, voxel size = $3.75 \times 3.75 \times 4\,\text{mm}^3$, 30 transverse slices without slice gap, flip angle = 90°, and a total of 255 volumes for each subject.

DATA PREPROCESSING

Data preprocessing was performed using the Statistical Parametric Mapping software (SPM8, http://www.fil.ion.ucl.ac.uk/spm). The first five volumes were discarded to ensure steady-state longitudinal magnetization. The remaining resting-state fMRI images were first corrected by the acquisition time delay among different slices, and then realigned to the first volume for head-motion correction. The dataset with translational or rotational parameters exceeding ±1 mm or ±1° would be excluded, according to our previous study on functional connectivity network (Liao et al., 2010). The images of remaining 71 participants were further spatially normalized into a standard stereotaxic space at $3 \times 3 \times 3\,\text{mm}^3$, using the Montreal Neurological Institute (MNI) template in SPM8. In order to avoid artificially introducing local spatial correlation, no spatial smoothing was applied, as previous studies suggested (Salvador et al., 2005; Achard et al., 2006; Achard and Bullmore, 2007; Liao et al., 2010). Since recent studies have showed that functional connectivity analysis is sensitive to gross head motion effects (Power et al., 2012; Van Dijk et al., 2012), we further evaluated the framewise displacement (FD) (Power et al., 2012) to express instantaneous head motion, and the threshold of 0.5 was suggested. The *mean* ± *SD* of FD over subjects was: 0.1080 ± 0.0159. Six subjects' FD values were beyond 0.5, but only in one frame for each subject. Scrubbing process was performed using toolbox "ArtRepair" in SPM8.

The mean time series of each ROI was corrected by a linear regression to remove the possible spurious variances including six head motion parameters acquired from the SPM8 preprocessing, the white matter (WM) and the ventricular brain signals averaged from a WM mask and a ventricular mask respectively (Fox et al., 2005; Salvador et al., 2005; Tian et al., 2006; Liao et al., 2010). The residuals of these regressions were temporally band-pass filtered ($0.01 < f < 0.08$ Hz) to reduce low-frequency drifts and physiological high-frequency respiratory and cardiac noise (Biswal et al., 1995), and linearly detrended for further functional connectivity and graph-theory analysis (Tian et al., 2006; Liao et al., 2010). The following approaches based on graph theory were performed by an in-house program coded in MATLAB (The Mathworks, Natick, MA).

COMPUTATION OF FUNCTIONAL CONNECTIVITY NETWORK

Node definition

To define the brain nodes, the anatomical parcellation was performed using the automated anatomical labeling (AAL) template, segmenting the images into 90 anatomical regions of interests (ROIs) (45 ROIs for each hemisphere). The representative time series in each ROI was obtained by averaging the fMRI time series across all voxels in the ROI.

Edge definition

To define the network edges, the residuals of the regression analysis were used to compute the Pearson's correlation, resulting in a 90×90 correlation matrix for each subject. A Fisher's r-to-z transformation was applied to the correlation matrices of all the subjects to improve the normality of the correlation coefficients (r) (Liu et al., 2008). The undirected edge e_{ij} between node i and node j is defined as:

$$e_{ij} = \begin{cases} 1 & \text{when } |r_{ij}| > T \\ 0 & \text{otherwise} \end{cases}$$

In general, if the absolute value of r_{ij} of a pair of brain regions, i and j, exceeds a predefined threshold T, an edge is assumed to exist; otherwise, no existence would be assumed (Liao et al., 2010).

GRAPH THEORETICAL ANALYSIS

Network metrics

The topological properties of the brain functional networks can be measured by both nodal and global network measures. In this study, we calculated the nodal measures including the degree K_i, the clustering coefficient C_i, the minimum path length L_i, the efficiency E_i, and the betweenness centrality BC_i of a node i; the global measures including the average degree K, the network efficiency involving the local efficiency E_{local} and the global efficiency E_{global}, the characteristic path length L, the clustering coefficient of a network C, the normalized clustering coefficient γ, the normalized characteristic path length λ, and the small-worldness σ.

Degree. The degree at each node, K_i, $i = 1, 2, \ldots, 90$, is defined as the number of nodes in a subgraph G_i, which is the graph including the nodes that are direct neighbors of node i. Briefly, K_i denotes to which extent the node is connected to the rest of the network (Bullmore and Sporns, 2009; Wang et al., 2010). A node with a higher degree has more connections (where each connection is counted once). The average degree K is the mean of K_i of all the nodes in the network.

Clustering coefficient. The absolute clustering coefficient C_i of a node is the ratio between the number of existing connections and the number of all possible connections in the subgraph G_i. C_i quantifies the level of local connectedness within a network (Bullmore and Sporns, 2009; Van Den Heuvel et al., 2009; He and Evans, 2010)

$$C_i = \frac{e_i}{K_i(K_i - 1)/2},$$

where e_i is the number of edges in the subgraph G_i. The clustering coefficient of the network C is the mean of C_i of all the nodes in the network.

Minimum path length. The nodal minimum path length L_i is defined as the mean shortest absolute path length of node i to other nodes in a network (Bullmore and Sporns, 2009), which quantifies the level of routing efficiency or the capability for parallel information propagation of a network (Van Den Heuvel et al., 2009; He and Evans, 2010; Liao et al., 2010)

$$L_i = \frac{1}{N-1} \sum_{i \neq j \in G} \min\{L_{i,j}\},$$

where min $\{L_{i,j}\}$ is the shortest absolute path length between node i and node j, and the absolute path length is the number of edges included in the path connecting two nodes. The characteristic path length L is the mean of L_i of all the nodes in the network.

Efficiency. The nodal efficiency E_i is the inverse of the harmonic mean of the length between node i and all other nodes in the network, to deal with the disconnected graphs, non-sparse graphs or both (Latora and Marchiori, 2001; Bassett and Bullmore, 2006; Wang et al., 2010)

$$E_i = \frac{1}{N-1} \sum_{\substack{j \in G \\ j \neq i}} \frac{1}{\min\{L_{i,j}\}}.$$

The global efficiency E_{global} of the network is the mean of E_i of all the nodes in the network.

In the subgraph G_i, we can calculate the local efficiency of node i as:

$$E_{i\_local} = \frac{1}{N_{G_i}(N_{G_i} - 1)} \sum_{\substack{j,k \in G_i \\ j \neq k}} \frac{1}{\min\{L_{j,k}\}}.$$

The local efficiency E_{local} of the network is then similarly defined as the mean of E_{i_local} of all the nodes in the network (Rubinov and Sporns, 2010).

Betweenness centrality. The betweenness centrality BC_i is defined as the fraction of all shortest paths in the network that pass through node i (Rubinov and Sporns, 2010). BC_i describes the central nodes that participate in many short paths within a network, and consequently act as important controls of information flow (Freeman, 1978)

$$BC_i = \frac{1}{(N-1)(N-2)} \sum_{\substack{j,k \in G \\ i \neq j \neq k}} \frac{\rho_{j,k}(i)}{\rho_{j,k}},$$

where $\rho_{j,k}$ is the number of shortest paths between node j and k; $\rho_{j,k}(i)$ is the number of shortest paths between j and k that pass through node i (Rubinov and Sporns, 2010).

Small-world parameters. Compared with random networks characterized by a low clustering coefficient and a typical short path length, networks with a small-world organization have a higher clustering coefficient and similar path length, i.e., $\gamma = C/C_{random} > 1$, $\lambda = L/L_{random} \approx 1$, namely normalized clustering coefficient and normalized characteristic path length, respectively (Watts and Strogatz, 1998). These two conditions can also be summarized into a quantitative measurement, $\sigma = \gamma/\lambda > 1$, namely small-worldness (Humphries et al., 2006; Wang et al., 2010). C_{random} and L_{random} were calculated as the averaged clustering coefficient and characteristic path length of a set of 100 random networks with the same degree distribution as that of the examined functional connectivity network (Van Den Heuvel et al., 2009; Liao et al., 2010). The random networks were generated based on a Markov-chain algorithm, according to our previous study (Liao et al., 2010).

Threshold selection

The threshold T was defined as the total number of edges in a graph divided by the maximum possible number of edges (Achard and Bullmore, 2007), namely wiring cost. We investigated the topological properties of brain functional network over a range of $T_{min} \leq T \leq T_{max}$. (1) T_{min} was selected by thresholding all networks to construct a sparse graph with the average degree $K \geq 2\times \log(N)$ (here $N = 90$ represents the number of nodes); (2) T_{max} was selected to ensure the small-worldness σ of the thresholded networks be larger than 1.1 for all participants (Liao et al., 2010; Zhang et al., 2011). The resultant threshold range of $0.10 \leq T \leq 0.31$ was used in our study. This range of sparsity allows the thresholded networks to be estimable for small-worldness and the number of spurious edges to be minimized (Watts and Strogatz, 1998; Achard and Bullmore, 2007; He et al., 2008; Zhang et al., 2011).

ASSOCIATION BETWEEN NETWORK ORGANIZATION AND PERSONALITY DIMENSIONS

All the nodal and global measures were thresholded repeatedly over the range of $0.1 \leq T \leq 0.31$ with an interval of 0.01, and the area under the curve (AUC) for each network metric was calculated, which provides a summarized scalar for topological characterization of brain networks independent of single threshold selection (Zhang et al., 2011). The partial correlation was then calculated between the AUC of each network metric and extraversion/neuroticism scores, with age and gender being covariates.

To assess the statistical significance of the correlation, the null distribution for each network metric was obtained by nonparametric permutation tests. Accordingly, 5000 subject specific random networks were generated at each threshold as null-model reference networks. The correlations between the AUC of each network metric and the personality scores were recalculated to obtain the null distribution. 1/number of regions was used as a false-positive correction, which implied that there was less than one false positive regional result per cortical map at this threshold (Lynall et al., 2010; Fornito et al., 2011).

LEAVE-ONE-OUT PREDICTION

To test the validity of the significantly correlated measures in predicting personality scores of extraversion and neuroticism, a leave-one-out cross-validation strategy was applied. The significantly correlated measures acted as explanatory variables in the linear regression models to predict the personality scores. The predicted results of all the subjects were assessed by calculating the Pearson's correlation between the predicted values and the original values. The precision of individual prediction was assessed by the average of the absolute relative errors between the predicted and original scores.

RESULTS

DESCRIPTIVE STATISTICS OF THE PERSONALITY DIMENSIONS

Table 2 describes the scores of the three personality dimensions from the EPQ-RSC questionnaire, and **Table 3** describes the correlations across the scores of the three dimensions. As two dimensions concerned in the present study, extraversion had a moderate negative correlation with neuroticism ($r = -0.238$, $p = 0.046$). The result was concordant with many prior studies, suggesting an inverse relationship between extraversion and neuroticism (Rusting and Larsen, 1997; Wright et al., 2006; Kim et al., 2008). Therefore, we added extraversion (or neuroticism) scores as covariate when calculating the partial correlation between neuroticism (or extraversion) and the AUC of each network metric, to obtain effects that were uniquely driven by each personality dimension.

Table 2 | Descriptive Statistics of the three personality dimensions of 71 participants.

Category	Data
Gender (male/female)	38/33
Age (years)	23.219 ± 2.031
Extraversion (E)	56.172 ± 8.703
Neuroticism (N)	43.048 ± 12.822
Psychoticism (P)	46.581 ± 8.229

Age and personality scores are displayed as mean ± SD.

THE ASSOCIATIONS BETWEEN NETWORK METRICS AND EXTRAVERSION

Among all the global measures of the network calculated in the present study, only the AUC of normalized clustering coefficient γ showed significant correlation with extraversion (**Figure 1**). As for the nodal measures, results indicated that only the AUC of BC_i showed significant correlations with extraversion. Extraversion significantly increased with BC_i in left INS, while significantly decreased with BC_i in bilateral MTG. **Figure 2** demonstrates the brain regions showing significant correlations between their BC_i and extraversion scores along with the corresponding correlation coefficients.

Figure 3 depicts the topological characteristics of network metrics which have significant associations with extraversion, as a function of wiring cost thresholds. The asterisk indicates the threshold where the significant correlation between the metric and extraversion was detected (permutation testing, $p < 1.90$). The inset figure indicates the correlation between the metric and extraversion at wiring cost = 0.22.

Table 3 | Correlations between scores of the three personality dimensions.

	P	*N*
N	0.106 (*p* = 0.379)	
E	−0.205 (*p* = 0.086)	−0.238 (*p* = 0.046*)

*E, extraversion; N, neuroticism; P, psychoticism. *p < 0.05.*

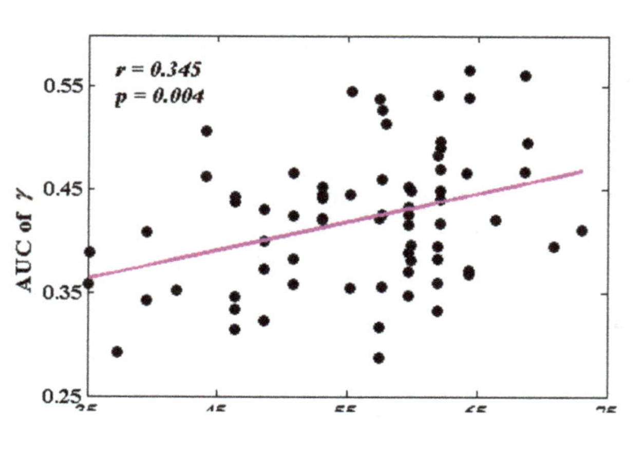

FIGURE 1 | The correlation between the area under the curve (AUC) of γ and extraversion scores ($p < 1.90$). AUC was calculated over the range of $0.1 \leq T \leq 0.31$ with an interval of 0.01.

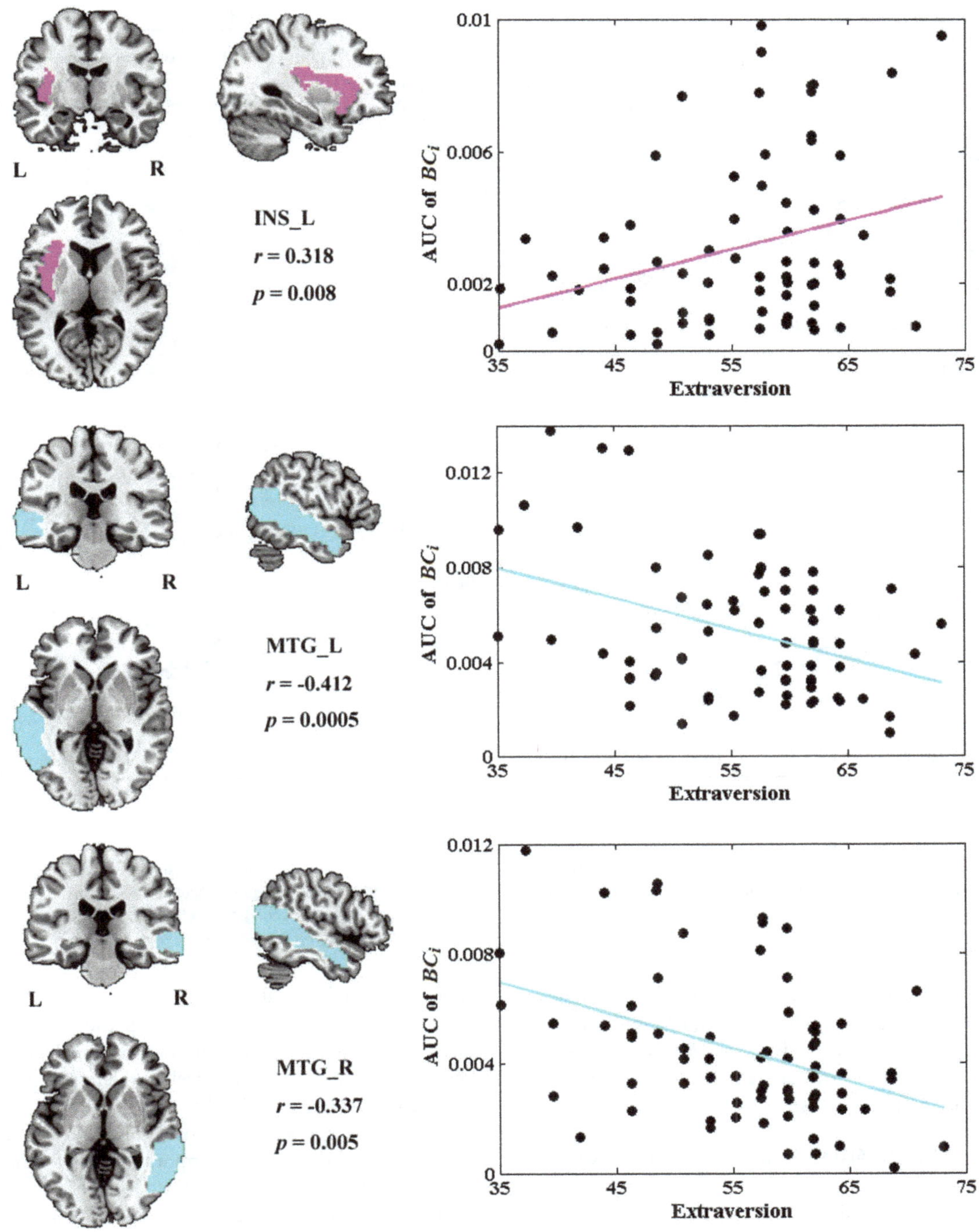

FIGURE 2 | The brain regions showing significantly correlations between AUC of BC_i and extraversion scores (p < 1.90). AUC was calculated over the range of $0.1 \leq T \leq 0.31$ with an interval of 0.01. The cyan color represents the negative correlations, while the magenta color represents the positive correlations. INS, insular; L, left; MTG, middle temporal gyrus; R, right.

THE ASSOCIATIONS BETWEEN NETWORK METRICS AND NEUROTICISM

No global measures showed significant correlation with neuroticism. Significant correlations were revealed in the AUC of BC_i, too. Neuroticism scores showed increased significant correlation with BC_i in right PreCG, right olfactory cortex (OLF), right caudate nucleus (CAU), and bilateral AMYG. No significantly negative correlation was found. **Figure 4** indicates the brain regions showing significant correlations between BC_i and neuroticism scores along with the corresponding correlation coefficients.

Figure 5 depicts the topological characteristics of BC_i as a function of wiring cost thresholds, in the brain regions whose BC_i

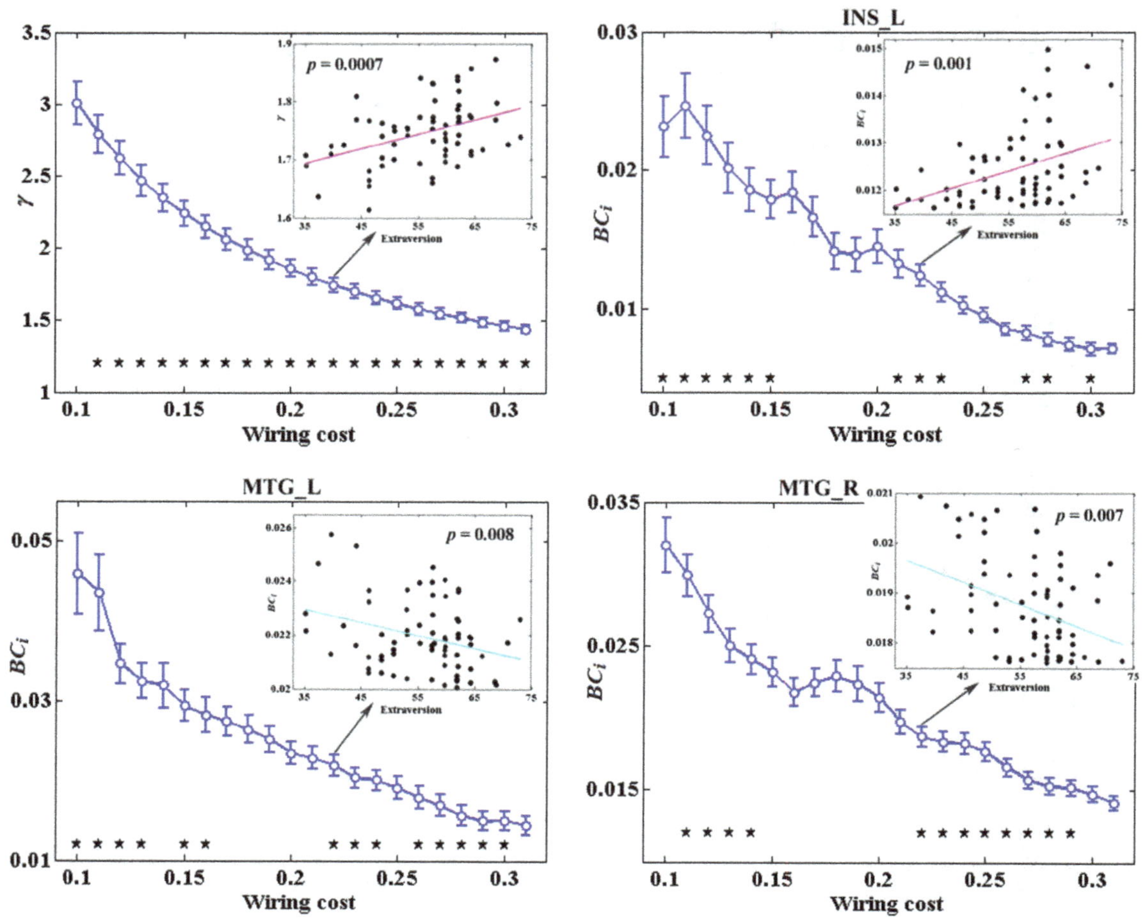

FIGURE 3 | The topological characteristics of network metrics which have significant associations with extraversion, as a function of wiring cost thresholds. The asterisk indicates the threshold where the significant correlation between the metric and extraversion was detected (permutation testing, $p < 1/90$). The inset figure indicates the correlation between the metric and extraversion at wiring cost = 0.22.

values have significant associations with neuroticism. The asterisk also indicates the threshold where the significant correlation between the metric and neuroticism was detected (permutation testing, $p < 1.90$). The inset figure indicates the correlation between the metric and neuroticism at wiring cost = 0.22.

THE PREDICTION OF PERSONALITY SCORES BY LEAVE-ONE-OUT APPROACH

Figure 6 shows the predicted and original pairs of extraversion (**Figure 6A**) and neuroticism (**Figure 6B**) scores, respectively. The Pearson's correlation coefficients of the predicted and original personality scores were 0.536 ($p = 0.146 \times 10^{-7}$) for extraversion, and 0.547 ($p = 0.784 \times 10^{-8}$) for neuroticism. The precisions of individual prediction were 11.4% for extraversion and 21.7% for neuroticism.

DISCUSSION

METHODOLOGICAL CONSIDERATIONS

The present study differed from our previous studies in both hypothesis and analysis methods. In the previous studies, the purpose was to identify the associations between the personality dimensions and the local synchronization of spontaneous BOLD activity (Wei et al., 2011), or between the personality dimensions and the fLFF in individual brain regions (Wei et al., 2012). Thereby the analysis method as well as the results obtained was at the functional segregation level.

Since the multiple spatially distinct brain regions are functionally connected with coherent temporal dynamics, the topological properties of the brain functional networks may predict individual differences in the two fundamental personality dimensions. To test this hypothesis, in the present study, we applied the graph theory method to explore the correlation between the network metrics in the resting-state brain network and the personality dimensions of extraversion and neuroticism at the functional integration level. To the best of our knowledge, the present study is among the first demonstrations of an association between personality dimensions and the properties of the resting-state functional network.

EXTRAVERSION AND THE NETWORK METRICS

The present results showed that compared to individuals with lower extraversion scores, individuals with higher extraversion

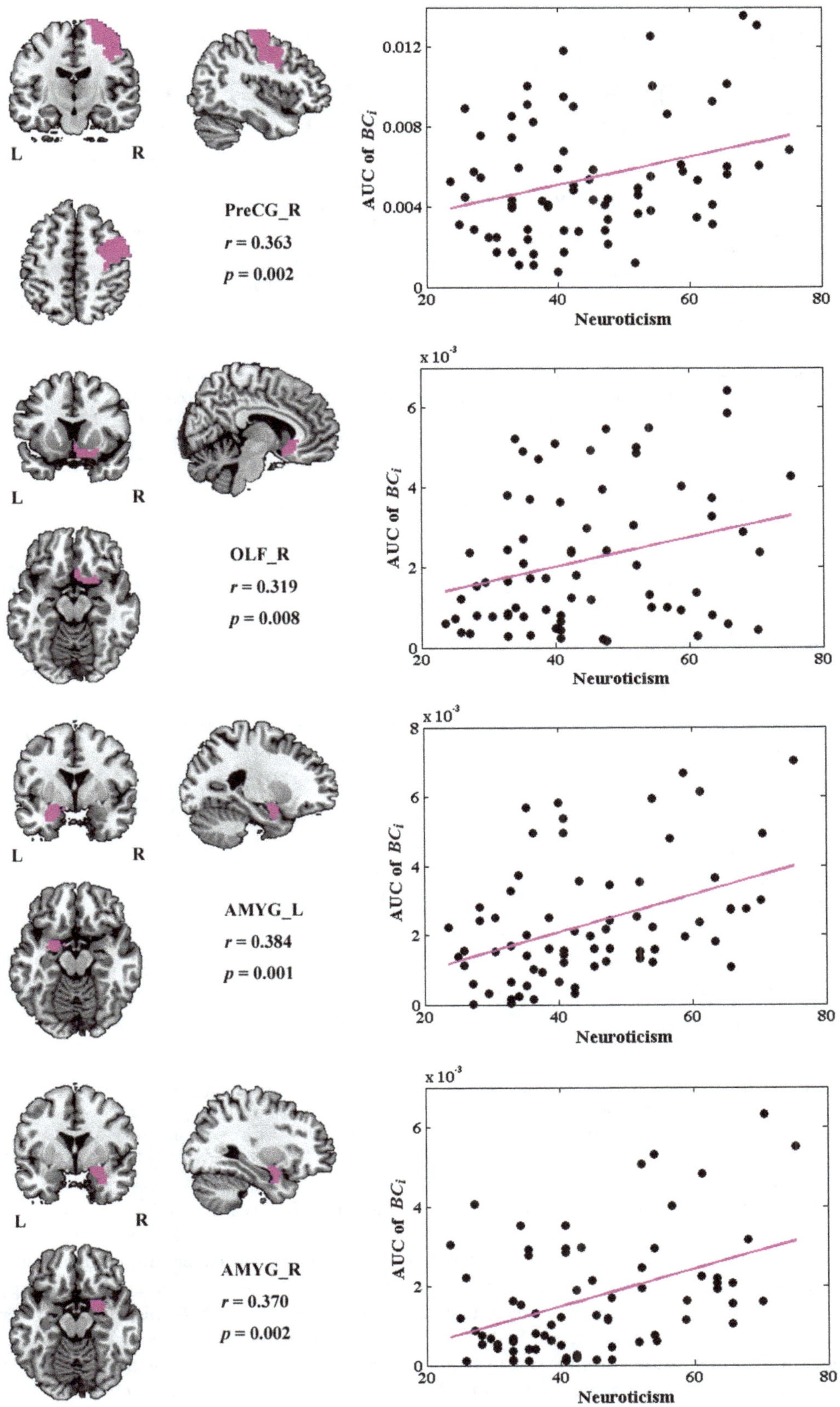

FIGURE 4 | Continued

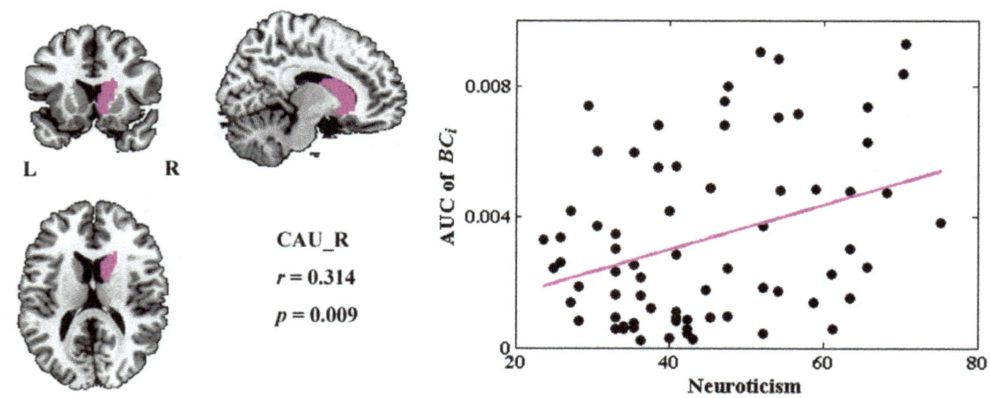

FIGURE 4 | The brain regions showing significantly correlations between AUC of BC_i and neuroticism scores ($p < 1.90$). AUC was calculated over the range of $0.1 \leq T \leq 0.31$ with an interval of 0.01. AMYG, amygdala; CAU, caudate nucleus; L, left; OLF, olfactory cortex; PreCG, precentral gyrus; R, right.

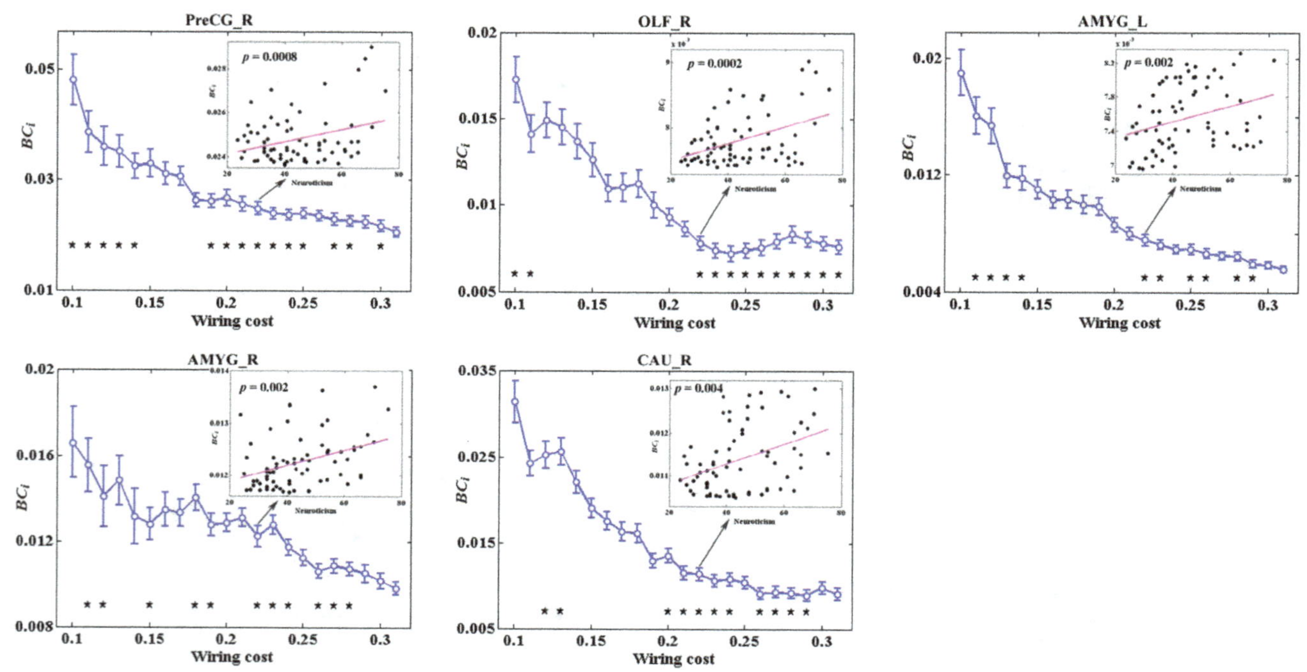

FIGURE 5 | The topological characteristics of BC_i as a function of wiring cost thresholds, in the brain regions whose BC_i values have significant associations with neuroticism. The asterisk also indicates the threshold where the significant correlation between the metric and neuroticism was detected (permutation testing, $p < 1/90$). The inset figure indicates the correlation between the metric and neuroticism at wiring cost = 0.22.

scores had larger AUC of normalized clustering coefficient γ. γ quantifies the extent of local cliquishness or local efficiency of information transfer of a network (He and Evans, 2010). Our results indicated that the whole functional brain networks of individuals with higher extraversion scores were more clustered than these of individuals with lower extraversion scores.

In Eysenck's biological theory of extraversion, extraverts have a higher threshold for cortical arousal, as they are assumed to be chronically "under-aroused" (Eysenck, 1967; Tran et al., 2006; Wilt and Revelle, 2009). It is this chronic intrinsic under-arousal which is thought to drive highly extraverted people to engage in typically extraverted behaviors in order to enhance their low arousal states (Eysenck, 1994; Kehoe et al., 2012). Thereby extraverts should, on average, respond more and faster than introverts (in order to increase their arousal) during performance tasks (Eysenck, 1994; Wilt and Revelle, 2009). Furthermore, this under-arousability enables extraverts to tolerate much higher levels of arousal than introverts, who withdraw to avoid further increases in arousal which they find difficult to withstand (Eysenck, 1967, 1994; Kehoe et al., 2012).

From a network perspective, compared to random network which has low clustering coefficient and short path length,

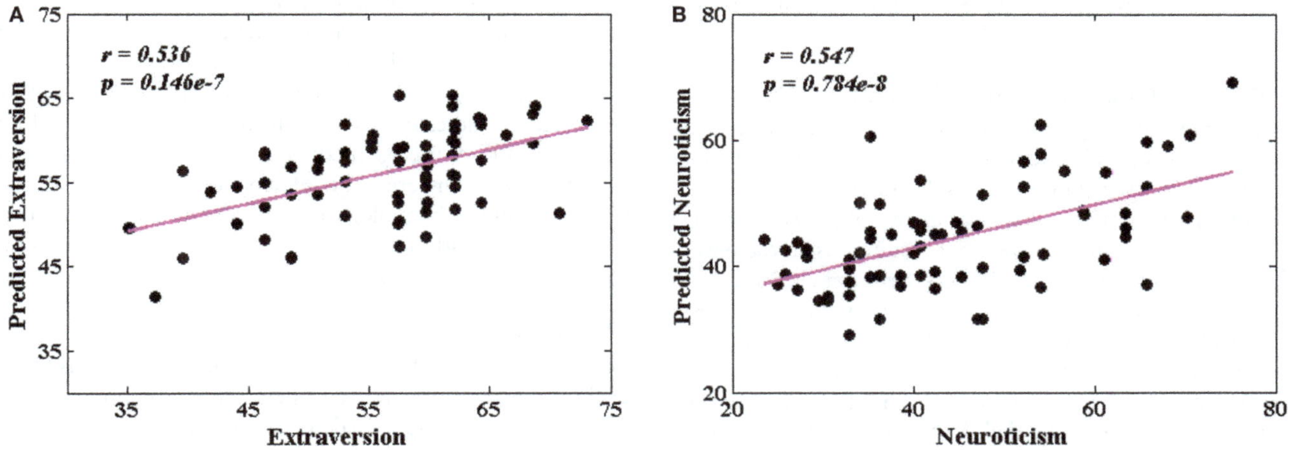

FIGURE 6 | The correlations between the predicted and original personality scores. (A) Extraversion scores ($r = 0.536$, $p = 0.146 \times 10^{-7}$); **(B)** neuroticism scores ($r = 0.547$, $p = 0.784 \times 10^{-8}$).

small-world network has higher clustering coefficient than a random network. The lower γ in the brain networks of introverts suggested that functional brain networks in introverts had a trend toward a randomized configuration. Random networks have less modularized information processing or fault tolerance compared with small-world networks (Latora and Marchiori, 2001; Zhang et al., 2011). A higher arousal threshold in cortex and higher level of arousal tolerance in extraverts could be interpreted by more clustered configuration in functional brain networks of extraverts.

As one of the nodal centrality metrics, increased BC_i suggested the strengthened roles of coordinating whole-brain networks (Zhang et al., 2011). The brain regions with relatively higher BC_i participate more in information transition and consequently act as important controls of information flow. The greater activation levels and lower arousal thresholds in these regions with higher BC_i may seem conceivable.

BC_i in left INS was found to be positively correlated with extraversion, whereas BC_i values in bilateral MTG were found to be negatively correlated with extraversion in this study.

INS is thought to play a central role for one's emotional processing (Iaria et al., 2008; Lamm and Singer, 2010) and is involved in various neuropsychiatric diseases such as mood disorders, depressive disorders, and panic disorders (Paulus and Stein, 2006; Nagai et al., 2007; Fitzgerald et al., 2008; Liu et al., 2010; Guo et al., 2011). There were many studies providing direct evidence for a link between INS activation and extraversion or extraversion-related dimension (Johnson et al., 1999; Omura et al., 2005a; Sollberger et al., 2009; Kehoe et al., 2012; Tamura et al., 2012). For example, a PET study showed the correlation between blood flow of INS and extraversion (Johnson et al., 1999). A fMRI study revealed that extraversion correlated with neural responses to positive word stimuli in bilateral INS (Omura et al., 2005a). A recent fMRI study suggested that INS activity may "mediate" the development of extraversion (Tamura et al., 2012). Our previous study found a positive association between extraversion and ReHo in INS. Positive correlation has also been found between extraversion and gray matter volume of INS in a morphometric study (Sollberger et al., 2009). The relation between BC_i and extraversion scores detected in INS in the present study further demonstrated that the regional characteristics of INS suggested individual differences in extraversion dimension. However, the positive correlation was unexpected according to Eysenck's predictions about this dimension. The expected negative correlations were revealed between extraversion and BC_i in bilateral MTG.

MTG was found to participate in both emotional processing and encoding tasks (Critchley et al., 2000; Dolcos et al., 2004; Olson et al., 2007). Abnormal functions of middle temporal areas in patients with borderline personality disorder (BPD) were reported both in resting MRI (Wolf et al., 2011) and emotional task MRI studies (Guitart-Masip et al., 2009). In normal late adolescents, fMRI study found correlations of age and extraversion with neural activation in MTG (Tamura et al., 2012). Our previous study also showed a negative association between extraversion and ReHo in MTG (Wei et al., 2011). These results demonstrated that MTG played a role in extraversion and the dysfunction of MTG was associated with personality disorders. Our study further showed the BC_i of bilateral MTG was negatively correlated with extraversion scores, suggesting that extraverts demonstrated lower levels of cortical arousal and higher arousal thresholds in bilateral MTG. This is consistent with Eysenck's arousal hypothesis of extraversion.

The results on the relationship between extraversion and arousal in specific brain regions some of which contradict Eysenck's predictions about this dimension while some of which agree with it have also been found in other studies (Kehoe et al., 2012; Wei et al., 2012). This may imply that the relationship between extraversion and arousal is a more complex story than that originally proposed by Eysenck (Kehoe et al., 2012). Researchers may face more complicated situations when looking into various brain regions. Further research is required to elucidate if and how arousal processing differences are a central feature of extraversion (Kehoe et al., 2012).

NEUROTICISM AND THE BETWEENNESS CENTRALITY

The other main finding of this study was significantly positive associations between BC_i and neuroticism scores in brain regions including right OLF, right CAU, and bilateral AMYG.

According to Eysenck's biological theory of personality, high levels of neuroticism are theorized to reflect increased reactivity of the limbic system (Eysenck, 1991, 1994; Kehoe et al., 2012). Our results provided some supporting evidence for this hypothesis, with individuals high in neuroticism showing higher BC_i values in right OLF, right CAU and bilateral AMYG. The limbic system supports a variety of functions involving motivation, emotion, learning, and memory. Especially, AMYG has been associated with anxiety and mood disorders, for which neuroticism is a risk factor (Haas et al., 2007). Individual differences in neuroticism, a dimension characterized by experiences of negative emotion, anxiety, and emotional lability (Cunningham et al., 2010), have been shown to correlate with greater AMYG activation during unpleasant picture stimuli (Harenski et al., 2009), during fear learning (Hooker et al., 2008), during trials of high emotional conflict (Haas et al., 2007), and greater amygdala-dorsolateral prefrontal cortex connectivity while viewing angry and fearful facial expressions (Cremers et al., 2010). All these studies suggested a greater activation levels in AMYG during stimuli in individuals with high neuroticism, which were concordant with Eysenck's arousal theory of neuroticism. Here, our results further demonstrated that in resting-state functional brain networks, individuals high in neuroticism exhibited higher BC_i values in AMYG as well as in OLF and CAU, suggesting greater activation levels and lower arousal thresholds in these regions in the resting brains of high neuroticism subjects.

Interestingly, most significantly correlated brain regions were located in the right hemisphere, suggesting the lateralization of these regions with regard to neuroticism. Electroencephalogram (EEG) researchers have found that dimensions related to the withdrawal aspect of neuroticism are associated with greater activation of right frontal lobe relative to left (Zuckerman, 2005; Shackman et al., 2009). The brain's right hemisphere appears to be preferentially involved in emotions and motivational states associated with withdrawal, whereas left hemisphere is preferentially involved in approach (Davidson, 2002; DeYoung, 2010). Our results provided neurofunctional evidence from the point of view of functional brain networks in resting-state.

THE PREDICTION OF PERSONALITY SCORES

In the present study, the leave-one-out cross-validation strategy was applied to test the validity of the significantly correlated measures in prediction personality scores. Our results showed very strong correlations between the original and predicted personality scores. The results suggested that statistically the functional brain network measures detected in our study did play roles in the prediction of personality. However, when considering the precision of individual prediction, the averages of the absolute relative errors for the prediction were 11.4% (range: 0.3–42.3%) for extraversion and 21.7% (range: 0.2–48.0%) for neuroticism. This implied the network measures alone were not able to precisely predict the individual personality. There have been some studies trying to predict individual personality from subjects' social behaviors (Bai et al., 2012) or emotional cognition tasks (Jackson, 2005). These studies combined with our findings shed light on the future work of precise prediction of personality, and further suggested that to integrate the information of individual's outer behaviors and inner topological properties of resting-state functional brain networks may give new clues to the neuropsychology of personality dimensions.

LIMITATIONS

Since this was an exploratory study, no prior hypothesis for the relation of a certain measure to personality was proposed. The false-positive correction used in the present study, which was 1/number of regions, was not as conservative as a Bonferroni or false discovery rate (FDR) correction (Lynall et al., 2010). Thereby type I error was not able to be strongly controlled in our analyses. In addition, whether extraversion/neuroticism is correlated with intelligence is still under controversial. Studies on the Big five model of personality and intelligence found associations between extraversion/neuroticism and intelligence. Extraversion and intelligence were found to be significantly negatively correlated (Ackerman and Heggestad, 1997; Wolf and Ackerman, 2005); however, further study argued extraversion might be related to some aspects of intelligence test-taking, rather than to actual intelligence (DeYoung, 2011). Neuroticism exhibited a small but reliable negative correlation with intelligence (Ackerman and Heggestad, 1997) though; this correlation was likely to be due to the mediation by test anxiety (Moutafi et al., 2006). Higher-order traits may exist above the Big Five, but they do not appear to be related to intelligence (DeYoung et al., 2008). In Eysenck's personality theory, he asserted that intelligence is unrelated to personality (Eysenck, 1994). A study assessing personality by EPQ_R demonstrated that affective dimensions of personality are independent of intelligence (Gray et al., 2005). Since the present study aimed to test the Eysenck's personality theory of cortical arousal on extraversion and neuroticism, personality traits was asserted to be unrelated to intelligence. Further investigations of the relations between intelligence and extraversion/neuroticism are required in future studies.

CONCLUSIONS

By applying the graph theoretical analysis to the resting-state fMRI data, the present study found that the normalized clustering coefficient values of the whole-brain functional networks were positively correlated with extraversion scores, suggesting an association between extraversion and the global network measure which quantifies the clustered configuration in the brain network. The more clustered configuration in brain functional network of extraverts may result in a higher arousal threshold in cortex and higher levels of arousal tolerance. However, extraversion scores were positively correlated with BC_i in right insula, while negatively correlated with BC_i in bilateral MTG, indicating that the relationship between extraversion and regional arousal is not as simple as that proposed by Eysenck. On the other hand, neuroticism scores showed consistently positive associations with BC_i in specific brain regions in the PreCG and limbic system, providing some supporting evidence for Eysenck's biological theory of neuroticism. Furthermore, the right lateralization of these regions with regard to neuroticism gave neurofunctional evidence to the preferential involvement of brain's right hemisphere in emotions and motivational states associated with withdrawal aspect of neuroticism.

ACKNOWLEDGMENTS

This work was supported by grants from the Natural Science Foundation of China (61035006, 91132721, and 61125304); Postdoctoral Science Foundation of China (20100481378) and Special Postdoctoral Science Foundation of China (2012T50772). The funders had no role in study design, data collection and analysis, decision to publish, or preparation of the manuscript.

REFERENCES

Achard, S., and Bullmore, E. (2007). Efficiency and cost of economical brain functional networks. *PLoS Comput. Biol.* 3:e17. doi: 10.1371/journal.pcbi.0030017

Achard, S., Salvador, R., Whitcher, B., Suckling, J., and Bullmore, E. (2006). A resilient, low-frequency, small-world human brain functional network with highly connected association cortical hubs. *J. Neurosci.* 26, 63–72. doi: 10.1523/JNEUROSCI.3874-05.2006

Ackerman, P. L., and Heggestad, E. D. (1997). Intelligence, personality, and interests: evidence for overlapping traits. *Psychol. Bull.* 121, 219–245. doi: 10.1037/0033-2909.121.2.219

Adelstein, J. S., Shehzad, Z., Mennes, M., Deyoung, C. G., Zuo, X. N., Kelly, C., et al. (2011). Personality is reflected in the brain's intrinsic functional architecture. *PLoS ONE* 6:e27633. doi: 10.1371/journal.pone.0027633

Bai, S., Zhu, T., and Cheng, L. (2012). Big-five personality prediction based on user behaviors at social network sites. *Comput. Soc.* arXiv:1204.4809.

Bassett, D. S., and Bullmore, E. (2006). Small-world brain networks. *Neuroscientist* 12, 512–523. doi: 10.1177/1073858406293182

Biswal, B., Yetkin, F. Z., Haughton, V. M., and Hyde, J. S. (1995). Functional connectivity in the motor cortex of resting human brain using echo-planar MRI. *Magn. Reson. Med.* 34, 537–541. doi: 10.3410/f.714597885.790202808

Bullmore, E., and Sporns, O. (2009). Complex brain networks: graph theoretical analysis of structural and functional systems. *Nat. Rev. Neurosci.* 10, 186–198. doi: 10.1038/nrn2575

Canli, T. (2004). Functional brain mapping of extraversion and neuroticism: learning from individual differences in emotion processing. *J. Pers.* 72, 1105–1132. doi: 10.1111/j.1467-6494.2004.00292.x

Canli, T., Zhao, Z., Desmond, J. E., Kang, E., Gross, J., and Gabrieli, J. D. (2001). An fMRI study of personality influences on brain reactivity to emotional stimuli. *Behav. Neurosci.* 115, 33–42. doi: 10.1037/0735-7044.115.1.33

Cremers, H. R., Demenescu, L. R., Aleman, A., Renken, R., Van Tol, M. J., Van Der Wee, N. J., et al. (2010). Neuroticism modulates amygdala-prefrontal connectivity in response to negative emotional facial expressions. *Neuroimage* 49, 963–970. doi: 10.1016/j.neuroimage.2009.08.023

Critchley, H., Daly, E., Phillips, M., Brammer, M., Bullmore, E., Williams, S., et al. (2000). Explicit and implicit neural mechanisms for processing of social information from facial expressions: a functional magnetic resonance imaging study. *Hum. Brain Mapp.* 9, 93–105.

Cunningham, W. A., Arbuckle, N. L., Jahn, A., Mowrer, S. M., and Abduljalil, A. M. (2010). Aspects of neuroticism and the amygdala: chronic tuning from motivational styles. *Neuropsychologia* 48, 3399–3404. doi: 10.1016/j.neuropsychologia.2010.06.026

Damoiseaux, J. S., Rombouts, S. A., Barkhof, F., Scheltens, P., Stam, C. J., Smith, S. M., et al. (2006). Consistent resting-state networks across healthy subjects. *Proc. Natl. Acad. Sci. U.S.A.* 103, 13848–13853. doi: 10.1073/pnas.0601417103

Davidson, R. J. (2002). Anxiety and affective style: role of prefrontal cortex and amygdala. *Biol. Psychiatry* 51, 68–80. doi: 10.1016/S0006-3223(01)01328-2

DeYoung, C. G. (2010). Personality neuroscience and the biology of traits. *Soc. Personal. Psychol. Compass* 4, 1165–1180. doi: 10.1111/j.1751-9004.2010.00327.x

DeYoung, C. G. (ed.). (2011). *Intelligence and Personality.* New York, NY: Cambridge University Press.

DeYoung, C. G., Peterson, J. B., Seguin, J. R., and Tremblay, R. E. (2008). Externalizing behavior and the higher order factors of the Big Five. *J. Abnorm. Psychol.* 117, 947–953. doi: 10.1037/a0013742

Dolcos, F., Labar, K. S., and Cabeza, R. (2004). Interaction between the amygdala and the medial temporal lobe memory system predicts better memory for emotional events. *Neuron* 42, 855–863. doi: 10.1016/S0896-6273(04)00289-2

Eguiluz, V. M., Chialvo, D. R., Cecchi, G. A., Baliki, M., and Apkarian, A. V. (2005). Scale-free brain functional networks. *Phys. Rev. Lett.* 94, 018102. doi: 10.1103/PhysRevLett.94.018102

Eisenberger, N. I., Lieberman, M. D., and Satpute, A. B. (2005). Personality from a controlled processing perspective: an fMRI study of neuroticism, extraversion, and self-consciousness. *Cogn. Affect. Behav. Neurosci.* 5, 169–181. doi: 10.3758/CABN.5.2.169

Eysenck, H. J. (1967). *The Biological Basis of Personality.* Springfield, IL: Charles C. Thomas.

Eysenck, H. J. (ed.). (1990). *Biological Dimensions of Personality.* New York, NY: Guilford Press.

Eysenck, H. J. (1991). *Manual of the Eysenck Personality Scales (EPS Adult).* London: Hodder and Stoughton.

Eysenck, H. J. (ed.). (1994). *Personality: Biological Foundations.* London: Academic Press.

Eysenck, H. J., and Eysenck, M. W. (eds.). (1985). *Personality and Individual Differences: a Natural Science Approach.* New York, NY; Plenum Press.

Fischer, H., Wik, G., and Fredrikson, M. (1998). Extraversion, Neuroticism and brain function: a PET study of personality. *Pers. Indiv. Differ.* 23, 345–352. doi: 10.1016/S0191-8869(97)00027-5

Fitzgerald, P. B., Laird, A. R., Maller, J., and Daskalakis, Z. J. (2008). A meta-analytic study of changes in brain activation in depression. *Hum. Brain Mapp.* 29, 683–695. doi: 10.1002/hbm.20426

Fornito, A., Yoon, J., Zalesky, A., Bullmore, E. T., and Carter, C. S. (2011). General and specific functional connectivity disturbances in first-episode schizophrenia during cognitive control performance. *Biol. Psychiatry* 70, 64–72. doi: 10.1016/j.biopsych.2011.02.019

Fox, M. D., and Raichle, M. E. (2007). Spontaneous fluctuations in brain activity observed with functional magnetic resonance imaging. *Nat. Rev. Neurosci.* 8, 700–711. doi: 10.1038/nrn2201

Fox, M. D., Snyder, A. Z., Vincent, J. L., Corbetta, M., Van Essen, D. C., and Raichle, M. E. (2005). The human brain is intrinsically organized into dynamic, anticorrelated functional networks. *Proc. Natl. Acad. Sci. U.S.A.* 102, 9673–9678. doi: 10.1073/pnas.0504136102

Freeman, L. C. (1978). Centrality in social networks: conceptual clarification. *Soc. Netw.* 1, 215–239. doi: 10.1016/0378-8733(78)90021-7

Friston, K. J., Buechel, C., Fink, G. R., Morris, J., Rolls, E., and Dolan, R. J. (1997). Psychophysiological and modulatory interactions in neuroimaging. *Neuroimage* 6, 218–229. doi: 10.1006/nimg.1997.0291

Gray, J. R., Burgess, G. C., Schaefer, A., Yarkoni, T., Larsen, R. J., and Braver, T. S. (2005). Affective personality differences in neural processing efficiency confirmed using fMRI. *Cogn. Affect. Behav. Neurosci.* 5, 182–190. doi: 10.3758/CABN.5.2.182

Greicius, M. D., Krasnow, B., Reiss, A. L., and Menon, V. (2003). Functional connectivity in the resting brain: a network analysis of the default mode hypothesis. *Proc. Natl. Acad. Sci. U.S.A.* 100, 253–258. doi: 10.1073/pnas.0135058100

Guitart-Masip, M., Pascual, J. C., Carmona, S., Hoekzema, E., Berge, D., Perez, V., et al. (2009). Neural correlates of impaired emotional discrimination in borderline personality disorder: an fMRI study. *Prog. Neuropsychopharmacol. Biol. Psychiatry* 33, 1537–1545. doi: 10.1016/j.pnpbp.2009.08.022

Guo, W. B., Sun, X. L., Liu, L., Xu, Q., Wu, R. R., Liu, Z. N., et al. (2011). Disrupted regional homogeneity in treatment-resistant depression: a resting-state fMRI study. *Prog. Neuropsychopharmacol. Biol. Psychiatry* 35, 1297–1302. doi: 10.1016/j.pnpbp.2011.02.006

Haas, B. W., Omura, K., Constable, R. T., and Canli, T. (2007). Emotional conflict and neuroticism: personality-dependent activation in the amygdala and subgenual anterior cingulate. *Behav. Neurosci.* 121, 249–256. doi: 10.1037/0735-7044.121.2.249

Hahn, T., Dresler, T., Ehlis, A. C., Pyka, M., Dieler, A. C., Saathoff, C., et al. (2012). Randomness of resting-state brain oscillations encodes Gray's personality trait. *Neuroimage* 59, 1842–1845. doi: 10.1016/j.neuroimage.2011.08.042

Harenski, C. L., Kim, S. H., and Hamann, S. (2009). Neuroticism and psychopathy predict brain activation during moral and nonmoral emotion regulation. *Cogn. Affect Behav. Neurosci.* 9, 1–15. doi: 10.3758/CABN.9.1.1

He, Y., Chen, Z., and Evans, A. (2008). Structural insights into aberrant topological patterns of large-scale cortical networks in Alzheimer's disease. *J. Neurosci.* 28, 4756–4766. doi: 10.1523/JNEUROSCI.0141-08.2008

He, Y., and Evans, A. (2010). Graph theoretical modeling of brain connectivity. *Curr. Opin. Neurol.* 23, 341–350. doi: 10.1097/WCO.0b013e32833aa567

Hooker, C. I., Verosky, S. C., Miyakawa, A., Knight, R. T., and D'Esposito, M. (2008). The influence of personality on neural mechanisms of observational fear and reward learning. *Neuropsychologia* 46, 2709–2724. doi: 10.1016/j.neuropsychologia.2008.05.005

Humphries, M. D., Gurney, K., and Prescott, T. J. (2006). The brainstem reticular formation is a small-world, not scale-free, network. *Proc. Biol. Sci.* 273, 503–511. doi: 10.1098/rspb.2005.3354

Hutcherson, C. A., Goldin, P. R., Ramel, W., McRae, K., and Gross, J. J. (2008). Attention and emotion influence the relationship between extraversion and neural response. *Soc. Cogn. Affect. Neurosci.* 3, 71–79. doi: 10.1093/scan/nsm040

Iaria, G., Committeri, G., Pastorelli, C., Pizzamiglio, L., Watkins, K. E., and Carota, A. (2008). Neural activity of the anterior insula in emotional processing depends on the individuals' emotional susceptibility. *Hum. Brain Mapp.* 29, 363–373. doi: 10.1002/hbm.20393

Jackson, C. J. (2005). How preferred ear for listening moderates emotional cognitions in the prediction of personality. *Laterality* 10, 305–320. doi: 10.1080/13576500442000102

Johnson, D. L., Wiebe, J. S., Gold, S. M., Andreasen, N. C., Hichwa, R. D., Watkins, G. L., et al. (1999). Cerebral blood flow and personality: a positron emission tomography study. *Am. J. Psychiatry* 156, 252–257.

Kehoe, E. G., Toomey, J. M., Balsters, J. H., and Bokde, A. L. (2012). Personality modulates the effects of emotional arousal and valence on brain activation. *Soc. Cogn. Affect. Neurosci.* 7, 858–870. doi: 10.1093/scan/nsr059

Kim, S. H., Hwang, J. H., Park, H. S., and Kim, S. E. (2008). Resting brain metabolic correlates of neuroticism and extraversion in young men. *Neuroreport* 19, 883–886. doi: 10.1097/WNR.0b013e328300080f

Kunisato, Y., Okamoto, Y., Okada, G., Aoyama, S., Nishiyama, Y., Onoda, K., et al. (2011). Personality traits and the amplitude of spontaneous low-frequency oscillations during resting state. *Neurosci. Lett.* 492, 109–113. doi: 10.1016/j.neulet.2011.01.067

Lamm, C., and Singer, T. (2010). The role of anterior insular cortex in social emotions. *Brain Struct. Funct.* 214, 579–591. doi: 10.1007/s00429-010-0251-3

Latora, V., and Marchiori, M. (2001). Efficient behavior of small-world networks. *Phys. Rev. Lett.* 87, 198701. doi: 10.1103/PhysRevLett.87.198701

Liao, W., Zhang, Z., Pan, Z., Mantini, D., Ding, J., Duan, X., et al. (2010). Altered functional connectivity and small-world in mesial temporal lobe epilepsy. *PLoS ONE* 5:e8525. doi: 10.1371/journal.pone.0008525

Liu, Y., Liang, M., Zhou, Y., He, Y., Hao, Y., Song, M., et al. (2008). Disrupted small-world networks in schizophrenia. *Brain* 131, 945–961. doi: 10.1093/brain/awn018

Liu, Z., Xu, C., Xu, Y., Wang, Y., Zhao, B., Lv, Y., et al. (2010). Decreased regional homogeneity in insula and cerebellum: a resting-state fMRI study in patients with major depression and subjects at high risk for major depression. *Psychiatry Res.* 182, 211–215. doi: 10.1016/j.pscychresns.2010.03.004

Lynall, M. E., Bassett, D. S., Kerwin, R., McKenna, P. J., Kitzbichler, M., Muller, U., et al. (2010). Functional connectivity and brain networks in schizophrenia. *J. Neurosci.* 30, 9477–9487. doi: 10.1523/JNEUROSCI.0333-10.2010

Matthews, G., and Gilliland, K. (1999). The personality theories of H.J. Eysenck and J.A. Gray: a comparative review. *Pers. Indiv. Differ.* 26, 583–626. doi: 10.1016/S0191-8869(98)00158-5

Moutafi, J., Furnham, A., and Tsaousis, I. (2006). Is the relationship between intelligence and trait neuroticism mediated by test anxiety? *Pers. Indiv. Differ.* 40, 587–597. doi: 10.1016/j.paid.2005.08.004

Nagai, M., Kishi, K., and Kato, S. (2007). Insular cortex and neuropsychiatric disorders: a review of recent literature. *Eur. Psychiatry* 22, 387–394. doi: 10.1016/j.eurpsy.2007.02.006

Olson, I. R., Plotzker, A., and Ezzyat, Y. (2007). The Enigmatic temporal pole: a review of findings on social and emotional processing. *Brain* 130, 1718–1731. doi: 10.1093/brain/awm052

Omura, K., Aron, A., and Canli, T. (2005a). Variance maps as a novel tool for localizing regions of interest in imaging studies of individual differences. *Cogn. Affect. Behav. Neurosci.* 5, 252–261. doi: 10.3758/CABN.5.2.252

Omura, K., Todd Constable, R., and Canli, T. (2005b). Amygdala gray matter concentration is associated with extraversion and neuroticism. *Neuroreport* 16, 1905–1908. doi: 10.1097/01.wnr.0000186596.64458.76

Paulus, M. P., and Stein, M. B. (2006). An insular view of anxiety. *Biol. Psychiatry* 60, 383–387. doi: 10.1016/j.biopsych.2006.03.042

Power, J. D., Barnes, K. A., Snyder, A. Z., Schlaggar, B. L., and Petersen, S. E. (2012). Spurious but systematic correlations in functional connectivity MRI networks arise from subject motion. *Neuroimage* 59, 2142–2154. doi: 10.1016/j.neuroimage.2011.10.018

Qian, M., Wu, G., Zhu, R., and Zhang, S. (2000). Development of the revised eysenck personality questionnaire short scale for Chinese (EPQ-RSC). *Acta. Psychol. Sinica* 32, 317–323.

Raichle, M. E., Macleod, A. M., Snyder, A. Z., Powers, W. J., Gusnard, D. A., and Shulman, G. L. (2001). A default mode of brain function. *Proc. Natl. Acad. Sci. U.S.A.* 98, 676–682. doi: 10.1073/pnas.98.2.676

Raichle, M. E., and Snyder, A. Z. (2007). A default mode of brain function: a brief history of an evolving idea. *Neuroimage* 37, 1083–1090. discussion: 1097–1089. doi: 10.1016/j.neuroimage.2007.02.041

Rauch, S. L., Milad, M. R., Orr, S. P., Quinn, B. T., Fischl, B., and Pitman, R. K. (2005). Orbitofrontal thickness, retention of fear extinction, and extraversion. *Neuroreport* 16, 1909–1912. doi: 10.1097/01.wnr.0000186599.66243.50

Rubinov, M., and Sporns, O. (2010). Complex network measures of brain connectivity: uses and interpretations. *Neuroimage* 52, 1059–1069. doi: 10.1016/j.neuroimage.2009.10.003

Rusting, C. L., and Larsen, R. J. (1997). Extraversion, neuroticism, and susceptibility to positive and negative affect: a test of two theoretical models. *Pers. Indiv. Differ.* 22, 607–612. doi: 10.1016/S0191-8869(96)00246-2

Salvador, R., Suckling, J., Coleman, M. R., Pickard, J. D., Menon, D., and Bullmore, E. (2005). Neurophysiological architecture of functional magnetic resonance images of human brain. *Cereb. Cortex* 15, 1332–1342. doi: 10.1093/cercor/bhi016

Shackman, A. J., McMenamin, B. W., Maxwell, J. S., Greischar, L. L., and Davidson, R. J. (2009). Right dorsolateral prefrontal cortical activity and behavioral inhibition. *Psychol. Sci.* 20, 1500–1506. doi: 10.1111/j.1467-9280.2009.02476.x

Sollberger, M., Stanley, C. M., Wilson, S. M., Gyurak, A., Beckman, V., Growdon, M., et al. (2009). Neural basis of interpersonal traits in neurodegenerative diseases. *Neuropsychologia* 47, 2812–2827. doi: 10.1016/j.neuropsychologia.2009.06.006

Sporns, O., Chialvo, D. R., Kaiser, M., and Hilgetag, C. C. (2004). Organization, development and function of complex brain networks. *Trends Cogn. Sci.* 8, 418–425. doi: 10.1016/j.tics.2004.07.008

Sporns, O., Tononi, G., and Edelman, G. M. (2000). Connectivity and complexity: the relationship between neuroanatomy and brain dynamics. *Neural Netw.* 13, 909–922. doi: 10.1016/S0893-6080(00)00053-8

Stam, C. J. (2004). Functional connectivity patterns of human magnetoencephalographic recordings: a 'small-world' network? *Neurosci. Lett.* 355, 25–28. doi: 10.1016/j.neulet.2003.10.063

Stam, C. J., and Reijneveld, J. C. (2007). Graph theoretical analysis of complex networks in the brain. *Nonlinear Biomed. Phys.* 1, 3. doi: 10.1186/1753-4631-1-3

Tamura, M., Moriguchi, Y., Higuchi, S., Hida, A., Enomoto, M., Umezawa, J., et al. (2012). Neural network development in late adolescents during observation of risk-taking action. *PLoS ONE* 7:e39527. doi: 10.1371/journal.pone.0039527

Tian, L., Jiang, T., Wang, Y., Zang, Y., He, Y., Liang, M., et al. (2006). Altered resting-state functional connectivity patterns of anterior cingulate cortex in adolescents with attention deficit hyperactivity disorder. *Neurosci. Lett.* 400, 39–43. doi: 10.1016/j.neulet.2006.02.022

Tran, Y., Craig, A., Boord, P., Connell, K., Cooper, N., and Gordon, E. (2006). Personality traits and its association with resting regional brain activity. *Int. J. Psychophysiol.* 60, 215–224. doi: 10.1016/j.ijpsycho.2005.05.008

Van Den Heuvel, M. P., Stam, C. J., Kahn, R. S., and Hulshoff Pol, H. E. (2009). Efficiency of functional brain networks and intellectual performance. *J. Neurosci.* 29, 7619–7624. doi: 10.1523/JNEUROSCI.1443-09.2009

Van Dijk, K. R., Sabuncu, M. R., and Buckner, R. L. (2012). The influence of head motion on intrinsic functional connectivity MRI. *Neuroimage* 59, 431–438. doi: 10.1016/j.neuroimage.2011.07.044

Wang, J., Zuo, X., and He, Y. (2010). Graph-based network analysis of resting-state functional MRI. *Front. Syst. Neurosci.* 4:16. doi: 10.3389/fnsys.2010.00016

Watts, D. J., and Strogatz, S. H. (1998). Collective dynamics of 'small-world' networks. *Nature* 393, 440–442. doi: 10.1038/30918

Wei, L., Duan, X., Yang, Y., Liao, W., Gao, Q., Ding, J. R., et al. (2011). The synchronization of spontaneous BOLD activity predicts extraversion and neuroticism. *Brain Res.* 1419, 68–75. doi: 10.1016/j.brainres.2011.08.060

Wei, L., Duan, X., Zheng, C., Wang, S., Gao, Q., Zhang, Z., et al. (2012). Specific frequency bands of amplitude low-frequency oscillation encodes personality. *Hum. Brain Mapp.* doi: 10.1002/hbm.22176. [Epub ahead of print].

Wilt, J., and Revelle, W. (2009). *Extraversion.* New York, NY: Guilford Press.

Wolf, M. B., and Ackerman, P. L. (2005). Extraversion and intelligence: a meta-analytic investigation. *Pers. Indiv. Differ.* 39, 531–542. doi: 10.1016/j.paid.2005.02.020

Wolf, R. C., Sambataro, F., Vasic, N., Schmid, M., Thomann, P. A., Bienentreu, S. D., et al. (2011). Aberrant connectivity of resting-state networks in borderline personality disorder. *J. Psychiatry Neurosci.* 36, 402–411. doi: 10.1503/jpn.100150

Wright, C. I., Feczko, E., Dickerson, B., and Williams, D. (2007). Neuroanatomical correlates of personality in the elderly. *Neuroimage* 35, 263–272. doi: 10.1016/j.neuroimage.2006.11.039

Wright, C. I., Williams, D., Feczko, E., Barrett, L. F., Dickerson, B. C., Schwartz, C. E., et al. (2006). Neuroanatomical correlates of extraversion and neuroticism. *Cereb. Cortex* 16, 1809–1819. doi: 10.1093/cercor/bhj118

Zhang, J., Wang, J., Wu, Q., Kuang, W., Huang, X., He, Y., et al. (2011). Disrupted brain connectivity networks in drug-naive, first-episode major depressive disorder. *Biol. Psychiatry* 70, 334–342. doi: 10.1016/j.biopsych.2011.05.018

Zuckerman, M. (ed.). (2005). *Psychobiology of Personality.* New York, NY: Cambridge University Press.

12

Decreased small-world functional network connectivity and clustering across resting state networks in schizophrenia: An fMRI classification tutorial

Ariana Anderson* and Mark S. Cohen

Department of Psychiatry and Biobehavioral Sciences, Center for Cognitive Neuroscience, University of California Los Angeles, Los Angeles, CA, USA

***Correspondence:**
*Ariana Anderson, Department of Psychiatry and Biobehavioral Sciences, Center for Cognitive Neuroscience, University of California Los Angeles, 760 Westwood Plaza, Suite 17-369, Los Angeles, CA 90095, USA
e-mail: ariana82@ucla.edu*

Functional network connectivity (FNC) is a method of analyzing the temporal relationship of anatomical brain components, comparing the synchronicity between patient groups or conditions. We use functional-connectivity measures between independent components to classify between Schizophrenia patients and healthy controls during resting-state. Connectivity is measured using a variety of graph-theoretic connectivity measures such as graph density, average path length, and small-worldness. The Schizophrenia patients showed significantly less clustering (transitivity) among components than healthy controls ($p < 0.05$, corrected) with networks less likely to be connected, and also showed lower small-world connectivity than healthy controls. Using only these connectivity measures, an SVM classifier (without parameter tuning) could discriminate between Schizophrenia patients and healthy controls with 65% accuracy, compared to 51% chance. This implies that the global functional connectivity between resting-state networks is altered in Schizophrenia, with networks more likely to be disconnected and behave dissimilarly for diseased patients. We present this research finding as a tutorial using the publicly available COBRE dataset of 146 Schizophrenia patients and healthy controls, provided as part of the 1000 Functional Connectomes Project. We demonstrate preprocessing, using independent component analysis (ICA) to nominate networks, computing graph-theoretic connectivity measures, and finally using these connectivity measures to either classify between patient groups or assess between-group differences using formal hypothesis testing. All necessary code is provided for both running command-line FSL preprocessing, and for computing all statistical measures and SVM classification within R. Collectively, this work presents not just findings of diminished FNC among resting-state networks in Schizophrenia, but also a practical connectivity tutorial.

Keywords: fMRI, classification, functional network connectivity, SVM, independent component analysis, *R*, Schizophrenia, small-world

1. INTRODUCTION

Functional Magnetic Resonance Imaging (fMRI) is a four-dimensional medical imaging modality that captures changes in blood oxygenation over time, an indirect measure of neuronal activation. Because fMRI scans are large, they are stored in specialized formats that make their direct access and manipulation difficult. Statistical analyses are therefore limited to the software the neuroscientist is able to use; pre-made routines are available to perform general analyses such as linear models, but the techniques and consequently the hypotheses that can be evaluated by them are limited and inflexible. Analyses are dependent upon the ability to create programs that not only can access directly subsets of the data, but also can be tailored to unique statistical analysis based on *a priori* hypotheses of the underlying neurological disorders.

An increasing focus is the classification of either mental disorders or states based on the fMRI signal variations within and among brain networks. One method of accomplishing this is through measurements of functional network connectivity (FNC), which infers differences in temporal brain connectivity that may depend on a disease or mental state (Biswal et al., 1995; van de Ven et al., 2004). FNC investigates temporal connectivity differences among either anatomical brain regions or functionally defined networks. Herein, we present a tutorial to perform FNC in *R* which can be altered easily for a unique hypothesis or dataset (Tabelow et al., 2011; R Development Core Team, 2012).

The methods we discuss here closely follows those presented in Anderson et al. (2010), which describes in full the motivation for, and findings of, using brain connectivity measures to classify between Schizophrenia patients and normal controls during rest. We demonstrate this procedure on a recently released dataset, publicly available for download at http://fcon_1000.projects.nitrc.org/indi/retro/cobre.html and studied previously in Calhoun et al. (2011), Hanlon et al. (2011), Mayer et al. (2012). This dataset, which we will refer to as the COBRE data, consists of 72 patients with Schizophrenia and 74 healthy controls, ranging in age from 18 to 65 years old. A full demographic table is provided in **Table 1**.

The code contained in this article is available through the Neuroimaging Informatics Tools and Resources Clearinghouse

Table 1 | COBRE FCON-1000 data demographics.

	N	Age (*SD*)	% Female	% Right-Handed
Schizophrenia	72	38.16 (13.89)	0.19	0.83
Patients	74	35.82 (11.58)	0.31	0.96

(NITRC) at http://www.nitrc.org/projects/fmriclassify/. NITRC is an NIH-sponsored project to categorize, compare, rate and distribute software and data, created by and for neuroimaging researchers. It contains both stand-alone programs and code snippets such as this project. Its usefulness is quite evident given the redundancies in research, where many labs develop independently routines to perform similar analysis techniques such as functional connectivity analysis. It is also useful for determining reproducibility, as users can test another's analysis on their own data to see if similar results are reached. This is particularly appropriate in fMRI analysis, where conclusions are often reached on quite small sample sizes since data are costly and difficult to obtain. The reader is encouraged to download and modify this code snippet from the NITRC website.

We demonstrate this analysis using preprocessing in FSL, which performs brain extraction [`bet` (Smith, 2002)] to remove non-brain tissue, motion-correction `mcflirt` (Jenkinson et al., 2002) to correct for subject movement within the scan, and ICA using `melodic` (Smith et al., 2004) with automatic component estimation. A full FSL tutorial is available at http://http://fsl.fmrib.ox.ac.uk/fslcourse/. We use independent component analysis (ICA) to identify networks within each patient and calculate properties of their temporal-connectivity, demonstrating this within FSL, implemented as "MELODIC", and within *R*. Using packages **vegan** (Oksanen et al., 2011) and **AnalyzeFMRI** (Bordier et al., 2009), we extract possible neurological networks and define distances among them as functional connectivity measures. This distance matrix is then converted into a graph structure, and properties of these connectivity graphs are computed using **igraph** (Csardi and Nepusz, 2006). We use this connectivity for classification with the Support Vector Machines (SVM) algorithm in the package **e1071** (Dimitriadou et al., 2010).

Because this analysis is heavily computational, we also demonstrate how to perform this same process in parallel using the package **parallel** (R Development Core Team, 2012). The ability to code this in *R* with minimal function calls, or changing of the original code, allows users to implement and test computationally intensive analyses efficiently and simply. Parallel computing is a specialized topic, and many researchers are uninterested in learning methods such as MPI to implement their analyses, as troubleshooting can often take as long as the time saved by running in parallel. Because of this, we demonstrate calling fork clusters within *R* to perform parallel analysis, without making major revisions to the code already created to run in serial. This supplementary section is listed in the *Appendix*. We additionally demonstrate in the *Appendix* using R to access fMRI data, including how to perform ICA using the package **AnalyzefMRI** (Bordier et al., 2009).

We begin with a description of our approach, and follow with an applications section where we provide and discuss the code necessary to accomplish these methods. In this tutorial we assume the reader has no specific knowledge of *R*, but does have general knowledge of basic programming techniques. An *R* tutorial is available at http://cran.r-project.org/doc/manuals/R-intro.html. We hard-code as little as possible to ensure minimal changes for a new users' analysis. As this analysis focuses on connectivity within subjects, spatial alignment across subjects is not necessary, although procedures such as motion correction and temporal filtering may be performed beforehand if desired. The **AnalyzeFMRI**, **vegan**, **igraph**, and **e1071** packages are used along with their dependencies, and must be pre-installed. These packages are available at http://cran.r-project.org/web/packages. The package **parallel** is a base package installed already within the latest *R* release. As the bulk of this code is constructed to classify between distance matrices, these routines can be adapted easily for a region of interest (ROI) analysis where distances are sought not between independent components, but instead between ROIs. More generally, these methods are applicable to longitudinal data analysis where the temporal correlations among units are indicative of a state or condition. Collectively, this article demonstrates code that can be adapted easily to new data for determining if functional connectivity differences exist between groups of fMRI scans, and is meant to serve as a bridge between neuroscientists interested in performing their own connectivity/classification analysis, and statisticians interested in seeing these methods applied to real-world data.

2. BACKGROUND

2.1. OVERVIEW OF fMRI

Function magnetic resonance imaging is a modality that measures brain activity over time. The fMRI Blood Oxygen Level Dependent (BOLD) signal is an indirect reflection of neuronal activity captured during an fMRI scan, and analysis is performed under the assumption that neuronal activity coincides with increased blood flow. The blood flow increase in response to neuronal activity is known as the hemodynamic response (Kim et al., 1999). When activation occurs within a region, oxygenated hemoglobin flows to that area to increase the local oxygen concentration. Deoxyhemoglobin has a faster MR signal decay rate (T2*) than oxyhemoglobin (Cohen and Bookheimer, 1994), so the signal from well-oxygenated regions results in a stronger MR signal intensity than areas lacking the increased blood flow. Areas with increased neuronal activity therefore give off a greater MRI signal, which indicates potential neural activity.

The four-dimensional fMRI picture can be used to discover anatomical regions specific to certain tasks such as language processing (Bookheimer, 2002), face recognition (Gauthier et al., 1999), or even to diagnose regional impairment specific to cognitive disorders such as Alzheimers disease, traumatic brain injury (TBI), or schizophrenia (Ford et al., 2003; Anderson et al., 2010). Such studies typically analyze regional blood flow to establish areas active during a task, or to compare regional blood oxygenation levels between two groups, such as Alzheimer's patients and normal controls, to find localized variation that could be the cause of cognitive impairment.

FNC is used to test the hypotheses that synchronicity across anatomically-defined brain regions or functionally-hypothesized networks are different, because of age, disease, or the task being performed. Connectivity differences are thought to underly many disorders such as autism (Koshino et al., 2005) and schizophrenia (Liang et al., 2006). More generally, temporal connectivity has been used to explore directed influences between neuronal populations in fMRI data (Roebroeck et al., 2005) using Granger causality, and to examine differences between schizophrenia patients compared to normal controls (Garrity et al., 2007; Jafri et al., 2008; Anderson et al., 2010; Yu et al., 2011) using cross-correlation measures. Within Schizophrenia, disrupted small-world properties were found compared to healthy controls among 90 cortical and subcortical regions (Liu et al., 2008). Increased regional functional connectivity in the 0.06–0.125 Hz interval were found in Schizophrenia, along with decreased strength by Bassett et al. (2008). Within the default mode network, abnormally high functional connectivity and altered temporal frequency have been found (Garrity et al., 2007; Whitfield-Gabrieli et al., 2009). Schizophrenia patients had higher correlations among seven selected resting-state networks than healthy controls (Jafri et al., 2008), and different topological measures were found between resting-state networks identified by group-ICA (Yu et al., 2011). Collectively, these works and others propose that within Schizophrenia, functional connectivity measures can be used to identify traits that are characteristic of the disease itself.

Because connectivity depends on how networks or regions are defined, and how the graphical properties of regions may be measured (Toppi et al., 2012; Zalesky et al., 2012), it is vital for researchers to be able to tailor connectivity analysis to their own data, to allow pre-existing knowledge or certain hypothesis to be tested. For example, Sato et al. (2010), implemented functional connectivity analysis among regions of interest, while Chu et al. (2011), analyzed connectivity among individual voxels. Similarly, Yu et al. (2011) analyzed FNC among group-ICA components, while we analyzed FNC among within-subject ICA components (Anderson et al., 2010).

2.2. fMRI CLASSIFICATION

The primary challenge of fMRI classification is the abundance of observations within a single scan, many of which are correlated strongly both in space and time. Although many of these voxels will be empty, they are not systematically empty across subjects as a result of differences in brain size and shape. Because many of these datapoints are redundant, dimension reduction techniques are used by creating statistical summaries of individual voxels (t-tests, correlation tests), isolating "regions of interests" (ROI) or neural hotspots on which discrimination could be performed, or implementing classical dimension reduction methods such as principal components analysis (PCA) to decompose the entire scan into orthogonal signal sources over time. Newer methods such as ICA (Hyvärinen and Oja, 2000) and Sparse Component Analysis (Georgiev et al., 2005) mimic the approach of PCA into decomposing the scan into a limited number of spatial networks operating over time, but alternatively impose assumptions such as statistical independence or sparsity to estimate the underlying signal sources.

Once the dimension reduction and feature extraction steps are complete, the reduced data are fed into classifiers such as SVM, random forests, and boosting algorithms. These classification techniques have been used previously to discriminate between Positron Emission Tomography (PET) scans of HIV positive and healthy individuals (Liow et al., 2000), to detect deceptive individuals within a group using fMRI (Lee et al., 2002; Fan et al., 2006), to separate drug-addicted patients from healthy controls using fMRI scans (Zhang and Samaras, 2005), and to discriminate between patients with Alzheimer's, schizophrenia, and TBI and healthy controls using fMRI scans (Ford et al., 2003).

In "leave one out" cross-validation, these classifiers often achieve around 90% accuracy, but because methods are constructed uniquely for each dataset they are difficult to validate across different patient groups, or even within the same patient group but with a new population. These studies are often performed on excessively small samples ($n \approx 20$). The reproducibility of such findings are often unverified, leaving open the criticism that superior classification accuracy is due to mere chance or model-mining, instead of underlying functional or anatomical differences between patient groups. It can be difficult to pool data taken across laboratories, because the scan parameters, resolution, and imaging sequences would have to be nearly equivalent. Because of this, the ability to evaluate models on different datasets would increase confidence in results, since the models acting on the same patient group should produce identical results, holding the scan environment constant.

2.3. R FOR fMRI

The *R* platform has important benefits for fMRI analyses because of its availability and functionality. *R* is free and open source, so licensing costs for research are not prohibitive and any researcher is able to install it easily. Because of this, sharing code to validate methods and reproduce findings is quite simple. *R* contains thousands of packages that can perform cutting-edge statistical and machine learning techniques; analyses and hypothesis are not limited by the available models. *R* allows the user direct contact with their data, with routines for fMRI that can efficiently extract single timeseries, volumes, or planes. This is of particular value because fMRI scans are encoded in specialized formats (ANALYZE or NIfTI) that are otherwise unaccessible. The ability to access directly the data combined with the high-level statistical methods available within the general *R* framework allows the user to construct his own methods unique to his hypothesis.

Finally, *R* contains packages to implement specifically fMRI analysis. There are routines pre-built into *R* for fMRI that can perform methods such as mixed effects analysis **3dMEMA** (Chen et al., 2010, 2012) to estimate the effect, which is implemented indirectly in *R* by sourcing through AFNI (http://afni.nimh.nih.gov/sscc/gangc/MEMA.html). The bread and butter of fMRI analysis, the general linear models (GLM) can be implemented in the package **fmri** (Polzehl and Tabelow, 2007), Bayesian multilevel modeling analysis in **cudaBayesreg** (Ferreira da Silva, 2011) and Granger Causality and structural equation modeling in **FIAR** (Roelstraete and Rosseel, 2011). Functional connectivity analysis also can be performed using the package **brainwaver**, where ROIs are analyzed for connectivity using wavelet analysis, and connections are trimmed with a hypothesis test (Achard et al., 2006). We refer the reader to a presentation at the useR! 2010 conference for a description of packages and options in *R* for fMRI analyses, at http://www.r-project.org/conferences/useR-2010/slides/Chen+Saad+Cox.pdf. Some packages require installing the most recent versions of `gfortran` and `tcltk` available for MacOS at http://cran.r-project.org/bin/macosx/tools/.

3. METHODS

In this section, we cover the specific methods used for FNC and fMRI classification presented in this paper. We first use the ICA dimension-reduction technique to decompose each scan into a set of spatial brain networks being modulated over time by associated timecourses. We then create functional connectivity matrices, by measuring the longitudinal correlations of the timecourses for each network. Next, each matrix is converted into a graph structure, and the connectivity properties of each graph are measured. Finally, these connectivity properties are used as features for an SVM classifier. We additionally use a t-test to evaluate whether the small-world connectivity of ICA networks is different between Schizophrenia patients and healthy controls. A flowchart depicting this process is shown in **Figure 1**.

3.1. ICA FOR fMRI

As fMRI is composed of recordings that are highly-redundant in both space and time, it is desirable to extract meaningful features prior to classification. This serves two purposes. Firstly, it lowers the noise by essentially tossing out signals that have no commonality with other signals. This is based on the assumption that noise is independent across observations; a signal seen only in a single location is more likely to be noise than a signal observed consistently throughout the brain. Secondly, reducing the scan to a manageable number of consistent signals reduces the tendency of overfitting in the classification process. The classification complexity is a function of the number of dimensions (features).

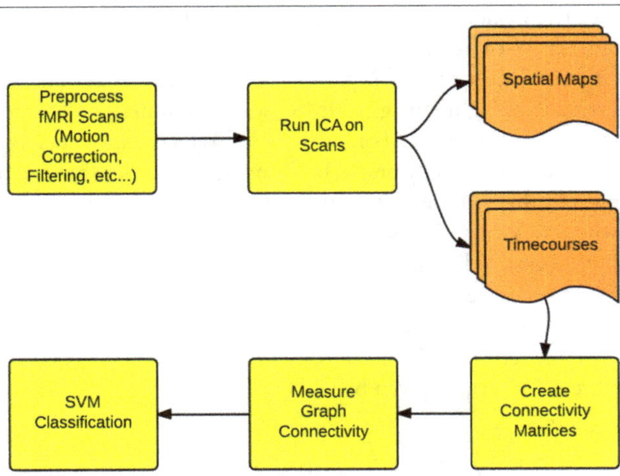

FIGURE 1 | Functional network connectivity (FNC) and classification: the first step in FNC is to define the scale of connectivity to observe. In this case, we use whole-brain networks obtained from ICA, but this analysis also can be implemented on the region-of-interest or the voxel scale. The connectivity is defined and measured to identify differences between either groups or conditions.

Although there are many methods of extracting common signals across the brain, ICA in particular has gained popularity in fMRI. It can isolate networks corresponding to neurological activity, as well as motion artifacts, where signals that operate most strongly on the peripheral regions along the scalp are taken to be motion. ICA has been validated through bootstrapping and clustering methods, identifying components that exist across subjects and scans that correspond to functionally identifiable brain networks (McKeown et al., 2003; Anderson et al., 2011). In this implementation we run ICA within subjects, rather than implementing a group-ICA which would have identified common networks across all subjects. This is based upon the hypothesis that there are a different set of networks operating within Schizophrenia, and assuming that the same exact networks operate within both patient groups would dampen any between-group differences.

Under the hypothesis that the activity of the brain is constructed of anatomical networks acting together to produce meaningful psychobehavioral cognitive states, the aggregate activity is decomposed into subcomponents in ICA. Prior to this, space is "unrolled" where the four dimensional scan (3 dimensions of space, 1 of time) are transformed into a matrix of dimension space by time, so that a scan array of dimension (X, Y, Z, T) would become a matrix of dimension $(T, X{*}Y{*}Z)$. An fMRI scan of time length T and spatial dimension S and can be expressed as a linear combination of $M < T$ components and the corresponding timeseries:

$$X_{ts} = \sum_{\mu=1}^{M} A_{t\mu} C_{\mu s}$$

where X_{ts} represents the raw scan intensity at timepoint $t \leq T$ and spatial location $s \leq S$, $A_{t\mu}$ is the amplitude of component μ at time t, and $C_{\mu s}$ is the spatial magnitude for component μ at spatial location s. An example of a spatial map output by *R* is shown in **Figure 2**.

The components c are estimated to be statistically independent as possible by solving instead the inverse problem via the FAST-ICA algorithm. To estimate the signal sources c in $x = Ac$, the inverse problem of $y = w'x$ is solved where w is a row of A^{-1}, or the inverse of the mixing matrix. Then $y = w'x \Rightarrow y = w'Ac$. Substituting $z = A'w$, $y = z'c$. W is optimized such that $y = w'x = z'c$ is as non-Gaussian as possible, leading to even *less* Gaussian sources c because of the Central Limit Theorem. Maximizing the kurtosis, minimizing the entropy, and maximizing the negentropy over w are all methods of finding the *least* Gaussian $y = w'x = z'c$.

$$Negentropy = J(y) = H(y_{Gauss}) - H(y)$$

$$H(y) = -\sum_{i} P(y = a_i) log[P(y = a_i)]$$

In the continuous case this becomes

$$H(y) = -\int f(y) log(f(y)) dy$$

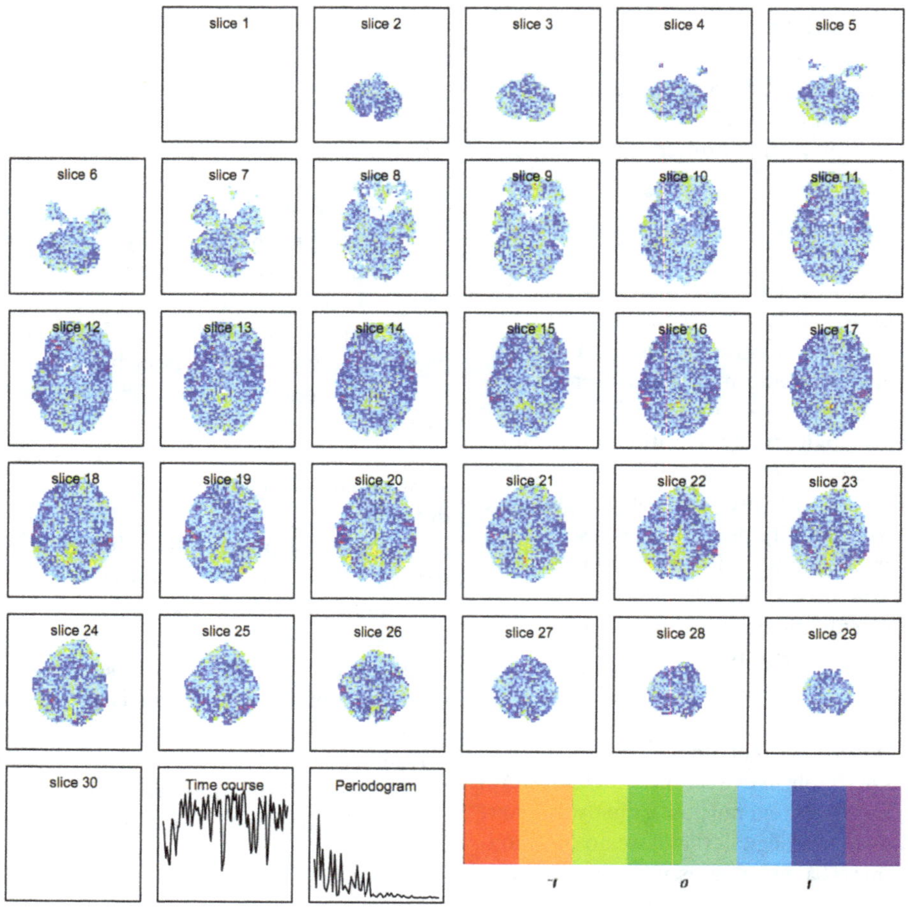

FIGURE 2 | Spatial map produced by independent components analysis within R. Each component is a set of spatially weighted regions modulated by the time course. The total longitudinal contribution of a component to the activity observed is the spatial map multiplied by the timecourse.

By default *R* and FSL use FAST-ICA. The default parameter setting in *R* is for parallel extraction, and also includes temporal normalization, 1000 maximum iterations for the algorithm using negentropy: $G(u) = \frac{1}{\alpha} log[cosh(\alpha u)]$ where $\alpha \in [1, 2]$ is the constant used for the negentropy approximation. An example of a ICA spatial map is shown in **Figure 2**.

We implement here spatial ICA the only option in FSL, which sought statistical independence of the spatial maps. We alternatively could have implemented temporal ICA, which would have maximized independence of the time-courses. A presentation of this using the **AnalyzeFMRI**, and a demonstration of how to implement temporal ICA within R using the **AnalyzeFMRI** is provided in (Bordier et al., 2011). We allowed the number of components to be determined within the data following (Allen et al., 2011).

3.2. CREATING FUNCTIONAL CONNECTIVITY MATRICES

A temporal interaction plot for a schizophrenia patient and a normal control is shown in **Figure 3**, showing the joint longitudinal activity by two components within each subject, (A_{μ_1}, A_{μ_2}). Since graphical interpretation is subjective, a fixed measure of this joint activity is established by computing a correlation-based distance metric. The distance function is a transformation of the maximal absolute cross-correlation between two timeseries. This computation is done for each possible pair of components within a subject, thus transforming the original fMRI scan into a matrix. This is a measure of the functional connectivity between components for a given subject, but is only one of many possible metrics that can be changed by the end user within this tutorial. This is but one example where *R* allows the user to change the methods according to the hypothesis and data being evaluated.

The cross-correlation function (CCF) between these timeseries is calculated over a range of temporal lags. We subtract the maximal absolute cross-correlation from 1 to create a pseudo distance measure, $d(A_{\mu_i}, A_{\mu_j})$, given by

$$d(A_{\mu_i}, A_{\mu_j}) = 1 - max[|CCF(A_{\mu_i}, A_{\mu_j}, l)|]$$

where

$$CCF(A_{\mu_i}, A_{\mu_j}, l) = \frac{E[(a_{\mu_i,t+l} - \overline{A_{\mu_i}})(a_{\mu_j,t} - \overline{A_{\mu_j}})]}{\sqrt{E[(a_{\mu_i,t} - \overline{A_{\mu_i}})^2]E[(a_{\mu_j,t} - \overline{A_{\mu_j}})^2]}} \quad (1)$$

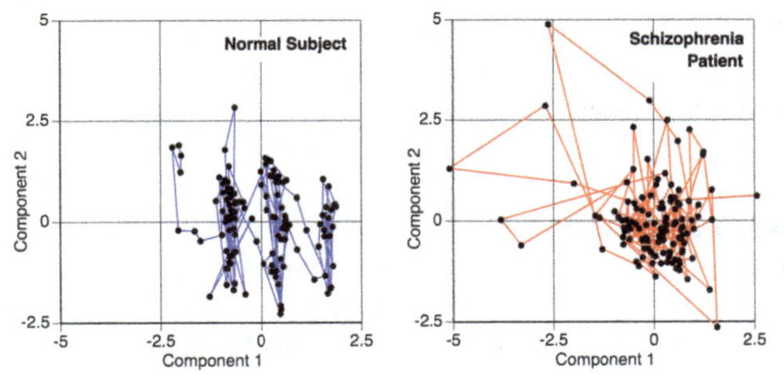

FIGURE 3 | Temporal activity plot of two primary components within a subject, depicting the relationship between two components over time. This phase space transition between pairs of components are measured for the functional connectivity analysis, to calculate the similarity of the components' behavior.

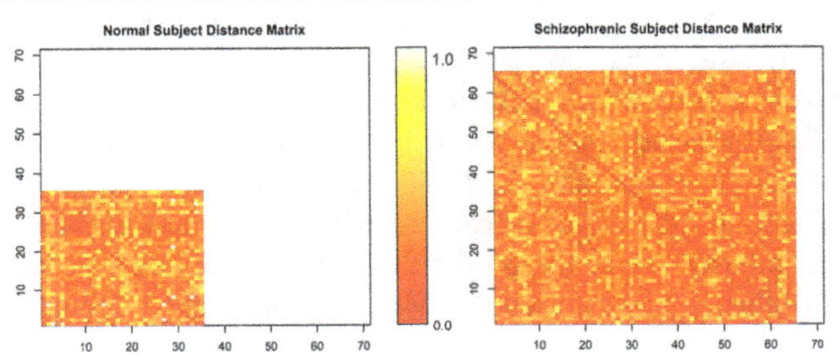

FIGURE 4 | Normalized distance matrices of two subjects, where rows and columns correspond to components within a subject and the intensity represents the functional connectivity between those components.

where l is the time lag separating the two timeseries A_{μ_i} and A_{μ_j}, and $\overline{A_{\mu_i}}$ is the mean of the entire timeseries $A_{\mu_i} = (a_{\mu_i,1}, a_{\mu_i,2}, \ldots, a_{\mu_i,T})$. The timeseries are calculated at lags ranging from 0 to 3 points (6 seconds), as higher lags results in fewer time points to calculate the correlation and a more noisy estimate, and also lacks biological plausibility given our current understanding of neurological coupling. Within *R*, the lag parameter is specified using `lag.max`.

The matrices by themselves are uninterpretable, since they are merely representations of a set of connected objects. An example of this is shown in **Figure 4**. Moreover, the rows and columns of these matrices, representing unique independent components within subjects, are themselves not comparable across subjects. Our ultimate goal is to measure this connectivity; not only how closely connected they are, but also how it changes with respect to patient diagnosis. For example, do all networks interact with all other networks? Are there subgraphs that are fragmented from the original graph? Does the number of steps to travel among nodes differ? Are some graphs more densely connected than others? To answer these questions, we must convert the connectivity matrices to graph objects, so we can use *R* packages designed purposefully for graph connectivity analysis.

3.3. GRAPH CREATION AND MEASUREMENT

Each matrix represents a structure of completely connected points on a high-dimensional manifold, where each point is an independent component and the distance between two points measures the similarity of their temporal activity. Every point is linked to every other point regardless of similarity. To create graphs out of the connectivity matrices, we prune weak connections among points and then embed the simplified structure into a lower-dimensional space using the ISOMAP procedure (Tenenbaum et al., 2000). Then, we measure the graph-theoretic connectivity to summarize the connections between resting-state networks.

3.3.1. Graph creation

Conceptually, any set of points contained in a distance matrix of dimension d can be embedded into a space of dimension $d-1$ without any information loss (preserving all the distances between points). Usually such a transformation assumes the space on which the points lie is linear. This, however, may not be the case. Consider if you were trying to measure the distance from Sacramento, California to Shanghai, China, using only the (x, y, z) grid coordinates of each city. The linear distance between the cities, while calculable, would assume that the correct path from Sacramento to Shanghai went through the core of the earth. Instead, a more reasonable way to measure the distance would be to travel along the flight-paths, from Sacramento to Los Angeles, Los Angeles to Tokyo, and finally from Tokyo to Shanghai. This method of measuring distance is known as the geodesic distance, or path-distance among points. It assumes that travel among distant points usually requires routing through intermediate nodes, as shown in **Figure 5**. It is this concept we will now use to sever weak connections and create graphs out of the matrices.

We transform each matrix into a graph structure using an initial geodesic distance calculation implemented in the function `isomap` in the library **vegan**. Weak ties among points are then severed; points can be connected if they are within a certain distance, ϵ, of each other ($|x-y| \leq \epsilon$), or they can be connected if they are within a set of k-nearest neighbors. The distances are recomputed after pruning, where the distance between connected points is the same as it was originally, but the new distance between unconnected points is computed as the shortest path through intermediary connecting nodes. Combined with multidimensional scaling to obtain a coordinate system for embedding, this procedure is called ISOMAP (Tenenbaum et al., 2000). An example of such a graph created by a geodesic distance transformation and a multidimensional scaling embedding is shown in **Figure 6**.

The two definitions of connectivity (nearest-neighbor vs. ϵ-distance) can lead to different results; establishing connectivity by ϵ-distance, also called edge density (sparsity), may lead to the graph becoming fragmented, with some portions of the graph having no connections, direct or indirect, to other subgraphs. This would be caused by some point(s) being too distant to others to maintain a connection with the main graph. This is an instance where the *a priori* knowledge about the disease may inform the parameter choices of the methods. In diseases such as Schizophrenia or autism, a hypothesis of disconnectivity may be tested directly by computing, for example, the fragmentation

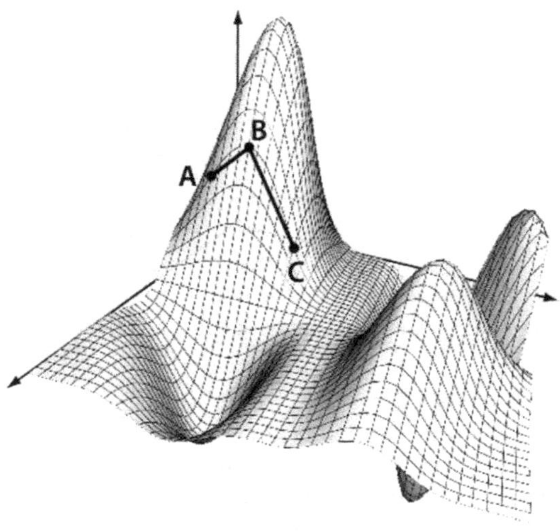

FIGURE 5 | Geodesic distance calculation. The distance between A and C is calculated as the manifold path distance from A to B to C, instead of the direct path from A to C. This eliminates the assumption that the points occupy a linear space when using a Euclidean distance.

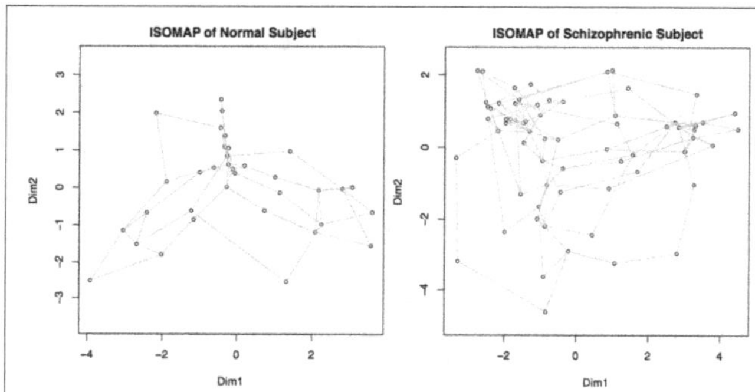

FIGURE 6 | Graphs representing connectivity of two subjects, obtained by converting the distance matrices for each subject into a structure where each node represents a component, and the distance between nodes represents the connectivity or similarity of their behaviors. Nodes close together demonstrate a higher functional connectivity measure. This map is obtained by recalculating the connectivity matrices using geodesic distances, and then embedding the points in a two dimensional space for plotting. Dim 1 and Dim 2 represent the weightings on the two primary dimensions, similar to multi-dimensional scaling.

rate of the patients versus controls. By allowing the user to choose these parameters within *R*, specific theories of neuropathology may be tested.

We threshold points as being connected using a modified nearest neighbor method. We select the k-nearest neighbors of all nodes to be connected by defining k as 10% of total components for that subject, or 2, whichever is greater. This enforces the graph be completely connected, unlike the edge density method. We select this parameter choice because we are using weighted graphs; edge density methods typically binarize the adjacency matrix by assigning weights above a given threshold a unit value, and a zero value to all below such as in Rubinov and Sporns (2010). Since we are using weighted graphs, we allow sufficiently "close" points to retain their given weights, and prune all other points which are not sufficiently close. This parameter could be investigated further, but because we are using these metrics for performing classification then optimizing the adjacency pruning method would lead to biased estimates of the accuracy.

3.3.2. Graph measurement

At this point, each brain scan has been transformed into a graphical structure, where each node represents a brain network and the connectivity between nodes represents the similarity in the activity of these networks. Each graph can then be summarized by its connectivity properties. There are many such measurements available within *R* within the package **igraph**. A tutorial by Gabor Csardi on Network Analysis with the package **igraph** is at http://igraph.sourceforge.net/igraphbook/. A description of network measures of brain connectivity is available at Rubinov and Sporns (2010), which describes in detail the graph-theoretic measures discussed only briefly here, and additionally describes other connectivity measures such as modularity. An additional connectivity measure which we used in a previous study to discriminate between Schizophrenia patients and healthy controls (Anderson et al., 2010) is the "eigenvector centrality," which can be computed here using the command `eigen(d)$values`.

Creating graphs out of each matrix using a non-linear distance metric such as the geodesic distance not only allows for a more efficient low-dimensional projection of the matrix, but also encourages the graph to be connected more efficiently by trimming poor connections while maintaining stronger ones. This fragmentation allows us to determine how many strong connections are within the subject, how many subnetworks (subgraphs) exist, what the sizes of these subnetworks are, and how efficiently the points are connected overall. These properties, all interrelated, give quantitative measurements of the connectivity that can be used to fingerprint the networking differences associated with different disorders. These individual metrics can be compared directly between groups if multiple comparisons are adjusted for.

Some of these available measures within **igraph** are:

- Average path length: average path length between all connected vertices.
- Clique number: number of elements in the largest subgraph.
- Graph density: ratio of the number of edges to the number of possible edges.
- Edge connectivity (also called graph adhesion): minimum number of edges needed to obtain a graph which is not strongly connected.
- Median closeness: median number of steps required to access every other vertex from a given vertex.
- Median Degree: median number of edges incident to a vertex, with loops being counted twice.
- Vertex Count: number of Vertices in the graph.
- Edge count: number of Edges in the graph.
- Maximum degree: maximum number of edges incident to a vertex, with loops being counted twice.
- Transitivity: probability that two vertices are connected. This is also called the *clustering coefficient*.

We use two of these measures to compute the *small-world* property generated by the Erdős-Renyi game (Erdős and Rényi, 1961). Alternative methods of computing this are presented by Rubinov and Sporns (2010). The small-world measure σ is computed as

$$\sigma = \frac{\gamma}{\lambda}$$

where γ is the ratio of the clustering coefficient of the real network to the mean of the clustering coefficient of n random networks with an equivalent number of edges and weights as the real (data-derived) network but randomly rewired. λ is the similar to γ but uses characteristic path length. The variable n is usually somewhere between 500 and 5000. Typically, biological networks have:

- $\gamma >> 1$, i.e., greater local clustering than a random network
- $\lambda \approx 1$, i.e., similar characteristic path length to a random network

Any network with $\sigma >> 1$ is considered to be "small world" (Humphries and Gurney, 2008).

3.4. CLASSIFICATION USING SVM

We have transformed each subject's fMRI scan into a graph, where the nodes of the graph represent functional networks and the distances between nodes represents the similarity of the activity of the nodes. We have measured the connectivity of these graphs, or the FNC. We now wish to use these connectivity features for classification. *R* has an immense number of libraries available for classification. Packages are continually being added that implement new machine learning algorithms, and packages for specific algorithms can be found at http://www.rseek.org. In this paper we use the basic SVM algorithm, included in the package **e1071**.

The SVM algorithm attempts to find a hyperplane that best separates different classes, using only the points contained in the margin (or region of overlap.) For a set of points (x_i, y_i) where $(x_i) \in R^n$ is the set of graph measurements for the graph G_i corresponding to subject i, a member of class $y_i \in (-1, 1)$ (patient or control), SVM will learn the hyperplane which best divides the classes $(-1, 1)$. If a hyperplane is modeled by $w \cdot x_i - b$ where w are the vectors normal to the hyperplanes, the parallel hyperplanes separating the observations can be defined by $w \cdot x_i - b \geq 1$ for $y_i = 1$ and $w \cdot x_i - b \leq -1$ for $y_i = -1$. The optimization problem becomes to maximize the distance between planes, $\frac{2}{\|w\|}$, such that $y_i(w \cdot x_i - b) \geq 1$

Using the graph properties (path length, clique number, etc...) as features, we can then perform classification between schizophrenia patients and healthy controls.

4. APPLICATIONS

4.1. PREPROCESSING AND COMPONENT EXTRACTION IN FSL

Our first step was to perform motion correction and skull-stripping on the fMRI data, and to run ICA within each scan to extract the networks of interest. We specifically use automatic component estimation in FSL because our previous research has suggested differences in the number of independent components for Schizophrenia patients and healthy controls. An example of an ICA map produced by FSL is shown in **Figure 7**.

Assuming the COBRE data has been downloaded and installed, then we can run FSL from the command line to process all scans, which includes motion correction, skull-stripping, smoothing with a 6 mm filter, high-filtering at 100 Hz, and finally running Melodic with automatic component estimation within each subject. This script is tailored to the COBRE data, and requires that the variable `STUDY_DIR` be changed for the users' specific path. Following this script the *melodic_mix* files containing the patients' ICA timecourses will all be located in the folder `./COBRE/COBRE_MELODIC`. To create a similar script for a new dataset, one can simply run Melodic from the GUI, and copy the command-line input from the *log* file.

```
#!/bin/sh
# Subject directories (Change Me)
STUDY_DIR="/u/home/of/my/COBRE";
#############
# CONSTANTS #
#############
subjects="0040000 0040005 0040010 0040015 0040020 0040025 0040030 0040035 0040040
0040045 0040050 0040055 0040060 0040065 0040070 0040075 0040080 0040085 0040090
```

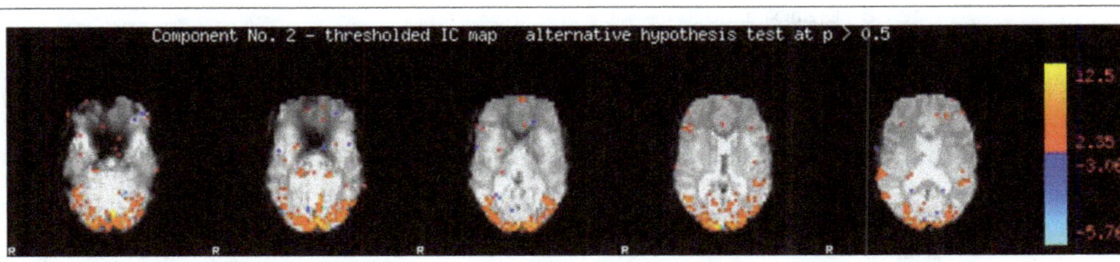

FIGURE 7 | Spatial map produced by independent components analysis in FSL.

```
0040095  0040100  0040105  0040110  0040115  0040120  0040125  0040130  0040135  0040140
0040145 0040001  0040006  0040011  0040016  0040021  0040026  0040031  0040036  0040041
0040046  0040051  0040056  0040061  0040066  0040071  0040076  0040081  0040086  0040091
0040096  0040101  0040106  0040111  0040116  0040121  0040126  0040131  0040136  0040141
0040146 0040002  0040007  0040012  0040017  0040022  0040027  0040032  0040037  0040042
0040047  0040052  0040057  0040062  0040067  0040072  0040077  0040082  0040087  0040092
0040097  0040102  0040107  0040112  0040117  0040122  0040127  0040132  0040137  0040142
0040147 0040003  0040008  0040013  0040018  0040023  0040028  0040033  0040038  0040043
0040048  0040053  0040058  0040063  0040068  0040073  0040078  0040083  0040088  0040093
0040098  0040103  0040108  0040113  0040118  0040123  0040128  0040133  0040138  0040143
0040004  0040009  0040014  0040019  0040024  0040029  0040034  0040039  0040044  0040049
0040054  0040059  0040064  0040069  0040074  0040079  0040084  0040089  0040094  0040099
0040104  0040109  0040114  0040119  0040124  0040129  0040134  0040139  0040144";

umask 0002;
######################
# PROCESSING COMMANDS #
######################

# Change to STUDY_DIR
cd $STUDY_DIR;
mkdir COBRE_MELODIC

# Loop through subjects
for i in $subjects; do
        if [ ! -f "$STUDY_DIR/COBRE_MELODIC/${i}_melodic_mix_new" ]; then
        cd $STUDY_DIR/${i}/session_1/rest_1
        rm -r *.ica*
        rm rest_mcf*
            rm prefiltered*
            rm filtered*
            mcflirt -in rest.nii.gz -out prefiltered_func_data_mcf -mats -rmsrel -rmsabs
            fslmaths prefiltered_func_data_mcf -Tmean mean_func
            bet2 mean_func mask -f 0.3 -n -m; immv mask_mask mask
            fslmaths prefiltered_func_data_mcf -mas mask prefiltered_func_data_bet
            fslstats prefiltered_func_data_bet -p 2 -p 98
            fslmaths prefiltered_func_data_bet -thr 100.8095459 -Tmin -bin mask -odt char
            fslstats prefiltered_func_data_mcf -k mask -p 50
            fslmaths mask -dilF mask
            fslmaths prefiltered_func_data_mcf -mas mask prefiltered_func_data_thresh
            fslmaths prefiltered_func_data_thresh -Tmean mean_func
            susan prefiltered_func_data_thresh 614.340225 2.12314225053 3 1 1
                        mean_func 614.340225 prefiltered_func_data_smooth
            fslmaths prefiltered_func_data_smooth -mas mask prefiltered_func_data_smooth
            fslmaths prefiltered_func_data_smooth -mul 12.2082189881 prefiltered_func_
                        data_intnorm
            fslmaths prefiltered_func_data_intnorm -bptf 25.0 -1 prefiltered_func_
                        data_tempfilt
            fslmaths prefiltered_func_data_tempfilt filtered_func_data
            fslmaths filtered_func_data -Tmean mean_func
            melodic -i filtered_func_data --nobet --bgthreshold=3 --tr=2.0000000000 -d 0
                        --mmthresh=0.5
            cp filtered_func_data.ica/melodic_mix
                        $STUDY_DIR/COBRE_MELODIC/${i}_melodic_mix_new
fi
done    #END "Loop through subjects..."
echo "Processing complete.";
```

4.2. GRAPH CREATION AND MEASUREMENT IN R

4.2.1. Computing functional network connectivity using lagged correlations

FNC requires breaking down the original temporal scans into a series of units modulated by time-series, where the correlations of the timeseries determines their similarity. We begin by calling the necessary libraries for this analysis:

```
> library(igraph)
> library(vegan)
> library(e1071)
```

For the COBRE data we can create the list of filenames using:

```
> setwd("/path/to/my/directory")
> filenames <-
            dir (pattern="melodic_mix_new")
```

Otherwise, we can read in the filenames from a text document using the scan() command.

With FSL the number of ICA components was determined uniquely for each subject. We first determine the number of components within each file to store within the vector, **s**.

```
> num_subjects <- length(filenames)
> s <- c(rep(0,num_subjects))
> for (i in 1:num_subjects)
{       s[i] <- dim((read.table(as.character
                (filenames[i]))))[2] }
```

We next read in each melodic_mix file and use these to create a distance matrix. We define the distance matrix as the maximal normed cross-correlation for a lag distance of 3. The distance between the timeseries for each component is calculated and stored in data_array_distance. The mapply function is used to apply the distance function to all elements in the upper-triangular part of the distance matrix, instead of using a nested for loop to calculate each item individually.

```
> data_array_distance <- array(NA, c(num_subjects, max(s), max(s)))
> for (i in 1:num_subjects)
{         ##Read in ICA results
        temp <- as.matrix(read.table(as.character(filenames[i])))
        for(j in 1:s[i])
        {         for(k in j:s[i])
                  {         data_array_distance[i,k,j] <- 1-max(abs(ccf(temp[,j], temp[,k],
                                        plot = FALSE, lag.max = 3)$acf))
                          data_array_distance[i,j,k] <- data_array_distance[i,k,j] }}
       diag(data_array_distance[i,,]) <- 0     }
```

At this point the fMRI scans of each subject have been converted: first by decomposing them into independent components, and then creating a functional connectivity matrix measuring the temporal connectivity among components within each subject. Every *melodic_mix* file has been converted into a functional connectivity distance matrix.

4.2.2. Graph creation and analysis

Next, we transform each matrix into a graph structure and measure the connectivity properties of each graphs. We first use the ISOMAP embedding algorithm to compute the distances among elements using the geodesic framework, and prune weak connections with package **vegan**. We then create a graph structure whose connectivity can be measured using functions in **igraph**. Because the data type output in **vegan** is different than the type needed for **igraph**, we create an internal conversion function named makegraph. This graphical structure uses weighted edges in a dissimilarity matrix, where '0' indicates that two points are not connected. Because of this, we use the inverse of the distance to define the weights between two vertices when the ISOMAP algorithm has computed they are connected.

```
> makegraph <- function(my_iso)
{         ##dim is dimension of matrix
          my_dist <- as.matrix(dist(my_iso
                                  $points[]))
          k <- dim(my_dist)[1]
          my_net <- matrix(0, nrow = k,
                                  ncol = k)
          which.rows <- my_iso$net[,1]
          which.cols <- my_iso$net[,2]
          for(j in 1:length(which.rows))
          {       my_net[which.rows[j],
                    which.cols[j]]
                    <- 1/my_dist[which.rows[j],
                    which.cols[j]]
                  my_net[which.cols[j],
                    which.rows[j]]
                    <- 1/my_dist[which.cols[j],
                    which.rows[j]]
                         }
          my_net          }
```

We next analyze the properties of these graphs. We create a function to calculate the coefficients γ and λ of a random graph. This is used to compute the *small worldness* of the actual graph proposed by the data. We call this function smallworld; it takes in 2 parameters: n = the number of vertices, and m = the number of edges. The value γ is a transitivity measure, of the probability that adjacent vertices are connected. This is sometimes called the *clustering coefficient.* This function is called later to compute the values γ and λ later for the randomly reconnected graph, and is averaged across 5000 random graphs. These values are used to form the ratio to calculate σ, the small-worldness measure.

```
> smallworld <- function(n,m)
{  smallworld <- matrix(nrow=5000,ncol=2)
    for(k in 1:5000)
    {    g   <-   erdos.renyi.game
                            (n,m, type="gnm")
        smallworld[k,1] <- transitivity(g)
        smallworld[k,2] <- average.path.
                               length(g)   }
    colMeans(smallworld)      }
```

We next run our geodesic-distance pruning procedure (ISOMAP) within **vegan**, convert the data structure using our function makegraph, and then measure the connectivity using **igraph**. We compute separately the small-world measure, σ, which is a vector output, by the routine called my_small_worldness. We threshold points as being connected using the k-nearest neighbors method.

We began with functional connectivity matrices, turned each matrix into a graph, and measured the connectivity of each graph. We used a total of 13 connectivity measures, include the small-world calculations. The feature vectors collectively form a feature matrix that will be used for classification in the following section.

4.3. SVM CLASSIFICATION IN R

In this section we demonstrate SVM Classification using the package **e1071** that contains an interface to the libsvm *C++* package by Chih-Chung Chang and Chih-Jen Lin. The *R* vignette (http://cran.r-project.org/web/packages/e1071/vignettes/svmdoc.pdf) details the functionality of this package, which includes many other classification routines besides SVM. The SVM method within this package has an optional benefit of cross-validation, which simplifies coding dramatically by implementing the training and testing steps within a single function call. In the following code we demonstrate classification of our feature vector using 10-fold cross-validation, but this is an adjustable parameter. There are many options within the svm() method that can be specified such as kernel choices, but we use the default parameters here ("radial basis function") for the sake of conciseness and clarity.

We create a vector my_cat with the response variables, in the case the patient diagnosis of each scan. This can alternatively be read in using the function read.table(). Because within the COBRE data two patients were disenrolled, we exclude those

```
> my_small_worldness <- matrix(NA, nrow = num_subjects, ncol = 1)
> my_feature_matrix <- matrix(NA, nrow = num_subjects, ncol = 12)
> randomsmallstore <- matrix(NA, nrow = num_subjects, ncol = 2)
> for(i in 1:num_subjects)
{  d <- matrix(data_array_distance[i,1:s[i],1:s[i]], nrow = s[i])
    my_iso <- isomap(d[1:s[i],1:s[i]],axes=3, k=max(floor(s[i]/10),2), ndim = 15,
        fragmentedOK=TRUE)
    my_net <- makegraph(my_iso)
    d2   <-   graph.adjacency(my_net )
    transitivity(d2)
    n=vcount(d2)
    m = ecount(d2)
    randomsmall  <- smallworld(n,m)
    sigma <- (transitivity(d2)/randomsmall[1])/(average.path.length(d2)/randomsmall[2])
    randomsmallstore[i,] <- c(randomsmall)
    my_small_worldness[i,] <- sigma
    my_net <- makegraph(my_iso)
    d2   <-   graph.adjacency(my_net, weighted = TRUE )
    my_feature_matrix[i,] <-c(average.path.length(d2),clique.number(d2),graph.density(d2),
        edge.connectivity(d2),median(closeness(d2)),median(graph.coreness(d2)),
        max(degree(d2)),median(degree(d2)),min(degree(d2)),vcount(d2),ecount(d2),
        transitivity(d2))     }
> my_feature_matrix <- cbind(my_feature_matrix,my_small_worldness)
```

Finally, we label the columns.

```
> colnames(my_feature_matrix) <- c("Average Path Length", "Clique Number","Graph Density",
    "Edge Connectivity", "Median Closeness", "Median Graph Coreness","Max Degree",
    "Median Degree",     "Min Degree",   "Vertex Count",  "Edge Count","Transitivity",
    "Small Worldness")
```

patients from this analysis. As R read in the list of files alphabetically and the COBRE demographic spreadsheet has patients entered in order of age, we reorganize the file formats to ensure that our patient labels read in from the spreadsheet match up with the data matrix already created.

```
> cobre <- read.csv
           ("COBRE_phenotypic_data.csv")
> cobre <- cobre[order(cobre[,1]),]
> my_cat <- cobre[,5]
> my_data_matrix <- my_feature_matrix
                    [my_cat!="Disenrolled",]
> my_cat <- my_cat[my_cat!="Disenrolled"]
> my_data_matrix <- cbind
                  (my_cat,my_data_matrix)
```

Finally, the library is loaded and the model is trained and tested using 10-fold cross-validation.

```
> my_svm <- svm(as.factor(my_cat)~.,
  data = as.data.frame(my_data_matrix),
  cross=10)
> pred <- fitted(my_svm)
```

The structure `my_svm` contains many details of the model. We can see the average cross-validation accuracy within each kth-fold using `my_svm$tot.accuracy`.

4.4. HYPOTHESIS TESTING

Alternatively, we can test for between-group differences using formal hypothesis testing. For example, if we wished to test the individual metrics between patients and controls, we could do so using:

```
> for(i in 2:14)
{  print(t.test(na.omit(my_data_matrix
                   [my_cat=="Patient",i]),
        na.omit(my_data_matrix[my_cat=
                      ="Control",i])))   }
```

All the computed graph-connectivity measures are correlated; for example, a graph with a low *median closeness* measure would imply that there is a short distance between two vertices, thus increasing the *transitivity*. Because of this, to compare the 13 measures we would have to adjust for multiple comparisons. Using a Bonferroni correction, only p-values below $0.05/13 = 0.0038$ would be considered significant.

5. RESULTS AND DISCUSSION

We briefly present here the results of this analysis.

Patients had a significantly lower clustering coefficient than healthy controls ($p < 0.05$, corrected). Lower clustering implies networks are less likely to be connected to each other in Schizophrenia, indicating that the networks are themselves less synchronized and more independent of each other. Patients had lower small-world measures of connectivity than healthy controls, although both groups exhibited small-world connectivity among independent components. This difference was not statistically significant when using unweighted graphs, but was statistically significant when using weighted graphs.

Using just the scripts provided here, our 10-fold cross-validation accuracy is 65%, compared to a chance accuracy of 50.7%. There are quite a number of things we could do to improve this accuracy, which we omitted intentionally here because they are outside the scope of this tutorial. We performed no quality-control on this data to exclude scans with excessive motion or scanner artifacts. We also took no measures to identify and exclude ICA networks that were related to motion, scanner noise, or physiological artifacts. We did not use any of the demographic information (patient gender, age, etc...) which would likely have improved accuracy, both by controlling for functional brain changes and also by controlling for sampling variation. For example, in this sample males were more likely to be Schizophrenia patients than females, so knowing this information would have permitted classification based upon this information, which is parallel to the actual functional connectivity analysis. Finally, we implemented only the basic SVM algorithm without any parameter tuning, and similarly did not optimize the definition of "connectivity" among points. Connectivity definitions have been shown previously to affect the final results, with different thresholds for connectivity having significant effects on the final graph-theoretic measurements (Toppi et al., 2012). Given the simplicity of our methods, it is perhaps somewhat remarkable that we were able to achieve the classification accuracy realized here and significant small-world differences between patients and controls.

6. CONCLUSION

Collectively, we have provided methods to determine whether functional connectivity differences exist between groups, and to demonstrate that the resting-state functional connectivity differences in schizophrenia can be useful for automated patient diagnosis. Functional connectivity measures can be used to discriminate between patients and controls, and schizophrenia patients show lowered clustering of networks than healthy controls, indicating that networks within Schizophrenia are more disconnected.

The analysis outlined here is intended to be adjusted and altered by the end user, even those who aren't regular users of *R*. The user has flexibility in altering parameters such as distance metrics, classification machines, and feature selection choices. For example, another method of implementing functional connectivity is through Granger causality among ROIs such as in Sato et al. (2010), whereas this presentation implements functional connectivity through correlations among functional networks determined by ICA. Other distance metrics could have been used, which would be optimal given the recent finding that using correlation metrics to compute distance automatically leads to non-random graphical structures (Zalesky et al., 2012). We performed SVM classification in *R*, a "black-box" model which ironically is remarkably simple to implement with a single function call to both train and test the model using cross-validation. Because *R* is an established package in the statistics research community, many newer machine learning procedures can easily be implemented to compare with more established classification machines.

This analysis and tutorial is not without limitations; primarily, we took no steps to identify and discard artifacts in the ICA data, which almost certainly would have increased the classification "accuracy" we obtained. This omission was intentional given the intentions of this tutorial; manually identifying artifacts within ICA is outside the scope of this manuscript, and other tutorials to perform to identify fMRI artifacts and clean data further are available elsewhere. We wish here to illustrate how functional connectivity can be measured in a graph-theoretic approach, and to provide a working framework for other researchers to alter and improve. Moreover, there are scripts available at http://www.nitrc.org/plugins/mwiki/index.php/fcon1000:ScriptUse to process this data and compute a variety of connectivity measures outside of the ICA-based measures presented here. These could be easily integrated with the methods outlined here to measure the connectivity properties once the connectivity matrices are established.

Although this analysis was created for analysis of fMRI data, more generally it applies to problems where the relationship among signal sources may determine the category to which an object belongs. The joint behavior of the signal sources (independent components) was observed as a graph object, where the distances between the sources represented the similarity of their behavior. Although second order measures were used to assess the functional connectivity (correlations), it is possible that as much discriminatory power exists using higher-order measurements that take into account the cohesiveness of triplets of components, or even more. Functional connectivity is one technique, of many, that should be assessed from multiple angles.

ACKNOWLEDGMENTS

We thank Dr. Xavier Quintana for his guidance during the original analysis, Dr. Ryan Rosario for an excellent tutorial on parallel analysis in *R* and Dr. Jesse Brown for helpful feedback, and NIH grant number R33DA026109 to Mark S. Cohen and the Burroughs Wellcome Fund Collaborative Research Travel Award to Ariana Anderson.

REFERENCES

Achard, S., Salvador, R., Whitcher, B., Suckling, J., and Bullmore, E. (2006). A resilient, low-frequency, small-world human brain functional network with highly connected association cortical hubs. *J. Neurosci.* 26, 63–72. doi: 10.1523/JNEUROSCI.3874-05.2006

Allen, E. A., Erhardt, E. B., Damaraju, E., Gruner, W., Segall, J. M., Silva, R. F., et al. (2011). A baseline for the multivariate comparison of resting-state networks. *Front. Syst. Neurosci.* 5:2. doi: 10.3389/fnsys.2011.00002

Anderson, A., Bramen, J., Douglas, P. K., Lenartowicz, A., Cho, A., Culbertson, C., et al. (2011). Large sample group independent component analysis of functional magnetic resonance imaging using anatomical atlas-based reduction and bootstrapped clustering. *Int. J. Imaging Syst. Technol.* 21, 223–231. doi: 10.1002/ima.20286

Anderson, A., Dinov, I. D., Sherin, J. E., Quintana, J., Yuille, A., and Cohen, M. S. (2010). Classification of spatially unaligned fMRI scans. *Neuroimage* 49, 2501–2519. doi: 10.1016/j.neuroimage.2009.08.036

Bassett, D. S., Bullmore, E., Verchinski, B. A., Mattay, V. S., Weinberger, D. R., and Meyer-Lindenberg, A. (2008). Hierarchical organization of human cortical networks in health and schizophrenia. *J. Neurosci.* 28, 9239–9248. doi: 10.1523/JNEUROSCI.1929-08.2008

Biswal, B., Yetkin, F. Z., Haughton, V. M., and Hyde, J. S. (1995). Functional connectivity in the motor cortex of resting human brain using echo-planar MRI. *Magn. Resona. Med.* 34, 537–541. doi: 10.1002/mrm.1910340409

Bookheimer, S. (2002). Functional MRI of language: new approaches to understanding the cortical organization of semantic processing. *Annu. Rev. Neurosci.* 25, 151–188. doi: 10.1146/annurev.neuro.25.112701.142946

Bordier, C., Dojat, M., and de Micheaux, P. L. (2011). Temporal and spatial independent component analysis for fMRI data sets embedded in the AnalyzeFMRI R package. *J. Stat. Soft.* 44, 1–24.

Bordier, C., Dojat, M., and de Micheaux, P. L. (2009). **AnalyzeFMRI**: an *R* package to perform statistical analysis on fmri datasets. *UseR 2009.* Software: R Package, AnalyzeFMRI, version 1.1-12.

Calhoun, V. D., Sui, J., Kiehl, K., Turner, J., Allen, E., and Pearlson, G. (2011). Exploring the psychosis functional connectome: aberrant intrinsic networks in schizophrenia and bipolar disorder. *Front. Psychiatry* 2:75. doi: 10.3389/fpsyt.2011.00075.

Chen, G., Saad, Z. S., and Cox, R. W. (2010). "Statistical analysis programs in *R* for fMRI data," in *UseR! 2010 Conference Proceedings.* Available online at: http://www.r-project.org/conferences/useR-2010/abstracts/Chen+Saad+Cox.pdf

Chen, G., Saad, Z. S., Nath, A. R., Beauchamp, M. S., and Cox, R. W. (2012). FMRI group analysis combining effect estimates and their variances. *Neuroimage* 60, 747–765. doi: 10.1016/j.neuroimage.2011.12.060

Chu, C., Handwerker, D. A., Bandettini, P. A., and Ashburner, J. (2011). "Measuring the consistency of global functional connectivity using kernel regression methods," in *Proceedings of the 2011 IEEE International Workshop on Pattern Recognition in NeuroImaging (PRNI)*, 41–44.

Cohen, M. S., and Bookheimer, S. Y. (1994). Localization of brain function using magnetic resonance imaging. *Trends Neurosci.* 17, 268–277. doi: 10.1016/0166-2236(94)90055-8

Csardi, G., and Nepusz, T. (2006). The **igraph** software package for complex network research. *InterJournal* Complex Systems, 1695.

Dimitriadou, E., Hornik, K., Leisch, F., Meyer, D., and Weingessel, A. (2010). ***e1071**: Misc Functions of the Department of Statistics (**e1071**), TU Wien.* R package version 1.5-24.

Erdős, P., and Rényi, A. (1961). On the strength of connectedness of a random graph. *Acta Math. Hung.* 12, 261–267. doi: 10.1007/BF02066689

Fan, Y., Shen, D., and Davatzikos, C. (2006). "Detecting cognitive states from fmri images by machine learning and multivariate classification," in *Proceedings of the Conference on Computer Vision and Pattern Recognition Workshop (CVPRW'06)*, 89–89.

Ferreira da Silva, A. R. (2011). CudaBayesreg: parallel implementation of a bayesian multilevel model for fMRI data analysis. *J. Stat. Soft.* 44, 1–24.

Ford, J., Farid, H., Makedon, F., Flashman, L. A., McAllister, T. W., Megalooikonomou, V., et al. (2003). "Patient classification of fMRI activation maps," in *Medical Image Computing and Computer-Assisted Intervention-MICCAI* (Berlin, Heidelberg: Springer), 58–65.

Garrity, A., Pearlson, G., McKiernan, K., Lloyd, D., Kiehl, K., and Calhoun, V. (2007). Aberrant default mode functional connectivity in schizophrenia. *Am. J. Psychiatry* 164, 450–457. doi: 10.1176/appi.ajp.164.3.450

Gauthier, I., Tarr, M. J., Anderson, A. W., Skudlarski, P., and Gore, J. C. (1999). Activation of the middle fusiform'face area'increases with expertise in recognizing novel objects. *Nat. Neurosci.* 2, 568–573. doi: 10.1038/9224

Georgiev, P. G., Theis, F. J., and Cichocki, A. (2005). Sparse component analysis and blind source separation of underdetermined mixtures. *IEEE Trans. Neural Netw.* 16, 992–996. doi: 10.1109/TNN.2005.849840

Hanlon, F. M., Houck, J. M., Pyeatt, C. J., Lundy, S. L., Euler, M. J., Weisend, M. P. (2011). Bilateral hippocampal dysfunction in schizophrenia. *Neuroimage* 58, 1158–1168. doi: 10.1016/j.neuroimage.2011.06.091

Humphries, M. D., and Gurney, K. (2008). Network small-world-ness: a quantitative method for determining canonical network equivalence. *PLoS ONE* 3:e0002051. doi: 10.1371/journal.pone.0002051

Hyvärinen, A., and Oja, E. (2000). Independent component analysis: algorithms and applications. *Neural Netw.* 13, 411–430. doi: 10.1016/S0893-6080(00)00026-5

Jafri, M. J., Pearlson, G. D., Stevens, M., and Calhoun, V. D. (2008). A method for functional network connectivity among spatially independent resting-state components in schizophrenia. *Neuroimage* 39, 1666–1681. doi: 10.1016/j.neuroimage.2007.11.001

Jenkinson, M., Bannister, P., Brady, M., and Smith, S. (2002). Improved optimization for the robust and accurate linear registration and motion correction of brain images. *Neuroimage* 17, 825–841. doi: 10.1006/nimg.2002.1132

Kim, S.-G., Rostrup, E., Larsson, H. B., Ogawa, S., and Paulson, O. B. (1999). Determination of relative cmro 2 from cbf and bold changes: significant increase of oxygen consumption rate during visual stimulation. *Magnet. Res. Med.* 41, 1152–1161.

Koshino, H., Carpenter, P. A., Minshew, N. J., Cherkassky, V. L., Keller, T. A., and Just, M. A. (2005). Functional connectivity in an fMRI working memory task in high-functioning autism. *Neuroimage* 24, 810–821. doi: 10.1016/j.neuroimage.2004.09.028

Lee, T. M., Liu, H.-L. Tan, L.-H., Chan, C. C., Mahankali, S., Feng, C.-M. et al. (2002). Lie detection by functional magnetic resonance imaging. *Hum. Brain Mapp.* 15, 157–164. doi: 10.1002/hbm.10020

Liang, M., Zhou, Y., Jiang, T., Liu, Z., Tian, L., Liu, H., et al. (2006). Widespread functional disconnectivity in schizophrenia with resting-state functional magnetic resonance imaging. *Neuroreport* 17, 209–213. doi: 10.1097/01.wnr.0000198434.06518.b8

Liow, J. S., Rehm, K., Strother, S. C., Anderson, R. R., Mørch, N., and Hansen, L. K. (2000). Comparison of voxel- and volume-of-interest-based analyses in FDG PET scans of HIV positive and healthy individuals. *J. Nuclear Med.* 41, 612–621. doi: 10.1093/brain/awn018

Liu, Y., Liang, M., Zhou, Y., He, Y., Hao, Y., Song, M., et al. (2008). Disrupted small-world networks in schizophrenia. *Brain* 131, 945–961.

Mayer, A. R., Ruhl, D., Merideth, F., Ling, J., Hanlon, F. M., Bustillo, J., et al. (2012). Functional imaging of the hemodynamic sensory gating response in schizophrenia. *Hum. Brain Mapp.* 34, 2302–2312. doi: 10.1002/hbm.22065

McKeown, M. J., Hansen, L. K., and Sejnowsk, T. J. (2003). Independent component analysis of functional mri: what is signal and what is noise? *Curr. Opin. Neurobiol.* 13, 620–629. doi: 10.1016/j.conb.2003.09.012

Oksanen, J., Blanchet, F. G., Kindt, R., Legendre, P., O'Hara, R. B., Simpson, G. L., et al. (2011). ***vegan:** Community Ecology Package* R package version 1.17-6.

Polzehl, J., and Tabelow, K. (2007). **fmri**: a package for analyzing fMRI data. *RNews* 7, 13–17.

R Development Core Team. (2012). *R: A Language and Environment for Statistical Computing.* Vienna: R Foundation for Statistical Computing. ISBN 3-900051-07-0.

Roebroeck, A., Formisano, E., and Goebel, R. (2005). Mapping directed influence over the brain using Granger causality and fMRI. *Neuroimage* 25, 230–242. doi: 10.1016/j.neuroimage.2004.11.017

Roelstraete, B., and Rosseel, Y. (2011). FIAR: an R package for analyzing functional integration in the brain. *J. Stat. Soft.* 44, 1–32.

Rubinov, M., and Sporns, O. (2010). Complex network measures of brain connectivity: uses and interpretations. *Neuroimage* 52, 1059–1069. doi: 10.1016/j.neuroimage.2009.10.003

Sato, J. R., Fujita, A., Cardoso, E. F., Thomaz, C. E., Brammer, M. J., and Amaro, E. (2010). Analyzing the connectivity between regions of interest: an approach based on cluster Granger causality for fMRI data analysis. *Neuroimage* 52, 1444–1455. doi: 10.1016/j.neuroimage.2010.05.022

Smith, S. M. (2002). Fast robust automated brain extraction. *Hum. Brain Mapp.* 17, 143–155. doi: 10.1002/hbm.10062

Smith, S. M., Jenkinson, M., Woolrich, M. W., Beckmann, C. F., Behrens, T. E. J., Johansen-berg, H, et al. (2004). Advances in functional and structural MR image analysis and implementation as *FSL Neuroimage* 23, 208–219. doi: 10.1016/j.neuroimage.2004.07.051

Tabelow, K., Clayden, J. D., Lafaye de Micheaux, P., Polzehl, J., Schmid, V. J., and Whitcher, B. (2011). Image analysis and statistical inference in neuroimaging with R. *Neuroimage* 55, 1686–1693. doi: 10.1016/j.neuroimage.2011.01.013

Tenenbaum, J. B., de Silva, V., and Langford, J. C. (2009). A global geometric framework for nonlinear dimensionality reduction. *Science* 290, 2319–2313. doi: 10.1126/science.290.5500.2319

Toppi, J., De Vico Fallani, F., Vecchiato, G., Maglione, A., Cincotti, F., Mattia, D., et al. (2012). How the statistical validation of functional connectivity patterns can prevent erroneous definition of small-world properties of a brain connectivity network. *Comput. Math. Methods Med.* 2012.

van de Ven, V. G. (2004). Functional connectivity as revealed by spatial independent component analysis of fMRI measurements during rest. *Hum. Brain Mapp.* 22, 165–178. doi: 10.1002/hbm.20022

Whitfield-Gabrieli, S., Thermenos, H. W., Milanovic, S., Tsuang, M. T., Faraone, S. V., McCarley, R. W., et al. (2009). Hyperactivity and hyperconnectivity of the default network in schizophrenia and in first-degree relatives of persons with schizophrenia. *Proc. Natl. Acad. Sci. U.S.A.* 106, 1279–1284. doi: 10.1073/pnas.0809141106

Yu, Q., Sui, J., Rachakonda, S., He, H., Gruner, W., Pearlson, G., et al. (2011). Altered topological properties of functional network connectivity in schizophrenia during resting state: a small-world brain network study. *PLoS ONE* 6:e25423. doi: 10.1371/journal.pone.0025423

Zalesky, A., Fornito, A., and Bullmore, E. (2012). On the use of correlation as a measure of network connectivity. *Neuroimage* 60, 2096–2106. doi: 10.1016/j.neuroimage.2012.02.001

Zhang, L., and Samaras, D. (2005). "Machine learning for clinical diagnosis from functional magnetic resonance imaging," in *IEEE Conference on Computer Vision and Pattern Recognition (CVPR)*, (San Diego, CA), 1211–1217.

APPENDIX

R FUNCTIONS AND FEATURES TUTORIAL

We begin by calling the library **AnalyzeFMRI** which must be pre-installed. When installing any package within the GUI, the option of "install dependencies" should be selected to install packages called by the main package. Once this package is installed, it is called, and the proper directory is navigated to. The current working directory can be obtained using `getwd()`. This directory needs to contain a list of scan names, `filenames.txt`, and the set of scans. We use here a scan produced by the FSL script supplied on the data available for download from NITRC.

```
> library(AnalyzeFMRI)
> rm(list = ls())
> setwd("/path/to/my/directory")
```

A scan can be read directly into *R*, and consequently held in memory, using

```
> myimage <- f.read.nifti.volume("rest_mcf_brain.nii")
```

We can get preliminary statistics using

```
> summary(myimage)
     Min.   1st Qu.    Median      Mean   3rd Qu.      Max.
   0.0000    0.0000    0.0000  129.0000    0.0006 1639.0000
```

We can access the header information using

```
> f.nifti.file.summary("rest_mcf_brain.nii")

        File name: rest_mcf_brain.nii
   Data Dimension: 4-D
      X dimension: 64
      Y dimension: 64
      Z dimension: 33
   Time dimension: 150 time points
Voxel dimensions: 3.75  x 3.75  x 4.55000019073486
        Data type:  (32 bits per voxel)
```

We can alternatively verify the dimensions of the scan using the command `dim`, since the image is held in memory.

```
> dim(myimage)
[1]  64  64  33 150
```

This image is stored as an array, which we can verify using

```
> is.array(myimage)
[1] TRUE
```

Functions such as `f.read.nifti.volume`, `f.read.nifti.ts`, and `f.read.nifti.slice.at.all.timepoints` can allow direct access to specific pieces of data. For example, if we wanted to access a single timeseries from the 4D scan at voxel location (30,30,10) *without* holding the entire scan in memory, we can do so by:

```
> f.read.nifti.ts("rest_mcf_brain.nii",30,30,10)
```

where the input parameters are the filename and the (x,y,z) coordinates of the voxel desired. We can also access this from the scan held in memory using `myimage[30,30,10,]` which is noticeably faster.

We next wish to perform ICA within *R*, but this is available only for Analyze format scans. We write out our scan as Analyze format with:

```
> f.write.analyze(myimage,file="rest_mcf_brain")
```

If we wish to see all the parameter options available for ICA, we can access this using

```
> help(f.ica.fmri)}
```

We next run ICA on the example fMRI scan.

```
> g <- f.ica.fmri("rest_mcf_brain.img", n.comp=20, alg.type = "deflation")
```

This performs ICA on the scan called "`rest_mcf_brain.img`", extracting 20 components and storing the results in the object `g`. It is necessary to state the number of components to be extracted with the parameter `ncomp`. The number of components is somewhat arbitrary; the ICA extraction is performed here using the deflation approach where components are individually estimated and then subtracted out, so limiting the number of components theoretically should not change the structure of the components that are extracted. We set the default value, (`num_components`), to 20 according to (**?**). Use `help(f.ica.fmri)` to see the full list of options within the function

There is also the option of using a GUI to run this analysis, using the command `f.ica.fmri.gui()`.

The object `g` contains several attributes:

```
> attributes(g)
$names
[1] "A"     "S"     "file" "mask"
```

The timeseries for the components are contained in `g$A`:

```
> dim(g$A)
[1] 150  20
```

The spatial maps are contained in the array `g$S`, the filename in `g$file`, and the mask (if used) in `g$mask`.

We can view a single component as shown in **Figure 2**, in this case the second of the set, by using

```
> f.plot.ica.fmri(g,2,cols=rainbow(100))
```

This image isn't thresholded, but can be roughly thresholded by adjusting the color options within `rainbow()`, by changing the number of colors to display to 3 and adjusting the saturation.

```
> f.plot.ica.fmri(g,2,cols=rainbow(3,alpha=.8))
```

We can also manually threshold using the spatial map `g$S[, , ,2]`. Here, we threshold the second component into the 10-th and 90-th percentile:

```
> g_thresholded <- g
> g_thresholded$S[,,,2][g$S[,,,2]>quantile(g$S[,,,2],probs=c(.1,.9))[2]] <- 3
> g_thresholded$S[,,,2][g$S[,,,2]<quantile(g$S[,,,2],probs=c(.1,.9))[2]] <- 2
> g_thresholded$S[,,,2][g$S[,,,2]<quantile(g$S[,,,2],probs=c(.1,.9))[1]] <- 1
```

The image can be written out using:

```
> f.write.analyze(g_thresholded$S[,,,2],file="MyThresholdedImage")
```

creating files called "MyThresholdedImage.img" and "MyThresholdedImage.hdr" in the working directory.

This concludes our example of the package **AnalyzefMRI**. This is not an exhaustive list of the functions available in this package, but a brief tutorial showing direct fMRI data access in R. For a full list of functions within this package, please see the manual at http://cran.r-project.org/web/packages/AnalyzeFMRI/AnalyzeFMRI.pdf.

ICA FOR fMRI IN R USING PREPROCESSED DATA

R can also perform ICA on Analyze format scans, so we demonstrate doing this in a loop. ICA within R uses the FAST-ICA algorithm, which is similar to FSL. This implementation will not work directly on the COBRE data since the function `f.ica.fmri` requires Analyze format data and the COBRE data is NIfTI, although the FSL command `fslchfiletype` will convert between the two formats. The filenames ("myfilename1.img") are written on a text file called filenames.txt, where each line contains a separate filename. The lines that will need to be changed for the user are as follows:

```
> setwd("/path/to/my/directory")
> filenames <- read.table("filenames.txt")
> filenames <- filenames[i,1]
We can alternatively create the list of filenames using:
> filenames <- dir(pattern="melodic_mix")
```

We then create a loop to read in our files, perform ICA on each scan using the function `f.ica.fmri()` within the library **AnalyzeFMRI**, extract the timeseries associated with the components, and create a distance matrix for each component.

```
> library(AnalyzeFMRI)
> num_subjects <- dim(filenames)[1]
> num_components <- 30
> data_array_distance <- array(NA, c(num_subjects, num_components, num_components))
> my_distance <-  function(x,y)
{   1-max(abs(ccf(x, y, plot = FALSE, lag.max = 3)$acf))    }

> for (i in 1:num_subjects)
{   #Perform ICA on each file
    temp <- f.ica.fmri(as.character(filenames[i,1]), n.comp = num_components,
                                                        alg.type="deflation")
    for(j in 1:num_components)
    {   j.vals <- rep(j,(num_components-j+1))
        k.vals <- (j:num_components)
        data_array_distance[i,j,j:num_components] <- c(mapply(x=j.vals,
            y=k.vals, function(x,y) my_distance(temp$A[,x],temp$A[,y])))
        data_array_distance[i,j:num_components,j]
                                      <- data_array_distance[i,j,j:num_components]   }
    diag(data_array_distance[i,,]) <- 0   }
```

This performs ICA on this i^{th} scan listed in `filenames.txt`, and stores the results into an object called `temp`. This object has several attributes, one of which is the timeseries associated with each component called `temp$A`.

PARALLEL ANALYSIS IN R

We now demonstrate parallel computing by using the base package **parallel** in R 2.1.4 as presented by http://www.bytemining.com/files/talks/larug/hpc2012/HPCinRrev2012.pdf which provides an extensive explanation of parallel data analysis using *R*. The package **cudaBayesreg** also provides parallel analysis of fMRI data using multi-level Bayesian modeling.

The package **parallel** wraps together packages **multicore** and **snow**. We assume the computing is being done on the local machine here with multiple cores, but these methods can easily be extended to run on a cluster. The number of available cores can be detected using Windows will report the number of logical CPUs, which may exceed the number of physical cores.

```
> library(parallel)
> mc  <-  detectCores()
> mc
[1] 2
```

To perform the parallel analysis, we create a new function `func_network_connectivity` which takes as an argument the file number, and performs within each scan the FNC analysis.

```
> data_array_distance <- array(NA, c(num_subjects, num_components, num_components))
> num_components <- 20
> func_network_connectivity <- function(i){
    temp <- f.ica.fmri(as.character(filenames[i,1]), n.comp = num_components)
    for(j in 1:num_components)
    {   j.vals <- rep(j,(num_components-j+1))
        k.vals <- (j:num_components)
        data_array_distance[i,j,j:num_components] <-
             c(mapply(x=j.vals,y=k.vals, function(x,y)
             1-max(abs(ccf(x, y, plot = FALSE, lag.max = 3)$acf)))
        data_array_distance[i,k.vals,j.vals] <- 1/data_array_distance[i,j,
             j:num_components]    }
    diag(data_array_distance[i,,]) <- 0
    d <- (data_array_distance[i,,])
    my_iso <- isomap(d,axes=1, ndim = 10,epsilon=median(d),
          fragmentedOK=TRUE)
    my_net <- makegraph(my_iso)
    d2  <-  graph.adjacency(my_net, weighted = TRUE )
    c(as.character(filenames[i,1]),average.path.length(d2),clique.number(d2),
         graph.density(d2),edge.connectivity(d2),median(closeness(d2)),
         median(graph.coreness(d2)),max(degree(d2)),median(degree(d2)),
         min(degree(d2)),vcount(d2),ecount(d2),transitivity(d2))  }
```

The new `func_network_connectivity` function is called by the parallel function `parLapply`, which is similar to `mapply` but operates in parallel. Using this, we perform ICA, establish functional connectivity and measure the graph structures in parallel. The function `makeForkCluster` is called to create multiple identical R processes on the same machine with a copy of the master workspace. This function will not work in Windows since Windows does not have a `fork` system call, so sockets must be used instead.

```
> cl <- makeForkCluster()
> clusterSetRNGStream (cl, 123)
> res   <-  parLapply(cl, seq_len(4), func_network_connectivity)
> stopCluster(cl)
```

13

GroupICA dual regression analysis of resting state networks in a behavioral variant of frontotemporal dementia

Riikka Rytty[1,2], Juha Nikkinen[3], Liisa Paavola[1,2], Ahmed Abou Elseoud[3], Virpi Moilanen[2], Annina Visuri[1], Osmo Tervonen[3], Alan E. Renton[4], Bryan J. Traynor[4], Vesa Kiviniemi[3†] and Anne M. Remes[5,6*†]

[1] *Department of Neurology, Institute of Clinical Medicine, University of Oulu, Oulu, Finland*
[2] *Department of Neurology, Oulu University Hospital, Oulu, Finland*
[3] *Department of Radiology, Institute of Clinical Medicine, University of Oulu, Oulu, Finland*
[4] *Neuromuscular Diseases Research Unit, Laboratory of Neurogenetics, National Institute on Aging, National Institutes of Health, Bethesda, MD, USA*
[5] *Department of Neurology, Institute of Clinical Medicine, University of Eastern Finland, Kuopio, Finland*
[6] *Department of Neurology, Kuopio University Hospital, Kuopio, Finland*

***Correspondence:**
Anne M. Remes, Department of Neurology, Institute of Clinical Medicine, University of Eastern Finland, Yliopistonranta 1, PO Box 1627, 70211 Kuopio, Finland
e-mail: anne.remes@uef.fi

† These authors have contributed equally to this work.

Functional MRI studies have revealed changes in default-mode and salience networks in neurodegenerative dementias, especially in Alzheimer's disease (AD). The purpose of this study was to analyze the whole brain cortex resting state networks (RSNs) in patients with behavioral variant frontotemporal dementia (bvFTD) by using resting state functional MRI (rfMRI). The group specific RSNs were identified by high model order independent component analysis (ICA) and a dual regression technique was used to detect between-group differences in the RSNs with $p < 0.05$ threshold corrected for multiple comparisons. A *y*-concatenation method was used to correct for multiple comparisons for multiple independent components, gray matter differences as well as the voxel level. We found increased connectivity in several networks within patients with bvFTD compared to the control group. The most prominent enhancement was seen in the right frontotemporal area and insula. A significant increase in functional connectivity was also detected in the left dorsal attention network (DAN), in anterior paracingulate—a default mode sub-network as well as in the anterior parts of the frontal pole. Notably the increased patterns of connectivity were seen in areas around atrophic regions. The present results demonstrate abnormal increased connectivity in several important brain networks including the DAN and default-mode network (DMN) in patients with bvFTD. These changes may be associated with decline in executive functions and attention as well as apathy, which are the major cognitive and neuropsychiatric defects in patients with frontotemporal dementia.

Keywords: default, resting state, functional MRI, dorsal attention network, frontotemporal dementia

INTRODUCTION

Frontotemporal lobar degeneration (FTLD) is a clinically and pathologically heterogeneous syndrome characterized by a progressive decline in behavior and/or language associated with degeneration of the frontal and anterior temporal lobes (Neary et al., 2005). FTLD is the second most frequent neurodegenerative disease leading to early onset dementia after Alzheimer's disease (AD). The most common clinical presentation of FTLD is behavioral-variant frontotemporal dementia (bvFTD). The prominent symptoms in bvFTD are a gradual decline in social behavior with loss of insight and decline in executive functions instead of typical memory problems.

Resting state functional MRI (rfMRI) can be used to study the intrinsic connectivity of brain networks in task-free settings by mapping temporally synchronous, spatially distributed, spontaneous low frequency (<0.08 Hz) blood oxygen level-dependent (BOLD) signal fluctuations (Fox and Raichle, 2007). rfMRI reports have revealed a number of functional networks in the brain, but mainly two major intrinsic connectivity networks, the default-mode network (DMN) and salience, have been studied in neurodegenerative diseases. The DMN is a posterior network that consists of the hippocampi, posterior cingulate cortex/precuneus, lateral parietal regions, and the rostromedial prefrontal cortex (Raichle et al., 2001). Regions of the DMN seem to participate in episodic memory and visuospatial imagery (Zhou et al., 2010). The salience network is a large anterior network that consists of the anterior cingulate cortex (ACC), orbital frontoinsula (FI), amygdala, and striatum and is related to socially-emotionally relevant information processing (Seeley et al., 2007a,b). Decreased connectivity in the DMN is consistently associated with AD (Greicius et al., 2004; Zhang et al., 2009; Gili et al., 2011), while reduction of connectivity in the salience network has been usually found in patients with bvFTD. However, the findings in patients with bvFTD are controversial (Zhou et al., 2010; Whitwell et al., 2011; Borroni et al., 2012). Disruption in other functional networks such as the dorsal attention network (DAN) has been found in AD (Li et al., 2012).

Previous rfMRI analyses have been done using relatively low model order (<30) independent component analysis (ICA) estimated from a single subject or group analyses (Zhou et al., 2010; Whitwell et al., 2011; Borroni et al., 2012). Detecting multiple networks from 1.5 T BOLD data from a single subject is not optimal in all occasions. Instead, group ICA offers much more robust delineation of identifiable networks (Kiviniemi et al., 2009; Smith et al., 2009; Abou-Elseoud et al., 2010). Also, the use of a higher model order in ICA detects more networks under detected at low model orders and introduces sub-network delineation of resting state networks (RSNs) at more detailed level separating noise more appropriately (Abou Elseoud et al., 2011, 2012). The problem with the more robust group ICA networks is still the challenge of acquiring accurate representations of networks from the individual level for a statistical group analysis.

The dual regression method has been introduced in order to overcome statistical inference problems (Filippini et al., 2009). Zuo and co-workers found that not only is the temporal concatenated ICA dual regression approach reliable, it produces more robust results than template matching ICA performed on an individual level (Zuo et al., 2010). This variability at the individual level seems to arise from the non-stationarity of the networks themselves, rather than the ICA method instability (Zuo et al., 2010; Kiviniemi et al., 2011; Hutchison et al., 2013). Moreover, group-level averaging seems to increase matching accuracy to RSN templates as well.

In order to obtain robust whole brain cortex network status with all relevant functional RSNs one still has to account for the multiple comparison problem introduced by the usage of several ICs. We have recently developed a *y*-concatenation method for correcting for multiple comparisons for multiple IC components as well as at the voxel level (Abou Elseoud et al., 2012). This correction enables the detection of statistically significant alterations between groups in all analysed RSNs of the brain cortex.

In bvFTD executive dysfunction is the prominent neuropsychological finding, and neurodegeneration is seen in frontal, temporal and insular areas including parts of the salience network (Neary et al., 1998, 2005; Rosen et al., 2002; Seeley et al., 2007a,b; Whitwell et al., 2009). Thus, we hypothesized to find decreased connectivity in the salience network associated with changes in executive networks. Our aim was to obtain a robust, fully data driven measure of the functional connectivity changes of all RSNs covering the whole brain. For this we performed time concatenated temporal ICA with a dual regression approach with y-concatenation statistics of bvFTD data compared to controls.

MATERIALS AND METHODS

PATIENTS

The patient group included 19 cases with bvFTD (nine male). A clinical diagnosis of bvFTD was made according to the criteria of Lund and Manchester (Neary et al., 1998; Rascovsky et al., 2011). Patients presenting other types of FTLD phenotype such as progressive aphasia and semantic dementia were excluded. All patients were examined in Oulu University Hospital at the Memory outpatient clinic of the Department of Neurology. The mean age at examination was 60.3 years (range 47–77 years). MMSE (Mini-Mental State Examination) score was on average 24.1 (17–30). Neuropsychological examination was performed within 6 months of the fMRI scan of each patient. Impairments in memory, language, executive, and visuospatial functions were then rated in three stages (absent, mild to moderate, severe). The declines in attention and executive functions were the most prominent findings in all of the patients, but there was also significant deterioration in other cognitive domains. Patients' reading and writing skills were normal. Dyspraxia was not present, and motor speed and control were at a normal level. Apathy was the most prevalent neuropsychiatric symptom (74%), but depression and irritability was also common (50%). The severity of the disease was rated as mild in nine patients, moderate in nine patients and severe in one patient (Piguet et al., 2011). Medications for neuropsychiatric symptoms were used in some of the patients (acetylcholinesterase inhibitors in three patients, memantine in two, neuroleptics in eight and valproate in three). Positive family history for any type of dementia was seen in 52.6% ($n = 10$) of patients. DNA samples were available from ten patients and five of them carried a C9ORF72 repeat expansion (Renton et al., 2011). Mutations in progranulin or microtubule-associated protein tau genes were not found in any of the patients.

Age and gender-matched controls ($n = 19$) were also examined. Mean age at examination was 57.8 years (range 50–70). No psychiatric or neurological disorders or medications affecting the central nervous system were allowed. Beck's depression inventory (BDI) score was mean 2.7 (range 0–10) and MMSE mean was 28.9 (range 26–30).

Written informed consent was obtained from all of the patients or their guardians. The research protocol was approved by the Ethics Committee of the Northern Ostrobothnia Hospital District.

IMAGING PROTOCOL

Resting-state BOLD data were collected on a GE Signa 1.5 T MRI scanner with an 8-channel parallel imaging-coil ASSET system (acceleration factor × 2) with an EPI GRE sequence (TR 1800 ms, TE 40 ms, 285 time points, 28 oblique axial slices, slice thickness 4 mm, inter-slice space 0.4 mm, covering the whole brain with an FOV of 25.6 cm × 25.6 cm with 64 × 64 matrix, and a flip angle of 90°). Hearing was protected using ear plugs and motion was minimized by using soft pads fitted over the ears. The subjects were instructed to simply lay still inside the scanner with their eyes closed, think of nothing in particular and not to fall asleep. High-resolution T1-weighted 3D FSPGR BRAVO images were taken in order to obtain anatomical images for co-registration of the fMRI data to the standard space coordinates and to investigate voxel-wise changes in the gray matter volume.

STRUCTURAL ANALYSIS

Structural data were analysed with FSL-VBM (www.fmrib.ox.ac.uk/fsl), a voxel-based morphometry style analysis (Ashburner and Friston, 2000; Good et al., 2001). Firstly, structural images were brain-extracted using BET (Smith, 2002). Next, tissue-type segmentation was carried out using FAST4 (Zhang et al., 2001). The resulting gray matter partial volume images were aligned to MNI152 standard space using nonlinear registration FNIRT in FSL (www.fmrib.ox.ac.uk/analysis/techrep), which uses a b-spline representation of the registration warp field (Rueckert et al., 1999). The resulting images were averaged to create a study-specific template, to which the native gray matter images were then non-linearly re-registered. The registered partial volume images were then modulated to correct for local expansion or contraction by dividing by the Jacobian of the warp field. The modulated segmented images were then smoothed with an isotropic Gaussian kernel with a sigma of 3 mm. Finally, voxelwise GLM was applied using FSL's randomize, which is a permutation-based non-parametric testing, correcting for multiple comparisons across space with $p < 0.05$ threshold.

fMRI DATA PRE-PROCESSING

Data pre-processing was carried out with FSL tools. Head motion in the fMRI data was corrected using multi-resolution rigid body co-registration of volumes, as implemented in the MCFLIRT software (Jenkinson et al., 2002). Brain extraction was carried out for motion corrected BOLD volumes with optimization of the deforming smooth surface model, as implemented in the BET software (Smith, 2002). This procedure was verified with visual inspection of the extraction result. The resulting image data was used as a mask for a secondary brain extraction. Multi-resolution affine co-registration as implemented in the FLIRT software was used to co-register fMRI volumes to 3D FSPGR volumes of the corresponding subjects and further the 3D FSPGR volumes to the MNI152 standard space. The images were transformed to 4 mm cubic voxels with 5 mm FWHM smoothing. There were no differences in head motion parameters in absolute [FTD (0.30 $\pm$ 0.12 mm) vs. control (0.26 $\pm$ 0.13 mm, t-test $p = 0.36$)] or relative [FTD (0.07 $\pm$ 0.03 mm) vs. controls (0.06 $\pm$ 0.03 mm, t-test $p = 0.34$)] between the study groups. Maximum absolute (2.9 mm) and relative (3.1 mm) head motion were below the voxel size in all subjects.

FUNCTIONAL CONNECTIVITY ANALYSIS

ICA analysis has been conducted as previously described (Abou Elseoud et al., 2011). Briefly, ICA analysis was carried out using FSL 4.1.4 MELODIC software implementing probabilistic independent component analysis (PICA) (Beckmann and Smith, 2004). A multisession temporal concatenation tool in MELODIC was used to perform PICA related pre-processing and data conditioning in the group analysis setting. Spatial ICA using 70 independent component maps (IC maps) was applied to detect RSNs from the control group. Control group data was chosen for two reasons: Firstly, our experience is that a combined groupICA having both cases and controls produces averaged maps of both groups which are then less sensitive in detecting differences between the groups in dual regression. Secondly, control data groupICA results are more robust match with previous healthy control data groupICA templates without disease-related alterations (Kiviniemi et al., 2009; Smith et al., 2009). Variance normalization was used. The IC maps were thresholded using an alternative hypothesis test based on fitting a Gaussian/gamma mixture model to the distribution of voxel intensities within spatial maps and controlling the local false-discovery rate at $P < 0.5$ (Beckmann and Smith, 2004; Beckmann et al., 2005). Thirty-six RSNs were identified as anatomically and functionally classical RSNs upon visual inspection by an experienced neuroradiologist (VK) using previously described criteria (Kiviniemi et al., 2009; Smith et al., 2009; Abou-Elseoud et al., 2010). The 36 RSNs are presented in **Figure 1**.

The analysis for the differences between groups was carried out using an FSL dual regression technique that allows for voxel-wise comparisons of resting-state fMRI (Filippini et al., 2009; Littow et al., 2010; Veer et al., 2010; Abou Elseoud et al., 2011). This involves (A) using the group-ICA spatial maps in a linear model fit against the separate fMRI data sets, resulting in matrices (time-course matrices) describing the temporal dynamics for each component and subject, and (B) using these time-course matrices to estimate subject-specific spatial maps. The ICA template for the dual regression was selected from the healthy control data. The dual regression analysis was performed both with and without variance normalization (FSL414 dual_regression command with des norm-option 1 or 0, respectively), since the results have a different emphasis on the spatial or amplitude of the BOLD signal depending on normalization (Allen et al., 2012a,b). With variance normalization, the dual regression reflects differences in both activity and spatial spread of the RSN. Without normalization, only spatial alterations are reflected in principle.

As a statistical analysis the different component maps are collected across subjects into single 4D files (1 per original ICA map) and tested voxel-wise for statistically significant differences between the groups using FSL randomize nonparametric permutation testing, with 5000 permutations, using a threshold-free cluster enhanced (TFCE) technique to control for multiple comparisons (Nichols and Holmes, 2002). The hypothesized differences between groups were calculated using a $p < 0.05$ threshold with voxel-wise changes in the FSL randomize tool. A newly developed inter-IC concatenation technique was used in order to control for multiple comparisons across the detected IC differences (Abou Elseoud et al., 2012). After discarding noise, motion and other artifact components, all the 36 RSN ICs were concatenated in the y-direction and fed to the FSL randomize tool as a joint dataset. After 5000 permutations the resulting datasets were separated with fslroi and thresholded for $p < 0.05$ correcting for type I error for the selected multiple ICs. As a new step, a gray matter regressor image was also fed in a similar fashion such that it was concatenated in the y-direction to control for gray matter differences with FSL randomize using—vxl and—vxf options.

The Juelich histological atlas incorporated in FSL and the Harvard-Oxford cortical and subcortical atlases (Harvard Center

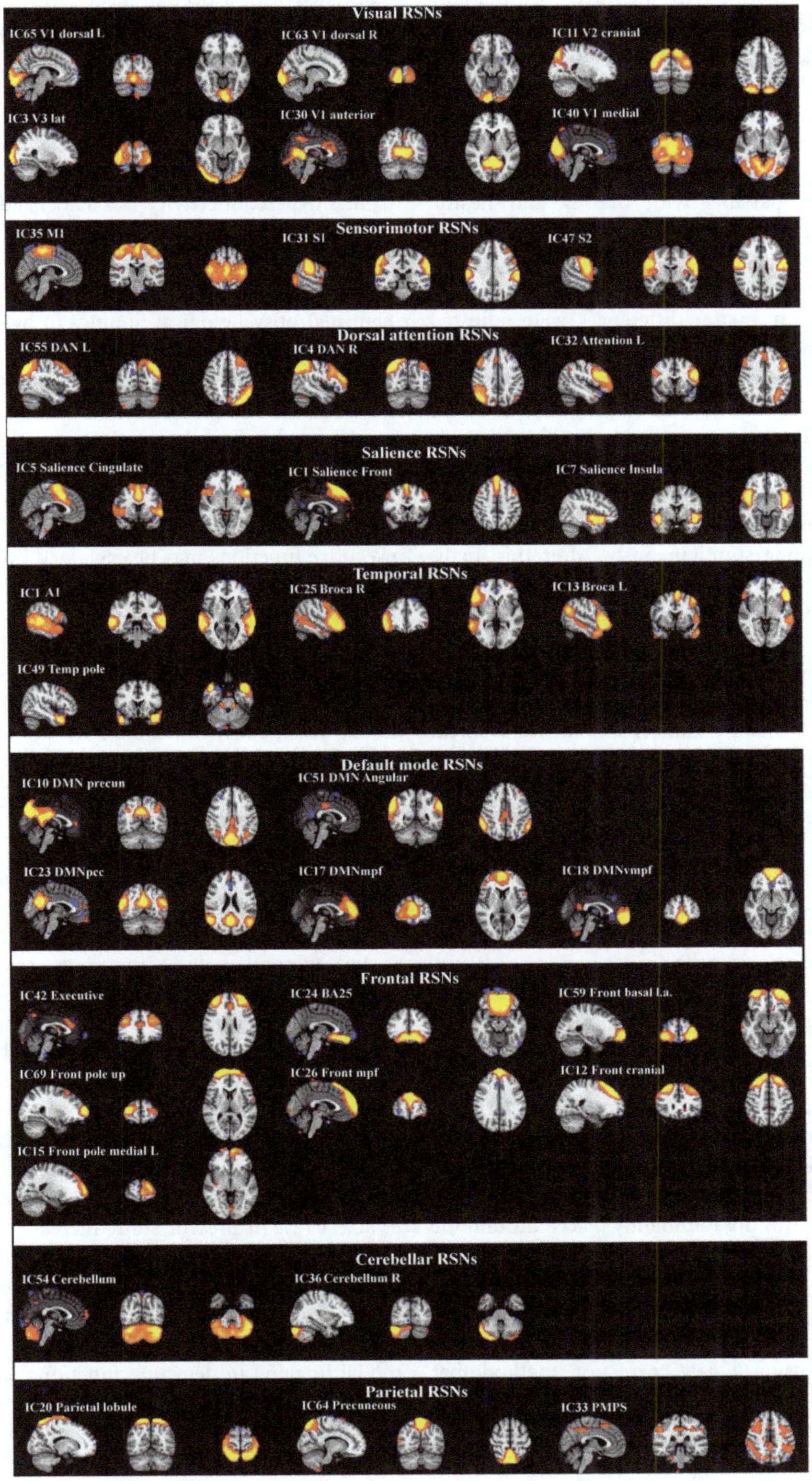

FIGURE 1 | Resting-state networks from the control group identified as anatomically and functionally classical RNSs and which were used for the dual regression analysis. The normal resting-state networks are shown in FSL red-yellow color encoding using a 3 < *z*-score < 9 threshold.

for Morphometric Analysis) which are provided with the FSL4 software were used to identify the anatomical characteristics of the resulting PICA maps. The FSL4 fslstats and fslmaths tools were used to calculate the number of non-zero voxels in the selected difference maps, and their *t*-score values.

RESULTS

The differences between patients with bvFTD and healthy controls were markedly smaller in the dual regression without variance normalization than with normalization. Thus, the differences between groups in the network shape seemed to be relatively limited when gray matter differences were adjusted. The variance normalized and non-normalized dual regression results suggest that the functional connectivity of the baseline RSNs is altered rather than the shape of the network in patients with bvFTD when compared with healthy controls. Based on this we further performed y-concatenation correction for multiple ICA components with the variance normalized (des norm = 1) results. We corrected for both multiple ICs and gray matter volume simultaneously. After this analysis, the number of ICs with significant differences reduced from fifteen detected after only voxel-level correction to six (**Table 1, Figure 2**).

Using this protocol, increased connectivity was found in several networks within patients with bvFTD compared to the control group. The most prominent enhancement was seen in the right frontotemporal area and insula (IC 25). Increased connectivity was also detected in the left DAN (IC 55), in the DMN (anterior paracingulate gyrus; IC 17) and in anterior parts of the frontal pole (IC 12). Minor changes were also seen in the visual network in the occipital region (IC 3) and in the premotor-postsensory network (IC 33).

The bvFTD group was divided into two separate groups according to the degree of severity of the disease, mild ($n = 9$) and moderate/severe ($n = 10$). There were no significant differences between mild and moderate to severe subgroups in functional connectivity.

In structural analysis, widespread gray matter atrophy was detected (**Table 2, Figure 3**). Atrophy was most prominent in the right temporal lobe in addition to the precuneus cortex and posterior cingulate gyrus. Mild atrophy was also detected in both hippocampi. After the adjustment for gray matter differences, the increased connectivity was predominantly placed around the atrophic area (**Figure 3**).

DISCUSSION

This is the first report of RSNs of the whole brain cortex in patients with bvFTD using a new correction method that allows the assessment of several brain networks. Connectivity changes as well as changes in the shape of the brain networks were analysed. The most extensive increase in connectivity was detected in the frontal poles bilaterally, in the right insular cortex and the ACC in several networks (IC 12, IC 17, IC 25). This area is associated with the human mirror neuron system and the von Economo cells, which are thought to be crucial in social cognition (Seeley et al., 2006, 2007a,b). These cells are destroyed in patients with bvFTD and atrophy in this area is associated with a decline in behavior and loss of empathy and insight in bvFTD. In a recent study, prefrontal hyperconnectivity has been associated with apathy in patients with bvFTD (Farb et al., 2012). Apathy was the most prevalent neuropsychiatric symptom in the present study and may be associated with hyperconnectivity in the prefrontal areas, which confirms the previous findings. Farb and colleagues also detected that prefrontal hyperconnectivity was associated with dementia severity, but this phenomenon was not seen in our patients (Farb et al., 2012).

Impairment in executive functions and attention are prominent neuropsychological findings in bvFTD patients. Significant increase in connectivity was detected in the left DAN (**Table 1, Figure 2**; IC 55). However, we did not detect any changes in the executive network itself (IC 42), which confirms the previous finding of normal executive networks in patients with bvFTD (Filippi et al., 2012). In previous studies the DAN has been found to be disrupted in AD, but not in bvFTD (Filippi et al., 2012; Li et al., 2012). Despite the normal executive network, a decline in executive functions may be explained by changes in the attention networks and the destruction of several frontal control networks (IC12, 17, 25).

Increased connectivity was also found in the frontal subnetwork of the DMN (IC 17). In several studies the disruption of the DMN is consistently associated with AD (Greicius et al., 2004; Zhang et al., 2009; Gili et al., 2011), but the findings are controversial in patients with bvFTD (Zhou et al., 2010; Whitwell et al., 2011; Borroni et al., 2012). In bvFTD, increased DMN connectivity has often been associated with decreased connectivity in the salience network (Zhou et al., 2010; Whitwell et al., 2011; Borroni et al., 2012; Farb et al., 2012). However, in the present study, decreased connectivity was not detected in the salience network even if increased connectivity in the DMN was found.

In structural analyses, the most prominent gray matter atrophy was detected in the right temporal region, precuneus, and posterior cingulate. Atrophy in the posterior cingulate is typically associated with AD and decreased connectivity in DMN. The research reports about gray matter atrophy in posterior brain areas in patients with bvFTD have been controversial. Broadly, precuneus and posterior cingulate seem to be preserved in bvFTD, however gray matter atrophy of these areas has been detected in some studies (Du et al., 2007; Zhou et al., 2010; Hartikainen et al., 2012). In present study increased functional connectivity was consistently located around the atrophic areas. The centrifugal disposition of increased functional connectivity around the atrophic areas suggests plasticity related shifting of function to areas still capable of functioning. It is noteworthy that multimodal imaging in detecting functional changes in diseases with abnormal anatomy is demanding. For example, how is the variance normalization of the BOLD signal affected by shifted and increased function; is it merely overlap of functional connectivity or plasticity effects? This question currently remains unanswered. In this study we were able to correct our results for both multiple comparisons related to the selecting of 36 RSNs and for gray matter differences known to exist in bvFTD.

We found only increased connectivity in patients with bvFTD compared to controls. Several factors may have an influence

Table 1 | Functional brain regions showing increased functional connectivity in patients with bvFTD compared to healthy controls.

		Voxel level correction								Inter-IC corrected y-concatenation for all RSNs									
IC	**RSN**	**voxels**	**max *X***	***Y***	***Z***	**min *T*-score**	**max *T*-score**	**mean *T*-score**	**Std**	**IC**	**voxels**	**max *X***	***Y***	***Z***	**min *T*-score**	**max *T*-score**	**mean *T*-score**	**Std**
IC01	Cranial salience, superior frontal gyrus	52	21	42	31	2.63	3.93	3.06	0.33									
IC03	Visual cortex 1–4	103	13	10	14	2.51	4.90	3.36	0.59	IC03	2	11	12	15	4.69	4.81	4.75	0.09
IC04	DAN R	158	9	18	28	2.31	5.26	2.86	0.49									
IC11	Visual cortex, inferior parietal lobule	4	17	9	24	3.59	4.44	3.91	0.35									
IC12	Bilateral frontal pole, middle frontal gyrus	733	29	35	25	1.93	4.86	2.71	0.57	IC12	268	30	38	31	2.60	4.52	3.16	0.38
IC17	Anterior paracingulate	387	22	44	17	2.07	5.05	2.65	0.48	IC17	7	22	45	17	3.76	4.33	4.05	0.21
IC21	Broca L	1369	34	41	14	1.90	5.28	2.91	0.67									
IC25	Insula, inferior frontal gyrus, middle temporal gyrus	1202	11	39	12	1.82	5.53	2.82	0.70	IC25	573	7	18	16	2.49	5.53	3.32	0.61
IC27	Pons, bilateral parahippocampus	7	23	12	21	3.73	4.22	3.97	0.21									
IC33	Premotor-presensory	555	11	32	27	1.91	5.46	2.54	0.49	IC33	2	17	33	30	5.01	5.30	5.16	0.21
IC35	Bilateral primary motor cortex	41	30	24	35	2.45	3.82	2.90	0.35									
IC41	Frontal pole R	508	10	42	13	2.03	6.14	3.20	0.84									
IC47	Primary somatosensory cortex	27	7	29	26	2.86	3.70	3.20	0.21									
IC51	Angular gyrus, bilateral supramarginal gyrus	217	6	22	22	2.40	4.89	3.01	0.47									
IC55	DAN L	956	35	16	24	1.85	5.13	2.53	0.54	IC55	260	24	11	27	2.54	4.58	3.05	0.42

Significant differences in functional connectivity were detected in fifteen RSNs by voxel level correction. By Inter-IC corrected y-concatenation for all RSNs significant differences in functional connectivity were detected in six RSNs. Significant differences are demonstrated by; the anatomical areas involved, number of voxels, MNI coordinates (in mm) of the involved anatomical areas, t-score and its standard deviation. Abbreviations: IC, independent component; R, right; L, left; DAN, dorsal attention network.

upon our results. We have used different data analysing methods compared to the previous rfMRI studies (Zhou et al., 2010; Whitwell et al., 2011; Borroni et al., 2012; Farb et al., 2012; Filippi et al., 2012). Higher model order (a.k.a 70) was used, which yields a more detailed RSN partition and reduces the presence of noise in the maps (Kiviniemi et al., 2009; Smith et al., 2009; Abou-Elseoud et al., 2010). Furthermore, global mean regression may be involved with unpredictable anti-correlations and this may also be one source of differences between our results and others' (Murphy et al., 2009). We also used a group ICA dual regression approach in this study. Matching individual level ICA maps is more prone to errors when compared to group map templates (Zuo et al., 2010). We also share this experience in this dataset. We analysed individual level ICA maps with low (20) model order, but had considerable difficulty in detecting a robustly identifiable salience and other high cognitive networks from individual ICA runs for each subject, especially when compared to group templates. This is not a problem of ICA *per se*, since it has been known to be robust in detecting fMRI sources (Kiviniemi et al., 2009; Smith et al., 2009). Actually, it may be the other way around; ICA is very sensitive to sparsity (Daubechies et al., 2009). On the individual level, the RSNs have marked spatiotemporal non-stationarity due to strong momentary neuronal avalanches (Chang and Glover, 2010; Kiviniemi et al., 2011; Hutchison et al., 2013; Liu and Duyn, 2013; Palva et al., 2013). The neuronal avalanches arising within RSN nodes have unique spatial connectivity distributions and match only with group level RSN templates when strongly averaged in both time and space (Zuo et al., 2010; Liu and Duyn, 2013). Dual regression maps may therefore provide a closer matching representation of an individual subject's RSN compared to ICA based maps.

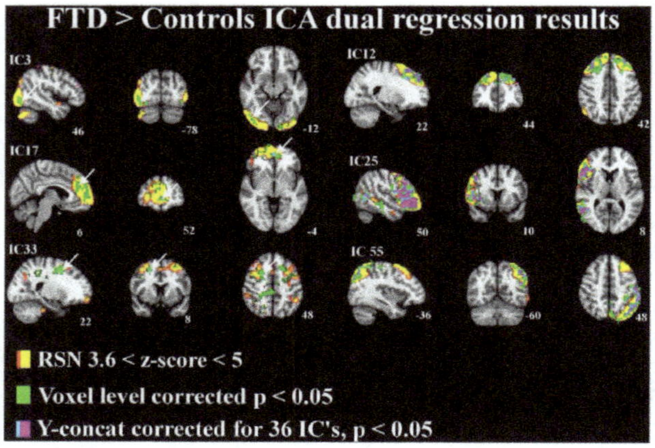

FIGURE 2 | Independent components (IC) with significant increase in functional connectivity in patients with bvFTD. The differences in resting state networks corrected for multiple comparison at voxel level in green and for y-concatenation correction for including all RSNs in lilac-blue, threshold $p < 0.05$. The differences between groups are also adjusted for gray matter differences. The involved RSN is presented in red-yellow color encoding with ($3.6 < z$-score < 6) threshold. Arrows in ICs 3, 17, and 33 indicate the y-concatenated results.

The advantage of the present method is the whole brain cortex coverage and higher hierarchical level of sub-networks (Kiviniemi et al., 2009; Abou-Elseoud et al., 2010; Littow et al., 2010). Moreover, the high model order enables increased accuracy of regressors of also the unwanted artifacts such as pulsating blood vessels, compartmental CSF pulsation/jet and motion artifacts that cannot be identified with other methods. The regression of these artifacts is crucial for the correct analysis of group differences in any kind of connectivity measurement. ICA dual regression offers a simultaneous data-driven regression of both artifacts and RSNs. Importantly, with group ICA, the effects of curved and often individually different cerebral artery and CSF

Table 2 | Regional atrophy detected by structural MRI.

Voxels	max_*Y*	min_*Z*	max_*Z*	Mean-*T*score	sem *T*-score	max *T*-score	Anatomical area
16479	72	−52	60	2.94	0.005	5.55	R middle and inferior temporal gyrus
15849	38	−50	72	2.94	0.006	6.38	L precuneus cortex, cingulate gyrus
422	58	−22	−6	2.62	0.016	3.58	L broca, frontal pole, inferior temporal gyrus
278	28	−30	0	3.40	0.045	5.76	L frontal pole, orbitofrontal, and subcallosal cortex
267	18	4	16	3.72	0.050	5.46	L insula, frontal and central opercular cortex, broca
82	−14	60	68	3.68	0.043	4.72	R premotor and motor cortex, precentral gyrus
52	12	−44	−26	2.34	0.020	2.74	R temporal pole, middle temporal gyrus
47	−8	38	46	2.52	0.039	3.24	L postcentral gyrus
42	28	−20	−16	2.39	0.026	2.85	R orbitofrontal cortex, frontal and temporal pole
28	26	−40	−34	2.55	0.062	3.29	R temporal pole
23	−20	48	56	3.43	0.031	3.75	L premotor and primary motor cortex, precentral gyrus
20	−32	−8	−2	3.43	0.048	3.87	R hippocampus, parahippocampal gyrus
19	−32	2	6	2.49	0.054	2.93	L superior and middle temporal gyrus
13	−80	12	14	2.21	0.010	2.28	L lateral occipital cortex

R, right; L, left.

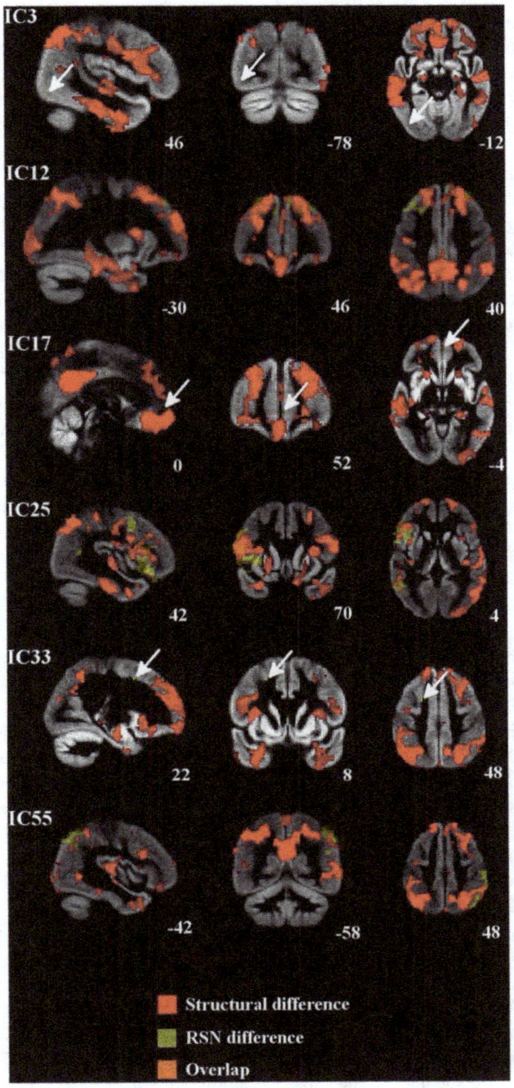

FIGURE 3 | Regional atrophy was detected in several frontal and temporal regions and also in the posterior cingulate cortex, occipital cortex, and occipital poles. Increased connectivity was constantly placed around the atrophied area. Atrophic regions are in red, difference in the RSNs are in yellow (bvFTD > controls) and overlapping areas are in orange color. Arrows in ICs 3, 17, and 33 indicate the difference in the RSN.

pulsations become separated by the best way within the analysed group as a whole, also with individual weighting in their time series. The adequate modeling of blood vessel noise may have an effect on the salience network results in the insular cortex near the medial cerebral artery branches. Advanced spiral in/out scanning sequences at the higher 3 T magnetic field are also likely to be more sensitive than conventional 1.5 T EPI sequences in providing frontal cortex/insular data at the individual level (Zhou et al., 2010; Whitwell et al., 2011; Farb et al., 2012; Filippi et al., 2012).

Despite careful diagnostics, long follow-up and genetic confirmation of bvFTD, it is possible that some patients with atypical AD may be included in the study cohort. The wide range in disease severity may affect the rfMRI results even though no difference was seen between the patient groups with different disease severity. Neuroleptic and cholinergic drugs may also modify results. However, there are no rfMRI data available concerning the effects of these drugs.

In conclusion, this is the first analysis of the whole brain cortex networks using high model order ICA in patients with bvFTD. Increased connectivity was seen in the left DAN and frontal control networks neighboring executive network, as well as the frontal poles and insula. These changes may explain bvFTD associated cognitive and neuropsychiatric symptoms. In general, the increase in functional connectivity centrifugally was surrounding the atrophied areas, which suggest plasticity related shifting of neuronal activity into intact brain structures.

ACKNOWLEDGMENTS

This work was supported by grants from the Finnish Academy [grants 117111 and 123772 (Vesa Kiviniemi)], Finnish Medical Foundation (Vesa Kiviniemi, Anne M. Remes), Finnish Neurological Foundation (Vesa Kiviniemi), KEVO grants from Oulu University Hospital (Vesa Kiviniemi, Anne M. Remes), National Graduate School of Clinical Investigation (Riikka Rytty), the Intramural Research Programs of the NIH, and National Institute on Aging (Z01-AG000949-02)(Bryan J. Traynor) the ALS Association, AriSLA, Packard Center for ALS research, FIGC, Microsoft Research (Bryan J. Traynor), and the Myasthenia Gravis Foundation (Bryan J. Traynor).

REFERENCES

Abou-Elseoud, A., Starck, T., Remes, J., Nikkinen, J., Tervonen, O., and Kiviniemi, V. (2010). The effect of model order selection in group PICA. *Hum. Brain Mapp.* 31, 1207–1216. doi: 10.1002/hbm.20929

Abou Elseoud, A., Littow, H., Remes, J., Starck, T., Nikkinen, J., Nissila, J., et al. (2011). Group-ICA model order highlights patterns of functional brain connectivity. *Front. Syst. Neurosci.* 5:37. doi: 10.3389/fnsys.2011.00037

Abou Elseoud, A., Nissila, J., Liettu, A., Remes, J., Jokelainen, J., Takala, T., et al. (2012). Altered resting-state activity in seasonal affective disorder. *Hum. Brain Mapp.* doi: 10.1002/hbm.22164. [Epub ahead of print].

Abou-Elseoud, A., Starck, T., Remes, J., Nikkinen, J., Tervonen, O., and Kiviniemi, V. (2010). The effect of model order selection in group PICA. *Hum. Brain Mapp.* 31, 1207–1216. doi: 10.1002/hbm.20929

Allen, E. A., Erhardt, E. B., Wei, Y., Eichele, T., and Calhoun, V. D. (2012a). Capturing inter-subject variability with group independent component analysis of fMRI data: a simulation study. *Neuroimage* 59, 4141–4159. doi: 10.1016/j.neuroimage.2011.10.010

Allen, E. A., Damaraju, E., Plis, S. M., Erhardt, E. B., Eichele, T., and Calhoun, V. D. (2012b). Tracking whole-brain connectivity dynamics in the resting State. *Cereb. Cortex.* doi: 10.1093/cercor/bhs352. [Epub ahead of print].

Ashburner, J., and Friston, K. J. (2000). Voxel-based morphometry-the methods. *Neuroimage* 11, 805–821. doi: 10.1006/nimg.2000.0582

Beckmann, C. F., DeLuca, M., Devlin, J. T., and Smith, S. M. (2005). Investigations into resting-state connectivity using independent component analysis. *Philos. Trans. R. Soc. Lond. B Biol. Sci.* 360, 1001–1013. doi: 10.1098/rstb.2005.1634

Beckmann, C. F., and Smith, S. M. (2004). Probabilistic independent component analysis for functional magnetic resonance imaging. *IEEE Trans. Med. Imaging*

23, 137–152. doi: 10.1109/TMI.2003.822821

Borroni, B., Alberici, A., Cercignani, M., Premi, E., Serra, L., Cerini, C., et al. (2012). Granulin mutation drives brain damage and reorganization from preclinical to symptomatic FTLD. *Neurobiol. Aging* 33, 2506–2520. doi: 10.1016/j.neurobiolaging.2011.10.031

Chang, C., and Glover, G. H. (2010). Time-frequency dynamics of resting-state brain connectivity measured with fMRI. *Neuroimage* 50, 81–98. doi: 10.1016/j.neuroimage.2009.12.011

Daubechies, I., Roussos, E., Takerkart, S., Benharrosh, M., Golden, C., D'Ardenne, K., et al. (2009). Independent component analysis for brain fMRI does not select for independence. *Proc. Natl. Acad. Sci. U.S.A.* 106, 10415–10422. doi: 10.1073/pnas.0903525106

Du, A., Schuff, N., Kramer, J., Rosen, H., Gorni-Tempini, M., Rankin, K., et al. (2007). Different regional patterns of cortical thinning in Alzheimer's disease and frontotemporal dementia. *Brain* 130, 1159–1166. doi: 10.1093/brain/awm016

Farb, N. A., Grady, C. L., Strother, S., Tang-Wai, D. F., Masellis, M., Black, S., et al. (2012). Abnormal network connectivity in frontotemporal dementia: evidence for prefrontal isolation. *Cortex* 49, 1856–1873. doi: 10.1016/j.cortex.2012.09.008

Filippi, M., Agosta, F., Scola, E., Canu, E., Magnani, G., Marcone, A., et al. (2012). Functional network connectivity in the behavioral variant of frontotemporal dementia. *Cortex.* doi: 10.1016/j.cortex.2012.09.017

Filippini, N., MacIntosh, B. J., Hough, M. G., Goodwin, G. M., Frisoni, G. B., Smith, S. M., et al. (2009). Distinct patterns of brain activity in young carriers of the APOE-epsilon4 allele. *Proc. Natl. Acad. Sci. U.S.A.* 106, 7209–7214. doi: 10.1073/pnas.0811879106

Fox, M. D., and Raichle, M. E. (2007). Spontaneous fluctuations in brain activity observed with functional magnetic resonance imaging. *Nat. Rev. Neurosci.* 8, 700–711. doi: 10.1038/nrn2201

Gili, T., Cercignani, M., Serra, L., Perri, R., Giove, F., Maraviglia, B., et al. (2011). Regional brain atrophy and functional disconnection across Alzheimer's disease evolution. *J. Neurol. Neurosurg. Psychiatry.* 82, 58–66. doi: 10.1136/jnnp.2009.199935

Good, C. D., Johnsrude, I. S., Ashburner, J., Henson, R. N., Friston, K. J., and Frackowiak, R. S. (2001). A voxel-based morphometric study of ageing in 465 normal adult human brains. *Neuroimage* 14, 21–36. doi: 10.1006/nimg.2001.0786

Greicius, M. D., Srivastava, G., Reiss, A. L., and Menon, V. (2004). Default-mode network activity distinguishes Alzheimer's disease from healthy aging: evidence from functional MRI. *Proc. Natl. Acad. Sci. U.S.A.* 101, 4637–4642. doi: 10.1073/pnas.0308627101

Hartikainen, P., Rasanen, J., Julkunen, V., Niskanen, E., Hallikainen, M., Kivipelto, M., et al. (2012). Cortical thickness in frontotemporal dementia, mild cognitive impairment, and Alzheimer's disease. *J. Alzheimers Dis.* 30, 857–874. doi: 10.3233/JAD-2012-112060

Hutchison, R. M., Womelsdorf, T., Allen, E. A., Bandettini, P. A., Calhoun, V. D., Corbetta, M., et al. (2013). Dynamic functional connectivity: promises, issues, and interpretations. *Neuroimage* 15, 360–378. doi: 10.1016/j.neuroimage.2013.05.079

Jenkinson, M., Bannister, P., Brady, M., and Smith, S. (2002). Improved optimization for the robust and accurate linear registration and motion correction of brain images.*Neuroimage* 17, 825–841. doi: 10.1006/nimg.2002.1132

Kiviniemi, V., Starck, T., Remes, J., Long, X., Nikkinen, J., Haapea, M., et al. (2009). Functional segmentation of the brain cortex using high model order group PICA. *Hum. Brain Mapp.* 30, 3865–3886. doi: 10.1002/hbm.20813

Kiviniemi, V., Vire, T., Remes, J., Abou Elseoud, A., Starck, T., Tervonen, O., et al. (2011). A sliding time-window ICA reveals spatial variability of the default mode Network in time. *Brain Connect.* 1, 339–347. doi: 10.1089/brain.2011.0036

Li, R., Wu, X., Fleisher, A. S., Reiman, E. M., Chen, K., and Yao, L. (2012). Attention-related networks in Alzheimer's disease: a resting functional MRI study. *Hum. Brain Mapp.* 33, 1076–1088. doi: 10.1002/hbm.21269

Littow, H., Elseoud, A., Haapea, M., Isohanni, M., Moilanen, I., Mankinen, K., et al. (2010). Age-related differences in functional nodes of the brain cortex - a high model order group ICA study. *Front. Syst. Neurosci.* 4:32. doi: 10.3389/fnsys.2010.00032

Liu, X., and Duyn, J. H. (2013). Time-varying functional network information extracted from brief instances of spontaneous brain activity. *Proc. Natl. Acad. Sci. U.S.A.* 110, 4392–4397. doi: 10.1073/pnas.1216856110

Murphy, K., Birn, R. M., Handwerker, D. A., Jones, T. B., and Bandettini, P. A. (2009). The impact of global signal regression on resting state correlations: are anti-correlated networks introduced? *Neuroimage* 44, 893–905. doi: 10.1016/j.neuroimage.2008.09.036

Neary, D., Snowden, J., and Mann, D. (2005). Frontotemporal dementia. *Lancet Neurol.* 4, 771–780. doi: 10.1016/S1474-4422(05)70223-4

Neary, D., Snowden, J. S., Gustafson, L., Passant, U., Stuss, D., Black, S., et al. (1998). Frontotemporal lobar degeneration: a consensus on clinical diagnostic criteria. *Neurology* 51, 1546–1554. doi: 10.1212/WNL.51.6.1546

Nichols, T. E., and Holmes, A. P. (2002). Nonparametric permutation tests for functional neuroimaging: a primer with examples. *Hum. Brain Mapp.* 15, 1–25. doi: 10.1002/hbm.1058

Palva, J. M., Zhigalov, A., Hirvonen, J., Korhonen, O., Linkenkaer-Hansen, K., and Palva, S. (2013). Neuronal long-range temporal correlations and avalanche dynamics are correlated with behavioral scaling laws. *Proc. Natl. Acad. Sci. U.S.A.* 110, 3585–3590. doi: 10.1073/pnas.1216855110

Piguet, O., Hornberger, M., Mioshi, E., and Hodges, J. R. (2011). Behavioural-variant frontotemporal dementia: diagnosis, clinical staging, and management. *Lancet Neurol.* 10, 162–172. doi: 10.1016/S1474-4422(10)70299-4

Raichle, M. E., MacLeod, A. M., Snyder, A. Z., Powers, W. J., Gusnard, D. A., and Shulman, G. L. (2001). A default mode of brain function. *Proc. Natl. Acad. Sci. U.S.A.* 98, 676–682. doi: 10.1073/pnas.98.2.676

Rascovsky, K., Hodges, J. R., Knopman, D., Mendez, M. F., Kramer, J. H., Neuhaus, J., et al. (2011). Sensitivity of revised diagnostic criteria for the behavioural variant of frontotemporal dementia. *Brain* 134, 2456–2477. doi: 10.1093/brain/awr179

Renton, A. E., Majounie, E., Waite, A., Simon-Sanchez, J., Rollinson, S., Gibbs, J. R., et al. (2011). A hexanucleotide repeat expansion in C9ORF72 is the cause of chromosome 9p21-linked ALS-FTD. *Neuron* 72, 257–268. doi: 10.1016/j.neuron.2011.09.010

Rosen, H. J., Gorno-Tempini, M. L., Goldman, W. P., Perry, R. J., Schuff, N., Weiner, M., et al. (2002). Patterns of brain atrophy in frontotemporal dementia and semantic dementia. *Neurology* 58, 198–208. doi: 10.1212/WNL.58.2.198

Rueckert, D., Sonoda, L. I., Hayes, C., Hill, D. L., Leach, M. O., and Hawkes, D. J. (1999).Nonrigid registration using free-form deformations: application to breast MR images. *IEEE Trans. Med. Imaging* 18, 712–721. doi: 10.1109/42.796284

Seeley, W. W., Carlin, D. A., Allman, J. M., Macedo, M. N., Bush, C., Miller, B. L., et al. (2006). Early frontotemporal dementia targets neurons unique to apes and humans. *Ann. Neurol.* 60, 660–667. doi: 10.1002/ana.21055

Seeley, W. W., Allman, J. M., Carlin, D. A., Crawford, R. K., Macedo, M. N., Greicius, M. D., et al. (2007a). Divergent social functioning in behavioral variant frontotemporal dementia and Alzheimer disease: reciprocal networks and neuronal evolution. *Alzheimer Dis. Assoc. Disord.* 21, S50–S57. doi: 10.1097/WAD.0b013e31815c0f14

Seeley, W. W., Menon, V., Schatzberg, A. F., Keller, J., Glover, G. H., Kenna, H., et al. (2007b). Dissociable intrinsic connectivity networks for salience processing and executive control. *J. Neurosci.* 27, 2349–2356. doi: 10.1523/JNEUROSCI.5587-06.2007

Smith, S. M. (2002). Fast robust automated brain extraction. *Hum. Brain Mapp.* 17, 143–155. doi: 10.1002/hbm.10062

Smith, S. M., Fox, P. T., Miller, K. L., Glahn, D. C., Fox, P. M., Mackay, C. E., et al. (2009). Correspondence of the brain's functional architecture during activation and rest. *Proc. Natl. Acad. Sci. U.S.A.* 106, 13040–13045. doi: 10.1073/pnas.0905267106

Veer, I. M., Beckmann, C. F., van Tol, M. J., Ferrarini, L., Milles, J., Veltman, D. J., et al. (2010). Whole brain resting-state analysis reveals decreased functional connectivity in major depression. *Front. Syst. Neurosci.* 4:41. doi: 10.3389/fnsys.2010.00041

Whitwell, J. L., Josephs, K. A., Avula, R., Tosakulwong, N., Weigand, S. D., Senjem, M. L., et al. (2011). Altered functional connectivity in asymptomatic MAPT subjects: a comparison to bvFTD.

Neurology 77, 866–874. doi: 10.1212/WNL.0b013e31822c61f2

Whitwell, J. L., Przybelski, S. A., Weigand, S. D., Ivnik, R. J., Vemuri, P., Gunter, J. L., et al. (2009). Distinct anatomical subtypes of the behavioural variant of frontotemporal dementia: a cluster analysis study. *Brain* 132, 2932–2946. doi: 10.1093/brain/awp232

Zhang, H. Y., Wang, S. J., Xing, J., Liu, B., Ma, Z. L., Yang, M., et al. (2009). Detection of PCC functional connectivity characteristics in resting-state fMRI in mild Alzheimer's disease. *Behav. Brain Res.* 197, 103–108. doi: 10.1016/j.bbr.2008.08.012

Zhang, Y., Brady, M., and Smith, S. (2001). Segmentation of brain MR images through a hidden Markov random field model and the expectation-maximization algorithm. *IEEE Trans. Med. Imaging* 20, 45–57. doi: 10.1109/42.906424

Zhou, J., Greicius, M. D., Gennatas, E. D., Growdon, M. E., Jang, J. Y., Rabinovici, G. D., et al. (2010). Divergent network connectivity changes in behavioural variant frontotemporal dementia and Alzheimer's disease. *Brain* 133, 1352–1367. doi: 10.1093/brain/awq075

Zuo, X. N., Kelly, C., Adelstein, J. S., Klein, D. F., Castellanos, F. X., and Milham, M. P. (2010). Reliable intrinsic connectivity networks: test-retest evaluation using ICA and dual regression approach. *Neuroimage* 49, 2163–2177. doi: 10.1016/j.neuroimage.2009.10.080

14

Graph theory reveals dysconnected hubs in 22q11DS and altered nodal efficiency in patients with hallucinations

Marie-Christine Ottet[1,2]*, Marie Schaer[1,3], Martin Debbané[1,4], Leila Cammoun[2], Jean-Philippe Thiran[2] and Stephan Eliez[1,5]

[1] Departement of Psychiatry, Office Médico-Pédagogique (OMP), University of Geneva School of Medicine, Geneva, Switzerland
[2] Signal Processing Laboratory (LTS5), Swiss Federal Institute of Technology (EPFL), Lausanne, Switzerland
[3] Department of Psychiatry, Stanford Cognitive and System Neuroscience Laboratory, Stanford University, Palo Alto, CA, USA
[4] Adolescence Clinical Psychology Research Unit, University of Geneva, Geneva, Switzerland
[5] Department of Genetic Medicine and Development, University of Geneva School of Medicine, Geneva, Switzerland

***Correspondence:**
Marie-Christine Ottet, Department of Psychiatry, Office Médico-Pédagogique, University of Geneva School of Medicine, Rue David-Dufour 1, Case postale 50, 1211 Geneva 8, GE, Switzerland
e-mail: marie-christine.ottet@unige.ch

Schizophrenia is postulated to be the prototypical dysconnection disorder, in which hallucinations are the core symptom. Due to high heterogeneity in methodology across studies and the clinical phenotype, it remains unclear whether the structural brain dysconnection is global or focal and if clinical symptoms result from this dysconnection. In the present work, we attempt to clarify this issue by studying a population considered as a homogeneous genetic sub-type of schizophrenia, namely the 22q11.2 deletion syndrome (22q11.2DS). Cerebral MRIs were acquired for 46 patients and 48 age and gender matched controls (aged 6–26, respectively mean age = 15.20 ± 4.53 and 15.28 ± 4.35 years old). Using the Connectome mapper pipeline (connectomics.org) that combines structural and diffusion MRI, we created a whole brain network for each individual. Graph theory was used to quantify the global and local properties of the brain network organization for each participant. A global degree loss of 6% was found in patients' networks along with an increased *Characteristic Path Length*. After identifying and comparing hubs, a significant loss of degree in patients' hubs was found in 58% of the hubs. Based on Allen's brain network model for hallucinations, we explored the association between local efficiency and symptom severity. Negative correlations were found in the Broca's area ($p < 0.004$), the Wernicke area ($p < 0.023$) and a positive correlation was found in the dorsolateral prefrontal cortex (DLPFC) ($p < 0.014$). In line with the dysconnection findings in schizophrenia, our results provide preliminary evidence for a targeted alteration in the brain network hubs' organization in individuals with a genetic risk for schizophrenia. The study of specific disorganization in language, speech and thought regulation networks sharing similar network properties may help to understand their role in the hallucination mechanism.

Keywords: DTI, small-world, network, Broca, psychosis, schizophrenia, human connectome, Wernicke

INTRODUCTION

22q11.2 deletion syndrome (22q11.2DS), also known as velo-cardio-facial syndrome (Shprintzen et al., 1978), is a well-established neurogenetic model for studying the pathogenesis of schizophrenia (Bassett and Chow, 1999). The prevalence rate of the 22q11DS population for developing schizophrenia is about 30%, making it the third highest risk rate after having an affected monozygotic twin (50% risk) or both parents being affected (46% risk) (McGuffin et al., 1995). Furthermore, 30–50% of non-schizophrenic 22q11DS individuals demonstrate sub-threshold symptoms of psychosis (Feinstein et al., 2002). Considering the genetic 22q11.2DS model as a homogenous sub-type may highlight the presence of neurodevelopmental biomarkers underlining the schizophrenic disorders.

As schizophrenia is a heterogeneous disorder previous literature on white matter has revealed highly variable alterations throughout the brain and a few replicated findings (see Fitzsimmons et al., 2013 for a recent review). Due to confounding factors such as duration of illness, medication, age sample or methodology, it remains unclear whether schizophrenia demonstrates localized alterations or a whole brain dysconnection. Graph theory provides promising tools to analyze both whole brain phenomenon using global network measurements, and specific properties using local network measurements (Bassett and Bullmore, 2009; He and Evans, 2010; Rubinov and Sporns, 2010). Few studies in schizophrenia have used the graph theory in structural magnetic resonance imaging. Bassett et al. (2008) characterized the cerebral gray matter volumetric covariation in a large sample (>200) of patients with schizophrenia compared to healthy controls. Although the small-world properties were preserved, a reduced network hierarchy with a loss of hubs was found in individuals with schizophrenia and more specifically in frontal (bilateral dorsolateral prefrontal cortex) areas (Bassett et al., 2008). Graph theory was also used in studies of functional connectivity in schizophrenia. Evidence of global rather than focal functional dysconnectivity grows in schizophrenia literature. Disruption of the small-world properties has been found in patients (Liu et al., 2008) as well as weaker connectivity and lower clustering coefficient (Yu et al., 2012), and hubs alteration (Yu et al., 2012, 2013). The functional connection of several specific regions has also been found such as the temporal lobe, the parietal lobe, the thalamus, hippocampus but more interestingly, functional integration between sub-networks (such as the semantic network, the default network) is impaired (see Zhang et al., 2012; Alexander-Bloch et al., 2013). Using diffusion images for reconstructing brain networks, van den Heuvel et al. (2010) replicated the observation that individuals with schizophrenia have preserved small-world properties and increased path length in frontal, temporal and occipital areas. Reduction of frontal hubs has also been demonstrated, involving the superior frontal and the anterior cingulate (van den Heuvel et al., 2010). Following Latora and Marchiori's conception of global and local efficiency measuring how well information is exchanged over the network (Latora and Marchiori, 2001), Wang et al. (2011) demonstrated that individuals with schizophrenia have a reduced global efficiency [reduced after controlling for the effect of age, gender and brain size (Wang et al., 2011)]. However, it remains unclear whether the network alterations are caused by the emergence of the schizophrenia disorder or if there is a predetermined network configuration that acts as a vulnerability factor for the later development of schizophrenia.

Amongst all the psychotic symptoms in the 22q11DS, hallucinations are often considered the most clinically salient signs of risk for psychosis (Debbané et al., 2006). Moreover, hallucinations constitute a valid early risk indicator for the development of schizophreniform disorders during adulthood (Poulton et al., 2000). As complex cognitive functions rely on a cerebral network involving several regions, (Sporns, 2010; Bassett and Gazzaniga, 2011) dysfunctions such as hallucination may result from abnormal topological connectivity between these areas (Lo et al., 2011). Structural and functional studies in individuals with schizophrenia suggest that several key regions play a role in the apparition of hallucinations and their severity [(see Allen et al., 2008) for a review]. In schizophrenic patients, reduction in the superior temporal gyrus (STG) gray matter volume has been associated with the severity of hallucinations (Flaum et al., 1995; Gaser et al., 2004; Onitsuka et al., 2004). Loss of gray matter volume in Broca's area has also been associated with this symptom (Gaser et al., 2004; Sumich et al., 2005). Several other brain areas, such as the insula (Shapleske et al., 2002), the thalamus (Neckelmann et al., 2006) and the supramarginal gyrus (Gaser et al., 2004), have been associated with the presence of hallucinations but have failed to show consistent volumetric reduction. Two network studies have explored the relationship between clinical symptoms of schizophrenia and brain network properties. Although van den Heuvel et al. (2010) found no significant association between the Positive and Negative Symptoms Scale (PNASS) (Kay et al., 1987) and topological features, Wang et al. (2011) showed a negative correlation between the PANSS (positive, negative and total scores) and global and local efficiency, meaning that the more severe the symptoms, the lower are both the local and the global topological efficiencies. Lower global efficiency and longer path length has also been related to higher score on the negative PANSS scale (Yu et al., 2011a,b).

The purpose of this present work is to study the global and local network features in a population at high genetic risk for schizophrenia (22q11.2DS) by focusing on the hierarchical structure of the brain network (hub topological configuration). Furthermore, we aim to explore the specific relationship between hallucination symptoms and the local efficiency of the related brain areas. According to Allen's model of brain regions involved in hallucinations (Allen et al., 2008), we suggest that the topological connectivity of the following regions—DLPFC, dorsal anterior cingulate, Broca's area, ventral anterior cingulate, orbitofrontal gyrus, and STG—will be associated with the severity of hallucinations in schizophrenia.

MATERIALS AND METHODS

PARTICIPANTS

All the participants underwent the same protocol, which included an MRI session for collecting a structural T1-weigthed image and a diffusion image along with an IQ measure with the Wechsler Intelligence Scale for Children-Third Edition revised (Wechsler, 1991) or the Wechsler Adult Intelligence Scale-III for adults (Wechsler, 1997). The participant or their parents signed consent forms containing information about the study and its purpose. The detailed protocol of the study was previously reviewed and accepted by the Institutional Review Board of Geneva University School of Medicine.

22q11.2DS GROUP

Forty-six participants with a 22q11.2DS aged between 6 and 26 (mean $= 15.20 \pm 4.53$), (23 males and 22 females) were recruited through parent associations in French speaking European countries. The 22q11.2 deletion was confirmed by a blood sample analyzed with the Quantitative Fluorescent Polymerase Chain Reaction (QF-PCR) performed on the deleted region. The average IQ was of 77.5 ± 16.6. All the patients were assessed by an experienced psychiatrist using the *Brief Psychiatric Rating Scale* (BPRS) (Leucht, 2005), the *Diagnostic Interview for children and adolescents* (DICA) (Reich, 2000) and the *Structured Clinical Interview for DSM-IV AXIS I Disorders* for adults (SCID) (First et al., 1996). Only one patient fulfilled the criteria for schizophrenia. The average BPRS hallucination subscale for the forty-six participants was 1.63 ± 1.12 and among them fourteen individuals reported to have verbal hallucination.

CONTROL GROUP

The participants from the control group were recruited among the siblings of the patients and in the community. The 48 control participants comprised 25 males and 24 females, aged from 7 to 24 (mean $= 15.28 \pm 4.35$). The average IQ was of 107 ± 18.12. None of the controls had present or past history of psychiatric or neurological disorders.

MRI CHARACTERISTICS

Using a Siemens Trio 3 Tesla scanner, we acquired a set of two cerebral MRIs for each participant. A T1-weighted sequence with a 3D volumetric pulse was collected using the following sequence: $TR = 2500$ ms, $TE = 3$ ms, flip angle = 8°, acquisition matrix of 256 × 256, field of view = 22 cm, slice thickness = 1.1 mm, 192 slices. The second MRI was a Diffusion Tensor Imaging (DTI) with the following parameters: number of directions = 30, $b = 1000$ s/mm^2, $TE = 82$ ms, $TR = [8300–8800]$ ms, flip angle = 90°, acquisition matrix of 128 × 128, field of view 25.6 cm, slice thickness = 2 mm.

IMAGE PROCESSING

The two acquired scans were processed for each participant using the Human Connectome Mapper (http://connectomics.org, Daducci et al., 2012). The software is a pipeline of several other software programs, combining each dedicated package for the purpose of creating an individual's connectome. For the T1-weigthed image, FreeSurfer software starts to remove all non-brain tissue, segmenting the image in order to extract the white matter, the sub-cortical gray matter volume and the cortical surface (Dale et al., 1999; Fischl et al., 1999). This step is performed using both intensity and continuity data through the whole 3D volume. The surfaces and volumes generated have been validated against histological studies (Rosas et al., 2002). However, these automatic steps need verification and manual correction if necessary. At the end of this process, three-dimensional volumes or surfaces and a cortical segmentation are available For the diffusion images, first we use a correction for the effect of head motion and distortion of eddy currents through an affine alignment using the FLIRT tool of the FSL-FDT software (Jenkinson and Smith, 2001). The realigned images are used to reconstruct the white matter macroscopic bundles using the streamline deterministic tractography of Diffusion Toolkit (http://trackvis.org/). The registration of the T1-weighted onto the diffusion images is an affine transformation using the *intensity-based linear registration* tool FLIRT. When combined, the intersection of the estimated fibers and the segmented regions creates a connectome which is represented by the connection matrix.

NETWORK MEASURES

Graph theory describes the human connectome as a network of nodes (in our case cortical regions) and edges (in our case white matter bundles) connecting two nodes. This network can be described either with weighted edges (where edges contain the information about the strength of the two nodes) or with binary edges (where only the existence of a link is represented). Therefore, two kinds of measurements are applicable: measurements on a binary network or on a weighted network. Following the purpose of the present study, which is to try to delineate the core organization of individuals with 22q11.2DS, we decided to explore the configuration of the binary network. Furthermore, binary network analyses have the advantage of showing a low variability in the network measures (Cheng et al., 2012).

In the present study, we used the tools for measuring network properties included in the brain connectivity toolbox developed for Matlab (https://sites.google.com/site/bctnet/) (see Rubinov and Sporns, 2010) for the description and mathematical formula of each measure. The first measurement step is the analysis of the global characteristics of the patients' and controls' networks, using the *Characteristic Path Length*, the *Mean Clustering Coefficient*, the *Global Transitivity*, the *Global Efficiency* and the *Global Degree*. In the context of the binary networks, the *Global Degree* represents the total number of edges (existing connections between two nodes) in the network. The *Mean Clustering Coefficient* measures the potential for functional segregation of the network and is calculated as the mean of the *clustering coefficient*, which is the fraction of the number of neighbors of a node that are also neighbors of each other (Watts and Strogatz, 1998). The *Characteristic Path Length* represents the average of the short path lengths of the network. The short path length is the number of edges that have to be crossed to go from one node to another. The *Characteristic Path Length* therefore measures the functional integration potential of a network. The normalized ratio between the *Mean Clustering Coefficient* and the *Characteristic Path Length* of a network gives the *Smallworldness* measure of the network (Watts and Strogatz, 1998; Humphries and Gurney, 2008). The *Smallworldness* measures the optimality between rapid communication throughout the network (functional integration) and the capacity to process locally based information (functional segregation) (Sporns and Honey, 2006). The optimal balance between the *Characteristic Path Length* and the *Mean Clustering Coefficient* can also be estimated by the *Global Efficiency* and the *local efficiency* (Latora and Marchiori, 2001). The *Global* and *local efficiency* measure how efficiently information is exchanged over the network, and respectively play similar roles to the *Characteristic Path Length* and the *clustering coefficient*.

The second analysis focuses on the hub configuration by ranking all of the nodes in the healthy control network on three local network measures, the *local degree*, the *clustering coefficient* and the *betweenness centrality*. The *local degree* measures a node's number of edges or neighbors. The *clustering coefficient* highlights a node's surrounding configurations by analyzing how many of its neighbors are also connected to each other. The *betweenness centrality* measures how many short path lengths pass through the node and is therefore a measure of node influence on the network (Rubinov and Sporns, 2010). By definition, the 20% highest ranking nodes for all 3 values are considered to be the network hubs (Sporns et al., 2007; Sporns, 2010; van den Heuvel et al., 2010; van den Heuvel and Sporns, 2011). The analysis then continues by comparing the hubs and node degrees between the 22q11.2DS group and the healthy control group.

The third step consists of exploring the relationship between Allen's model's network characteristics (*local efficiency*) and the clinical measures such as the presence and severity of hallucinations (BPRS). According to Allen's model of hallucinations, the DLPFC, dorsal anterior cingulate, Broca's area, ventral anterior cingulate, orbitofrontal gyrus, the supplementary motor area and STG are the brain regions involved in hallucinations. These regions are not represented in the same way in the Freesurfer Desikan parcellation scheme: region that corresponds the most to the DLPFC is the rostral middle frontal parcel; for the superior temporal gyrus it is the superior temporal parcel and the transverse temporal parcel; for the ventral and dorsal anterior cingulated it is respectively the rostral anterior parcel and the caudal anterior cingulate parcel; the inferior frontal gyrus including Broca's area refers to the pars triangularis parcel, the pars opercularis parcel and the pars orbitalis parcel; and the orbito frontal gyrus corresponds to the lateral orbito-frontal parcel and the medial orbito-frontal parcel (see **Figure 1**). We decided not to include the supplementary motor area, as it is equally spread over three Freesurfer's regions (the caudal middle frontal, the superior frontal and the precentral).

As Latora and Marchiori (2001) demonstrated, the local efficiency measures the functional segregation of one node when this particular node is removed from the sub-network. This measure represents the level of local information-processing. More precisely the local efficiency measures the functional segregation which means the capacity of locally processed information. In the case of hallucination, Allen et al. postulated a neuroanatomical model, composed of several cortical regions where their dysfunctional interplay fosters the hallucination emergence. Therefore, we wanted to see if the local capacity of this sub-network to process the information was related to the emergence and the severity of the hallucination.

In order to analyze the efficiency of communication in Allen's theoretical network, we compared the local efficiency value of each node between patients and healthy participants. Then, in the patients' networks, we analyzed the relationship between each node's efficiency and the BPRS hallucination subscale. For the ten regions, an outlier analysis was applied on the efficiency measurement and the correlation was controlled for age and gender.

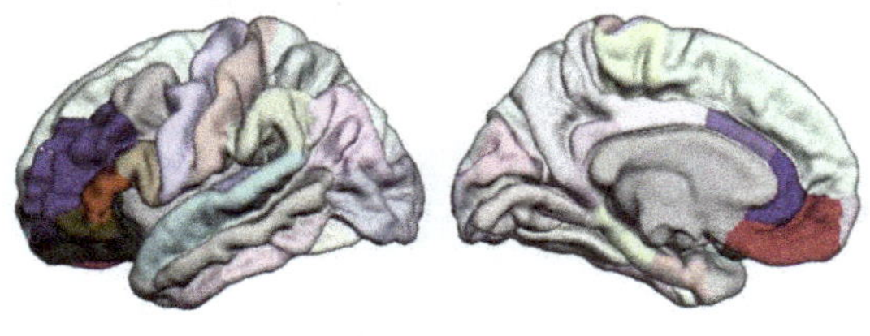

FIGURE 1 | Among the Desikan parcellation scheme, the regions elected as similar to Allen's model areas are the represented in full color and the remainder parcels are in faded color. On the lateral view: the superior temporal is cyan, the rostral middle frontal is purple, the lateral orbitofrontal is dark green, the pars orbitalis is khaki, the pars triangularis is dark orange, and the pars opercularis is beige. On the medial view, the medial orbitofrontal is fuchsia, the rostral anterior cingulate is dark purple, and the caudal cingulate is parme.

SIMULATION METHOD

As previous literature in the 22q11.2DS demonstrated that the brains of patients with 22q11.2DS show a 10% volumetric reduction (Eliez et al., 2000; Kates et al., 2001), which has an impact on the number of fibers (~10% less fibers) (Ottet et al., 2013), in the current study we simulated a random 10% reduction on the controls' connectome. This simulation enables a determination of whether the network measures applied for comparing both groups are biased by the reduction of the number of fibers or not. Using Matlab, we randomly subtracted one fiber at a time until 10% of the total number of fibers in the network were removed. This procedure was replicated for each healthy control connectome before applying the global network measurements.

RESULTS

GLOBAL NETWORK MEASURES

All the global network results comparing patients, controls and simulated networks can be found in **Table 1**.

The one tailed t-test comparison between the number of fibers contained in the patients' network and the controls' network revealed a significant loss of 10% of fibers ($p < 0.001$). The same test was applied between the patients' and the simulated network revealing that the significance was no longer preserved ($p = 0.59$). Although the simulated network didn't show any difference in the number of fibers compared to the patient group, the number of edges demonstrated a connectivity reduction of 6% ($p < 0.005$). Similarly, the *Global Efficiency* was significantly reduced in the brain network of the patients ($p = 0.0117$). No difference was observed in *the Mean Clustering Coefficient* between the two groups. Although the *Characteristic Path Length* was increased for the patient group ($p = 0.04$), the *Smallworldness* measure did not differ significantly between the two groups ($p = 0.368$).

HUB ANALYSIS

To determine which of the 83 nodes are hubs in the healthy control network, each node was ranked on 3 local network measures: the *local degree*, the *betweenness centrality* and the *clustering*

Table 1 | Mean, standard deviation and significant differences in the brain network global measures for participants with 22q11.2DS, healthy participants and simulated networks.

Global network measures	22q11.2DS		Control		p	Simulated		p
	Mean	Std	Mean	Std		Mean	Std	
Total number of fibers	42087	6608	46764	7343	**0.0005**	42385	5098	0.59
Total number of edges	1269.8	167.5	1354.5	132.4	**0.0038**	1354.5	132.4	**0.0038**
Characteristic path length	2.1652	0.1640	2.1150	0.1069	**0.0402**	2.1150	0.1069	**0.0402**
Mean clustering coefficient	0.7319	0.0295	0.7345	0.0234	0.3224	0.7345	0.0234	0.3224
Global efficiency	0.5238	0.0335	0.5372	0.0221	**0.0117**	0.5372	0.0221	**0.0117**
Smallworldness	1.6837	0.0859	1.68961	0.0783	0.368	1.68961	0.0783	0.368

The first p column from the left reports in bold the significant value (p < 0.05) of the comparison between the 22q11.2DS and control network. The second reports in bold the significant values (p < 0.05) when comparing the 22q11.2DS with the simulated network.

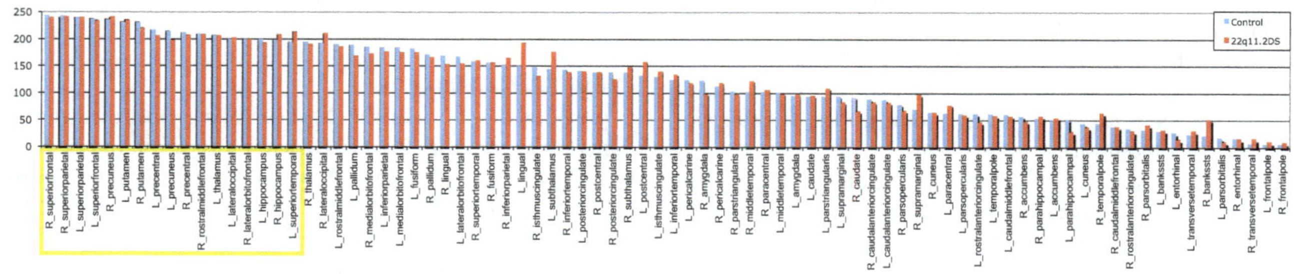

FIGURE 2 | Final ranking of the 82 gray matter regions in the healthy controls' brain. The 17 nodes with the highest rank highlighted in yellow, are considered as the connector hubs of the network. In blue is represented the repartition of the final ranking for the control and in red for the 22q11.2DS.

coefficient. According to the literature, hubs are defined as nodes that demonstrate a high degree, a high centrality and a low clustering coefficient. A ranking score was attributed to each of the nodes for the three measures previously discussed and averaged for the 48 healthy controls. The highest connected and the most central node scored 83 and the least connected and least central node scored 1. Inversely the least clustered node scored 83 and the most clustered scored 1. The final classification is the addition of the three scores, in which the top 20% are considered as the connector hubs of the network (see yellow bars in **Figure 2**). Although the stem node was the highest node on the final classification, we did not consider it as a hub because it is not a gray matter region (therefore all subsequent analyses considered 82 regions and not 83). Twelve out of 17 hubs were represented on both hemispheres in the superior frontal, the hippocampus, the superior parietal, the precuneus, the precentral and the putamen. In the right hemisphere two supplementary hubs are found, the rostral middle frontal and the lateral orbito-frontal. In the left hemisphere, three supplementary hubs were found, the superior temporal the lateral occipital and the thalamus.

DEGREE ANALYSIS

The results demonstrated that 26 nodes out of 82 (33%) in the patients' networks have a significantly reduced degree after FDR correction (pFDR $= 0.0149$). The names of the brain regions affected are listed in **Table 2**. Only one node showed an increased degree in the patients' networks: the right supramarginal region.

When analyzing how many of the hubs are altered, we noted that 10 out of 17 hubs (58%) were reduced in the patients network (see **Figure 3**). Conversely only 16 non-hubs out of 65 (25%) were reduced (see **Table 2**). Therefore, the percentage of affected hubs is more than double that of affected non-hub nodes. The 10 affected hubs are the bilateral hippocampus, superior parietal and precentral regions, right rostral middle frontal, superior frontal, precuneus and left thalamus.

EFFICIENCY AND HALLUCINATIONS

Following Allen's brain network model, the efficiency of ten nodes of the left hemisphere was correlated with the BPRS hallucination subscale. After controlling for age and gender, three of them showed a significant association with the presence and/or severity of the symptoms. Both the pars triangularis parcel and the transverse temporal parcel demonstrated a negative correlation with the symptom's scale (respectively $R = -0.312$, $p = 0.04$, *uncorrected* and $R = -0.354$, $p = 0.023$, *uncorrected*). Inversely, the rostral middle frontal shows a positive correlation with the symptom's scale ($R = 0.373$, $p = 0.014$, *uncorrected*) (see **Figure 4**).

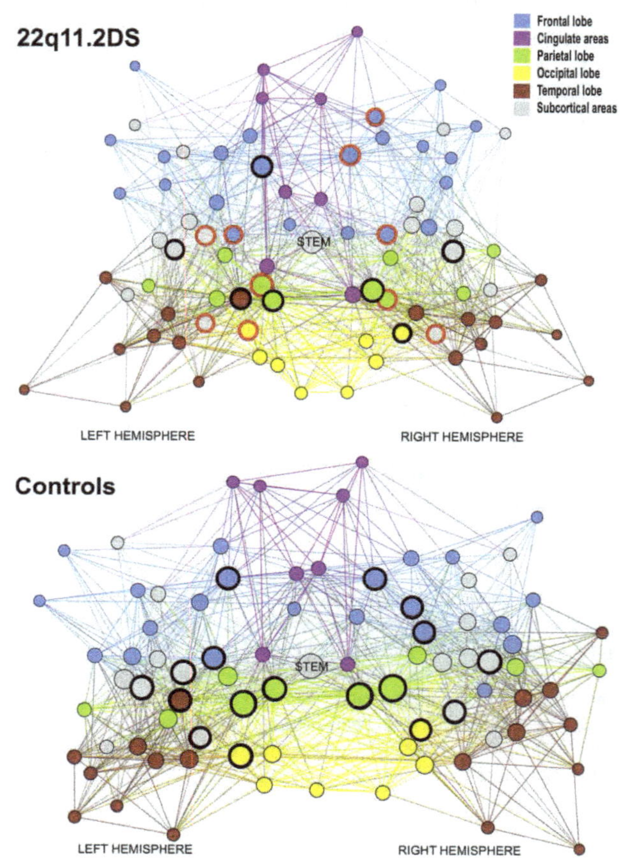

FIGURE 3 | Graph representation of the mean brain network for patients and controls using Gephi (http://gephi.org/) to produce optimal visualization of all the nodes and connections embedded in the networks. The circled nodes are the hubs of the network. The red circles are altered hubs and the black circles are preserved hubs. Every nodes contained in the same lobe or cerebral structure has the same color, blue for the node of the frontal lobe, magenta for the cingulate areas, green for the parietal lobe, yellow for the occipital lobe, brown for the temporal lobe and gray for the subcortical areas. The size of the nodes indicates their degree level.

Table 2 | List of the 26 nodes out of 82 that are significantly different in the patients' network after FDR correction, and indication as being hubs or not.

Parcel name	Control mean degree	Std	22q11DS mean degree	Std	FDR corrected (0.014883)	Hub
R_medialorbitofrontal	16.70	4.36	14.39	4.66	0.00733	No
R_parsopercularis	11.97	3.32	10.04	3.18	0.00245	No
R_rostralmiddlefrontal	21.5	4.52	19.45	3.63	0.00903	Yes
R_superiorfrontal	28.31	3.38	26.30	3.98	0.00492	Yes
R_precentral	23.41	3.96	21.26	3.79	0.00422	Yes
R_caudalantcingulate	10.68	2.41	9.23	2.17	0.00148	No
R_superiorparietal	31	4.35	27.82	6.01	0.00208	Yes
R_inferiorparietal	18.81	5.09	16.71	3.97	0.01451	No
R_precuneus	28.29	3.99	25.45	5.62	0.00290	Yes
R_lateraloccipital	21.70	5.24	18.69	5.74	0.00463	No
R_lingual	18.70	5.27	15.71	5.35	0.00382	No
R_parahippocampal	9.58	3.40	8.06	2.60	0.00874	No
R_inferiortemporal	18.37	5.15	16.10	4.77	0.01488	No
R_hippocampus	21.70	3.36	19.23	3.70	0.00051	Yes
L_parsopercularis	11.91	3.21	9.97	3.44	0.00291	No
L_precentral	24	3.55	20.69	3.36	6.14E-06	Yes
L_superiorparietal	31.91	5.03	28.97	6.19	0.00658	Yes
L_inferiorparietal	21.66	4.27	18.84	4.17	0.00085	No
L_pericalcarine	15.43	4.23	12.89	6.16	0.01064	No
L_lingual	16.52	5.41	13.67	5.06	0.00498	No
L_fusiform	19.18	4.11	14.95	3.34	2.04E-07	No
L_parahippocampal	9.02	3.32	7.52	3.20	0.01432	No
L_middletemporal	16.12	3.96	13.56	4.50	0.00215	No
L_thalamus	24.37	3.00	22.47	3.66	0.00356	Yes
L_caudate	13.81	3.07	11.60	2.86	0.00026	No
L_hippocampus	20.60	3.64	18.02	3.86	0.00062	Yes

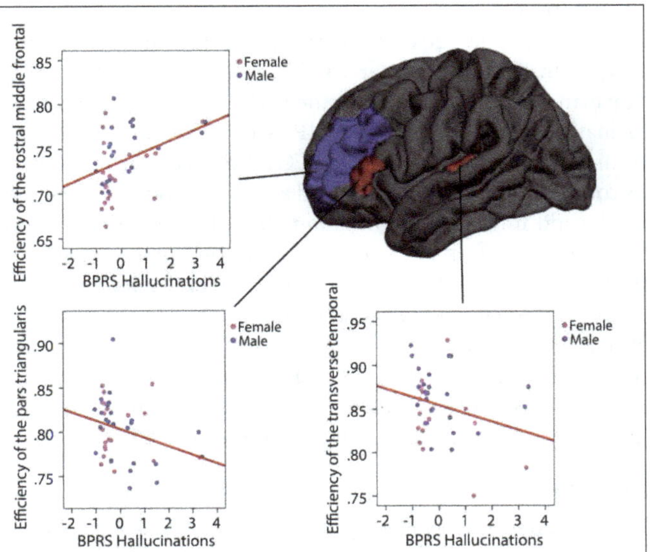

FIGURE 4 | Correlations between the BPRS hallucination subscale and the network efficiency in individuals with 22q11.2DS after age and gender correction. On the left hemisphere, the red regions (pars triangularis and transverse temporal) represent a negative correlation and the blue region (rostral middle frontal) represents a positive correlation.

The level of IQ, an additional controlling variable, was introduced, but nevertheless the significance for the three correlations survived.

DISCUSSION

Using white matter deterministic tractography and gray matter surface-based parcellation to reconstruct the brain connectome, the present work is the first study that analyzes the brain connectome in the 22q11.2DS in the light of the graph theory framework. In line with previous white matter studies in the 22q11DS, we found a 10% reduction in the number of fibers in the brain connectome of patients with 22q11DS (Eliez et al., 2000; Kates et al., 2001; Gothelf et al., 2011; Ottet et al., 2013). We also observed a 6% reduction of connectivity in patients, which means that 6% of the edges of the patients' network were missing. The simulation analysis demonstrated that the initial 10% fiber loss was not the cause of the 6% connectivity loss. This global dysconnection found in our analyses sustains the dysconnection hypothesis in schizophrenia (Friston and Frith, 1995; Stephan et al., 2009).

Despite the observed global disconnection, graph theoretical analysis comparing individuals with a high risk of developing schizophrenia (22q11.2DS) and healthy controls revealed that the smallworldness property of the patients' brain network was still preserved. However, a longer path length, similar to a lower global efficiency, demonstrates that the functional integration [capacity to transmit information more directly, with less interference or attenuation (Latora and Marchiori, 2001)] is reduced in 22q11.2 deletion syndrome. Although the global clustering coefficient is not significantly different from the healthy controls, the small-world brain organization of patients with 22q11.2DS tends to be closer to a regular network organization, in which the functional segregation (capacity to process specialized information, organized in clusters) is preserved but the functional integration is not optimum. Our study is in line with the previous network analysis on non-syndromic schizophrenia patients where a longer *Characteristic Path Length* has been systematically found (van den Heuvel et al., 2010; Zalesky et al., 2010b; Wang et al., 2011).

In the present work, local connectivity analysis allowed localization of the network nodes that were significantly altered in the patients' network. Every lobe and sub-cortical structure had one or more disconnected nodes sustaining the hypothesis that there is a widespread impact on the brain network in schizophrenia (Fornito et al., 2012). However, among the nodes that had a lower connectivity in patients, the proportion of affected hubs compared to non-affected hubs (58%) is interesting. Similarly in schizophrenia, previous findings shows a loss of hub connectivity specifically in frontal lobes (van den Heuvel et al., 2010). Our finding shed light on a possible targeted alteration of cerebral hubs in the 22q11.2DS that may also have some relevance for schizophrenia. Network hubs have special integrative or control functions as their privileged position in the hierarchical organization is postulated to be a key element for large-scale cognitive abilities. Because of their high centrality and influence any perturbation in a hub would heavily impact brain network function (Sporns et al., 2007). The major hub connectivity alteration in individuals with 22q11.2DS may explain their mild cognitive impairments, but also the cognitive collapse seen in schizophrenia during and after their first psychotic episode.

Schizophrenia is a disease with multifactorial etiologies. However, among the multiple causes, genetic factors play an important role (Stephan et al., 2006). Studying brain alterations in populations with high risk or ultra-high risk of developing schizophrenia could break out the predetermining cerebral organization leading to the development of psychosis (Cannon et al., 2007). To the best of our knowledge, no study to date has measured the network properties of white matter connectivity using graph theory in adolescents at risk for schizophrenia. However, a recent study by Shi et al. (2012) demonstrates a significant reduction of global efficiency, an increased global Characteristic Path Length, less hub nodes and lower edge "global efficiency" in neonates' brain networks having a mother with schizophrenia or a schizoaffective disorder. These results suggest that the topological abnormalities in individuals carrying a familial genetic risk for schizophrenia can already be observed a few weeks after birth (Shi et al., 2012). As the 22q11.2 deletion syndrome is commonly considered as a high risk population for schizophrenia (Bassett and Chow, 1999), our study adds some evidence to the hypothesis that early alterations in a cerebral network organization due to genetic factors may partially drive the development of schizophrenia and psychotic symptoms such as hallucinations.

Indeed, the graph theory of large-scale brain networks postulates that cognitive abilities arise from several cerebral regions interacting together (Bressler and Menon, 2010). In our graph network study, we explored the relationship between the alterations of a topological network property and a cognitive dysfunction. Our analyses revealed that the local efficiency value within three parcels of the left hemisphere, namely Broca's area (pars triangularis), Wernicke's area (transverse temporal) and the dorsolateral prefrontal cortex (DLPFC) (rostral middle frontal), correlated significantly with clinical ratings of hallucination severity. Efficiency values in Broca and Wernicke's areas suggested that, as local connections within these parcels decreased, the severity of hallucinatory phenomena increased in our 22q11DS sample. Given the implication of these areas in language production and comprehension, our results suggest that impairments in the different components of language processing in 22q11DS may significantly contribute to the expression of hallucinations. These findings are consistent with previously reported associations between a decrease in verbal IQ and psychotic symptoms (Gothelf et al., 2005; Debbané et al., 2006), and further suggest that local network connectivity in key language areas of the brain contributes to hallucinations in this deletion syndrome (Gothelf et al., 2011).

Hallucination severity further correlated positively with efficiency within the dorsolateral prefrontal parcel. The DLPFC region is one of the most consistently examined regions in MRI studies involving individuals with schizophrenia (Lewis et al., 2004) because of its implications at different levels of impairments, from working memory and executive functions to dopaminergic system malfunction (Tanaka, 2006). Neuromodulation of the DLPFC activity and its role in regulation of thought content is hypothesized to depend on its connectivity patterns with surrounding regions (Arnsten et al., 2012). In this perspective, our results may suggest that an atypically high local efficiency in 22q11DS works against the DLPFC's connectivity with surrounding parcels that modulate its activity. This impairment may thus increase the propensity to experience hallucinations. Future functional MRI studies should examine the connectivity dynamics of the DLPFC more specifically to evaluate its contributions to symptoms such as hallucinations. Overall, our results add important information about the relevance of brain topological network organization to previous longitudinal investigations in 22q11DS that have linked cerebral integrity of gray matter in the DLPFC to the development of psychosis (Gothelf et al., 2005; Schaer et al., 2009; Gothelf et al., 2011). Further research is necessary to understand the maturational dynamics between gray and white matter, and how these may interact to increase the potential for psychotic symptoms in 22q11DS.

LIMITATIONS

In this study, Graph theory principles were applied for the first time on a population with 22q11.2DS bringing new insight on the alterations in their brain organization that could in turn lead to schizophrenia symptoms. Nevertheless, the present work shows some limitations.

Although we choose the recommended ratio between scan timing, voxel size and the number of directions, the same limitations found in every DTI and tractography study remain present. Listed in detail in (Bammer et al., 2003), the major limitations are the absence of *in vitro* validation studies and the distance-related effect of the tractography [see the limitation section in (Ottet et al., 2013)]. This distance related effect biases the number of fibers included in a bundle. Nevertheless, as the present work used unweighted (binary) network analysis, we do not take in consideration the number of fibers, therefore the latter issue is not expected to influence our analyses.

The comparison of brain networks when assessing their properties with graph theory measures, is very sensitive with regard to two constitutive elements, first the choice of the nodes and second the connection density. The first limitation relies on the choice of the cortical parcellation and its scale. Indeed, the choice of a network node is a critical step (He and Evans, 2010). Zalesky et al. (2010a,b) demonstrated the strong influence on network measures of different choices of parcellation scales and diffusion imaging, which impairs the comparability and the constituency across studies (Zalesky et al., 2010a). A wider discrepancy arises when comparing two different parcellation scales (80 vs. 4000 nodes) and/or when comparing two different diffusion imaging techniques [High angular (HARDI) diffusion vs. DTI]. The analyses in our study do not suffer from this issue as we compared our patients' cerebral diffusion image with the same sequence in healthy control cerebral images. Furthermore, for both patients and controls we used the same connectome processing pipeline including the parcellation scheme, which demonstrated a good to excellent test-retest reliability on graph network measures (Owen et al., 2013). Therefore, the comparison between the two populations of the global and local network measures does not suffer from this kind of issue.

Nevertheless, the Desikan parcellation scheme we chose for processing our participants' brain may yield an issue. Although this parcellation is based on the primary and secondary sulci delineation which confers a very high reliability across humans brains (Desikan et al., 2006), the size of the parcels differ importantly. Thus, when delineating the hubs of the network, the very large parcels display a higher degree value, which is one of the three measures used to rank the nodes onto the hub scale. This concern is valid for the two other measures used for delineating the hubs (clustering coefficient and the centrality). However, the hubs we found were highly consistent with previous literature. Indeed, Li et al. (2011) evaluated as the highest reliable hubs the bilateral putamen, bilateral superior frontal and left precuneus among three tractography methods (Li et al., 2011). van den Heuvel and Sporns (2011) found that bilaterally, the precuneus, superior frontal and superior parietal, hippocampus, putamen and thalamus were hubs of structural derived networks (van den Heuvel and Sporns, 2011). Amongst all the hubs delineated in our study, only the bilateral precentral could have been elected because of its large size.

The second limitation concerns the difference in the number of connections that exist between the control and patient networks. This discrepancy may bias the topological measurements and may result in the significant findings. As van Wijk et al. shows in 2010, there is no way to rule out these differences without introducing another bias.

CONCLUSION

In the present study, the targeted dysconnectivity of the hubs in a population considered as a model for schizophrenia (22q11.2DS) suggests the existence of an early alteration in the cerebral network organization that is due to genetic factors which may partially drive the development of schizophrenia and psychotic symptoms. Furthermore, altered local efficiency in areas responsible for language processing (Broca and Wernicke) sheds light on the implication of structural network organization in the severity of hallucinations. Further research is needed to understand the interaction between structural networks and psychotic symptoms.

ACKNOWLEDGMENTS

This research was funded by the Swiss National Research Fund, with funds to Dr. Stephan Eliez (3200-063135.00/1, 3232-063134.00/1, PP0033-102864 and 32473B-121996), and by the National Center of Competence in Research (NCCR) "SYNAPSY—The Synaptic Bases of Mental Diseases" financed by the Swiss National Science Foundation (nu 51AU40_125759) and by the Center for Biomedical Imaging (CIBM) of the Geneva-Lausanne Universities and the EPFL, as well as the foundations Leenaards and Louis-Jeantet. The authors would also like to warmly thank all the participants and their family for volunteering in this study. We also greatly thank Sarah Menghetti for organizing and collecting data, and Jason Last for proof reading this manuscript. Our thank goes also to François Lazeyras, Frank Henri, Yohann Ouvrier-Buffet.

REFERENCES

Alexander-Bloch, A., Giedd, J. N., and Bullmore, E. (2013). Imaging structural co-variance between human brain regions. *Nat. Rev. Neurosci.* 14, 322–336. doi: 10.1038/nrn3465

Allen, P., Larøi, F., McGuire, P. K., and Aleman, A. (2008). The hallucinating brain: a review of structural and functional neuroimaging studies of hallucinations. *Neurosci. Biobehav. Rev.* 32, 175–191. doi: 10.1016/j.neubiorev.2007.07.012

Arnsten, A. F. T., Wang, M. J., and Paspalas, C. D. (2012). Neuromodulation of thought: flexibilities and vulnerabilities in prefrontal cortical network synapses. *Neuron* 76, 223–239. doi: 10.1016/j.neuron.2012.08.038

Bammer, R., Acar, B., and Moseley, M. E. (2003). *In vivo* MR tractography using diffusion imaging. *Eur. J. Radiol.* 45, 223–234. doi: 10.1016/S0720-048X(02)00311-X

Bassett, A. S., and Chow, E. W. (1999). 22q11 deletion syndrome: a genetic subtype of schizophrenia. *Biol. Psychiatry* 46, 882–891. doi: 10.1016/S0006-3223(99)00114-6

Bassett, D. S., and Bullmore, E. T. (2009). Human brain networks in health and disease. *Curr. Opin. Neurol.* 22, 340–347. doi: 10.1097/WCO.0b013e32832d93dd

Bassett, D. S., Bullmore, E., Verchinski, B. A., Mattay, V. S., Weinberger, D. R., and Meyer-Lindenberg, A. (2008). Hierarchical organization of human cortical networks in health and schizophrenia. *J. Neurosci.* 28, 9239–9248. doi: 10.1523/JNEUROSCI.1929-08.2008

Bassett, D. S., and Gazzaniga, M. S. (2011). Understanding complexity in the human brain. *Trends Cogn. Sci. (Regul Ed)* 15, 200–209. doi: 10.1016/j.tics.2011.03.006

Bressler, S. L., and Menon, V. (2010). Large-scale brain networks in cognition: emerging methods and principles. *Trends Cogn. Sci. (Regul. Ed.)* 14, 277–290. doi: 10.1016/j.tics.2010.04.004

Cannon, T. D., Cornblatt, B., and McGorry, P. (2007). Introduction: the empirical status of the ultra high-risk (prodromal) research paradigm.

Schizophr. Bull. 33, 661–664. doi: 10.1093/schbul/sbm031

Cheng, H., Wang, Y., Sheng, J., Kronenberger, W. G., Mathews, V. P., Hummer, T. A., et al. (2012). Characteristics and variability of structural networks derived from diffusion tensor imaging. *Neuroimage* 61, 1153–1164. doi: 10.1016/j.neuroimage.2012.03.036

Daducci, A., Gerhard, S., Griffa, A., Lemkaddem, A., Cammoun, L., Gigandet, X., et al. (2012). The connectome mapper: an open-source processing pipeline to map connectomes with MRI. *PLoS ONE* 7:e48121. doi: 10.1371/journal.pone.0048121

Dale, A. M., Fischl, B., and Sereno, M. I. (1999). Cortical surface-based analysis i. segmentation and surface reconstruction. *Neuroimage* 194, 179–194. doi: 10.1006/nimg.1998.0395

Debbané, M., Glaser, B., David, M. K., Feinstein, C., and Eliez, S. (2006). Psychotic symptoms in children and adolescents with 22q11.2 deletion syndrome: neuropsychological and behavioral implications. *Schizophr. Res.* 84, 187–193. doi: 10.1016/j.schres.2006.01.019

Desikan, R. S., Ségonne, F., Fischl, B., Quinn, B. T., Dickerson, B. C., Blacker, D., et al. (2006). An automated labeling system for subdividing the human cerebral cortex on MRI scans into gyral based regions of interest. *Neuroimage* 31, 968–980. doi: 10.1016/j.neuroimage.2006.01.021

Eliez, S., Schmitt, J. E., White, C. D., and Reiss, A. L. (2000). Children and adolescents with velocardiofacial syndrome: a volumetric MRI study. *Am. J. Psychiatry* 157, 409–415. doi: 10.1176/appi.ajp.157.3.409

Feinstein, C., Eliez, S., Blasey, C., and Reiss, A. L. (2002). Psychiatric disorders and behavioral problems in children with velocardiofacial syndrome: usefulness as phenotypic indicators of schizophrenia risk. *Biol. Psychiatry* 51, 312–318. doi: 10.1016/S0006-3223(01)01231-8

First, M. B., Spitzer, R. L., Gibbon, M., and Williams, J. B. W. (1996). *Structured Clinical Interview for DSM-IV Axis I Disorders, Clinician Version (SCID-CV)*. Washington, D.C: American Psychiatric Press, Inc.

Fischl, B., Sereno, M. I., and Dale, A. M. (1999). Cortical surface-based analysis ii.inflation flattening and a surface-based coordinate system. *Neuroimage* 207, 195–207. doi: 10.1006/nimg.1998.0396

Fitzsimmons, J., Kubicki, M., and Shenton, M. E. (2013). Review of functional and anatomical brain connectivity findings in schizophrenia. *Curr. Opin. Psychiatry* 26, 172–187. doi: 10.1097/YCO.0b013e32835d9e6a

Flaum, M., Oandapos;Leary, D. S., Swayze, V. W., Miller, D. D., Arndt, S., and Andreasen, N. C. (1995). Symptom dimensions and brain morphology in schizophrenia and related psychotic disorders. *J. Psychiatr. Res.* 29, 261–276. doi: 10.1016/0022-3956(94)00046-T

Fornito, A., Zalesky, A., Pantelis, C., and Bullmore, E. T. (2012). Schizophrenia, neuroimaging and connectomics. *Neuroimage* 62, 2296–2314. doi: 10.1016/j.neuroimage.2011.12.090

Friston, K. J., and Frith, C. D. (1995). Schizophrenia: a disconnection syndrome? *Clin. Neurosci.* 3, 89–97.

Gaser, C., Nenadic, I., Volz, H. P., Büchel, C., and Sauer, H. (2004). Neuroanatomy of "hearing voices": a frontotemporal brain structural abnormality associated with auditory hallucinations in schizophrenia. *Cereb. Cortex* 14, 91–96. doi: 10.1093/cercor/bhg107

Gothelf, D., Furfaro, J. A., Penniman, L. C., Glover, G. H., and Reiss, A. L. (2005). The contribution of novel brain imaging techniques to understanding the neurobiology of mental retardation and developmental disabilities. *Ment. Retard. Dev. Disabil. Res. Rev.* 11, 331–339. doi: 10.1002/mrdd.20089

Gothelf, D., Hoeft, F., Ueno, T., Sugiura, L., Lee, A. D., Thompson, P., et al. (2011). Developmental changes in multivariate neuroanatomical patterns that predict risk for psychosis in 22q11.2 deletion syndrome. *J. Psychiatr. Res.* 45, 322–331. doi: 10.1016/j.jpsychires.2010.07.008

He, Y., and Evans, A. (2010). Graph theoretical modeling of brain connectivity. *Curr. Opin. Neurol.* 23, 341–350. doi: 10.1097/WCO.0b013e32833aa567

Humphries, M. D., and Gurney, K. (2008). Network "small-world-ness": a quantitative method for determining canonical network equivalence. *PLoS ONE* 3:e0002051. doi: 10.1371/journal.pone.0002051

Jenkinson, M., and Smith, S. (2001). A global optimisation method for robust affine registration of brain images. *Med. Image Anal.* 5, 143–156. doi: 10.1016/S1361-8415(01)00036-6

Kates, W. R., Burnette, C. P., Jabs, E. W., Rutberg, J., Murphy, A. M., Grados, M., et al. (2001). Regional cortical white matter reductions in velocardiofacial syndrome: a volumetric MRI analysis. *Biol. Psychiatry* 49, 677–684. doi: 10.1016/S0006-3223(00)01002-7

Kay, S. R., Fiszbein, A., and Opler, L. A. (1987). The positive and negative syndrome scale (PANSS) for schizophrenia. *Schizophr. Bull.* 13, 261–276. doi: 10.1093/schbul/13.2.261

Latora, V., and Marchiori, M. (2001). Efficient behavior of small-world networks. *Phys. Rev. Lett.* 87:198701. doi: 10.1103/PhysRevLett.87.198701

Leucht, S. (2005). Clinical implications of brief psychiatric rating scale scores. *Br. J. psychiatry* 187, 366–371. doi: 10.1192/bjp.187.4.366

Lewis, D. A., Cruz, D., Eggan, S., and Erickson, S. (2004). Postnatal development of prefrontal inhibitory circuits and the pathophysiology of cognitive dysfunction in schizophrenia. *Ann. N.Y. Acad. Sci.* 1021, 64–76. doi: 10.1196/annals.1308.008

Li, L., Rilling, J. K., Preuss, T. M., Glasser, M. F., and Hu, X. (2011). The effects of connection reconstruction method on the interregional connectivity of brain networks via diffusion tractography. *Hum. Brain Mapp.* 33, 1894–1913. doi: 10.1002/hbm.21332

Liu, Y., Liang, M., Zhou, Y., He, Y., Hao, Y., Song, M., et al. (2008). Disrupted small-world networks in schizophrenia. *Brain* 131, 945–961. doi: 10.1093/brain/awn018

Lo, C.-Y. Z., He, Y., and Lin, C.-P. (2011). Graph theoretical analysis of human brain structural networks. *Rev. Neurosci.* 22, 1–13. doi: 10.1515/RNS.2011.039

McGuffin, P., Owen, M. J., and Farmer, A. E. (1995). Genetic basis of schizophrenia. *Lancet* 346, 678–682. doi: 10.1016/S0140-6736(95)92285-7

Neckelmann, G., Neckelmann, D. A. G., Specht, K., Lund, A., Ersland, L., Smievoll, A. I., et al. (2006). MR Morphometry Ananlsysis of gray matter volume reduction in schizophrenia: association with hallucinations. *Int. J. Neurosci.* 116, 9–23. doi: 10.1080/00207450690962244

Onitsuka, T., Shenton, M. E., Salisbury, D. F., Dickey, C. C., Kasai, K., Toner, S. K., et al. (2004). Middle and inferior temporal gyrus gray matter volume abnormalities in chronic schizophrenia: an MRI study. *Am. J. Psychiatry* 161, 1603–1611. doi: 10.1176/appi.ajp.161.9.1603

Ottet, M.-C., Schaer, M., Cammoun, L., Schneider, M., Debbané, M., Thiran, J.-P., et al. (2013). Reduced fronto-temporal and limbic connectivity in the 22q11.2 deletion syndrome: vulnerability markers for developing schizophrenia? *PLoS ONE* 8:e58429. doi: 10.1371/journal.pone.0058429

Owen, J. P., Ziv, E., Bukshpun, P., Pojman, N., Wakahiro, M., Berman, J., et al. (2013). Test-retest reliability of computational network measurements derived from the structural connectome of the human brain. *Brain Connect.* 3, 160–176. doi: 10.1089/brain.2012.0121

Poulton, R., Caspi, A., Moffitt, T. E., Cannon, M., Murray, R., and Harrington, H. (2000). Children's self-reported psychotic symptoms and adult schizophreniform disorder: a 15-year longitudinal study. *Arch. Gen. Psychiatry* 57, 1053–1058. doi: 10.1001/archpsyc.57.11.1053

Reich, W. (2000). Diagnostic interview for children and adolescents (DICA). *J. Am. Acad. Child Adolesc. Psychiatry* 39, 59–66. doi: 10.1097/00004583-200001000-00017

Rosas, H. D., Liu, A. K., Hersch, S., Glessner, M., and Ferrante, R. J. (2002). Regional and progressive thinning of the cortical ribbon in Huntington' s disease. *Neurology* 05886, 695–701. doi: 10.1212/WNL.58.5.695

Rubinov, M., and Sporns, O. (2010). Complex network measures of brain connectivity: uses and interpretations. *Neuroimage* 52, 1059–1069. doi: 10.1016/j.neuroimage.2009.10.003

Schaer, M., Debbané, M., Bach Cuadra, M., Ottet, M.-C., Glaser, B., Thiran, J.-P., et al. (2009). Deviant trajectories of cortical maturation in 22q11.2 deletion syndrome (22q11DS): a cross-sectional and longitudinal study. *Schizophr. Res.* 115, 182–190. doi: 10.1016/j.schres.2009.09.016

Shapleske, J., Rossell, S. L., Chitnis, X. A., Suckling, J., Simmons, A., Bullmore, E. T., et al. (2002). A computational morphometric MRI study of schizophrenia: effects of hallucinations. *Cereb. Cortex* 12, 1331–1341. doi: 10.1093/cercor/12.12.1331

Shi, F., Yap, P.-T., Gao, W., Lin, W., Gilmore, J. H., and Shen, D. (2012). Altered structural connectivity in neonates at genetic risk for schizophrenia: a combined study using morphological and white matter networks. *Neuroimage* 62, 1622–1633. doi: 10.1016/j.neuroimage.2012.05.026

Shprintzen, R. J., Goldberg, R. B., Lewin, M. L., Sidoti, E. J., Berkman, M. D., Argamaso, R. V., et al. (1978). A new syndrome involving cleft palate, cardiac anomalies, typical facies, and learning disabilities: velo-cardio-facial syndrome. *Cleft Palate J.* 15, 56–62.

Sporns, O. (2010). *Networks of the Brain.* MA: MIT Press. Available online at: http://books.google.com/books?id=v1DBKE7-UrYCandamp;printsec=frontcoverandamp;dq=intitle:Networks+of+the+Brainandamp;hl=andamp;cd=1andamp;source=gbs_api

Sporns, O., and Honey, C. J. (2006). Small worlds inside big brains. *Proc. Natl. Acad. Sci. U.S.A.* 103, 19219–19220. doi: 10.1073/pnas.0609523103

Sporns, O., Honey, C. J., and Kötter, R. (2007). Identification and classification of hubs in brain networks. *PLoS ONE* 2:e1049. doi: 10.1371/journal.pone.0001049

Stephan, K. E., Baldeweg, T., and Friston, K. J. (2006). Synaptic plasticity and dysconnection in schizophrenia. *Biol. Psychiatry* 59, 929–939. doi: 10.1016/j.biopsych.2005.10.005

Stephan, K. E., Friston, K. J., and Frith, C. D. (2009). Dysconnection in schizophrenia: from abnormal synaptic plasticity to failures of self-monitoring. *Schizophr. Bull.* 35, 509–527. doi: 10.1093/schbul/sbn176

Sumich, A., Chitnis, X. A., Fannon, D. G., O'Ceallaigh, S., Doku, V. C., Faldrowicz, A., et al. (2005). Unreality symptoms and volumetric measures of Heschl's gyrus and planum temporal in first-episode psychosis. *Biol. Psychiatry* 57, 947–950. doi: 10.1016/j.biopsych.2004.12.041

Tanaka, S. (2006). Dopaminergic control of working memory and its relevance to schizophrenia: a circuit dynamics perspective. *Neuroscience* 139, 153–171. doi: 10.1016/j.neuroscience.2005.08.070

van den Heuvel, M. P., Mandl, R. C. W., Stam, C. J., Kahn, R. S., and Hulshoff Pol, H. E. (2010). Aberrant frontal and temporal complex network structure in schizophrenia: a graph theoretical analysis. *J. Neurosci.* 30, 15915–15926. doi: 10.1523/JNEUROSCI.2874-10.2010

van den Heuvel, M. P., and Sporns, O. (2011). Rich-club organization of the human connectome. *J. Neurosci.* 31, 15775–15786. doi: 10.1523/JNEUROSCI.3539-11.2011

van Wijk, B. C. M., Stam, C. J., and Daffertshofer, A. (2010). Comparing brain networks of different size and connectivity density using graph theory. *PLoS ONE* 5:e13701. doi: 10.1371/journal.pone.0013701

Wang, Q., Su, T.-P., Zhou, Y., Chou, K.-H., Chen, I.-Y., Jiang, T., et al. (2011). Anatomical insights into disrupted small-world networks in schizophrenia. *NeuroImage* 59, 1085–1093. doi: 10.1016/j.neuroimage.2011.09.035

Watts, D. J., and Strogatz, S. H. (1998). Collective dynamics of "small-world" networks. *Nature* 393, 440–442. doi: 10.1038/30918

Wechsler, D. (1991). *Wechsler Intelligence Scale for Children.* San Antonio, TX: The Psychological Corporation.

Wechsler, D. (1997). *Wechsler Adult Intelligence Scale.* San Antonio, TX: Administration and Scoring Manual.

Yu, Q., Allen, E., Sui, J., Arbabshirani, M., Pearlson, G., and Calhoun, V. (2012). Brain connectivity networks in schizophrenia underlying resting state functional magnetic resonance imaging. *Curr. Top. Med. Chem.* 12, 2415–2425. doi: 10.2174/156802612805289890

Yu, Q., Plis, S. M., Erhardt, E. B., Allen, E. A., Sui, J., Kiehl, K. A., et al. (2011a). Modular organization of functional network connectivity in healthy controls and patients with schizophrenia during the resting state. *Front. Syst. Neurosci.* 5:103. doi: 10.3389/fnsys.2011.00103

Yu, Q., Sui, J., Rachakonda, S., He, H., Gruner, W., Pearlson, G., et al. (2011b). Altered topological properties of functional network connectivity in schizophrenia during resting state : a small-world brain network study. *PLoS ONE* 6:e25423. doi: 10.1371/journal.pone.0025423

Yu, Q., Sui, J., Liu, J., Plis, S. M., Kiehl, K. A., Pearlson, G., et al. (2013). Disrupted correlation between low frequency power and connectivity strength of resting state brain networks in schizophrenia. *Schizophr. Res.* 143, 165–171. doi: 10.1016/j.schres.2012.11.001

Zalesky, A., Fornito, A., Harding, I. H., Cocchi, L., Yücel, M., Pantelis, C., et al. (2010a). Whole-brain anatomical networks: does the choice of nodes matter? *Neuroimage* 50, 970–983. doi: 10.1016/j.neuroimage.2009.12.027

Zalesky, A., Fornito, A., Seal, M. L., Cocchi, L., Westin, C. F., Bullmore, E. T., et al. (2010b). Disrupted axonal fiber connectivity in schizophrenia. *Biol. Psychiatry* 69, 80–89. doi: 10.1016/j.biopsych.2010.08.022

Zhang, Y., Lin, L., Lin, C.-P., Zhou, Y., Chou, K.-H., Lo, C.-Y., et al. (2012). Abnormal topological organization of structural brain networks in schizophrenia. *Schizophr. Res.* 141, 109–118. doi: 10.1016/j.schres.2012.08.021

15

Age-related changes in brain structural covariance networks

Xinwei Li*[1,2]*, Fang Pu*[2]*, Yubo Fan*[2]*, Haijun Niu*[1,2]*, Shuyu Li*[1,2]* and Deyu Li*[2]

[1] *State Key Laboratory of Software Development Environment, Beihang University, Beijing, China*
[2] *Key Laboratory for Biomechanics and Mechanobiology of Ministry of Education, Department of Biomedical Engineering, School of Biological Science and Medical Engineering, Beihang University, Beijing, China.*

***Correspondence:**
Shuyu Li and Deyu Li, Key Laboratory for Biomechanics and Mechanobiology of Ministry of Education, School of Biological Science and Medical Engineering, Beihang University, No. 37 Xueyuan Road, Haidian District, Beijing 100191, China.
e-mail: shuyuli@buaa.edu.cn; deyuli@buaa.edu.cn

Previous neuroimaging studies have suggested that cerebral changes over normal aging are not simply characterized by regional alterations, but rather by the reorganization of cortical connectivity patterns. The investigation of structural covariance networks (SCNs) using voxel-based morphometry is an advanced approach to examining the pattern of covariance in gray matter (GM) volumes among different regions of the human cortex. To date, how the organization of critical SCNs change during normal aging remains largely unknown. In this study, we used an SCN mapping approach to investigate eight large-scale networks in 240 healthy participants aged 18–89 years. These participants were subdivided into young (18–23 years), middle aged (30–58 years), and older (61–89 years) subjects. Eight seed regions were chosen from widely reported functional intrinsic connectivity networks. The voxels showing significant positive associations with these seed regions were used to describe the topological organization of an SCN. All of these networks exhibited non-linear patterns in their spatial extent that were associated with normal aging. These networks, except the primary motor network, had a distributed topology in young participants, a sharply localized topology in middle aged participants, and were relatively stable in older participants. The structural covariance derived using the primary motor cortex was limited to the ipsilateral motor regions in the young and older participants, but included contralateral homologous regions in the middle aged participants. In addition, there were significant between-group differences in the structural networks associated with language-related speech and semantics processing, executive control, and the default-mode network (DMN). Taken together, the results of this study demonstrate age-related changes in the topological organization of SCNs, and provide insights into normal aging of the human brain.

Keywords: connectivity, structural covariance network, normal aging, neuroimaging, sensorimotor, neurocognition

INTRODUCTION

The majority of neuroimaging studies of aging have reported a consistent pattern of gray matter (GM) volumetric reductions in the human cortex, involving mainly prefrontal regions, parietal, and temporal association cortices, and the insula and cingulum (Resnick et al., 2003; Sowell et al., 2003; Raz et al., 2005; Du et al., 2006; Terribilli et al., 2011). However, more and more studies have demonstrated that cerebral changes with normal aging are not simply characterized by regional alterations but rather by the reorganization of cortical connectivity patterns (O'Sullivan et al., 2001; Koch et al., 2010; Wu et al., 2011b; Zhu et al., 2012). Using diffusion tensor imaging (DTI), several studies have consistently reported a diffuse loss of axonal integrity in senior populations (Salat et al., 2005; Pagani et al., 2008; Madden et al., 2009), which allowed for inferences regarding changes of structural connectivity in older people compared with younger adults. Building on complex network analysis methods, Gong et al. (2009) reported a reduction in overall cortical connectivity, decreased local efficiency, and a shift in regional efficiency from parietal and occipital to frontal and temporal neocortex in older brains.

The investigation of structural covariance networks (SCNs) using structural magnetic resonance imaging (sMRI) is another useful method to explore structural brain networks. This approach mainly characterizes the pattern of structural covariance in GM morphology (e.g., volume, thickness and surface area) between brain regions using a general linear model (GLM) framework (Mechelli et al., 2005; Lerch et al., 2006; Nosarti et al., 2010; Zielinski et al., 2010; Montembeault et al., 2012; Soriano-Mas et al., 2012). Many studies have demonstrated underlying relationships among brain areas using structural correlation by sMRI, anatomical connectivity by DTI, and functional correlation by resting-state functional MRI. For example, He and colleagues found that structural networks based on cortical thickness measurements were compatible with known functional networks (He et al., 2007). Greicius et al. measured functional connectivity using independent component analysis and anatomical connectivity using DTI and found there existed white matter tract structural connections between functionally connected regions (Greicius et al., 2009). A recent study reported agreement in the correlations in GM thickness and underlying fiber connections across brain areas, but more information was included for the thickness network than the fiber network (Gong et al., 2012). In addition, Seeley and colleagues demonstrated that SCNs using voxel-based morphometry (VBM) were able to recapitulate the functional connectivity network topologies (Seeley et al., 2009). The covariance of different cortical regions in their GM volumes was considered to be the result of mutual trophic influences (Ferrer et al., 1995) or common experience-related plasticity (Draganski et al., 2004; Mechelli et al., 2004). The consistency among these three networks provides substantial support for SCNs serving a measure of network integrity in cross-sectional studies.

Of note, the analysis of SCNs using VBM has been successfully applied to map the eight SCNs and explore how neural systems build large-scale structural covariance during development (Zielinski et al., 2010). One previous aging study using structural covariance approaches compared two populations (younger vs. older subjects) and reported reduced structural associations in order adults, specifically in high-order cognitive networks (Montembeault et al., 2012). However, because subjects in only two age categories were involved in that experiment, it could not determine the aging trajectories of these sensorimotor and high-order cognitive networks. Zielinski et al. (2010) found that there were non-linear trajectories of primary visual, auditory, and sensorimotor networks during development. Moreover, these networks were provisionally established by early childhood, but underwent significant expansion in early adolescence before contraction or pruning in late adolescence. Many studies have shown that age-related atrophy of some neural regions follows variable, non-linear patterns (Allen et al., 2005; Kennedy et al., 2009; Terribilli et al., 2011). However, it remains unknown whether and how age-related changes of primary sensorimotor and high-order cognitive SCNs exhibit non-linear trajectories during normal aging.

Here, we used an SCN mapping approach to investigate eight large-scale networks in 240 healthy participants aged 18–89. These participants were subdivided into young (18–23 years), middle aged (30–58 years), and older (61–89 years) subjects. Given that SCNs subserving language, social–emotional, and executive control functions have shown gradual deterioration through normal aging, we expected to observe age-related trajectories in the deterioration of these large-scale networks. To test our hypothesis, we first investigated the aging trajectories of three sensorimotor and five high-order cognitive SCNs in three groups composed of an equal number of subjects at different ages, and then compared these SCNs differences between the groups.

MATERIALS AND METHODS

PARTICIPANTS

Three hundred sixteen right-handed, healthy subjects were selected from the Open Access Series of Imaging Studies (OASIS) cross-sectional database (http://www.oasis-brains.org) (Marcus et al., 2007). Data from seven subjects were excluded from further analysis because of poor image quality or image preprocessing. Because of relatively few subjects aged 30–60 years, we first selected 80 subjects from this age range as the middle-aged group (30 males and 50 females). Then, we selected 80 separate subjects around 75 years of age as the old group. Finally, we selected the youngest 80 subjects matched for gender as the young group. The names and characteristics of the groups are shown in **Table 1**. All subjects were evaluated using the Mini-Mental State Examination (MMSE) (Folstein et al., 1975) and Clinical Dementia Rating (CDR) scales (Morris, 1993; Morris et al., 2001). MMSE scores were higher than 29, and CDR scores were all zero. For demographic data on all subjects, see Marcus et al. (2007). This dataset has been used in several previous studies (Bakkour et al., 2009; Fjell et al., 2009; Salat et al., 2009; Li et al., 2011).

IMAGE ACQUISITION

For each subject, three to four individual T1-weighted magnetization-prepared rapid gradient echo (MP-RAGE) images were acquired on a 1.5T Vision scanner (Siemens, Erlangen, Germany) within a single session. Head movement was minimized with cushioning and a thermoplastic face-mask. Images were motion corrected and averaged to create a single image with a high contrast-to-noise ratio. MP-RAGE parameters were empirically optimized for gray/white contrast: $TR = 9.7$ ms; $TE = 4$ ms; flip angle $= 10°$; slice number $= 128$; resolution $= 256 \times 256$ (1×1 mm); thickness $= 1.25$ mm.

IMAGE PREPROCESSING

Structural MR images were processed using a technical computing software program (MATLAB 2010; The MathWorks Inc., Natick, Mass) and Statistical Parametric Mapping software (SPM 8; The Wellcome Department of Imaging Neuroscience, London, UK). Following the inspection of image artifacts, image preprocessing was performed with the VBM8 toolbox (http://dbm.neuro.uni-jena.de/vbm/). Briefly, all native-space MRIs were segmented to extract GM based on an adaptive maximum *a posteriori* technique (Rajapakse et al., 1997) and partial volume estimation method (Tohka et al., 2004) without the need for *a priori* tissue probability information. In addition, a spatially adaptive non-local denoising filter (Manjon et al., 2010) and a hidden Markov random field model (Rajapakse et al., 1997) were applied to minimize the level of noise in the resulting GM segments. Subsequently, the high-dimensional DARTEL (diffeomorphic anatomical registration using exponentiated lie algebra) approach provided non-linear deformation to normalize the images to the DARTEL template in Montreal Neurological Institute (MNI) space, which was derived from 550 healthy control subjects (Ashburner, 2007). Non-brain tissue was also

Table 1 | Characteristics of the subjects in this study.

Group ID	Age (mean ± SD)	Number of subjects
Young (Y)	18–23 (20.66 ± 1.47)	80 (F:50/M:30)
Middle-aged (M)	30–58 (47.43 ± 8.23)	80 (F:50/M:30)
Old (O)	61–89 (73.75 ± 7.12)	80 (F:55/M:25)

Abbreviations: F, female; M, male.

removed. Additionally, the Jacobian determinants derived from the spatial normalization were used to modulate the GM value for each voxel to preserve the total amount of GM from the original images (Good et al., 2001). We used non-linear components only, which allowed us to analyze relative (i.e., corrected for individual brain size) differences in regional GM volume. Finally, the resulting modulated and normalized images were smoothed with a 12 mm full width at half maximum isotropic Gaussian kernel.

EXTRACTION OF SEED VOLUMES

To assess the structural covariance pattern of each large-scale network, we extracted individual GM volumes from eight seed regions of interest (ROIs). These ROIs included the primary visual, auditory, and motor cortex, as well as language-related speech and semantic areas, areas related to salience and executive control, and the default-mode network (DMN). We based our ROIs on previous studies (Zielinski et al., 2010; Montembeault et al., 2012). For each region, seeds were defined with the MarsBar ROI toolbox (http://marsbar.sourceforge.net/) as 4-mm radial spheres centered at the following MNI coordinates: right calcarine sulcus (9, −81, 7), right Heschl's gyrus (46, −18, 10), right precentral gyrus (28, −16, 66), left inferior frontal gyrus, pars opercularis (IFGo) (−50, 18, 7), left temporal pole (−38 10, −28), right frontoinsular cortex (38, 26, −10), right dorsolateral prefrontal cortex (DLPFC) (44, 36, 20), and right angular gyrus (46, −59, 23). In addition, we selected contralateral seeds by changing the sign on each seed's x coordinate to perform similar SCNs analyses (**Table A1**, and **Figure A1**).

STATISTICAL ANALYSIS

A voxel-wise statistical analysis was performed on the GM images using the GLM as applied in SPM8. Eight multiple regression models were used to test the strength of the structural covariance between each seeds and all other regions across whole-brain GM for each age group. In each regression model, the extracted mean GM volume from each ROI was entered as a covariate of interest, and gender as a confounding covariate. Because of the unequal sample size across the genders, we removed the effects of gender on the SCN patterns in the correlation analysis. These statistical analyses identified voxels that had a positive covariance with each *a priori* selected ROI in each group. The resulting correlation maps were using height and extent thresholds at $P < 0.05$ with family-wise error (FWE) correction. They were displayed on the MNI template to allow qualitative comparisons between the age groups using BrainNet Viewer software (http://www.nitrc.org/projects/bnv/). To quantify differences in normal aging trajectories across networks, we calculated the total number of significant positive ipsilateral, contralateral, and whole-brain voxels and plotted these across the age groups.

To further examine the effects of age on specific regional covariance, we performed between-group difference analyses of SCN patterns for any two groups according to the scientific literature (Lerch et al., 2006). For any pair of voxels in two groups, their structural correlation may have different slopes, and the difference in slope may represent the difference in their structural association. The difference in slope was tested using a classic interaction linear model:

$$V_i = \beta_0 + \beta_1 V_j + \beta_2 \text{Group} + \beta_3 (V_j \times \text{Group}) + \varepsilon$$

where V_i and V_j represented the GM volumes of a pair of voxels in two groups. The Group component was modeled using treatment contrasts, and significance tested using the Student's t statistic. Specific t-value contrasts were established to map the voxels that expressed a significantly different structural association between any two groups. The threshold for the resulting statistical parametric maps was given at $P < 0.05$ for the height and extent thresholds, with FWE multiple comparisons correction.

RESULTS

For each network, the age-related SCN trajectory was identified by the spatial extent of each SCN. These results were demonstrated by functional domain, as described in the following sections. We also explored regions that significantly differed in their structural associations between any two groups.

PRIMARY SENSORY AND MOTOR NETWORKS

Seeds within primary visual cortex (right calcarine sulcus) produced SCNs with a relatively preserved pattern (**Figure 1**). However, there were small changes in the distributions of the covariance maps. In the young and middle-aged groups, the covariance regions mainly included the bilateral calcarine sulcus, lingual gyrus, cuneus and right lateral occipital gyrus, whereas only included bilateral calcarine sulcus, lingual gyrus, and cuneus in the old group. Primary auditory cortex (i.e., the right Heschl's gyrus) covaried with the bilateral insula and precuneus, the right posterior cingulate cortex (PCC), parahippocampus, and inferior frontal gyrus, and the left orbital-frontal cortex in the young participants, and underwent significant contraction in the middle-aged and old groups to include only the bilateral insula regions. There was a flat transition in the covariance maps during aging. Primary motor cortex (right precentral gyrus) correlated with the ipsilateral precentral regions in the young participants, which progressed at middle age to include the contralateral precentral and supplementary motor areas. In old participants, these structural associations were similar to the young participants.

In addition, within the primary sensory and motor networks, there were no significant differences observed in the structural association between any two groups when we compared the slopes of the structural associations on a voxel-by-voxel basis.

LANGUAGE-RELATED SPEECH AND SEMANTIC NETWORKS

The two language-related speech and semantic networks followed similar variation patterns (**Figure 2**). From the young participants to the middle group, the covariance regions showed abrupt decreases. They then showed smaller changes at the following ages. For the language-related speech network, the covariance map involved the bilateral anterior insula, medial frontal, cingulate cortex, and temporal regions in the young participants, and then contracted to include seed autocorrelation in the older participants. The semantic regions correlated with the bilateral

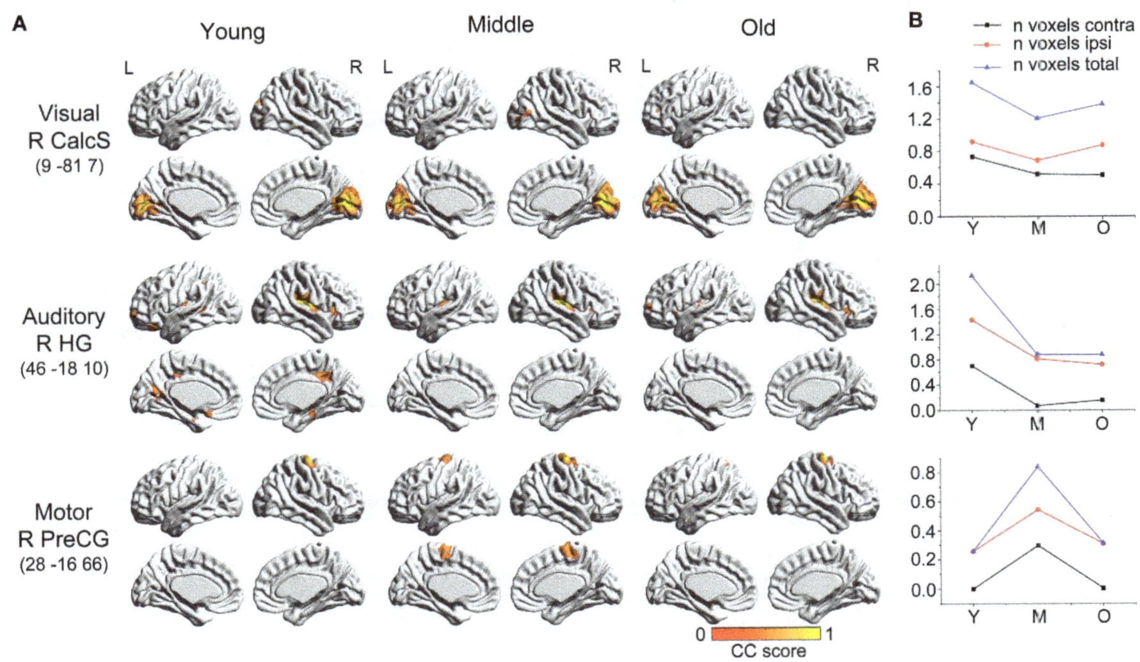

FIGURE 1 | Age-related changes in primary sensory and motor structural covariance networks. (A) Statistical maps of regions significantly correlated with the seed region in each group. The results are presented as correlation coefficient values ($P < 0.05$, FWE corrected). **(B)** The plots of voxel counts by group indicate small covariance changes throughout the life-span. The y-axis represents the voxel number ($\times 10^4$). Abbreviations: Calcs, calcarine sulcus; HG, Heschl's gyrus; PreCG, precentral gyrus; R, right; L, left; Y, young group; M, middle-aged group; O, old group; CC, correlation coefficient.

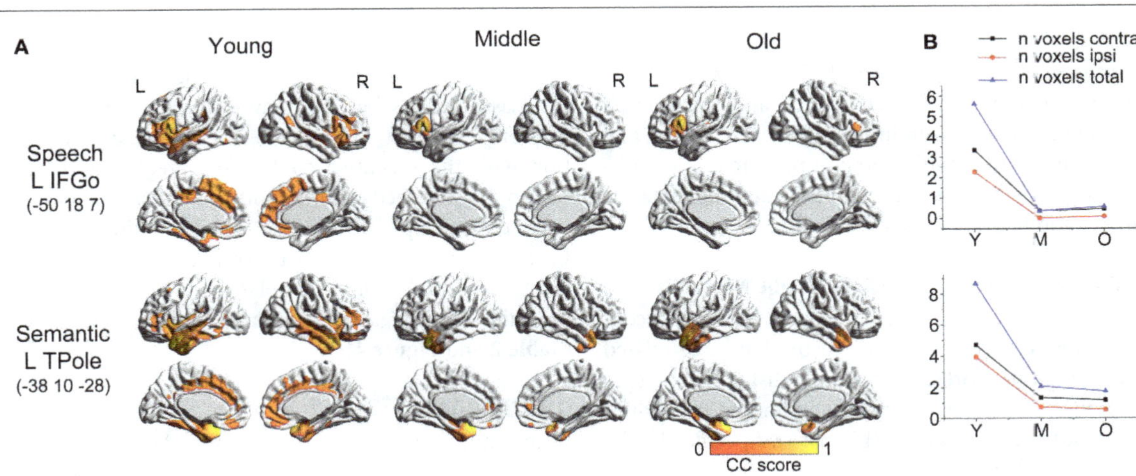

FIGURE 2 | Age-related changes in speech and semantic structural covariance networks. (A) Statistical maps of regions significantly correlated with the seed region in each group. The results are presented as correlation coefficient values ($P < 0.05$, FWE corrected). **(B)** The plots of voxel counts by group indicate abrupt contraction in the middle-aged group and mild changes in the old group. The y-axis represents the voxel number ($\times\times 10^4$). Abbreviations: IFGo, inferior frontal gyrus, pars opercularis; TPole, temporal pole; L, left; R, right; Y, young group; M, middle-aged group; O, old group; CC, correlation coefficient.

temporal cortices, cingulate gyrus, insula and frontal regions in the young participants, and shrank sharply to include only the anterior temporal cortices during normal aging.

Comparing the other SCNs, language-related speech and semantic networks showed more age-related changes. Specifically, the left supplementary motor and superior temporal areas showed significant positive associations with the speech seed region in young adults, whereas this covariance disappeared in the middle-aged group (**Table 2** and **Figure 3**). Decreased positive associations between the left superior temporal region and left temporal pole were found in the middle-aged group compared with the young group (**Table 2** and **Figure 4**). There were

Table 2 | Contrast analysis of structural covariance network trajectories.

Network	Contrast	x	y	z	Region	BA	Voxel size	maxT
DMN (R ANG)	Y > M	27	65	1	R PFC	10	181	4.97
	Y > O	−3	−10	40	L PCC	23/24/31	1100	5.34
		−6	33	25	L ACC	32	110	4.43
Speech (L IFGo)	Y > M	−3	12	52	L SMA	6/8	3498	5.35
		−51	−16	−11	L STC	21/22	741	4.77
		54	−28	3	R STC	21/22	630	4.52
	Y > O	−10	35	25	L ACC	8/9/32	3235	5.82
		−5	29	52	L SFC			5.28
		−4	−21	37	L PCC	24/31	218	4.29
Semantic (L TPole)	Y > M	−54	−15	−11	L STC	22	114	4.31
	Y > O	10	−34	36	R PCC	23/31	978	5.33
		−40	−3	10	L Insula	13	217	4.72
		26	33	−21	R OFC	11	200	4.33
Executive (R DLPFC)	Y > O	−4	−22	43	L PCC	24/31	419	4.99

The regions listed showed significant between-group differences ($P < 0.05$, FWE corrected). x, y, z coordinates are reported in standard MNI space. Abbreviations: DMN, default-mode network; ANG, angular gyrus; IFGo, inferior frontal gyrus, pars opercularis; TPole, temporal pole; DLPFC, dorsolateral prefrontal cortex; PFC, prefrontal cortex; PCC, posterior cingulate cortex; ACC, anterior cingulate cortex; SMA, supplementary motor area; STC, superior temporal cortex; SFC, superior frontal cortex; OFC, orbitofrontal cortex; R, right; L, left; Y, young group; M, middle-aged group; O, old group; BA, Brodmann area.

significant positive associations between the left anterior and the PCC and left IFG in the young participants, and this covariance became a negative correlation in the old group (**Table 2** and **Figure 4**). When compared with the old group, there was a significant positive association between the right PCC and the semantic seed region in the young participants (**Table 2** and **Figure 5**).

SALIENCE, EXECUTIVE CONTROL, AND DEFAULT-MODE NETWORKS

The three networks associated with social–emotional and cognitive function showed similar patterns to the language-related speech and semantic networks, with more distributed structural covariance in the young participants and limited covariance patterns throughout the later stages (**Figure 5**). Specifically, the right frontoinsular cortex anchored covariance maps included extensive areas of the bilateral lateral and medial frontal cortex, temporal cortices, and cingulate regions. This SCN underwent significant shrinkage in the middle-aged group to include only bilateral insular regions. In the older subjects, this network somewhat extended to include the bilateral medial prefrontal regions. The right DLPFC seed covaried with the bilateral frontal, temporal, and cingulate cortices in the young participants, but shrank into a more focal distribution in the middle-aged and older subjects. A seed in right angular gyrus produced an aging SCN, including the bilateral angular gyrus, middle temporal, cingulum, and prefrontal regions in the young participants, and contracting to include the bilateral PCC and angular gyrus in the middle-aged group, and only the bilateral angular gyrus in the old group.

There were no significant differences observed in the structural associations between any two groups within the salience network. The left PCC showed a significant positive association with the executive control seed region and right angular region (DMN seed) in the young adults, whereas this covariance disappeared in the old group (**Table 2** and **Figure 5**). Furthermore, a less robust positive association between the right prefrontal region and DMN seed region was found in the middle-aged group compared with the young participants (**Table 2** and **Figure 4**).

DISCUSSION

In this study, we investigated the age-related trajectories of eight large-scale networks using an SCN mapping approach in three distinct age groups. All networks exhibited non-linear patterns across normal aging in terms of the spatial extent of the network. Except for the primary motor network, these networks showed a more distributed topology in young participants, which shrank sharply to a more localized topology in the middle-aged group, and maintained this localized topology in the old group. Primary sensory and motor networks showed fewer age-related changes compared with high-order cognitive networks. Moreover, there were significant between-group differences in language-related speech and semantic networks, the executive control network, and the DMN. Taken together, our results provide evidence of variations in the topological organization of SCNs during normal aging.

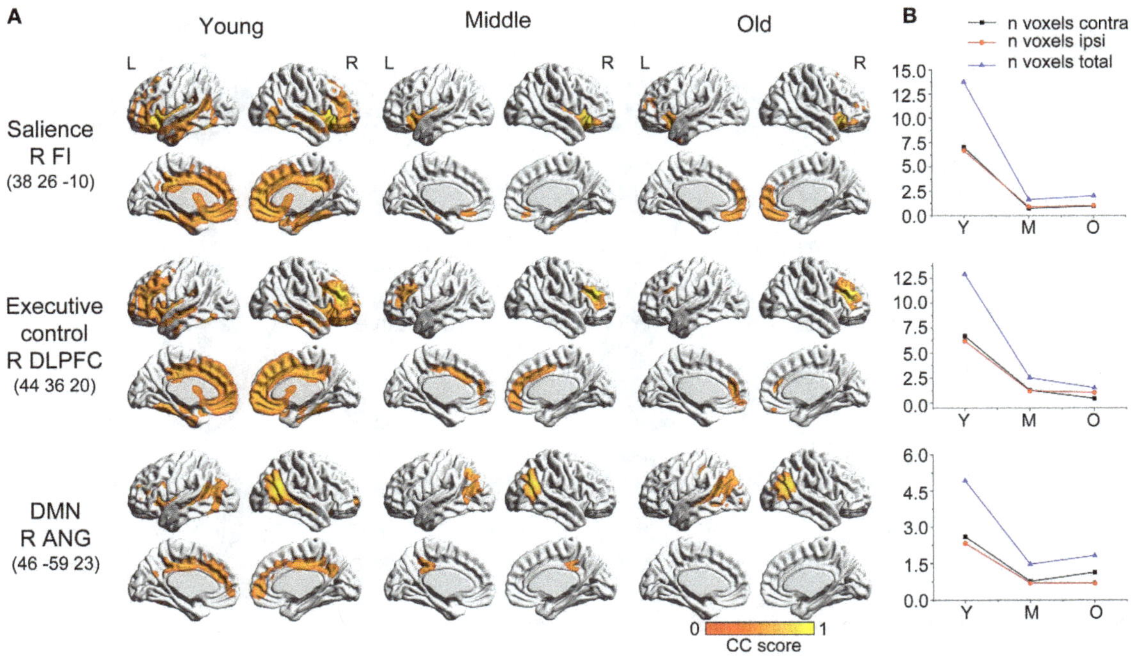

FIGURE 3 | Age-related changes in salience, executive control, and default-mode structural covariance networks. (A) Statistical maps of regions significantly correlated with the seed region in each group. The results are presented as correlation coefficient values ($P < 0.05$, FWE corrected). **(B)** The plots of voxel counts by group indicate abrupt contraction in the middle-aged group and mild changes in the old group. The y-axis represents the voxel number ($\times 10^4$). Abbreviations: DMN, default-mode network; DLPFC, dorsolateral prefrontal cortex; FI, frontoinsular cortex; ANG, angular gyrus; R, right; L, left; Y, young group; M, middle-aged group; O, old group; CC, correlation coefficient.

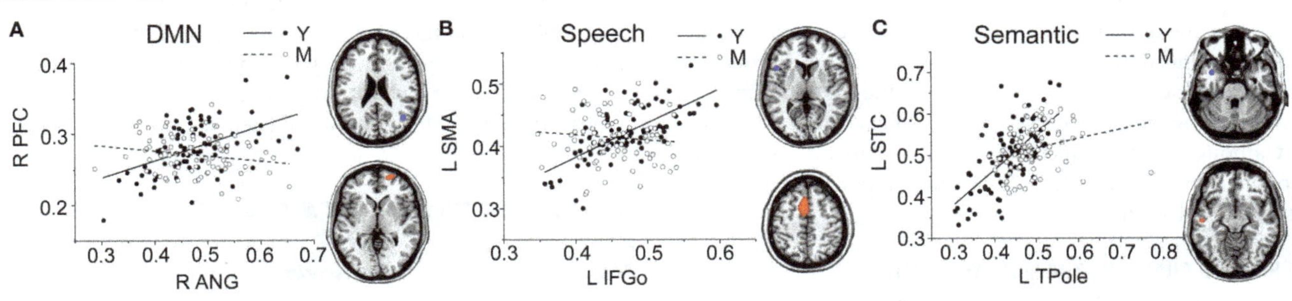

FIGURE 4 | Group differences for the young vs. the middle-aged subjects. Significant between-group differences within the DMN **(A)**, speech **(B)**, and semantic **(C)** structural covariance networks were found. For each network, the region of interest (upper) and region showing the most significant structural association (lower) are presented on the right, and a plot of slop differences between the seed region and a 4-mm radius sphere centered on the peak voxel are presented in the left. Voxels with $P_{FWE} < 0.05$ are displayed. Abbreviations: DMN, default-mode network; ANG, angular gyrus; IFGo, inferior frontal gyrus, pars opercularis; TPole, temporal pole; PFC, prefrontal cortex; SMA, supplementary motor area; STC, superior temporal cortex; R, right; L, left; Y, young group; M, middle-aged group.

COMPARISON OF STRUCTURAL COVARIANCE NETWORKS AND OTHER NETWORKS

The cerebral cortex is organized into networks of functionally complementary areas. New advances in modern neuroimaging techniques and quantitative analysis of complex networks have made the investigation of brain network topological organization possible. DTI is a useful tool for non-invasively mapping cortico-cortical anatomical connections by examining axonal integrity. Insight into the structural covariance of GM morphology (e.g., volume, thickness, and surface area) between brain regions is provided by sMRI. Resting-state fMRI has allowed for assessments of the strength of functional connections within a network by quantifying correlated activity [i.e., spontaneous, low-frequency fluctuations in the blood oxygen level-dependent (BOLD) signal] between brain regions at rest.

The current studies have demonstrated the underlying relationships among structural correlations, anatomical connectivity, and functional correlations. For example, structural networks based on cortical thickness measurements were consistent with known functional networks (He et al., 2007). A recent study

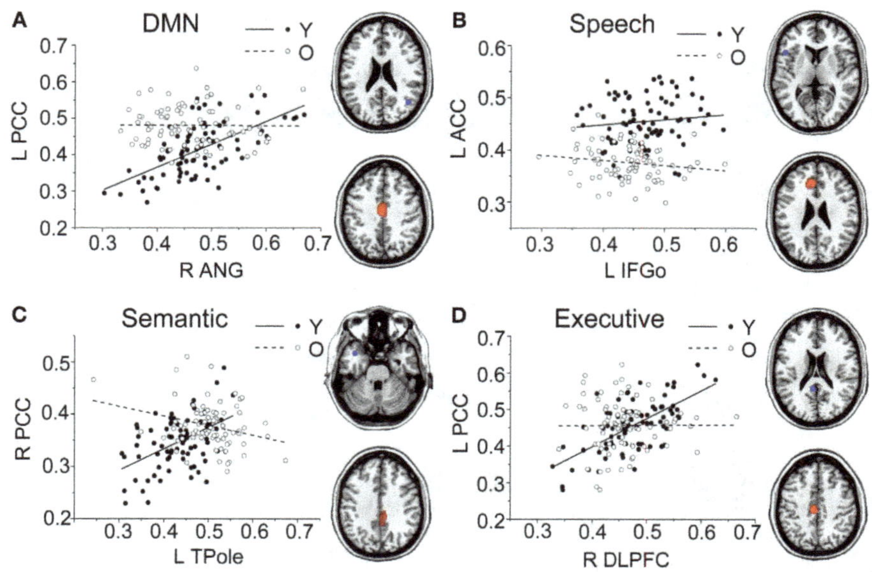

FIGURE 5 | Group differences for the young vs. the old subjects. Significant between-group differences within the DMN **(A)**, speech **(B)**, semantic **(C)**, and executive **(D)** structural covariance networks were found. For each network, the region of interest (upper) and region showing the most significant structural association (lower) are presented on the right, and a plot of slop differences between the seed region and a 4-mm radius sphere centered on the peak voxel are presented in the left. Voxels with $P_{FWE} < 0.05$ are displayed. Abbreviations: DMN, default-mode network; ANG, angular gyrus; IFGo, inferior frontal gyrus, pars opercularis; TPole, temporal pole; DLPFC, dorsolateral prefrontal cortex; PCC, posterior cingulate cortex; ACC, anterior cingulate cortex; R, right; L, left; Y, young group; O, old group.

reported agreement in the correlations in GM thickness and underlying fiber connections across brain areas, but more information was included for the thickness correlation network than the fiber connection network (Gong et al., 2012). In addition, SCNs determine using VBM recapitulated the canonical intrinsic connectivity networks topologies (Seeley et al., 2009). The consistency among the SCNs and other networks provides substantial support for the use of SCNs as a measure of network integrity for cross-sectional studies.

AGE-RELATED CHANGING TRAJECTORY OF SCNs

In this study, we employed three age groups to map the trajectory of SCN changes over age. Except the primary motor network, these SCNs appeared the similar non-linear pattern that had a distributed topology in young participants, a sharply localized topology in middle aged participants, and were relatively stable in older participants. This trajectory was similar to age-related changes of integrated local efficiency of brain network (Wu et al., 2011b). They employed the graph theory analysis method and reported that the local efficiency in the young group was significantly larger than those of the middle and old groups, whereas no significant difference was found between the middle and old groups. The shrinkage of SCNs as well as the reduction of local efficiency might be explained by the regionally distributed pattern of GM atrophy (Bergfield et al., 2010). As for primary motor network, we found inverted V-curve tendency among three age groups in the SCN of primary motor cortex. The previous study reported increased inter-regional correlations between bilateral primary motor cortex in the aging brain (Chen et al., 2011). In our study, we found the structural covariance of primary motor cortex between two hemispheres in the middle group. Alternatively, we found that the volume of right precentral gyrus reduced with age increasing (**Figure A2**), which might reflect a compensation mechanism that a network may need to work harder by becoming overactive due to regional volumetric atrophy with the network (Reuter-Lorenz and Cappell, 2008).

INTRAGROUP PATTERNS AND BETWEEN-GROUP DIFFERENCES OF SCNs

Primary sensory and motor networks

In this study, we found that seeds within the primary visual, auditory, and motor cortices produced SCNs with smaller spatial extents (i.e., total voxel count exhibiting a significant correlation at the corrected threshold) compared with other networks. This is consistent with previous work (Lerch et al., 2006) with mapped anatomical correlations across cerebral cortex (MACACC) using cortical thickness. Similarly, they used the number of cortical region showing significant correlations with seed region to describe the strength of MACACC. They found the primary motor, sensorimotor, and visual areas had the lowest strengths of correlation, whereas the association cortices had the highest strength. This could be explained by the functions of association cortices, because these cortices receive and integrate inputs from multiple cortical and non-cortical sources, and distribute information to multiple areas.

In addition, primary sensory and motor networks showed fewer age-related changes compared with high-order cognitive networks. There were no significant differences observed in the structural association between any two groups when the slopes of the structural associations were contrasted on a voxel-by-voxel basis within the primary sensory and motor networks. This finding is in line with a recent study (Montembeault et al., 2012) in which between-group differences were only observed in high-order cognitive SCNs between young and old subjects, rather than primary sensory and motor networks.

Language-related speech and semantic networks

The language-related speech and semantic networks showed significant age-related changes, with a more localized topology with increasing age. These results could account for the decline of language abilities across in normal aging. Federmeier and colleagues observed age-related changes in the timing with which message-level information impacted semantic analysis using event-related potentials, which indicated that aging affects high-order language processes (Federmeier et al., 2003). Wierenga and colleagues also reported that healthy older adults had increased difficulty in word retrieval with unchanged semantic knowledge (Wierenga et al., 2008).

Within the language-related speech SCN, a reduced structural association was observed the between inferior frontal gyrus and the supplementary motor area in the middle-aged group compared with the young participants. The speech SCN linked the language and motor systems that enable speech fluency (Seeley et al., 2009). This reduced structural covariance may explain the decline of motor speech skills with the transference of language to a speech code in older adults. Similarly, there was a significant decrease in the covariance between the seed region and the anterior cingulate cortex (ACC) in the old group compared with the young participants. This could be related to the functional degradation of these areas. Takahashi et al. reported that significant age-related reductions in regional cerebral blood flow in the left IFG and the bilateral medial frontal gyri and ACC using single-photon emission tomography (Takahashi et al., 2005). In addition, as the ACC plays a critical role in the control of speech responses (Paus et al., 1993), this reduced covariance may explain some speech difficulties in senior populations.

In semantic SCN analysis, a reduced structural association between the left temporal pole and left superior temporal cortex was found in the middle-aged group compared with the young participants. Many studies have shown that the superior temporal cortex is associated with understanding spoken words (Demonet et al., 1992; Chao et al., 2002; Okada and Hickok, 2006). Thus, this reduced structural association may be related to a decline in auditory word comprehension with increasing age. In the comparisons of the young and old participants, the main differences we found were in the structural associations between the left temporal pole and PCC. The results of functional neuroimaging studies in young, healthy adults provide compelling evidence for the involvement of the PCC in memory retrieval. For example, PCC activation was elicited during recognition of thematic narrative information learned during training sessions (Maguire et al., 1999). The reduced structural association between these two regions may explain the decline of semantic memory in senior populations.

Salience, executive control, and default-mode networks

The three high-order cognitive SCNs showed a similar pattern to the language SCNs, showing a distributed topology in young participants that shrank sharply to a localized topology in the middle-aged group, and maintained a localized topology in the old group. Cepeda and colleagues found age-related decline of executive control processes by examining task-switching performance (Cepeda et al., 2001). Kelly and colleagues also demonstrated the stability of executive control decreased in older subjects (West et al., 2002). Several studies have shown that the DMN is altered in old subjects (Andrews-Hanna et al., 2007; Koch et al., 2010; Sambataro et al., 2010), especially in anterior regions (Damoiseaux et al., 2008). Similarly, Chen et al. found the decreased inter-regional correlations with the DMN module (Chen et al., 2011). Cognitive decline with age, such as cognitive control (Persson et al., 2007) and working memory (Sambataro et al., 2010), is associated with decreased DMN connectivity.

In the executive-control SCN analysis, the main differences we found were in the structural association between the right DLPFC and PCC, which exhibited a positive correlation in the young participants and no association in the old group. The DLPFC shows increased activity when experimental stimuli are presented, and is thought to support on-task processing in attention tasks. The PCC, in contrast, shows decreased activity during stimulus presentation, and is thought to support off-task processing in attention tasks. Some studies have reported that activity in the DLPFC shows a negative correlation with activity in the PCC during the resting state (Greicius et al., 2003; Fransson, 2005), and the negative coupling between these regions is lower in older adults (Sambataro et al., 2010). Our findings are inconsistent with functional connectivity between these areas, which should be further investigated in future studies.

Finally, for the DMN, we found a reduction in the structural association between the right angular gyrus and right prefrontal cortex from the young to the middle-aged participants. In the comparison of the young and old group, we found age-related differences in the structural association between the right angular gyrus and PCC. Similarly, Wu and colleagues reported that the left angular gyrus has a significantly reduced correlation with the PCC in older compared with younger participants in a resting-state fMRI study (Wu et al., 2011a). As the PCC is a prominent region within the DMN, the reduced structural association between the seed regions and the PCC indicates that the DMN SCN shrinks with age.

LATERALITY OF THE SCNs

We found similar SCNs across both hemispheres (**Figure A1**), consistent with previous SCN analyses of the developing brain (Zielinski et al., 2010). However, the auditory and speech networks showed a notable exception. The SCN derived from the left seed of Heschl's gyrus was distinctly smaller than the one derived from the right seed. In contrast, the SCN derived from the left seed of the IFGo was distinctly larger than the one derived from the right seed, which may explain why speech networks are left-dominated (Powell et al., 2006; Xiang et al., 2010).

FURTHER CONSIDERATIONS

To build upon this study, several issues need to be addressed. First, we assigned subjects in their 30s to the middle-aged group because there were fewer subjects in their 40s and 50s in our sample. This resulted in wide age range in the middle-aged group. In future, this age range should be refined by including more subjects. Second, a previous study has reported the brain functional connectivity pattern could be affected by the sex factor (Biswal et al., 2010). In future, it is interesting to explore the sexual differences when the SCNs change with age. Third, it should be highlighted that this study used ROIs based on previous studies (Zielinski et al., 2010; Montembeault et al., 2012). Future studies using ROIs extracted from ICNs of the same subjects may obtain more accurate definitions of seed regions.

CONCLUSIONS

In this study, we used an SCN mapping approach to investigate eight large-scale networks in a large cohort of healthy participants. Our results show age-related changes in the topological organization of SCNs and provide insights into the normal aging process of the human brain.

ACKNOWLEDGMENTS

This work was supported by the National Science Foundation of China (Nos. 81171403, 81071212, and 30700182) and the State Key Laboratory of Software Development Environment (No. SKLSDE-2011ZX-10).

REFERENCES

Allen, J. S., Bruss, J., Brown, C. K., and Damasio, H. (2005). Normal neuroanatomical variation due to age: the major lobes and a parcellation of the temporal region. *Neurobiol. Aging* 26, 1245–1260.

Andrews-Hanna, J. R., Snyder, A. Z., Vincent, J. L., Lustig, C., Head, D., Raichle, M. E., et al. (2007). Disruption of large-scale brain systems in advanced aging. *Neuron* 56, 924.

Ashburner, J. (2007). A fast diffeomorphic image registration algorithm. *Neuroimage* 38, 95–113.

Bakkour, A., Morris, J. C., and Dickerson, B. C. (2009). The cortical signature of prodromal AD: regional thinning predicts mild AD dementia. *Neurology* 72, 1048–1055.

Bergfield, K. L., Hanson, K. D., Chen, K., Teipel, S. J., Hampel, H., Rapoport, S. I., et al. (2010). Age-related networks of regional covariance in MRI gray matter: reproducible multivariate patterns in healthy aging. *Neuroimage* 49, 1750–1759.

Biswal, B. B., Mennes, M., Zuo, X. N., Gohel, S., Kelly, C., Smith, S. M., et al. (2010). Toward discovery science of human brain function. *Proc. Natl. Acad. Sci. U.S.A.* 107, 4734–4739.

Cepeda, N. J., Kramer, A. F., and Gonzalez De Sather, J. (2001). Changes in executive control across the life span: examination of task-switching performance. *Dev. Psychol.* 37, 715.

Chao, L. L., Weisberg, J., and Martin, A. (2002). Experience-dependent modulation of category-related cortical activity. *Cereb. Cortex* 12, 545–551.

Chen, Z. J., He, Y., Rosa-Neto, P., Gong, G. L., and Evans, A. C. (2011). Age-related alterations in the modular organization of structural cortical network by using cortical thickness from MRI. *Neuroimage* 56, 235–245.

Damoiseaux, J., Beckmann, C., Arigita, E. J. S., Barkhof, F., Scheltens, P., Stam, C., et al. (2008). Reduced resting-state brain activity in the "default network" in normal aging. *Cereb. Cortex* 18, 1856–1864.

Demonet, J. F., Chollet, F., Ramsay, S., Cardebat, D., Nespoulous, J. L., Wise, R., et al. (1992). The anatomy of phonological and semantic processing in normal subjects. *Brain* 115, 1753–1768.

Draganski, B., Gaser, C., Busch, V., Schuierer, G., Bogdahn, U., and May, A. (2004). Neuroplasticity: changes in grey matter induced by training. *Nature* 427, 311–312.

Du, A. T., Schuff, N., Chao, L. L., Kornak, J., Jagust, W. J., Kramer, J. H., et al. (2006). Age effects on atrophy rates of entorhinal cortex and hippocampus. *Neurobiol. Aging* 27, 733–740.

Federmeier, K. D., Van Petten, C., Schwartz, T. J., and Kutas, M. (2003). Sounds, words, sentences: age-related changes across levels of language processing. *Psychol. Aging* 18, 858.

Ferrer, I., Blanco, R., Carulla, M., Condom, M., Alcantara, S., Olive, M., et al. (1995). Transforming growth factor-alpha immunoreactivity in the developing and adult brain. *Neuroscience* 66, 189–199.

Fjell, A. M., Westlye, L. T., Amlien, I., Espeseth, T., Reinvang, I., Raz, N., et al. (2009). High consistency of regional cortical thinning in aging across multiple samples. *Cereb. Cortex* 19, 2001–2012.

Folstein, M. F., Folstein, S. E., and McHugh, P. R. (1975). "Mini-mental state". A practical method for grading the cognitive state of patients for the clinician. *J. Psychiatr. Res.* 12, 189–198.

Fransson, P. (2005). Spontaneous low-frequency BOLD signal fluctuations: an fMRI investigation of the resting-state default mode of brain function hypothesis. *Hum. Brain Mapp.* 26, 15–29.

Gong, G., He, Y., Chen, Z. J., and Evans, A. C. (2012). Convergence and divergence of thickness correlations with diffusion connections across the human cerebral cortex. *Neuroimage* 59, 1239–1248.

Gong, G., Rosa-Neto, P., Carbonell, F., Chen, Z. J., He, Y., and Evans, A. C. (2009). Age- and gender-related differences in the cortical anatomical network. *J. Neurosci.* 29, 15684–15693.

Good, C. D., Johnsrude, I. S., Ashburner, J., Henson, R. N., Friston, K. J., and Frackowiak, R. S. (2001). A voxel-based morphometric study of ageing in 465 normal adult human brains. *Neuroimage* 14, 21–36.

Greicius, M. D., Krasnow, B., Reiss, A. L., and Menon, V. (2003). Functional connectivity in the resting brain: a network analysis of the default mode hypothesis. *Proc. Natl. Acad. Sci. U.S.A.* 100, 253.

Greicius, M. D., Supekar, K., Menon, V., and Dougherty, R. F. (2009). Resting-state functional connectivity reflects structural connectivity in the default mode network. *Cereb. Cortex* 19, 72–78.

He, Y., Chen, Z. J., and Evans, A. C. (2007). Small-world anatomical networks in the human brain revealed by cortical thickness from MRI. *Cereb. Cortex* 17, 2407–2419.

Kennedy, K. M., Erickson, K. I., Rodrigue, K. M., Voss, M. W., Colcombe, S. J., Kramer, A. F., et al. (2009). Age-related differences in regional brain volumes: a comparison of optimized voxel-based morphometry to manual volumetry. *Neurobiol. Aging* 30, 1657–1676.

Koch, W., Teipel, S., Mueller, S., Buerger, K., Bokde, A., Hampel, H., et al. (2010). Effects of aging on default mode network activity in resting state fMRI: does the method of analysis matter? *Neuroimage* 51, 280–287.

Lerch, J. P., Worsley, K., Shaw, W. P., Greenstein, D. K., Lenroot, R. K., Giedd, J., et al. (2006). Mapping anatomical correlations across cerebral cortex (MACACC) using cortical thickness from MRI. *Neuroimage* 31, 993–1003.

Li, S., Xia, M., Pu, F., Li, D., Fan, Y., Niu, H., et al. (2011). Age-related changes in the surface morphology of the central sulcus. *Neuroimage* 58, 381–390.

Madden, D. J., Bennett, I. J., and Song, A. W. (2009). Cerebral white matter integrity and cognitive aging: contributions from diffusion tensor imaging. *Neuropsychol. Rev.* 19, 415–435.

Maguire, E. A., Frith, C. D., and Morris, R. (1999). The functional neuroanatomy of comprehension and memory: the importance of prior knowledge. *Brain* 122, 1839–1850.

Manjon, J. V., Coupe, P., Marti-Bonmati, L., Collins, D. L., and Robles, M. (2010). Adaptive non-local means denoising of MR images with spatially varying noise levels. *J. Magn. Reson. Imaging* 31, 192–203.

Marcus, D. S., Wang, T. H., Parker, J., Csernansky, J. G., Morris, J. C., and Buckner, R. L. (2007). Open Access Series of Imaging Studies (OASIS): cross-sectional MRI data in young, middle aged, nondemented, and demented older adults. *J. Cogn. Neurosci.* 19, 1498–1507.

Mechelli, A., Crinion, J. T., Noppeney, U., O'Doherty, J., Ashburner, J., Frackowiak, R. S., et al. (2004). Neurolinguistics: structural plasticity in the bilingual brain. *Nature* 431:757. doi: 10.1038/431757a

Mechelli, A., Friston, K. J., Frackowiak, R. S., and Price, C. J. (2005). Structural covariance in the human cortex. *J. Neurosci.* 25, 8303–8310.

Montembeault, M., Joubert, S., Doyon, J., Carrier, J., Gagnon, J. F., Monchi, O., et al. (2012). The impact of aging on gray matter structural covariance networks. *Neuroimage* 63, 754–759.

Morris, J. C. (1993). The Clinical Dementia Rating (CDR): current version and scoring rules. *Neurology* 43, 2412–2414.

Morris, J. C., Storandt, M., Miller, J. P., McKeel, D. W., Price, J. L., Rubin, E. H., et al. (2001). Mild cognitive impairment represents early-stage Alzheimer disease. *Arch. Neurol.* 58, 397–405.

Nosarti, C., Mechelli, A., Herrera, A., Walshe, M., Shergill, S. S., Murray, R. M., et al. (2010). Structural covariance in the cortex of very preterm adolescents: a voxel-based morphometry study. *Hum. Brain Mapp.* 32, 1615–1625.

Okada, K., and Hickok, G. (2006). Identification of lexical-phonological networks in the superior temporal sulcus using functional magnetic resonance imaging. *Neuroreport* 17, 1293–1296.

O'Sullivan, M., Jones, D. K., Summers, P. E., Morris, R. G., Williams, S. C., and Markus, H. S. (2001). Evidence for cortical "disconnection" as a mechanism of age-related cognitive decline. *Neurology* 57, 632–638.

Pagani, E., Agosta, F., Rocca, M. A., Caputo, D., and Filippi, M. (2008). Voxel-based analysis derived from fractional anisotropy images of white matter volume changes with aging. *Neuroimage* 41, 657–667.

Paus, T., Petrides, M., Evans, A. C., and Meyer, E. (1993). Role of the human anterior cingulate cortex in the control of oculomotor, manual, and speech responses: a positron emission tomography study. *J. Neurophysiol.* 70, 453–469.

Persson, J., Lustig, C., Nelson, J. K., and Reuter-Lorenz, P. A. (2007). Age differences in deactivation: a link to cognitive control? *J. Cogn. Neurosci.* 19, 1021–1032.

Powell, H., Parker, G. J. M., Alexander, D. C., Symms, M. R., Boulby, P. A., Wheeler-Kingshott, C. A. M., et al. (2006). Hemispheric asymmetries in language-related pathways: a combined functional MRI and tractography study. *Neuroimage* 32, 388–399.

Rajapakse, J. C., Giedd, J. N., and Rapoport, J. L. (1997). Statistical approach to segmentation of single-channel cerebral MR images. *IEEE Trans. Med. Imaging* 16, 176–186.

Raz, N., Lindenberger, U., Rodrigue, K. M., Kennedy, K. M., Head, D., Williamson, A., et al. (2005). Regional brain changes in aging healthy adults: general trends, individual differences and modifiers. *Cereb. Cortex* 15, 1676–1689.

Resnick, S. M., Pham, D. L., Kraut, M. A., Zonderman, A. B., and Davatzikos, C. (2003). Longitudinal magnetic resonance imaging studies of older adults: a shrinking brain. *J. Neurosci.* 23, 3295–3301.

Reuter-Lorenz, P. A., and Cappell, K. A. (2008). Neurocognitive aging and the compensation hypothesis. *Curr. Dir. Psychol. Sci.* 17, 177–182.

Salat, D. H., Greve, D. N., Pacheco, J. L., Quinn, B. T., Helmer, K. G., Buckner, R. L., et al. (2009). Regional white matter volume differences in nondemented aging and Alzheimer's disease. *Neuroimage* 44, 1247–1258.

Salat, D. H., Tuch, D. S., Greve, D. N., van der Kouwe, A. J., Hevelone, N. D., Zaleta, A. K., et al. (2005). Age-related alterations in white matter microstructure measured by diffusion tensor imaging. *Neurobiol. Aging* 26, 1215–1227.

Sambataro, F., Murty, V. P., Callicott, J. H., Tan, H. Y., Das, S., Weinberger, D. R., et al. (2010). Age-related alterations in default mode network: impact on working memory performance. *Neurobiol. Aging* 31, 839.

Seeley, W. W., Crawford, R. K., Zhou, J., Miller, B. L., and Greicius, M. D. (2009). Neurodegenerative diseases target large-scale human brain networks. *Neuron* 62, 42–52.

Soriano-Mas, C., Harrison, B. J., Pujol, J., Lopez-Sola, M., Hernandez-Ribas, R., Alonso, P., et al. (2012). Structural covariance of the neostriatum with regional gray matter volumes. *Brain Struct. Funct.* doi: 10.1007/s00429-012-0422-5. [Epub ahead of print].

Sowell, E. R., Peterson, B. S., Thompson, P. M., Welcome, S. E., Henkenius, A. L., and Toga, A. W. (2003). Mapping cortical change across the human life span. *Nat. Neurosci.* 6, 309–315.

Takahashi, K., Yamaguchi, S., Kobayashi, S., and Yamamoto, Y. (2005). Effects of aging on regional cerebral blood flow assessed by using technetium Tc 99 m hexamethylpropyleneamine oxime single-photon emission tomography with 3D stereotactic surface projection analysis. *AJNR Am. J. Neuroradiol.* 26, 2005–2009.

Terribilli, D., Schaufelberger, M. S., Duran, F. L., Zanetti, M. V., Curiati, P. K., Menezes, P. R., et al. (2011). Age-related gray matter volume changes in the brain during non-elderly adulthood. *Neurobiol. Aging* 32, 354–368.

Tohka, J., Zijdenbos, A., and Evans, A. (2004). Fast and robust parameter estimation for statistical partial volume models in brain MRI. *Neuroimage* 23, 84–97.

West, R., Murphy, K. J., Armilio, M. L., Craik, F. I. M., and Stuss, D. T. (2002). Lapses of intention and performance variability reveal age-related increases in fluctuations of executive control. *Brain Cogn.* 49, 402–419.

Wierenga, C. E., Benjamin, M., Gopinath, K., Perlstein, W. M., Leonard, C. M., Rothi, L. J. G., et al. (2008). Age-related changes in word retrieval: role of bilateral frontal and subcortical networks. *Neurobiol. Aging* 29, 436–451.

Wu, J. T., Wu, H. Z., Yan, C. G., Chen, W. X., Zhang, H. Y., He, Y., et al. (2011a). Aging-related changes in the default mode network and its anti-correlated networks: a resting-state fMRI study. *Neurosci. Lett.* 504, 62–67.

Wu, K., Taki, Y., Sato, K., Kinomura, S., Goto, R., Okada, K., et al. (2011b). Age-related changes in topological organization of structural brain networks in healthy individuals. *Hum. Brain Mapp.* 33, 552–568.

Xiang, H. D., Fonteijn, H. M., Norris, D. G., and Hagoort, P. (2010). Topographical functional connectivity pattern in the perisylvian language networks. *Cereb. Cortex* 20, 549.

Zhu, W., Wen, W., He, Y., Xia, A., Anstey, K. J., and Sachdev, P. (2012). Changing topological patterns in normal aging using large-scale structural networks. *Neurobiol. Aging* 33, 899–913.

Zielinski, B. A., Gennatas, E. D., Zhou, J., and Seeley, W. W. (2010). Network-level structural covariance in the developing brain. *Proc. Natl. Acad. Sci. U.S.A.* 107, 18191–18196.

APPENDIX

Table A1 | Contrast analysis of structural covariance network trajectories derived from contralateral seeds.

Network	Contrast	*x*	*y*	*z*	Region	BA	Voxel size	maxT
DMN (R ANG)	Y > O	36	24	−20	R IFC	47	1149	5.56
		−36	15	−23	L TPole	38/47	808	5.15
		−44	42	−3	L IFC	47	128	4.53
		4	−27	42	R PCC	24/31	139	4.5
Speech (L IFGo)	Y > M	−50	−55	22	L ANG	39	57	4.23
	Y > O	4	−54	28	R PCC	7/31	2443	5.4
Semantic (L TPole)	Y > M	62	−21	−23	R ITC	20	200	4.38
	Y > O	28	35	−6	R IFC	11/47	361	4.93
		−30	−36	−15	L FG	37	138	4.41
Salience (R FI)	Y > O	5	−47	36	R PCC	23/31/32	1575	5.64
		−39	−3	7	L Insula	13	166	4.65
		−26	−35	−22	L FG	37	392	4.67
Auditory (R HG)	Y > M	26	44	−24	R OFC	11	906	5.30
	Y > O	−8	21	34	L ACC	24/32	864	4.86

The regions listed showed significant between-group differences ($P < 0.05$, FWE corrected). x, y, z coordinates are reported in standard MNI space. Abbreviations: DMN, default-mode network; ANG, angular gyrus; IFGo, inferior frontal gyrus, pars opercularis; TPole, temporal pole; FI, frontoinsular cortex; HG, Heschl's gyrus; IFC, inferior frontal cortex; PCC, posterior cingulate cortex; ITC, inferior temporal cortex; FG, fusiform gyrus; OFC, orbitofrontal cortex; ACC, anterior cingulate cortex; R, right; L, left; Y, young group; M, middle-aged group; O, old group; BA, Brodmann area.

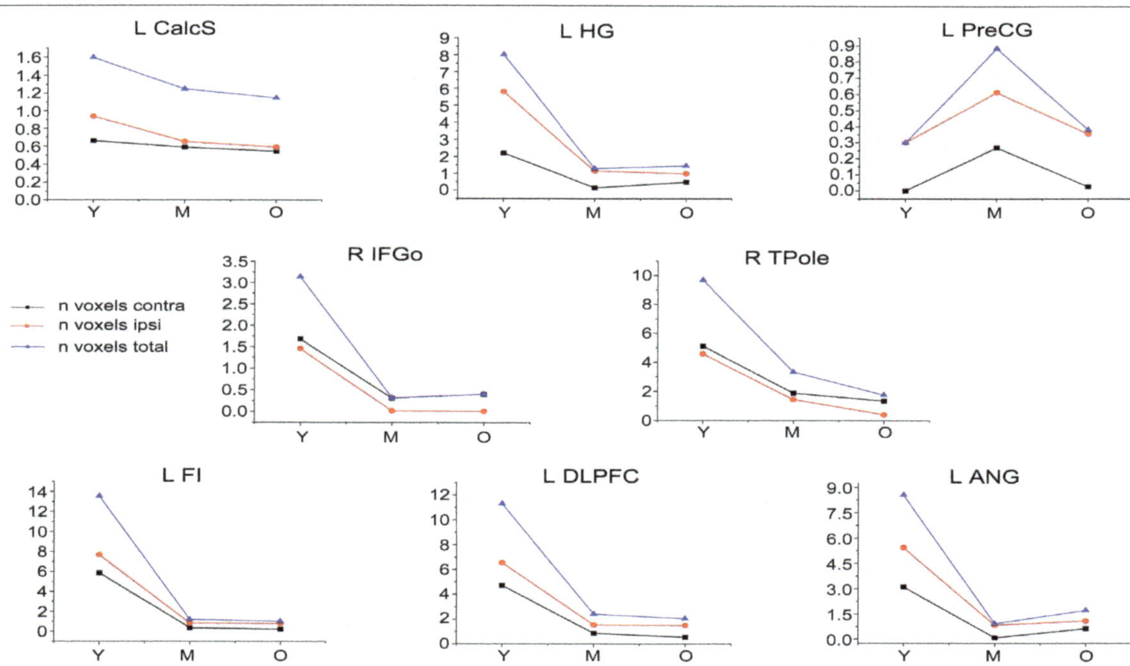

FIGURE A1 | Trajectories of the structural covariance networks derived from contralateral seeds. The plots of voxel counts by group ($P < 0.05$, FWE) indicate a similar pattern to the ipsilateral seed, except for the auditory and speech networks, which show differences in their spatial extents. The y-axis represents the voxel number ($\times 10^4$).

Abbreviations: Calcs, calcarine sulcus; HG, Heschl's gyrus; PreCG, precentral gyrus; IFGo, inferior frontal gyrus, pars opercularis; TPole, temporal pole; ANG, angular gyrus; DLPFC, dorsolateral prefrontal cortex; FI, frontoinsular cortex; R, right; L, left; Y, young group; M, middle-aged group; O, old group.

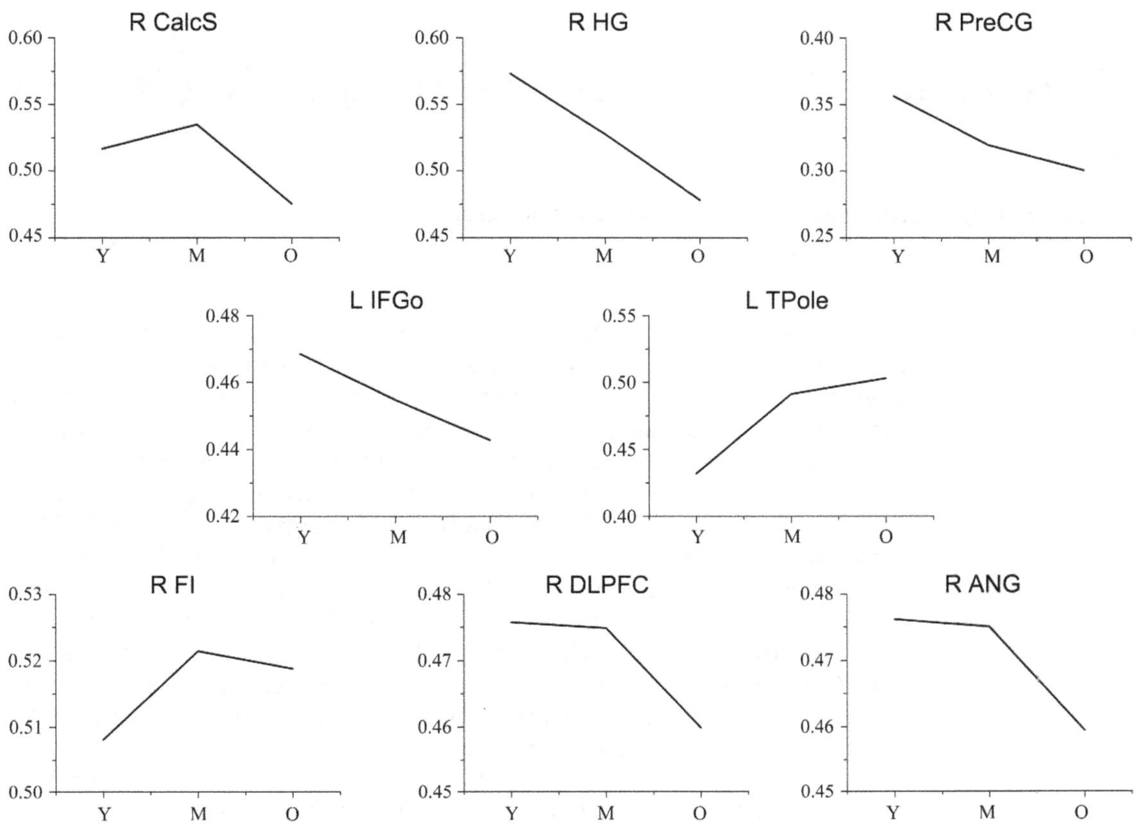

FIGURE A2 | Trajectories of the gray matter volume for each seed. The y-axis represents the mean gray matter volume for each age group. Abbreviations: Calcs, calcarine sulcus; HG, Heschl's gyrus; PreCG, precentral gyrus; IFGo, inferior frontal gyrus, pars opercularis; TPole, temporal pole; ANG, angular gyrus; DLPFC, dorsolateral prefrontal cortex; FI, frontoinsular cortex; R, right; L, left; Y, young group; M, middle-aged group; O, old group.

16

PANDA: A pipeline toolbox for analyzing brain diffusion images

Zaixu Cui, Suyu Zhong, Pengfei Xu, Yong He and Gaolang Gong*

State Key Laboratory of Cognitive Neuroscience and Learning, Beijing Normal University, Beijing, China

Correspondence:
Gaolang Gong, State Key Laboratory of Cognitive Neuroscience and Learning, Beijing Normal University, #19 Xinjiekouwai Street, Beijing 100875, China.
e-mail: gaolang.gong@bnu.edu.cn

Diffusion magnetic resonance imaging (dMRI) is widely used in both scientific research and clinical practice in *in-vivo* studies of the human brain. While a number of post-processing packages have been developed, fully automated processing of dMRI datasets remains challenging. Here, we developed a MATLAB toolbox named "Pipeline for Analyzing braiN Diffusion imAges" (PANDA) for fully automated processing of brain diffusion images. The processing modules of a few established packages, including FMRIB Software Library (FSL), Pipeline System for Octave and Matlab (PSOM), Diffusion Toolkit and MRIcron, were employed in PANDA. Using any number of raw dMRI datasets from different subjects, in either DICOM or NIfTI format, PANDA can automatically perform a series of steps to process DICOM/NIfTI to diffusion metrics [e.g., fractional anisotropy (FA) and mean diffusivity (MD)] that are ready for statistical analysis at the voxel-level, the atlas-level and the Tract-Based Spatial Statistics (TBSS)-level and can finish the construction of anatomical brain networks for all subjects. In particular, PANDA can process different subjects in parallel, using multiple cores either in a single computer or in a distributed computing environment, thus greatly reducing the time cost when dealing with a large number of datasets. In addition, PANDA has a friendly graphical user interface (GUI), allowing the user to be interactive and to adjust the input/output settings, as well as the processing parameters. As an open-source package, PANDA is freely available at http://www.nitrc.org/projects/panda/. This novel toolbox is expected to substantially simplify the image processing of dMRI datasets and facilitate human structural connectome studies.

Keywords: PANDA, diffusion MRI, DTI, pipeline, diffusion metrics, structural connectivity, network, connectome

INTRODUCTION

Diffusion magnetic resonance imaging (dMRI) has become one of the most popular MRI techniques for brain research. dMRI can be used to quantify white matter (WM) property and to virtually reconstruct WM pathways in the living brain (Le Bihan, 2003). Given its unique merits, dMRI has been extensively applied to the study of WM connectivity in both normal and abnormal conditions, leading to a substantial enhancement in our understanding of the role of WM, particularly in brain diseases (Johansen-Berg and Rushworth, 2009).

One popular application of dMRI is to extract various diffusion metrics [e.g., fractional anisotropy (FA) and mean diffusivity (MD)] that putatively reflect WM integrity (Basser and Pierpaoli, 1996; Pierpaoli and Basser, 1996; Beaulieu, 2002). These metrics can be further applied to identify differences in WM integrity across subjects. To perform this type of analysis, multiple sequential image-processing steps (e.g., eddy-current correction, tensor calculation, metric calculation, and normalization) are required. Currently, a number of packages, such as FMRIB Software Library (FSL) (Smith et al., 2004) and DTI-Studio (Jiang et al., 2006), provide a set of functions that can carry out these jobs. However, these packages typically perform the processing step-by-step and subject-by-subject. Obviously, this processing pattern is inefficient, as users have to wait until the preceding steps or until each subject is completely finished before initiating the next step or subject. In addition, this pattern requires a large amount of manual operation, which potentially increases the possibility of processing errors caused by manual mistakes. To date, a toolbox supporting fully automated processing of raw dMRI datasets to diffusion metrics that are ready for statistical analysis is still lacking.

Another popular application of dMRI is to virtually reconstruct WM tracts, referred to as diffusion tractography (Mori et al., 1999; Behrens et al., 2007). Previous studies using diffusion tractography mainly focus on a few specific WM tracts. Recently, accurately constructed entire brain anatomical networks (i.e., the connectome) based on diffusion tractography have attracted a lot of attention (Behrens and Sporns, 2012) and are the key target of the ongoing human connectome project (http://humanconnectome.org/). While the framework for constructing anatomical networks of the human brain (i.e., definition of network nodes and edges) has been established (Hagmann et al., 2008; Gong et al., 2009a,b), it is mainly implemented in-house. The community is in urgent need of a fully automated public tool that can construct anatomical brain networks using dMRI datasets.

Currently, there have been a few packages such as MIPAV (McAuliffe et al., 2001), JIST (Lucas et al., 2010), Nipype (Gorgolewski et al., 2011), and LONI (Dinov et al., 2009), which aim to facilitate automated processing of neuroimaging dataset.

Essentially, these packages provide environments for constructing analysis workflows with a number of pre-included processing modules from existing tools (e.g., Camino, FSL, AFNI, FreeSurfer, and SPM), and therefore various automated processing pipelines (e.g., a dMRI processing pipeline) can be developed within these environments. In order to construct pipelines with these packages, users need to choose processing modules and define dependencies and parameters themselves. It is noted that, if particular processing modules are not encapsulated [e.g., JIST does not include Tract-Based Spatial Statistics (TBSS) analysis], users have to develop their own modules and further incorporate them into the environment. While these powerful and sophisticated packages make it possible to generate a dMRI processing pipeline, they are favored by developers, and not end users without programming skills. A ready-for-use pipeline tool for dMRI processing is highly desired, particularly for end users.

Here, we present a MATLAB toolbox named PANDA (a Pipeline for Analyzing braiN Diffusion imAges) for a comprehensive pipeline processing of dMRI dataset, aiming to facilitate image processing for the across-subject analysis of diffusion metrics and brain network constructions. Of note, the processing pipelines in this toolbox have been completely set up, allowing the end-users of dMRI to process the data immediately. Moreover, the processing procedures within this pipeline were carefully designed to follow the recommended practice as possible (Jones et al., 2012). After the user sets the input/output and processing parameters through the friendly graphical user interface (GUI), PANDA fully automates all processing steps for datasets of any number of subjects, and results in data pertaining to many diffusion metrics that are ready for statistical analysis at three levels (Voxel-level, ROI-level, and TBSS-level). Additionally, anatomical brain networks can be automatically generated using either deterministic or probabilistic tractography techniques. Particularly, PANDA can run processing jobs in parallel with multiple cores either in a single computer or within a distributed computing environment using a Sun Grid Engine (SGE) system, thus allowing for maximum usage of the available computing resources.

To assess the usability and validity of PANDA, we apply PANDA to study the age effect (i.e., old vs. young) on the diffusion metrics of WM as well as the topological properties of the WM network. According to previous findings, decreased WM anisotropy and weakened network efficiency are expected in old individuals.

MATERIALS AND METHODS

PANDA was developed by using MATLAB under an Ubuntu Operating System. A number of processing functions from FSL (Smith et al., 2004), Pipeline System for Octave and Matlab (PSOM) (Bellec et al., 2012), Diffusion Toolkit (Wang et al., 2007), and MRIcron (http://www.mccauslandcenter.sc.edu/mricro/mricron/) were called by PANDA. Here, we will describe the procedures of pipeline processing in PANDA, followed by an introduction to the realization of pipelines.

PANDA PROCESSING PROCEDURES

The main procedure of PANDA is shown in **Figure 1** and includes three steps: (1) preprocessing; (2) producing diffusion metrics (ready for statistical analysis); and (3) constructing networks.

Preprocessing

Converting DICOM files into NIfTI images. The input files of PANDA can be in either DICOM or NIfTI format. If the input files are in NIfTI format, this conversion step will be skipped. Otherwise, DICOM files will be converted into NIfTI format during this step. The *dcm2nii* tool embedded in MRIcron accomplished this task.

Estimating the brain mask. This step yields the brain mask by using the *bet* command of FSL (Smith, 2002). The brain mask is required for the subsequent processing steps. Here, the b0 image without diffusion weighting was used for the estimation.

Cropping the raw images. To reduce the memory cost and speed up the processing in subsequent steps we cut off the non-brain space in the raw images, leading to a reduced image size. The acquired brain mask was used to determine the borders of the brain along the three dimensions. The *fslroi* command of FSL was then applied to remove the non-brain spaces.

Correcting for the eddy-current effect. Eddy-current induced distortion of diffusion weighted images (DWI), as well as simple head-motion during scanning, can be corrected by registering the DW images to the b0 image with an affine transformation. To achieve this, the *flirt* command of FSL was used. Notably, this registering procedure was applied to all images, with the b0 image of first acquisition used as the target if multiple DWI acquisitions were scanned. It is worth mentioning that while the *eddy_correct* command of FSL is not called here, the result of this step is exactly the same as the output of *eddy_correct*. Basically, PANDA just splits the 4D file (the input file of *eddy_correct*) into a number of 3D files and then performed the affine-registration exactly like *eddy_correct*. The purpose of this implementation is to avoid the large memory demand when the 4D file size is huge. Finally, the gradient direction of each DWI volume was rotated according to the resultant affine transformations (Leemans and Jones, 2009).

Averaging multiple acquisitions. This step will be skipped if there is only one DWI acquisition. Otherwise, after eddy-current correction, the aligned multiple DWI was averaged by calling the *fslmaths* command of FSL.

Calculating diffusion tensor (DT) metrics. This step involves a voxel-wise calculation of the tensor matrix and the DT metrics, including FA, MD, axial diffusivity (AD), and radial diffusivity (RD) (Pierpaoli and Basser, 1996; Song et al., 2002). The *dtifit* command of FSL was applied.

Producing diffusion metrics that are ready for statistical analysis

Normalizing. To allow for comparison across subjects, location correspondence has to be established. To end this, registration of all the individual images to a standardized template is always applied. Here, PANDA non-linearly registered individual

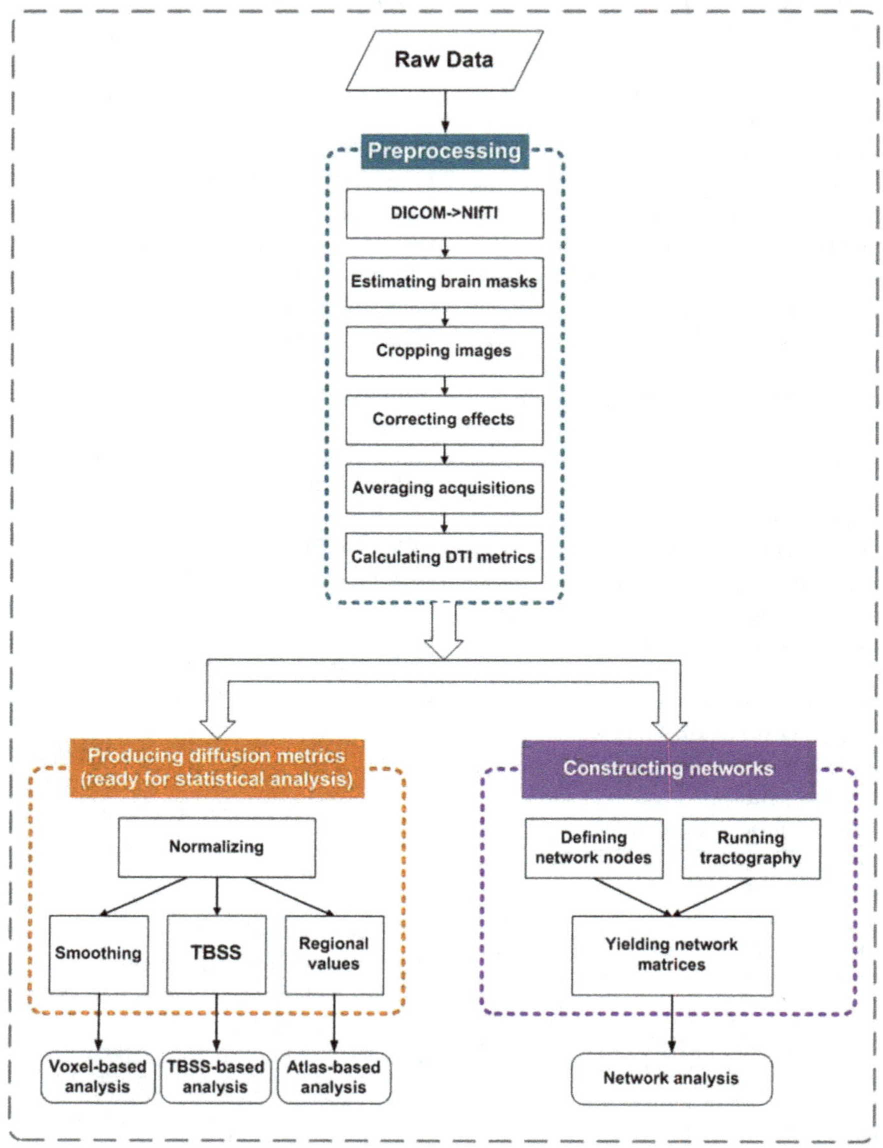

FIGURE 1 | Main procedure for pipeline processing of dMRI datasets in PANDA. The procedure includes three parts: (1) preprocessing; (2) producing diffusion metrics that are ready for statistical analysis; and (3) constructing networks.

FA images of native space to the FA template in the MNI space by calling the *fnirt* command of FSL. The resultant warping transformations were then used to resample the images of the diffusion metrics (i.e., FA, MD, AD, and RD) into the MNI space with a customized spatial resolution (e.g., 1 × 1 × 1 mm or 2 × 2 × 2 mm). This resampling step was implemented by the *applywarp* command of FSL.

Output for voxel-based analysis. The resultant images of the diffusion metrics in the standard space are ready for voxel-based statistical analysis. However, in the framework of voxel-based analysis, these images are typically smoothed to some degree, which can reduce the effect of image noise and misalignment between subjects. Accordingly, PANDA smoothed the images with a given Gaussian kernel, which was realized by calling the *fslmaths* command of FSL. The smoothed diffusion metric images can then be directly used for voxel-based statistical analysis with any preferred tools, e.g., FSL (http://www.fmrib.ox.ac.uk/fsl/), SPM (http://www.fil.ion.ucl.ac.uk/spm/), or AFNI (http://afni.nimh.nih.gov/afni/).

Output for atlas-based analysis. In addition to the popular voxel-based method of analysis, diffusion metrics can be analyzed at the level of region of interests (ROI), which may provide better statistical sensitivity in some cases (Faria et al., 2010). Recently, a few WM atlases (e.g., the ICBM-DTI-81 WM labels atlas and the JHU WM tractography atlas) have been proposed (Mori et al., 2008). These WM atlases in the standard space allow for parcellation of the entire WM into multiple ROIs, each representing a labeled region in the atlas. To support ROI-based analysis, PANDA calculates the regional diffusion metrics (i.e., FA, MD, AD, and RD) by averaging the values within each region of the WM atlases. These resultant ROI-based data (saved as text files) can be statistically analyzed with SPSS (http://www-01.ibm.com/software/analytics/spss/) and other statistical packages.

Output for TBSS-based analysis. The TBSS framework avoids the necessity of choosing a spatial smoothing procedure during voxel-based analysis and may provide better sensitivity and interpretability when it is applied to multi-subjects dMRI datasets (Smith et al., 2006). To support this type of analysis, PANDA follows the standard TBSS framework. Firstly, the mean of all the aligned FA images was created and skeletonized, resulting in a mean FA skeleton. Secondly, the diffusion metric data from individual subjects were projected onto the skeleton. Finally, individual images with data on the skeleton were created. The resultant images can be directly used for voxel-wise statistical analysis on the skeleton. Here, the *fslmaths* and *tbss_skeleton* commands of FSL were employed.

Constructing networks

Two basic elements are required for a network: a node and a connection. Thus, the central tasks for constructing brain networks are: (1) defining network nodes and (2) defining connections between nodes. The schematic flowchart of network construction is demonstrated in **Figure 2**.

Defining network nodes. Typically, the entire brain is divided into multiple regions using a prior gray matter (GM) atlas, where each region represents a network node (Bullmore and Sporns, 2009). However, the prior atlases are generally defined in the standard space and need to be transformed to the native dMRI space of each individual. To address this, PANDA uses the framework

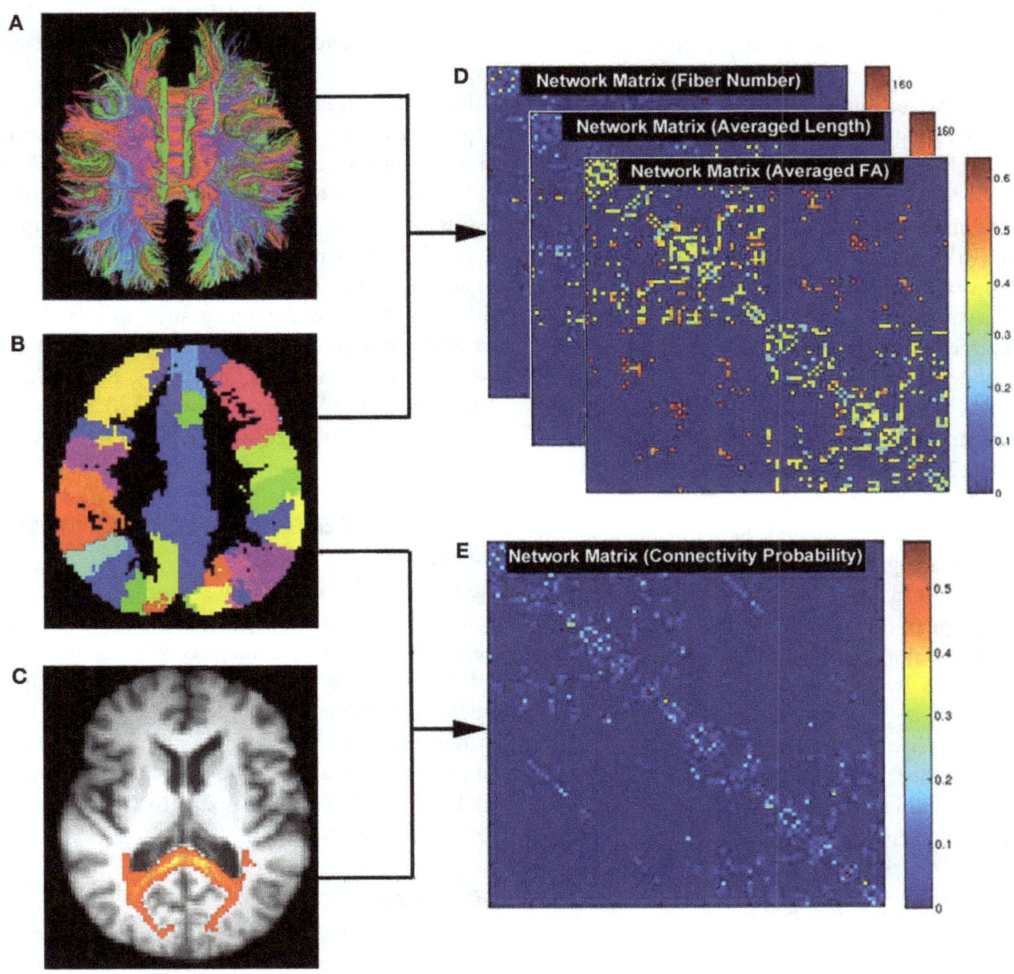

FIGURE 2 | Flowchart for constructing anatomical brain networks using diffusion tractography in PANDA. (A) White matter tracts reconstructed using deterministic tractography. **(B)** Parcellation of gray matter in diffusion space. Each color represents a node in a brain network. **(C)** White matter connectivity maps using FSL probabilistic tractography. **(D)** Three resultant network matrices weighted by fiber number, averaged length, and averaged FA. **(E)** The network matrix weighted by connectivity probability.

proposed by Gong et al. (2009a). Specifically, the individual FA image in native space was co-registered to its corresponding structural image (i.e., T1-weighted) using an affine transformation. The individual structural image was then non-linearly registered to the ICBM152 template. Based on the resultant transformations in these two steps, an inverse warping transformation from the standard space to the native dMRI space can be obtained. Prior atlases in the standard space were then inversely warped back to individual native space by applying this inverse transformation. Currently, PANDA provides two well-defined atlases: the Automated Anatomical Labeling (AAL) (Tzourio-Mazoyer et al., 2002) atlas and the Harvard-Oxford atlas (HOA) (http://www.cma.mgh.harvard.edu/fslatlas.html). Notably, users can import customized atlases into PANDA to define the network nodes. During this step, the *flirt*, *fnirt*, *inwarp*, and *applywarp* commands of FSL were used.

Constructing networks using deterministic tractography. In general, deterministic tractography assumes a deterministic fiber orientation at every location during tracking, typically ending up with 3D trajectories for reconstructed WM tracts. Here, the *dti_recon* and *dti_tracker* commands of the Diffusion Toolkit (http://trackvis.org/dtk/) were called to reconstruct all possible fibers within the brain by seeding from all the WM voxels. For every pair of brain nodes/regions defined above, fibers with two end-points located in their respective masks were considered to link the two nodes. Based on the linking fibers, PANDA calculated three basic weighted matrices: *number-weighted matrix* (M^N), *FA-weighted matrix* (M^{FA}), and *length-weighted matrix* (M^L). In the matrices, each row or column represents a brain region/node. The values of the elements $M(i, j)^N$, $M(i, j)^{FA}$, and $M(i, j)^L$ represent the number, averaged FA and averaged length of linking fibers between node i and node j, respectively. The resultant matrices were saved as a MATLAB data file and can be directly used for topological analysis with graph theoretic approaches (Bullmore and Sporns, 2009; Bullmore and Bassett, 2011).

Constructing networks using probabilistic tractography. In contrast, probabilistic tractography typically runs the tracking procedure many times, and fiber orientation is determined probabilistically. This type of tractography may improve tracking sensitivity, particularly for non-dominant fibers. The probabilistic tractography proposed by Behrens et al. (2003, 2007) has been implemented in FSL and is called by PANDA for network construction. This process involves two steps as follows:

BedpostX. Using the Markov Chain Monte Carlo sampling technique, this module estimated the local probability distribution of fiber direction at each voxel, a prerequisite for running subsequent probabilistic tractography (Behrens et al., 2003). In PANDA, bedpostX was realized by calling the *xfibres* command of FSL.

Probabilistic Tractography and Network Construction. Network construction using FSL-based probabilistic tractography has been previously described (Gong et al., 2009b). Briefly, for each defined brain region/node, probabilistic tractography was performed by seeding from all voxels of this region. For each voxel, 5000 fibers were sampled. To achieve this, the *probtrackx* command of FSL was called. The connectivity probability from the seed region i to another region j was defined by the number of fibers passing through region j divided by the total number of fibers sampled from region i. The connectivity probability of each node to the other nodes within the brain network can be calculated by repeating the tractography procedure for all nodes. This leads to an individual-specific weighted matrix, whose rows and columns represent the brain nodes and whose elements represent the connectivity probability between nodes. This matrix can also be directly used for various network analyses.

REALIZATION OF PIPELINES

PSOM is a flexible framework for the implementation of pipelines in the form of Octave or Matlab scripts (Bellec et al., 2012), and was employed to build up the processing pipeline in our study. Here, a pipeline refers to a collection of jobs with a well identified set of options that use files for inputs and outputs. The entire processing flow of PANDA includes 41 steps, each of which is a job within the PANDA pipeline. Notably, more steps can be added if new functions or processing steps are included. The workflow of the current PANDA pipeline showing all the jobs and their associated dependencies is illustrated in Appendix A.

In particular, PANDA was designed to allow for jobs running in parallel either on a single computer with multiple cores or on a computing cluster. Notably, the PANDA processing steps are parallelizable at multiple levels. For example, the same processing steps (i.e., preprocessing) for a group of subjects can be parallelized, since the steps are independent across subjects. In addition, for the same subject, different processing steps without between-dependency such as *producing diffusion metrics* and *brain parcellation* can be parallelized as well. Finally, a few very time-consuming steps (i.e., *BedpostX* and *Probabilistic Tractography and Network Construction*) have been internally parallelized. The parallelizing strategies in PANDA are demonstrated in **Figure 3**.

TESTING THE AGE EFFECT ON WM CONNECTIVITY BY USING PANDA

Subjects

The test included data from 23 young adults (males, 11; females, 12; age, 17–24 years) and 17 elderly individuals (males, 8; females, 9; age, 54–77 years). All subjects were recruited from the campus and the local community. Subjects with a history of neurological or psychiatric disorders were excluded from this study. Written informed consent was obtained from each subject, and the protocol was approved by the Ethics Committee of the State Key Laboratory of Cognitive Neuroscience and Learning, Beijing Normal University.

MRI acquisition

All scans were performed using the 3-T Siemens Tim Trio MRI scanner in the Imaging Center for Brain Research, Beijing Normal University. Diffusion MRI was acquired using a single-shot echo-planar imaging-based sequence with following parameters: coverage of the whole brain; slice thickness, 2 mm; no gap; 68 axial slices; repetition time (TR), 9000 ms; echo time (TE), 92 ms; flip angle, 90°; 66 non-linear diffusion weighting directions with

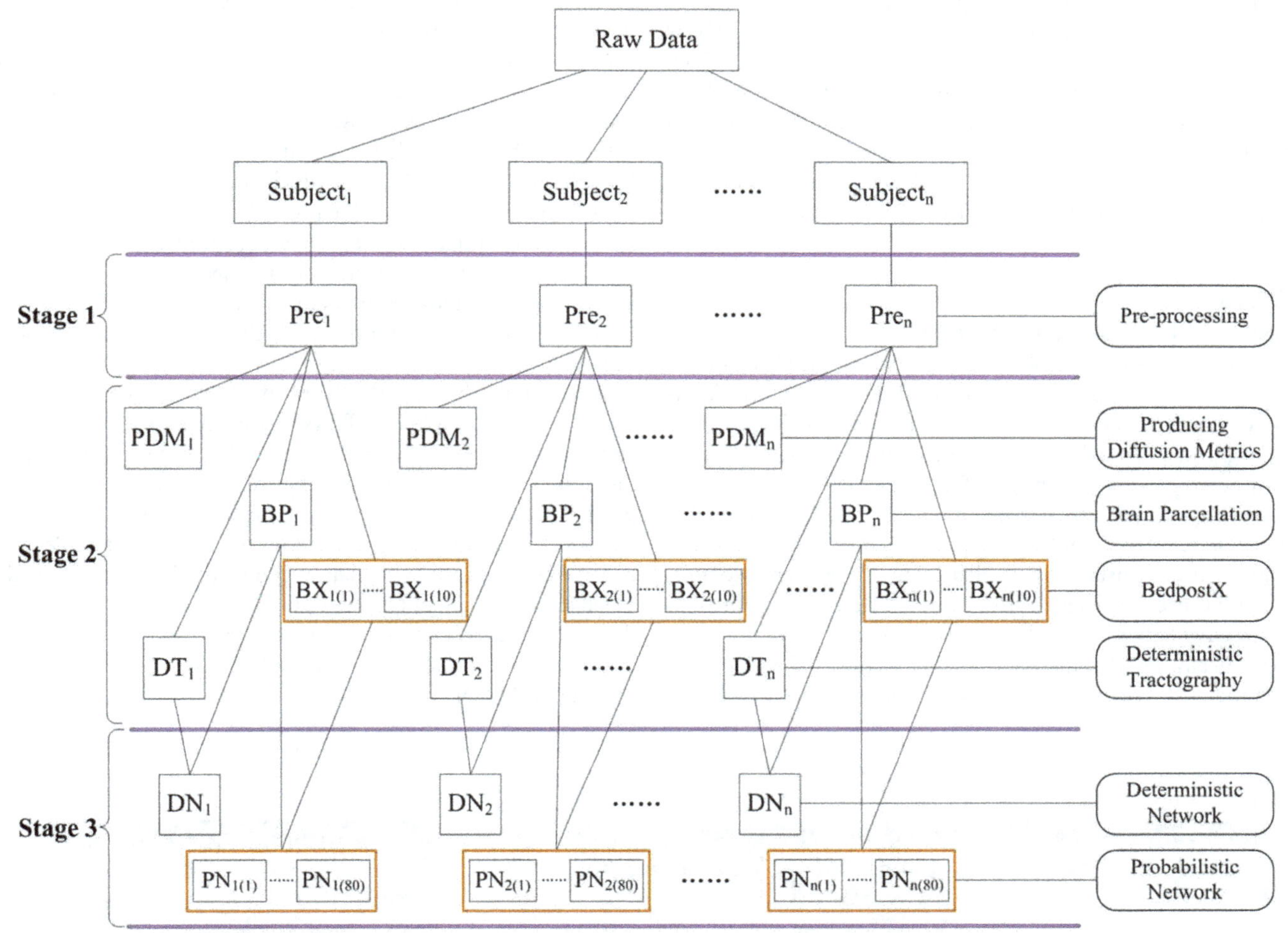

FIGURE 3 | The schematic parallelizing strategy of PANDA. For example, pre-processing steps in Stage 1 are parallelizable across subjects. Independent processing steps from the same subject or across subjects in Stage 2 and Stage 3 can be parallelized as well. In addition, *BedpostX* and *Probabilistic Network Construction* have been internally parallelized, as indicated by orange boxes.

$b = 1000\,\text{s/mm}^2$ and one image without diffusion weighting (i.e., $b = 0\,\text{s/mm}^2$); 4 repetitive acquisitions; acquisition matrix, 128×124; field of view (FOV), $256 \times 248\,\text{mm}^2$; resolution, $2 \times 2 \times 2\,\text{mm}$. Three-dimensional T1-weighted images with high resolution were obtained using a three-dimensional magnetization prepared rapid gradient echo (MP-RAGE) sequence with the following parameters: 1 mm slice thickness without gap; 176 sagittal slices; TR, 1900 ms; TE, 3.44 ms; flip angle, 9°; acquisition matrix, 256×256; FOV, $256 \times 256\,\text{mm}^2$; resolution, $1 \times 1 \times 1\,\text{mm}$.

Image processing

The whole pipeline procedure of PANDA was run on all dMRI datasets with an in-house computing cluster of 6 nodes, each with 30GB of memory and 12 Intel Xeon E5649 2.53 GHz cores. For each pipeline step, default parameters were chosen.

Network topology

Graph theoretical approaches have been applied to characterize the topology of brain networks that are derived from neuroimaging data (Bullmore and Sporns, 2009). Here, we focus on two topological network parameters: global efficiency and local efficiency. Global efficiency was defined as the average of the inverse of the "harmonic mean" of the characteristic path length, which represents global information transferring ability within the network (Latora and Marchiori, 2001). Local efficiency quantifies the ability of the network fault tolerant, corresponding to the efficiency of the information flow between nodal neighbors. Specifically, local efficiency was defined as the average of nodal local efficiency that is computed as the global efficiency of the subgraph composed by its nearest neighbors (Latora and Marchiori, 2001).

Statistical analysis

For diffusion metric, we tested the group difference on FA across the entire WM. Specifically, normalized and smoothed (6 mm Gaussian kernel) FA images produced by PANDA were employed for this voxel-based analysis. A general linear model (GLM) with gender being taken as a covariate was applied to each WM voxel. For multiple comparison correction, false discovery ratio (FDR) was applied, and $p < 0.01$ was considered as significant.

For each subject, the FA-weighted matrix generated from PANDA was selected for topological analysis. Each matrix is 78 × 78 and represents the WM network of cerebral cortex. Each row or column of the matrix represents a cortical region of the AAL template (Gong et al., 2009a,b). The global efficiency and local efficiency were then calculated. To test the group effect on the global and local efficiency, a GLM with gender and brain size as covariates was applied, and $p < 0.05$ was chosen as the significant level.

RESULTS

AN INTEGRATED MATLAB TOOLBOX: PANDA

An integrated MATLAB toolbox named PANDA has been developed for fully automated processing of dMRI datasets, which is an open-source package and is freely available at http://www.nitrc.org/projects/panda. An online discussion forum (http://www.nitrc.org/forum/forum.php?forumid=2731) and a mailing list (http://www.nitrc.org/mailman/listinfo/panda-commits) have been registered for PANDA, and technical supports and updates will be constantly provided by the developers. Notably, PANDA has been packaged with PSOM, MRIcron, and Diffusion Toolkit. Only FSL is required to be installed separately.

Specifically, PANDA includes a main function and a set of separate modules/utilities. Using the main function, PANDA can run pipeline processing for any number of subjects, after raw dMRI datasets are loaded into the program. This running mode will finish all processing steps and end up with all outputs as described in "Materials and Methods." In contrast, the utilities can be used separately for specific processing steps (e.g., DICOM conversion, TBSS, and brain parcellation). Particularly, PANDA has a very friendly GUI (**Figure 4**), with which users can perform various interactions with the embedded functions, e.g., setting inputs or outputs and configuring the processing parameters. In addition, PANDA can provide the status of the ongoing pipeline processing in real-time, allowing users to monitor progress through the GUI. The detailed descriptions for GUIs of PANDA are included in Appendix B.

As provided by PSOM (Bellec et al., 2012), PANDA has a number of advantages as follows: (1) it can run jobs in parallel either in a single computer with multiple cores or in a computing cluster; (2) it can generate log files and keep track of the pipeline execution; (3) if the program terminates before finishing, users can load a configuration file, click "RUN," and PANDA will restart from the termination point; (4) if users re-run the pipelines after changing some options, PANDA will only restart the procedures related to these options; and (5) the jobs will run in the background and PANDA & MATLAB can be closed after clicking the "RUN" button.

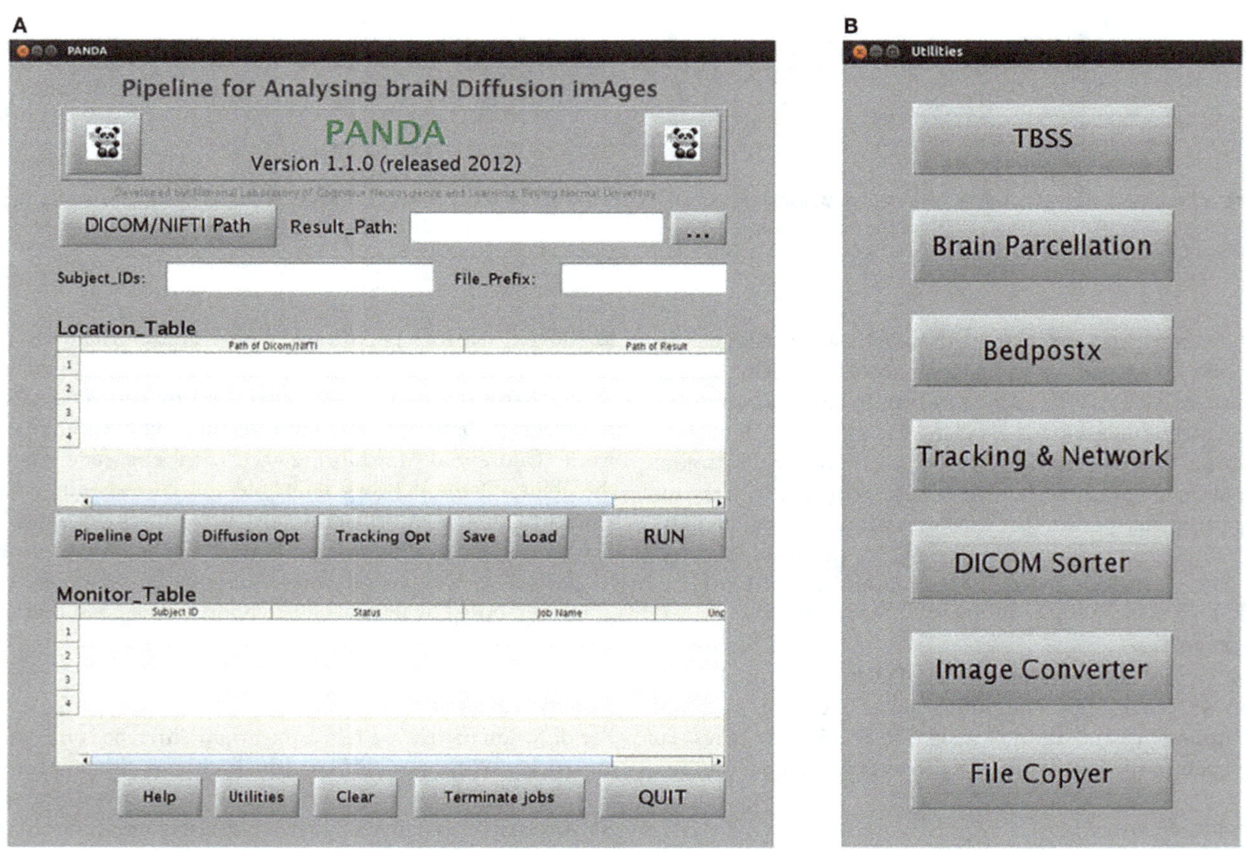

FIGURE 4 | A snapshot of the GUIs of PANDA. (A) The main GUI for loading dataset and monitoring job status. **(B)** The GUI for initiating separate utilities.

RESULTANT FILES OF PANDA

For each subject, PANDA generates six folders containing resultant files, as listed in **Table 1**. Specifically, the *native_space* folder consists of all images and files in the native space. The files in the *quality_control* folder include 2D snapshot pictures of FA, T1, normalized FA, and normalized T1, which can be quickly viewed to check the quality of the data and related registrations (**Figure 5**). All files of the diffusion metrics that are ready for statistical analysis are stored in the folder named *standard_space*. The *trackvis* folder consists of resultant files generated by the "Diffusion Toolkit" for deterministic tractography, which can be opened with Trackvis. The *native_space.bedpostx* folder contains the resultant files of bedpostX that are required for FSL probabilistic tractography. Finally, the MATLAB files containing the network matrices with different weighting (i.e., fiber number, averaged FA, averaged length, and connectivity probability) are stored in the folder named *network*.

TIME COST

To provide information about the time cost of PANDA procedures, a few baseline running-time tests were conducted. Specifically, two dMRI datasets with different acquisition schemes (dataset I: 64 directions, 4 repetitive acquisitions, resolution: $2 \times 2 \times 2$ mm; dataset II: 30 directions, 2 repetitive acquisitions, resolution: $2.2 \times 2.2 \times 2.2$ mm) were tested under four conditions (one subject with four cores; one subject with eight cores; two subjects with four cores; two subjects with eight cores). The results are listed in **Table 2**.

Obviously, the running time depends on dMRI scanning schemes. More DWI directions and more repetitive acquisitions will result in longer running time of *preprocessing* and *bedpostX*. Our results further demonstrated that the running-time for multiple subjects with multiple cores in PANDA can be effectively saved, due to the parallelized processing. For example, finishing the pre-processing steps for two subjects costs almost the same time as for one subject (**Table 2**). In addition, since the *bedpostX* has been parallelized internally, finishing *bedpostX* with eight cores cost only half of time as cost with four cores (**Table 2**).

THE AGE EFFECT ON WM CONNECTIVITY USING PANDA

As expected, voxel-based comparison revealed a distributed FA decreases ($p < 0.01$, FDR corrected) throughout the brain in the old group. Specifically, FA was mainly affected in the bilateral superior longitudinal fasciculus, uncinate fasciculus, internal capsules, external capsules, fornices, and corpus callosum (**Figure 6**).

Moreover, we observed group differences in topological efficiencies of WM network of cerebral cortex. As demonstrated in **Figure 7**, the global efficiency of the WM network showed a significant reduction in the old group ($p = 0.03$) after controlling for gender and brain size, and the local efficiency exhibited only a trend of reduction ($p = 0.16$).

DISCUSSION

In this study, we have developed a MATLAB toolbox named PANDA for comprehensively processing dMRI datasets. The key advantage of PANDA is that it fully automates all the processing steps of dMRI datasets for any number of subjects. PANDA can yield diffusion metric data that is ready for statistical analysis at three levels (voxel-level, atlas-level, and TBSS-level), and can generate anatomical networks/matrices of the entire brain using either deterministic or probabilistic diffusion tractography.

Table 1 | Folders produced by PANDA.

Folder name	Files
native_space	Text files of bvals and bvecs
	Native-space images of DWI, b0, brain mask, FA, MD, AD, RD, and parcellation mask
quality_control	Snapshot pictures of native FA, native T1, normalized FA, and normalized T1
standard_space	Normalized images of FA, MD, AD, and RD (ready for voxel-based analysis)
	Text files of regional FA, MD, AD, and RD (ready for ROI-based analysis)
	Images of skeletonized FA, MD, AD, and RD (ready for TBSS analysis)
trackvis	Trackvis-related resultant files (for deterministic tractography)
native_space bedpostx	BedpostX-related resultant files (for probabilistic tractography)
network	MATLAB files containing network matrices weighted by fiber number, averaged FA, averaged length (from deterministic tractography), and connectivity probability (from probabilistic tractography)

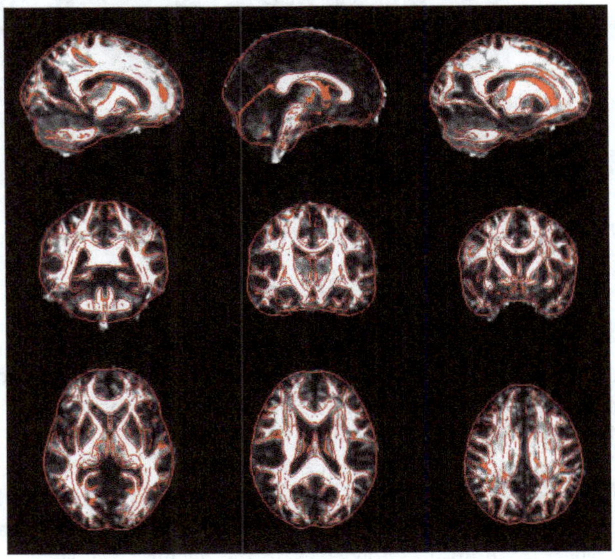

FIGURE 5 | Snapshot pictures for quality control of FA normalization. The normalized FA is overlaid with image edges that were derived from the FA template. These pictures can be quickly viewed to check the quality of normalization.

Table 2 | Baseline time cost of pipeline processing on dataset I (64 DWI directions, 4 repetitive acquisitions, resolution: 2 × 2 × 2 mm) and dataset II (30 DWI directions, 2 repetitive acquisitions, resolution: 2.2 × 2.2 × 2.2 mm) with PANDA.

Dataset I Dataset II	Time cost (h)			
	One subject Four cores	**One subject Eight cores**	**Two subjects Four cores**	**Two subjects Eight cores**
Preprocessing and producing data that is ready for statistical analysis	0.883 0.167	0.900 0.150	0.917 0.217	0.900 0.183
Brain parcellation (for network node definition)	0.167 0.133	0.167 0.133	0.167 0.183	0.150 0.183
Deterministic tractography and network construction (AAL template 90)	0.067 0.017	0.050 0.017	0.050 0.033	0.067 0.033
BedpostX	3.667 1.467	2.317 0.883	7.117 2.933	4.233 1.650
Probabilistic tractography and network construction (AAL template 90)	6.017 3.283	3.683 1.917	11.883 6.583	6.750 3.633

The processing was performed using a local workstation with 30 GB of memory and Intel Xeon E5649 2.53 GHz cores. Four conditions were tested: one subject with four cores; two subjects with four cores; one subject with eight cores; two subjects with eight cores.

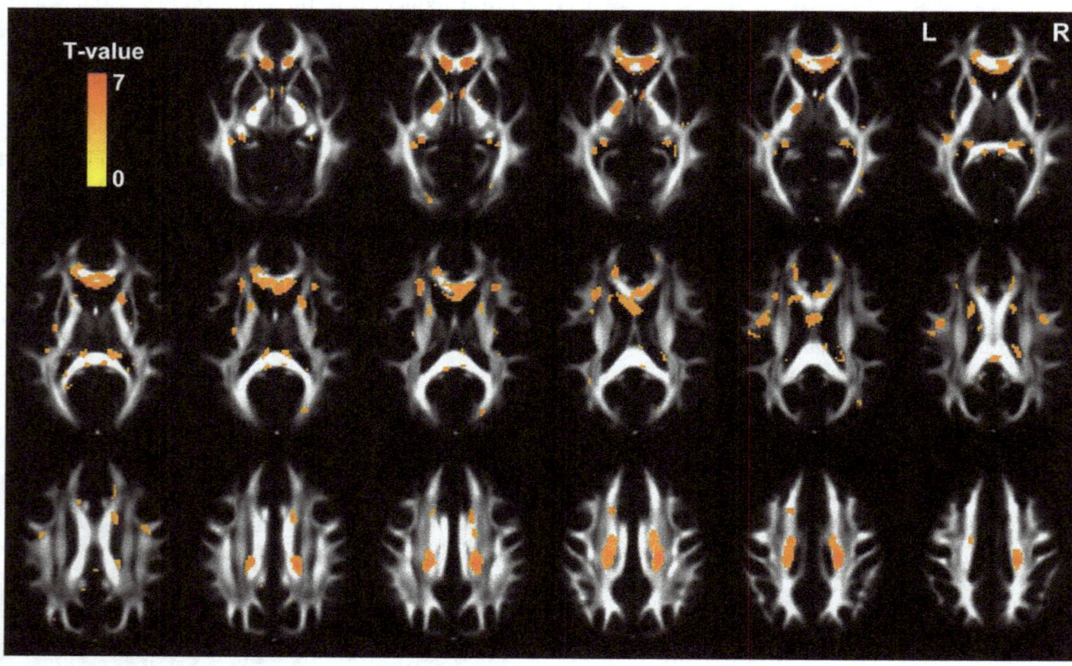

FIGURE 6 | The statistical map showing significant FA decreases in old group ($p < 0.01$, FDR corrected). The hot color represents *t* values for the age effect.

A fully automated pipeline naturally makes the data processing efficient, at the same time reducing potential mistakes by avoiding manual processing of individual steps. While constructing a dMRI processing pipeline with MIPAV (McAuliffe et al., 2001), JIST (Lucas et al., 2010), Nipype (Gorgolewski et al., 2011), or LONI (Dinov et al., 2009) is possible, it requires prior knowledge on pipeline design and programming skills related to these packages. In addition, knowledge on the details of all steps for processing dMRI dataset is required, which might be another challenge for end users. To provide a ready-for-use pipeline tool for end users, PANDA was developed, making it possible to process dMRI datasets immediately with established pipelines.

Notably, there exist differences in the processing procedures across existing dMRI packages, and some important processing steps might be overlooked (Jones et al., 2012). These issues have been well discussed by a few recent articles (Jones and Cercignani, 2010; Jones et al., 2012). The processing pipelines of PANDA have tried to follow the best practice as possible. For example, the adjustment of diffusion gradient directions after eddy-current correction, which has been frequently missed (Leemans and Jones, 2009; Jones et al., 2012), has been included in the PANDA pipeline. In future versions, PANDA will keep being updated to include processing steps of the best practice at the moment.

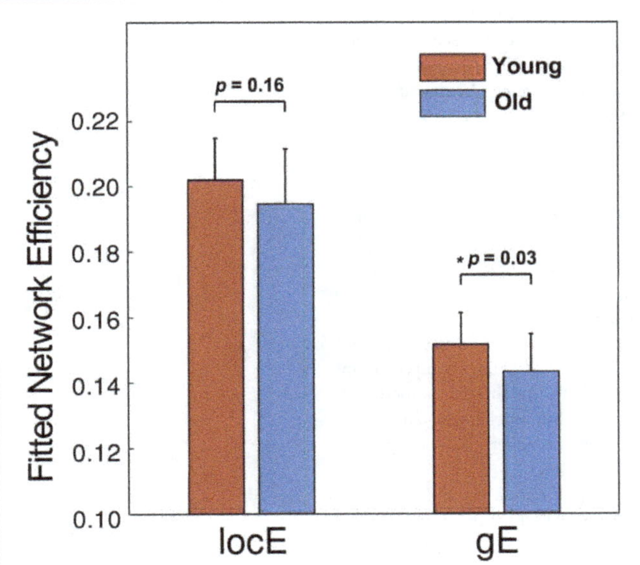

FIGURE 7 | The group comparison of network efficiency. The old group showed a significant reduction of global efficiency and a trend of reduction in local efficiency.

Another advantage of PANDA is that both sequential and parallel processing modes are supported, which makes it possible to take full advantage of available computing resources. The parallel environment can be either a single computer with multiple cores or a computing cluster, which increasingly enters into labs around the world. As shown in **Figure 3**, the PANDA processing have been parallelized as much as possible, and can thus reduce the time cost substantially under a parallel processing mode. For instance, the running time for pre-processing two subjects is almost the same as for one subject by using a workstation with four cores.

Finally, PANDA has a very friendly GUI (**Figure 4**), allowing the advanced users to select the desired options for each processing step. Depending on the datasets, users may change the options of some processing steps to optimize the processing quality. The reference data, e.g., image templates for normalization or prior atlases for node definition, can also be replaced by customized data, making it possible for processing dMRI data of non-human (e.g., primate) brains.

In the present study, we applied PANDA to produce results for testing the age effect on WM diffusion metrics as well as topological properties of the WM network. Significant FA reductions during aging were found in the bilateral uncinate fasciculus, superior longitudinal fasciculus, external capsules, fornices and corpus callosum, which are highly consistent with previous findings (Bennett et al., 2010; Michielse et al., 2010). In addition, significant reduction of global efficiency and a trend of reduction of local efficiency were observed in the old group. These topological changes are largely compatible with our previous results that are based on a larger dataset (Gong et al., 2009b). The declined WM connectivity and topology may underlie various patterns of cognitive decline during normal aging. The results for this specific study prove the usability and validity of the PANDA processing.

PANDA is of great applicability in the area of connectivity neuroscience. For example, this tool can be applied to dMRI datasets that are collected to study various connectivity hypotheses. Also, the effects of dMRI processing parameters or steps on the final connectivity results can be easily tested by using PANDA. Recently, the term "connectome" has been proposed to advocate efforts for comprehensively mapping and analyzing brain connectivity and networks (Sporns et al., 2005), and dMRI has been taken as a primary technique for structural macro-connectome (Behrens and Sporns, 2012). This will lead to a large number of dMRI datasets in the foreseeable future (http://humanconnectome.org/). To process these connectome dataset, PANDA has unique advantages, as it can handle the large number of datasets very efficiently because of its parallelizing strategies. Meanwhile, it can automatically provide important metrics of interest (e.g., diffusion metrics of brain connectivity and brain network matrices) for connectome studies. Therefore, PANDA can potentially make contributions to the study of the human connectome in the near future.

In summary, PANDA can substantially facilitate/simplify image processing in a dMRI-related study, and can provide measures for WM connectivity and network analysis. It has an extendable design framework, and new functions or utilities can and will be added in the future.

ACKNOWLEDGMENTS

The authors sincerely thank all the developers of FSL, PSOM, Diffusion Toolkit, and MRIcron, whose functions are called by PANDA. In addition, the authors thank Dr. Pierre Bellec for his support when implementing PSOM to PANDA, and thank Dr. Yanchao Bi for English editing. This work was supported by the National Science Foundation of China (No. 31000499, 81271649, 81030028), the Beijing Nova Program (No. Z121110002512032), the 973 program (No. 2013CB837300), and Open Research Fund of the State Key Laboratory of Cognitive Neuroscience and Learning.

REFERENCES

Basser, P. J., and Pierpaoli, C. (1996). Microstructural and physiological features of tissues elucidated by quantitative-diffusion-tensor MRI. *J. Magn. Reson. B* 111, 209–219.

Beaulieu, C. (2002). The basis of anisotropic water diffusion in the nervous system – a technical review. *NMR Biomed.* 15, 435–455.

Behrens, T. E. J., and Sporns, O. (2012). Human connectomics. *Curr. Opin. Neurobiol.* 22, 144–153.

Behrens, T., Berg, H. J., Jbabdi, S., Rushworth, M., and Woolrich, M. (2007). Probabilistic diffusion tractography with multiple fibre orientations: what can we gain? *Neuroimage* 34, 144–155.

Behrens, T., Woolrich, M., Jenkinson, M., Johansen-Berg, H., Nunes, R., Clare, S., et al. (2003). Characterization and propagation of uncertainty in diffusion-weighted MR imaging. *Magn. Reson. Med.* 50, 1077–1088.

Bellec, P., Lavoie-Courchesne, S., Dickinson, P., Lerch, J. P., Zijdenbos, A. P., and Evans, A. C. (2012). The pipeline system for Octave and Matlab (PSOM): a lightweight scripting framework and execution engine for scientific workflows. *Front. Neuroinform.* 6:7. doi: 10.3389/fninf.2012.00007

Bennett, I. J., Madden, D. J., Vaidya, C. J., Howard, D. V., and Howard, J. H. Jr. (2010). Age-related differences in multiple measures of white matter integrity: a diffusion tensor imaging study of healthy aging. *Hum. Brain Mapp.* 31, 378–390.

Bullmore, E., and Sporns, O. (2009). Complex brain networks: graph theoretical analysis of structural and functional systems. *Nat. Rev. Neurosci.* 10, 186–198.

Bullmore, E. T., and Bassett, D. S. (2011). Brain graphs: graphical models of the human brain connectome. *Annu. Rev. Clin. Psychol.* 7, 113–140.

Dinov, I. D., Van Horn, J. D., Lozev, K. M., Magsipoc, R., Petrosyan, P., Liu, Z., et al. (2009). Efficient, distributed and interactive neuroimaging data analysis using the LONI pipeline. *Front. Neuroinform.* 3:22. doi: 10.3389/neuro.11.022.2009

Faria, A. V., Zhang, J., Oishi, K., Li, X., Jiang, H., Akhter, K., et al. (2010). Atlas-based analysis of neurodevelopment from infancy to adulthood using diffusion tensor imaging and applications for automated abnormality detection. *Neuroimage* 52, 415–428.

Gong, G., He, Y., Concha, L., Lebel, C., Gross, D. W., Evans, A. C., et al. (2009a). Mapping anatomical connectivity patterns of human cerebral cortex using *in vivo* diffusion tensor imaging tractography. *Cereb. Cortex* 19, 524–536.

Gong, G. L., Rosa, P., Carbonell, F., Chen, Z. J., He, Y., and Evans, A. C. (2009b). Age- and gender-related differences in the cortical anatomical network. *J. Neurosci.* 29, 15684–15693.

Gorgolewski, K., Burns, C. D., Madison, C., Clark, D., Halchenko, Y. O., Waskom, M. L., et al. (2011). Nipype: a flexible, lightweight and extensible neuroimaging data processing framework in python. *Front. Neuroinform.* 5:13. doi: 10.3389/fninf.2011.00013

Hagmann, P., Cammoun, L., Gigandet, X., Meuli, R., Honey, C. J., Wedeen, V. J., et al. (2008). Mapping the structural core of human cerebral cortex. *PLoS Biol.* 6:e159. doi: 10.1371/journal.pbio.0060159

Jiang, H., Van Zijl, P., Kim, J., Pearlson, G. D., and Mori, S. (2006). DtiStudio: resource program for diffusion tensor computation and fiber bundle tracking. *Comput. Methods Programs Biomed.* 81, 106–116.

Johansen-Berg, H., and Rushworth, M. F. S. (2009). Using diffusion imaging to study human connectional anatomy. *Annu. Rev. Neurosci.* 32, 75–94.

Jones, D. K., and Cercignani, M. (2010). Twenty-five pitfalls in the analysis of diffusion MRI data. *NMR Biomed.* 23, 803–820.

Jones, D. K., Knosche, T. R., and Turner, R. (2012). White matter integrity, fiber count, and other fallacies: the do's and don'ts of diffusion MRI. *Neuroimage* doi: 10.1016/j.neuroimage.2012.06.081. [Epub ahead of print].

Latora, V., and Marchiori, M. (2001). Efficient behavior of small-world networks. *Phys. Rev. Lett.* 87, 198701.

Le Bihan, D. (2003). Looking into the functional architecture of the brain with diffusion MRI. *Nat. Rev. Neurosci.* 4, 469–480.

Leemans, A., and Jones, D. K. (2009). The B-matrix must be rotated when correcting for subject motion in DTI data. *Magn. Reson. Med.* 61, 1336–1349.

Lucas, B. C., Bogovic, J. A., Carass, A., Bazin, P. L., Prince, J. L., Pham, D. L., et al. (2010). The Java Image Science Toolkit (JIST) for rapid prototyping and publishing of neuroimaging software. *Neuroinformatics* 8, 5–17.

McAuliffe, M. J., Lalonde, F. M., McGarry, D., Gandler, W., Csaky, K., and Trus, B. L. (2001). "Medical image processing, analysis and visualization in clinical research," in *Proceedings of the 14th IEEE Symposium on Computer-Based Medical Systems*, (Bethesda, USA), 381–386.

Michielse, S., Coupland, N., Camicioli, R., Carter, R., Seres, P., Sabino, J., et al. (2010). Selective effects of aging on brain white matter microstructure: a diffusion tensor imaging tractography study. *Neuroimage* 52, 1190–1201.

Mori, S., Crain, B. J., Chacko, V., and Van Zijl, P. (1999). Three-dimensional tracking of axonal projections in the brain by magnetic resonance imaging. *Ann. Neurol.* 45, 265–269.

Mori, S., Oishi, K., Jiang, H., Jiang, L., Li, X., Akhter, K., et al. (2008). Stereotaxic white matter atlas based on diffusion tensor imaging in an ICBM template. *Neuroimage* 40, 570–582.

Pierpaoli, C., and Basser, P. J. (1996). Toward a quantitative assessment of diffusion anisotropy. *Magn. Reson. Med.* 36, 893–906.

Smith, S. M. (2002). Fast robust automated brain extraction. *Hum. Brain Mapp.* 17, 143–155.

Smith, S. M., Jenkinson, M., Johansen-Berg, H., Rueckert, D., Nichols, T. E., Mackay, C. E., et al. (2006). Tract-based spatial statistics: voxelwise analysis of multi-subject diffusion data. *Neuroimage* 31, 1487–1505.

Smith, S. M., Jenkinson, M., Woolrich, M. W., Beckmann, C. F., Behrens, T., Johansen-Berg, H., et al. (2004). Advances in functional and structural MR image analysis and implementation as FSL. *Neuroimage* 23, S208.

Song, S. K., Sun, S. W., Ramsbottom, M. J., Chang, C., Russell, J., and Cross, A. H. (2002). Dysmyelination revealed through MRI as increased radial (but unchanged axial) diffusion of water. *Neuroimage* 17, 1429–1436.

Sporns, O., Tononi, G., and Kötter, R. (2005). The human connectome: a structural description of the human brain. *PLoS Comput. Biol.* 1:e42. doi: 10.1371/journal.pcbi.0010042

Tzourio-Mazoyer, N., Landeau, B., Papathanassiou, D., Crivello, F., Etard, O., Delcroix, N., et al. (2002). Automated anatomical labeling of activations in SPM using a macroscopic anatomical parcellation of the MNI MRI single-subject brain. *Neuroimage* 15, 273–289.

Wang, R., Benner, T., Sorensen, A. G., and Wedeen, V. J. (2007). Diffusion toolkit: a software package for diffusion imaging data processing and tractography. *Proc. Intl. Soc. Mag. Reson. Med.* 15, 3720.

APPENDICES

APPENDIX A

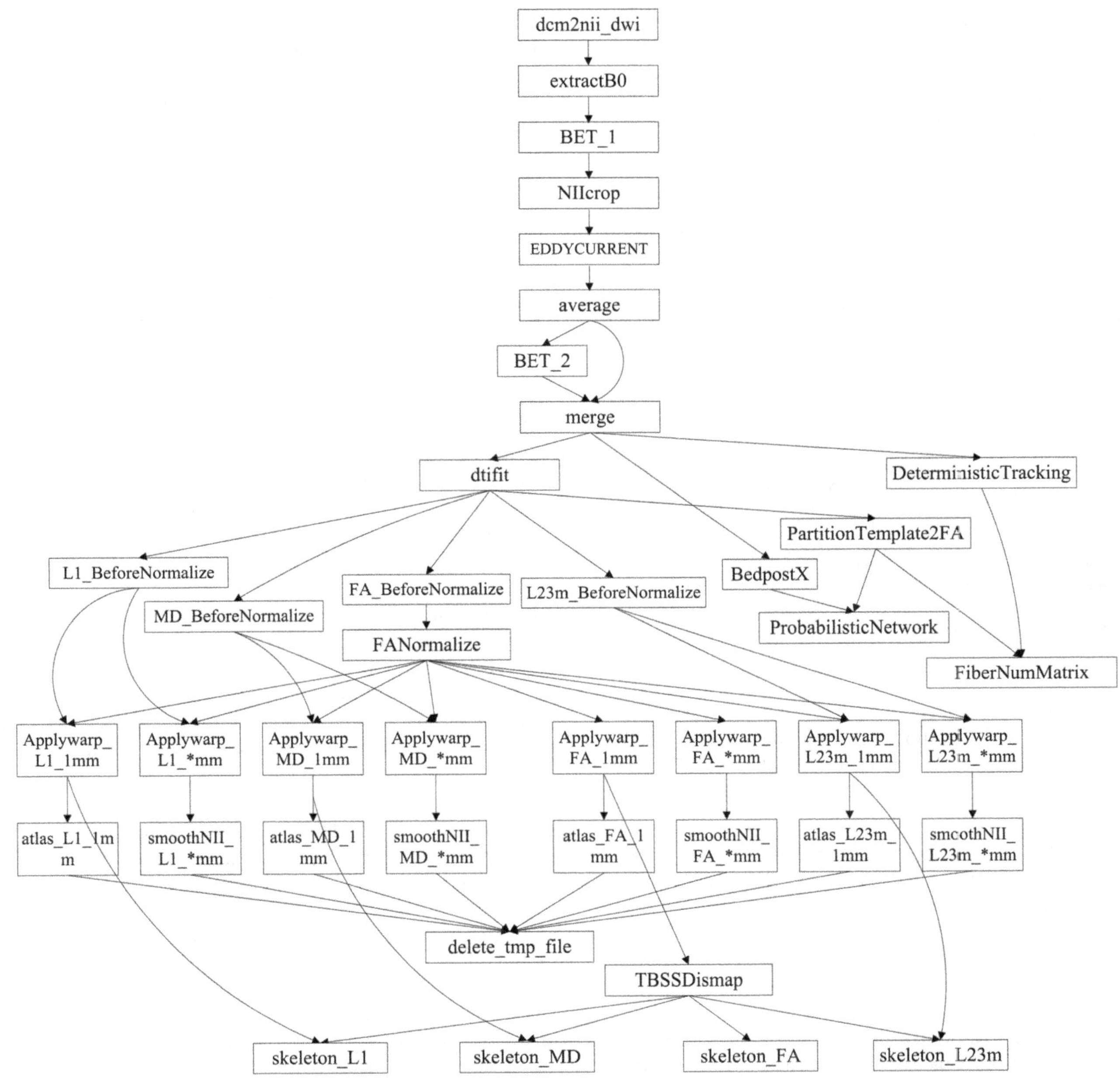

FIGURE A1 | Implementation of the PANDA pipeline. The entire process of the PANDA pipeline was divided into 41 steps. Arrows indicate dependencies: A→B means that B cannot start until A is finished.

APPENDIX B: GUIs OF PANDA

Main function

The main GUI of PANDA is shown in **Figure B1**. Users are required to set up inputs and configure outputs through this GUI. Specifically, the data inputs are folders, each containing files in either DICOM or NIfTI format, for each subject. The output configuration includes: (1) a main output folder that contains subject-specific subfolders of results; (2) digital subject IDs; and (3) a prefix. The IDs and prefixes are used to name the resultant subfolder or files for each subject. In addition, users may change the pipeline options (**Figure B2A**), diffusion options (**Figure B2B**), and tracking options (**Figure B2C**). The default setting for these options will be used if no changes are made.

Once all required settings are established, users simply click the "RUN" button to start the processing. PANDA will automatically finish all the sequential jobs and yield files containing

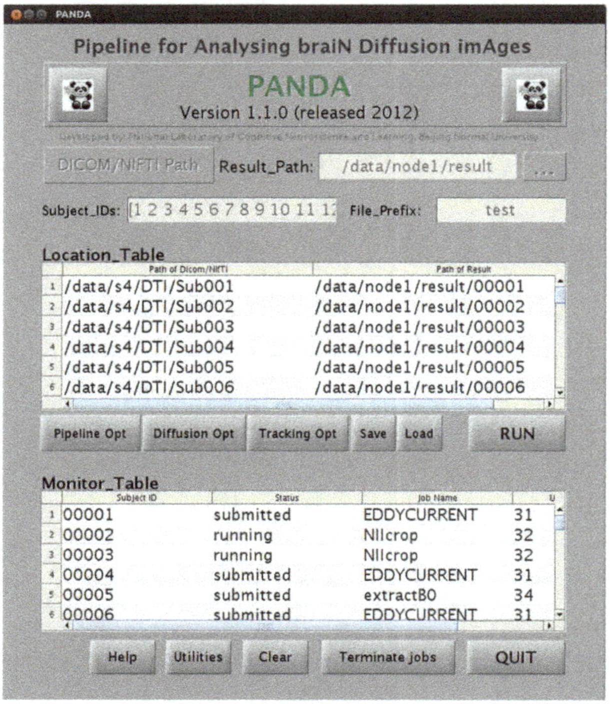

FIGURE B1 | A snapshot of the main GUI while PANDA is running. The GUI allows for (1) inputting raw dMRI datasets and configuring processing parameters and (2) monitoring the progress of data processing in real-time.

diffusion metrics and anatomical brain networks, as described in the "Materials and Methods." During processing, the status of jobs can be checked in the monitor table of the GUI (**Figure B1**).

Separate utilities

TBSS. As shown in **Figure B3A**, this utility is for separate TBSS procedures, which require all images of FA and other diffusion metrics to be aligned in the MNI space. With correct input settings, this module will automatically generate individual images with data on the skeleton for all subjects. Statistical analyses can be directly applied to the resultant images.

Brain parcellation (node definition). This utility is used to separately define the brain network nodes. The sub-GUI is shown in **Figure B3B**. This module requires FA images of native space and skull-stripped T1 images as inputs. A prior atlas in the MNI space should also be specified. The results of this utility are individual atlas images in the dMRI native space for all subjects. These images can be directly loaded by the utility "Tracking & Network."

Bedpostx. As shown in **Figure B4A**, this utility allows for the estimation of voxel-wise local probability distributions of fiber orientation for a set of subjects, which is typically very time-consuming. The input for each subject should be a folder containing four files as listed: (1) a 4D image named *data.nii.gz* containing diffusion-weighted volumes and volumes without diffusion weighting; (2) a 3D binary brain mask volume named *nodif_brain_mask.nii.gz*; (3) a text file named *bvecs* containing gradient directions for diffusion weighted volumes; and (4) a text file named *bvals* containing the b-values that were applied to each volume acquisition. This module will generate a separate folder containing all the files that are required for subsequent probabilistic tractography.

Tracking & Network. This utility can separately construct anatomical brain networks based on tractography. The sub-GUI is shown in **Figure B4B**. For a deterministic tractography-based network, a folder with four files described in the section "Bedpostx" together with an individual-specific atlas image generated by the utility "Brain Parcellation" are required. For a probabilistic tractography-based network, the resultant folder of the utility "Bedpostx" and the individual-specific atlas image should be the inputs. As described in the "Materials and Methods," this module will generate network matrices that are saved in a MATLAB data file.

DICOM sorter. This handy utility, as shown in **Figure B5A**, can automatically sort multiple DICOM files in the same folder into sequence-specific or subject-specific sub-folders, based on the header information of the DICOM files. This is particularly useful when the DICOM files from different sequences or subjects are saved in the same folder, which happens very often.

Image converter. The NIfTI format can be a pair of files (hdr/img), a single file (nii), or a compressed file (nii.gz). A NIfTI file may be required in a certain file type, e.g., *.nii or *.hdr/img. As shown in **Figure B5B**, this utility can convert NIfTI pair format (hdr/img), NIfTI format (nii), and NIfTI GZ format (nii.gz) file types.

File copier. This utility can copy a large number of files located in different source folders into the same target folder. The sub-GUI is shown in **Figure B5C**. After PANDA processing, each subject will have unique folders containing the resultant files. "File Copier" can easily copy the same types of resultant files (e.g., aligned FA images) of all the subjects to one target folder, which might be helpful for further statistical analysis or other purposes.

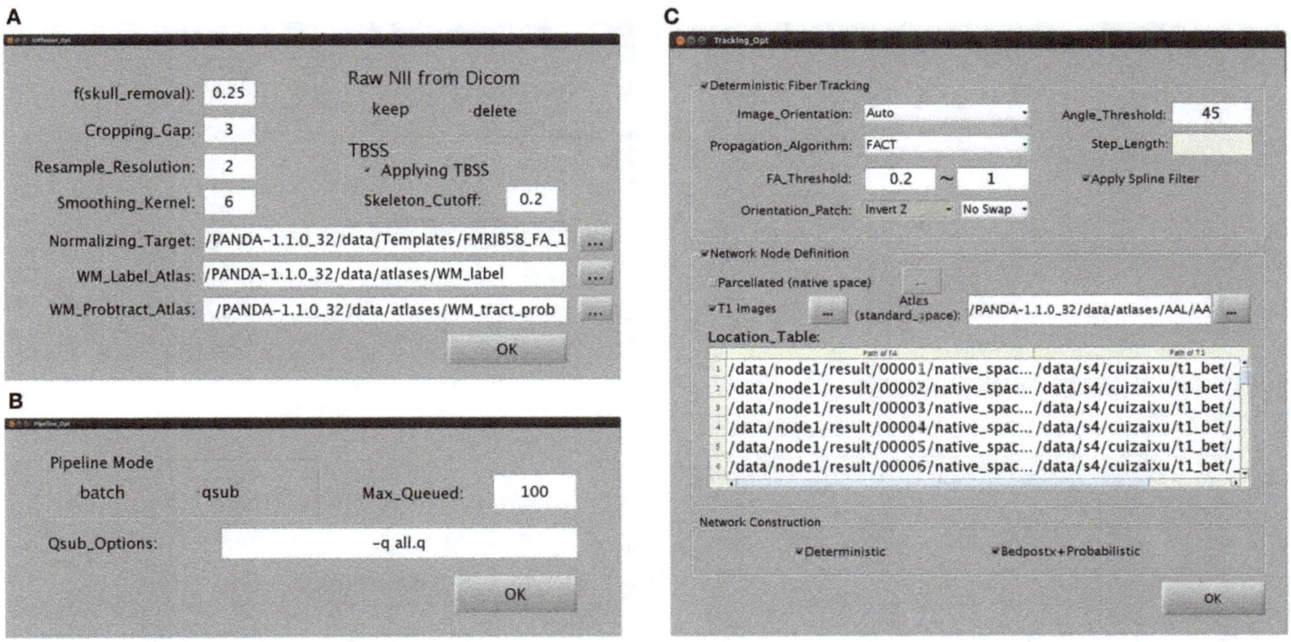

FIGURE B2 | Snapshots of the GUI for configuring the processing parameters. (A) A snapshot of the GUI for changing the preprocessing parameters and for producing diffusion metrics that are ready for statistical analysis. **(B)** A snapshot of the GUI for changing the computing modes of PANDA. **(C)** A snapshot of the GUI for changing the parameters used to construct anatomical brain networks.

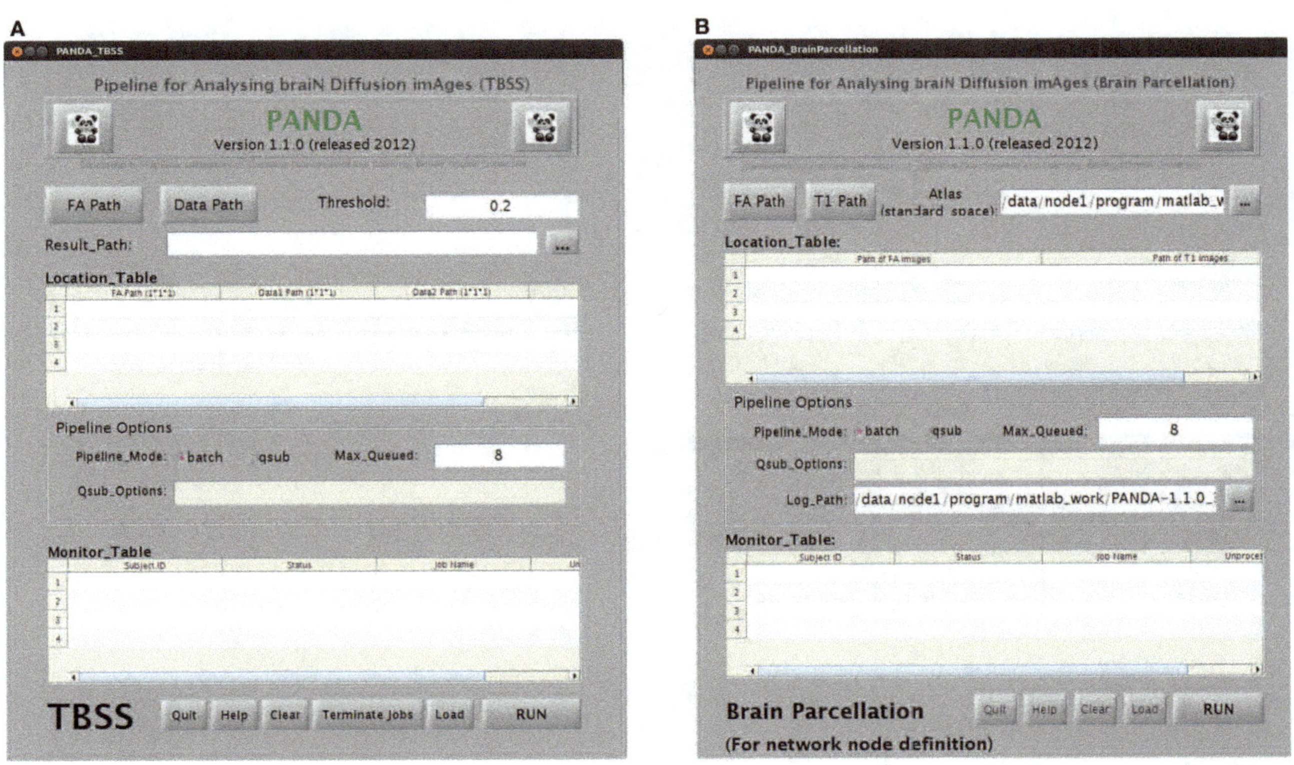

FIGURE B3 | GUIs for the utilities "TBSS" and "brain parcellation" in PANDA. (A) The utility for TBSS analysis. **(B)** The utility for brain parcellation.

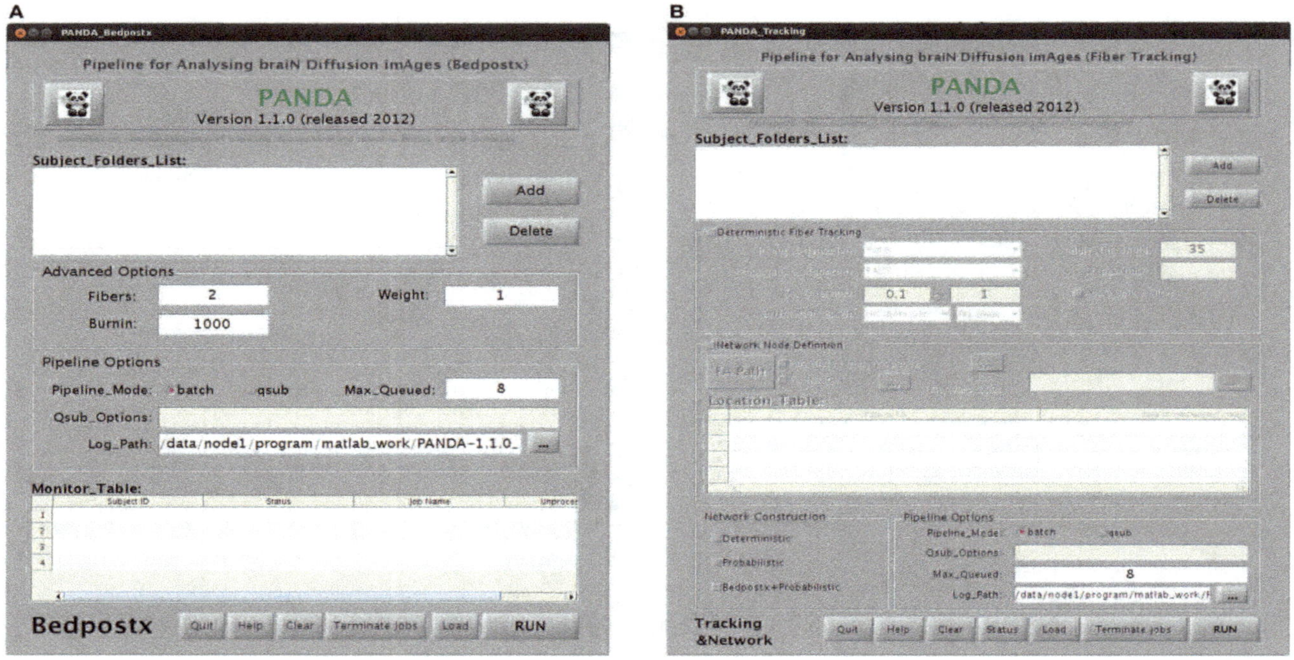

FIGURE B4 | GUIs for the utilities "Bedpostx" and "Tracking & Network" in PANDA. (A) The utility for Bedpostx. **(B)** The utility for tractography and network construction.

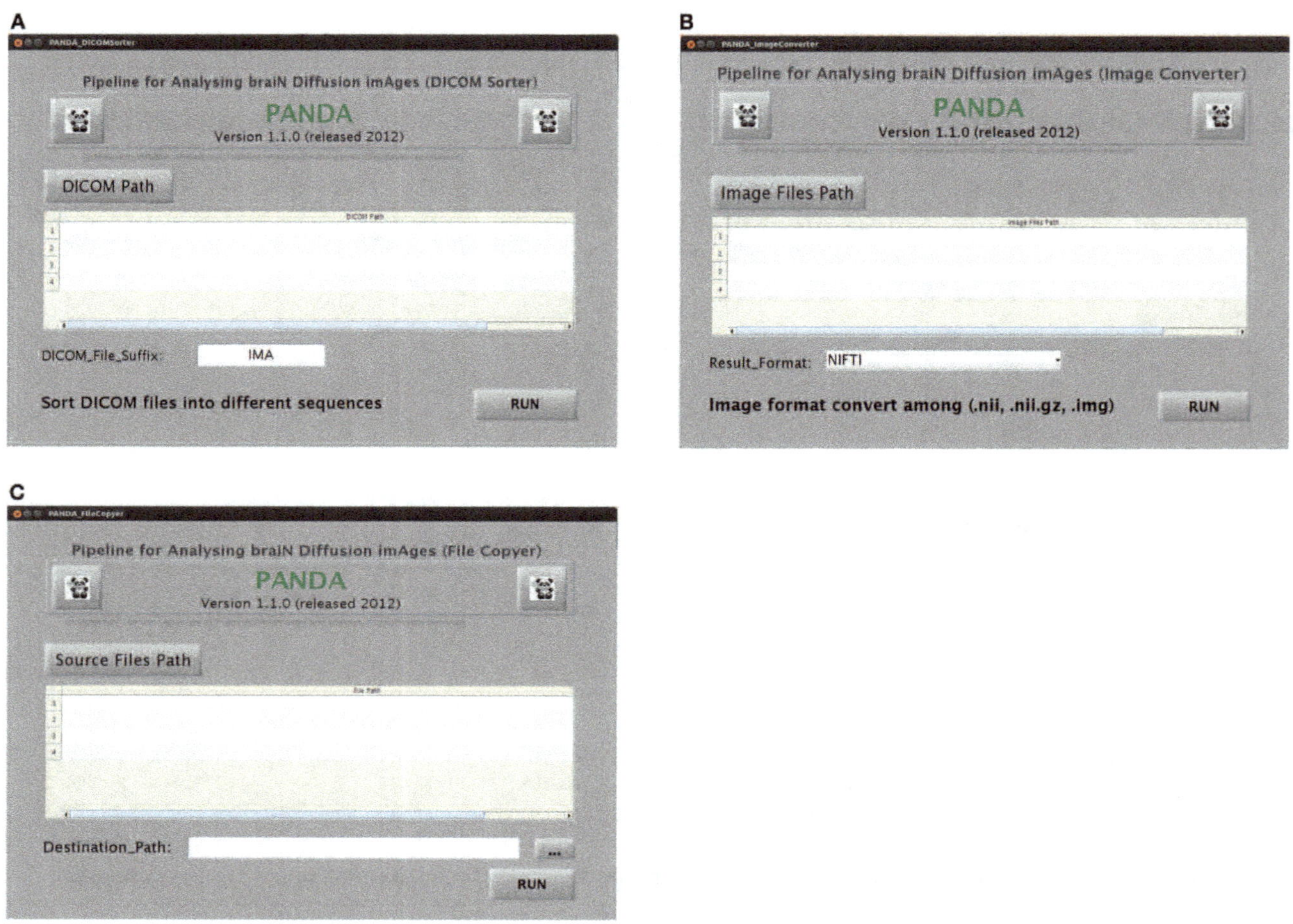

FIGURE B5 | GUIs for the utilities "DICOM Sorter," "Image Converter," and "File Copier" in PANDA. (A) The utility for DICOM Sorter. **(B)** The utility for Image Converter. **(C)** The utility for File Copier.

17

A longitudinal study of structural brain network changes with normal aging

Kai Wu[1,2]*, Yasuyuki Taki[1,3,4], Kazunori Sato[1], Haochen Qi[2], Ryuta Kawashima[4,5,6] and Hiroshi Fukuda[1]

[1] *Department of Nuclear Medicine and Radiology, Institute of Development, Aging and Cancer, Tohoku University, Sendai, Japan*
[2] *Department of Biomedical Engineering, School of Materials Science and Engineering, South China University of Technology, Guangzhou, China*
[3] *Division of Medical Image Analysis, Department of Community Medical Supports, Tohoku Medical Megabank Organization, Tohoku University, Sendai, Japan*
[4] *Division of Developmental Cognitive Neuroscience, Institute of Development, Aging and Cancer, Tohoku University, Sendai, Japan*
[5] *Smart Ageing International Research Centre, Institute of Development, Aging and Cancer, Tohoku University, Sendai, Japan*
[6] *Department of Functional Brain Imaging, Institute of Development, Aging and Cancer, Tohoku University, Sendai Japan*

***Correspondence:**
Kai Wu, Department of Nuclear Medicine and Radiology, Institute of Development, Aging and Cancer, Tohoku University, Seiryo-Machi 4-1, Smart Ageing Research Building, Sendai 980-8575, Japan.
e-mail: kai.wu.22@gmail.com

The aim of this study was to investigate age-related changes in the topological organization of structural brain networks by applying a longitudinal design over 6 years. Structural brain networks were derived from measurements of regional gray matter volume and were constructed in age-specific groups from baseline and follow-up scans. The structural brain networks showed economical small-world properties, providing high global and local efficiency for parallel information processing at low connection costs. In the analysis of the global network properties, the local and global efficiency of the baseline scan were significantly lower compared to the follow-up scan. Moreover, the annual rate of change in local and global efficiency showed a positive and negative quadratic correlation with the baseline age, respectively; both curvilinear correlations peaked at approximately the age of 50. In the analysis of the regional nodal properties, significant negative correlations between the annual rate of change in nodal strength and the baseline age were found in the brain regions primarily involved in the visual and motor/control systems, whereas significant positive quadratic correlations were found in the brain regions predominately associated with the default-mode, attention, and memory systems. The results of the longitudinal study are consistent with the findings of our previous cross-sectional study: the structural brain networks develop into a fast distribution from young to middle age (approximately 50 years old) and eventually became a fast localization in the old age. Our findings elucidate the network topology of structural brain networks and its longitudinal changes, thus enhancing the understanding of the underlying physiology of normal aging in the human brain.

Keywords: structural brain network, economical small-world, normal aging, longitudinal study, regional gray matter volume

INTRODUCTION

Recent advances in generating a network map of the human brain, known as the human connectome, provided new insights into structural and functional connectivity patterns of the human brain (Sporns et al., 2005; Bullmore and Bassett, 2011; Sporns, 2011a,b). The quantitative analysis of the structural and functional systems of the human brain, based largely on graph theory, reveal the topological properties of complex networks, such as economical small-world properties, highly connected hubs, and modularity (Bullmore and Sporns, 2009; He and Evans, 2010; Wig et al., 2011). Prodigious efforts in the study of the human connectome have greatly expanded our knowledge of the topological principles of brain network organization in the healthy, developing, aging, and diseased brains (Bassett and Bullmore, 2009; Uddin et al., 2010; Lo et al., 2011; Xia and He, 2011; Xie and He, 2011; Greicius and Kimmel, 2012; Sun et al., 2012).

It has been well-established that advanced aging is accompanied by cognitive decline, even in the absence of disease. Cognitive deficits in normal aging might arise from anatomical changes in specific brain regions or alterations of the structural and functional associations between distinct brain regions (Andrews-Hanna et al., 2007). Normal aging has been proven to be associated with changes in both functional (Achard and Bullmore, 2007; Meunier et al., 2009; Wang et al., 2010, 2012; Meier et al., 2012; Spreng and Schacter, 2012) and structural (Gong et al., 2009; Montembeault et al., 2012; Wu et al., 2012; Zhu et al., 2012) brain networks. However, these findings were revealed by cross-sectional studies, and few studies using a longitudinal design have been applied to investigate human brain networks with normal aging. Several Alzheimer's disease Neuroimaging Initiative (ADNI) studies have shown longitudinal changes in default mode network (DMN) regions, including the medial temporal lobe and posterior cingulate cortex (PCC), as patients progress into Alzheimer's disease (AD) and through its later stages (Risacher et al., 2010; Li et al., 2012). Thus, we hypothesized that significant longitudinal changes might occur in the topological properties of structural brain networks with normal aging.

By applying a longitudinal design over 6 years in a large number of healthy subjects aged 21–80, our previous studies have indicated the following: significant correlations between the annual percentage change in the ratio of gray matter and the age at baseline (Taki et al., 2011a), as well as significant correlations between the annual rate of regional gray matter volume change in many brain regions and the age at baseline (Taki et al., 2012a). In the present study, we aimed to investigate structural brain networks with normal aging by applying the above-mentioned longitudinal design. Structural brain networks have been constructed from inter-regional correlation of morphological measurements [e.g., cortical thickness (He et al., 2007), regional gray matter volume (RGMV) (Bassett et al., 2008), and surface area (Sanabria-Diaz et al., 2010)] in structural magnetic resonance imaging (sMRI) data. Recently, many studies have investigated the topological organization of structural brain networks in health [e.g., healthy subjects with normal aging (Montembeault et al., 2012; Wu et al., 2012; Zhu et al., 2012)] and disease [e.g., AD (He et al., 2008), multiple sclerosis (He et al., 2009), schizophrenia (Bassett et al., 2008), and breast cancer (Hosseini et al., 2012)]. In this study, we divided 380 healthy subjects into 29 age-specific groups using a sliding boxcar grouping ordered by baseline age. A structural brain network consisting of 90 regions was constructed by computing the correlation matrix of the RGMV across subjects within each age group in both the baseline and follow-up scans. We then computed both global and regional network properties in the structural brain networks and compared their differences between baseline and follow-up. Finally, to characterize the longitudinal changes of structural brain networks with normal aging, the correlations between the baseline age and the annual rate of change in both global and regional network properties were analyzed.

MATERIALS AND METHODS

SUBJECTS

The subjects were normal, community-dwelling Japanese subjects recruited by the Aoba Brain Imaging Project (Sato et al., 2003). Subject recruitment was described previously (Taki et al., 2011a,b,c, 2012a,b). Briefly, we performed longitudinal follow-up (Aoba2) scans of 442 subjects who were selected from 1604 participants in the baseline (Aoba1) scan. In both the baseline and follow-up scans, we excluded those subjects who had a past or present history of malignant tumors, head traumas, cerebrovascular diseases, epilepsy, or psychiatric diseases. After the interview, brain MR images were obtained from each subject. The MR images were inspected by 2–3 well-trained radiologists. Images with any of the following findings were excluded from this study: head injuries, brain tumors, hemorrhage, major and lacunar infarctions, or moderate to severe white matter hyperintensities. Thus, the final sample consisted of 380 participants (157 men/223 women). The mean ± standard deviation (SD) interval between baseline and follow-up was 7.41 ± 0.54 years (range, 6.1–9.0). The mean ± SD age of the participants at baseline was 51.1 ± 11.7 years old (range, 21–80).

A total of 11 subjects (mean age = 65.3 years; range, 57.7–73.4 years at follow-up; 3 men/8 women) were scanned twice on the same day to obtain an estimation of the measurement reliability. We observed no significant differences in the gray matter volume or intracranial volume between the baseline and follow-up scans. The details of the measurement reliability are reported elsewhere (Taki et al., 2011a).

After a full explanation of the purpose and procedures of the study, written informed consent according to the Declaration of Helsinki (1991) was obtained from each subject prior to MRI scanning. Approval for these experiments was obtained from the institutional review board of Tohoku University.

IMAGE ACQUISITION

All images were collected using the same 0.5-T MR scanner (Signa contour; GE-Yokogawa Medical Systems, Tokyo, Japan) for both the baseline and follow-up studies. The scanner was routinely calibrated using the same standard GE phantom between baseline and follow-up. During the course of this study, no major hardware upgrade occurred. At baseline and follow-up, all subjects were scanned with identical pulse sequences: 124 contiguous, 1.5-mm-thick axial planes of three-dimensional T1-weighted images (spoiled gradient recalled acquisition in steady state: repetition time, 40 ms; echo time, 7 ms; flip angle, 30; voxel size, 1.02 mm × 1.02 mm × 1.5 mm).

MEASUREMENTS OF REGIONAL GRAY MATTER VOLUME

After the image acquisition, the RGMV for each subject was measured using statistical parametric mapping 2 (SPM2) (Wellcome Department of Cognitive Neurology, London, UK) (Friston et al., 1995) in Matlab (MathWorks, Natick, MA). First, the T1-weighted MR images were transformed to the same stereotactic space by registering each of the images to the ICBM 152 template (Montreal Neurological Institute, Montreal, Canada), which approximates the Talairach space (Jean Talairach, 1988). Then, tissue segmentation from the raw images to the gray matter, white matter, cerebrospinal fluid space, and non-brain tissue was performed using the SPM2 default segmentation procedure. We applied these processes using the "cg_vbm_optimized" MATLAB function (http://dbm.neuro.uni-jena.de/vbm.html). WFU_PickAtlas software was employed to label the regions in the gray matter images, providing a method for generating ROI masks based on the Talairach Daemon database (Lancaster et al., 2000; Maldjian et al., 2003, 2004). To calculate the regional gray matter volume (RGMV) for each subject, we parcellated the entire gray matter into 45 separate regions for each hemisphere (90 regions in total, see **Table 1**) defined by the Automated Anatomical Labeling (AAL) atlas (Tzourio-Mazoyer et al., 2002).

CONSTRUCTION OF STRUCTURAL BRAIN NETWORKS

We applied the methodology described in our previous studies (Wu et al., 2011, 2012) to construct structural brain networks. Briefly, we computed a correlation matrix using the measurement of RGMV across a group of subjects. In this study, we created 29 age groups using a sliding boxcar grouping (Fair et al., 2009) in the order of baseline age (i.e., Group1: subjects 1–100, Group2: subjects 11–110, Group3: subjects 21–120, ... Group 29: subjects 281–380). Similarly, 29 age groups in the follow-up scan were also created, which corresponded to the age groups in the baseline scan. For each age group, a linear regression

Table 1 | Regions of interest included in AAL-atlas.

Lobes	Regions	Abbreviations	Lobes	Regions	Abbreviations
Frontal	Precentral gyrus	PreCG	Temporal	Hippocampus	HIP
	Superior frontal gyrus (dorsal)	SFGdor		Parahippocampal gyrus	PHG
	Orbitofrontal cortex (superior)	ORBsup		Amygdala	AMYG
	Middle frontal gyrus	MFG		Fusiform gyrus	FFG
	Orbitofrontal cortex (middle)	ORBmid		Heschl gyrus	HES
	Inferior frontal gyrus (opercular)	IFGoperc		Superior temporal gyrus	STG
	Inferior frontal gyrus (triangular)	IFGtriang		Temporal pole (superior)	TPOsup
	Orbitofrontal cortex (inferior)	ORBinf		Middle temporal gyrus	MTG
	Rolandic operculum	ROL		Temporal pole (middle)	TPOmid
	Supplementary motor area	SMA		Inferior temporal gyrus	ITG
	Olfactory	OLF	Occipital	Calcarine cortex	CAL
	Superior frontal gyrus (medial)	SFGmed		Cuneus	CUN
	Orbitofrontal cortex (medial)	ORBmed		Lingual gyrus	LING
	Rectus gyrus	REC		Superior occipital gyrus	SOG
	Anterior cingulate gyrus	ACG		Middle occipital gyrus	MOG
	Middle cingulate gyrus	MCG		Inferior occipital gyrus	IOG
Parietal	Posterior cingulate gyrus	PCG	Subcortical	Caudate	CAU
	Postcentral gyrus	PoCG		Putamen	PUT
	Superior parietal gyrus	SPG		Pallidum	PAL
	Inferior parietal lobule	IPL		Insula	INS
	Supramarginal gyrus	SMG		Thalamus	THA
	Angular gyrus	ANG			
	Precuneus	PCUN			
	Paracentral lobule	PCL			

analysis was performed on the RGMV to remove the effects of the total gray matter volume, age, sex, and age-by-sex interaction. Thus, the residuals of this regression were employed as the substitute for the raw RGMV and denoted as the corrected RGMV (cRGMV). We then computed the Pearson correlation coefficient between cRGMV across 100 subjects included in one group to construct an interregional correlation matrix ($N \times N$, where N is the number of gray matter regions; here, $N = 90$). Each element of the correlation matrix represents the structural connectivity between two regions. For example, the bilateral precentral gyrus (PreCG) showed strong correlations in Group 1 in both the baseline and follow-up scans (**Figure 1A**), indicating high connectivity between the same region in the bilateral hemispheres; however, the correlation between the left PreCG and the left opercular part of the inferior frontal gyrus (IFGoperc) in Group 1 was stronger in the follow-up scan compared to the baseline scan (**Figure 1B**). A correlation matrix (r_{ij}, $N \times N$) can be converted to a weighted and undirected network G using a cost threshold approach (t, $0 < t < 1$), which can normalize all networks to have the same number of edges or wiring cost and, thus, provide an avenue to detect changes in topological organization with aging (Achard and Bullmore, 2007).

$$G(i,j) = \begin{cases} 1, & |r_{ij}| \geq r_t \\ 0, & |r_{ij}| < r_t \end{cases}$$

Finally, we constructed a structural brain network for each of the 29 age groups in both the baseline and follow-up scans.

GRAPH THEORETICAL ANALYSIS

To ensure that the resulting brain networks are sparse, fully connected, and distinguishable from degree-matched random and regular networks, we adopted a range of cost thresholds ($0.11 \leq t \leq 0.25$, step $= 0.01$) to calculate the topological properties of structural brain networks (Bassett et al., 2008; Liu et al., 2008; Wang et al., 2009b; Wu et al., 2012). Small-world efficiency metrics (local efficiency, *LE*, and global efficiency, *GE*) were computed to characterize the global network properties of the structural brain networks. The node strength (*NS*) was used to examine regional nodal properties because of its high test-retest reliability (Wang et al., 2011). Here, both global and regional network metrics are briefly described as follows (Rubinov and Sporns, 2010) and were calculated using the Brain Connectivity Toolbox (www.brain-connectivity-toolbox.net).

The global efficiency of the graph G can be computed as (Latora and Marchiori, 2001):

$$GE(G) = \frac{1}{N(N-1)} \sum_{i \neq j \in G} \frac{1}{d_{ij}},$$

where d_{ij} is the shortest path length between nodes i and j. The path length between nodes i and j is defined as the sum of the edge lengths along this path, where each edge's length was obtained by computing the reciprocal of the edge weight, $1/w_{ij}$. Thus, the shortest path length d_{ij} is the length of the path

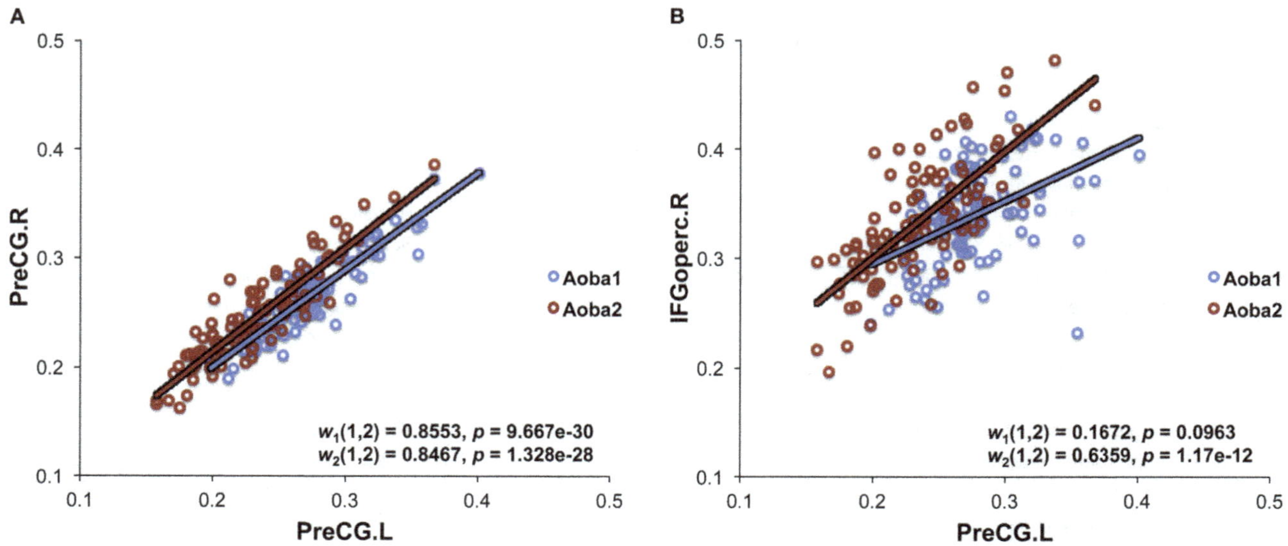

FIGURE 1 | Structural connectivity derived from the measurement of regional gray matter volume. (A) The structural connectivity between the bilateral precentral gyrus (PreCG). **(B)** The structural connectivity between left PreCG and the left opercular part of the inferior frontal gyrus (IFGoperc). The plots indicate Pearson's correlation coefficients [$w_N(i, j)$] between two brain regions (i and j) using the measurement of regional gray matter volume, which was corrected by a linear regression analysis to remove the effects of total gray matter volume, age, sex, and age-by-sex interaction. The data from both the baseline (Aoba1, $N = 1$) and follow-up (Aoba2, $N = 2$) scans are shown.

with the shortest length between nodes i and j. The local efficiency of the graph G is defined as (Latora and Marchiori, 2001):

$$LE(G) = \frac{1}{N}\sum_{i\in G} GE(Gi),$$

where $GE(G_i)$ is the global efficiency of G_i, the subgraph of the neighbors of node i. The small-world efficiency metrics (GE and LE) of real brain networks were compared with 1000 random networks (G_{rand}) that preserved the degree and weight distributions of real networks (Maslov and Sneppen, 2002). A real brain network is considered to be a small-world network if it shows similar global efficiency but much higher local efficiency than its matched random networks (Latora and Marchiori, 2001).

The node strength (NS_i) for a given node i is defined as the sum of all of the edge weights between this node and all of the other nodes in the network. Regions with a high nodal strength indicate high interconnectivity with other regions.

Regarding the structural brain network for each age group, we averaged the global and regional network metrics (LE, GE, and NS) over the range of cost thresholds ($0.11 \leq t \leq 0.25$) to obtain the summary network metrics (Bassett et al., 2008). To investigate the longitudinal changes of network properties, the annual rate of change in the summary network metrics (ARC_X) was defined as:

$$ARC\_X = \frac{X_2 - X_1}{\text{Age}_2 - \text{Age}_1},$$

where X_1 and X_2 are the summary network metrics at baseline and follow-up, respectively; and Age_1 and Age_2 are the mean age of 100 subjects included in the age group at baseline and follow-up, respectively. The ARC_X value indicates the differences in summary network metrics between the baseline and follow-up scans, normalized by the interval of age.

STATISTICAL ANALYSIS

To analyze the differences in the summary global network properties (e.g., LE and GE) of the same age group between two scans (e.g., Group 1 at baseline vs. Group 1 at follow-up), a non-parametric permutation test method was applied (Bullmore et al., 1999; He et al., 2008; Wu et al., 2012). Moreover, a paired t-test was performed to determine whether there were significant longitudinal changes in each summary network metric (LE, GE, and NS) between all age groups at baseline and those at follow-up. To evaluate correlations between the longitudinal changes in network properties and the baseline age, we performed multiple linear regression analyses with the annual rate of change in the summary network metrics as the dependent variables and the baseline age as the independent variable. Here, three multiple linear regressions (Model I, II, and III) modeling mean value, age, age^2, and age^3 as predictors were applied to detect the linear, quadratic, and cubic changes with the baseline age. We then determined the best model among the three regressions using Akaike's information criterion (AIC) (Akaike, 1974).

$$ARC\_X = \text{mean} + a \times \text{Age}_1 + e \qquad \text{(I)}$$

$$ARC\_X = \text{mean} + a_1 \times \text{Age}_1 + a_2 \times \text{Age}_1^2 + e \qquad \text{(II)}$$

$$ARC\_X = \text{mean} + a_1 \times \text{Age}_1 + a_2 \times \text{Age}_1^2 + a_3 \times \text{Age}_1^3 + e \qquad \text{(III)}$$

For the regression analysis of regional nodal property, we only included regions with significant differences in the summary regional network metric (e.g., *NS*) between the baseline and follow-up scans by the paired *t*-test ($p < 0.05$, FDR-corrected).

RESULTS

ECONOMICAL SMALL-WORLD PROPERTIES AND LONGITUDINAL CHANGES

The structural brain networks of the age-specific groups exhibited economical small-world properties, showing higher local efficiency but similar global efficiency compared to the matched random networks (Latora and Marchiori, 2001). This finding is illustrated in **Figure 2**, where we plot the local and global efficiency of the structural brain networks of the age-specific groups from both the baseline and follow-up scans against those of the matched random networks. Moreover, significant differences (a non-parametric permutation test; $p < 0.05$) in the summary local efficiency were found in several age groups across the baseline age but those in the summary global efficiency were found in the middle age groups (**Figure 3**). For all age groups, the structural brain networks from the baseline scan showed significantly lower local efficiency (a paired *t*-test; *t*-value = 8.446; $p < 10^{-4}$) and global efficiency (a paired *t*-test; *t*-value = 10.478; $p < 10^{-4}$) compared to those from the follow-up scan. The annual rate of change in local efficiency (*ARC_LE*) and global efficiency (*ARC_GE*) showed a positive quadratic (*F*-value = 3.622, $p = 0.041$) and a negative quadratic (*F*-value = 3.506, $p = 0.045$) correlation with the baseline age, respectively (**Figures 3A,B**). The curvilinear correlations peaked at the baseline ages of 45.49 years and 50.95 years, respectively.

REGIONAL NODAL PROPERTIES AND LONGITUDINAL CHANGES

We found significant correlations between the annual rate of change in node strength (*ARC_NS*) and the baseline age in many brain regions, which showed significant differences in the node strength (a paired *t*-test; $p < 0.05$, FDR-corrected) between the baseline and follow-up scans. Specifically, significant negative correlations ($p < 0.05$) between the *ARC_NS* and the baseline age were found in several brain regions that were primarily related to the visual system [e.g., the bilateral middle occipital gyrus (MOG) and right inferior temporal gyrus (ITG)] and the motor/control system [e.g., the left postcentral gyrus (PoCG), left superior parietal gyrus (SPG), right medial part of superior frontal gyrus (SFGmed), and right middle cingulate gyrus (MCG)] (**Table 2**, **Figure 4**). Significant positive quadratic correlations ($p < 0.05$) between the *ARC_NS* and the baseline age were found in several brain regions that were mainly associated with the default-mode system [e.g., the left anterior cingulate gyrus (ACG) and right medial part of the orbitofrontal cortex (ORBmed)], the attention system [e.g., the right middle frontal gyrus (MFG), right IFGoperc, and bilateral inferior parietal lobule (IPL)], and the memory system [e.g., the right parahippocampal gyrus (PHG), left amygdala (AMYG), and bilateral putamen (PUT)] (**Table 3**, **Figure 4**); the significant positive quadratic correlations peaked at a baseline age of 51.17–54.87 years (**Table 3**). The regional nodal properties of these brain regions were visualized in anatomical space (**Figure 4A**) and mapped onto the cortical surface (**Figure 4B**) using the BrainNet Viewer (http://www.nitrc.org/projects/bnv/).

DISCUSSION

To our knowledge, this is the first study to investigate longitudinal changes in the topological organization of structural brain networks in a large number of healthy individuals. We found that the structural brain networks of age-specific groups exhibit economical small-world properties. *ARC_LE* and *ARC_GE* showed

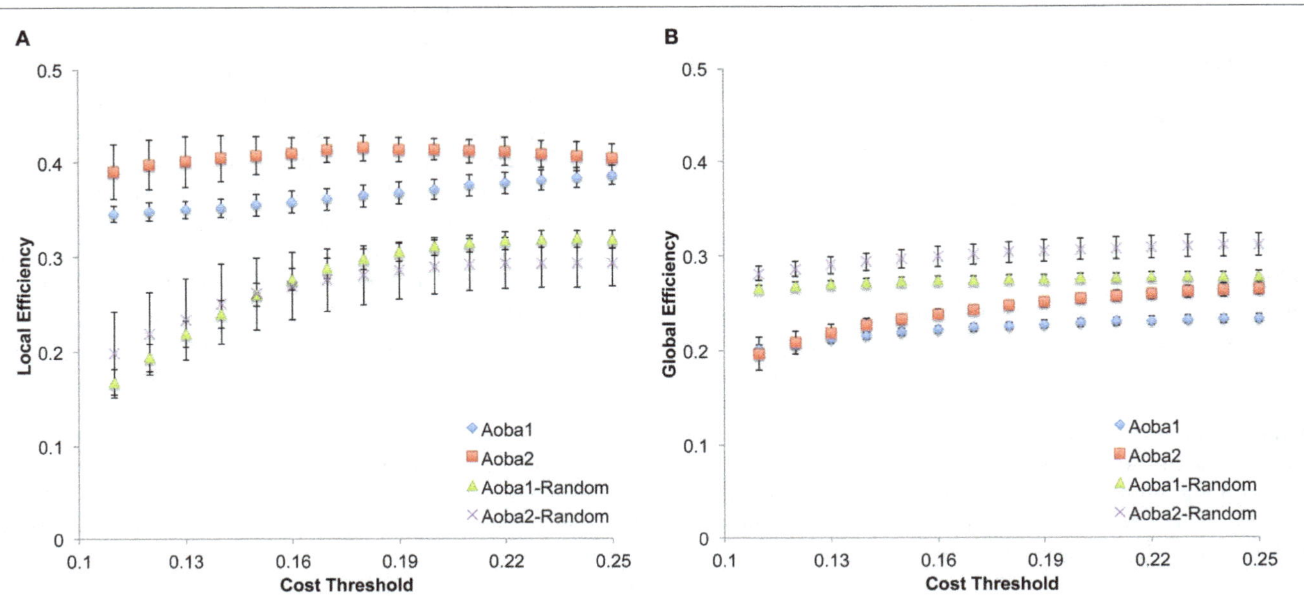

FIGURE 2 | Small-world efficiency properties in structural brain networks. (A) Local efficiency calculated under the cost threshold range of 0.11–0.25. **(B)** Global efficiency calculated under the cost threshold range of 0.11–0.25. Aoba1-Random and Aoba2-Random correspond to the matched random networks for the structural brain network in Aoba1 and Aoba2, respectively.

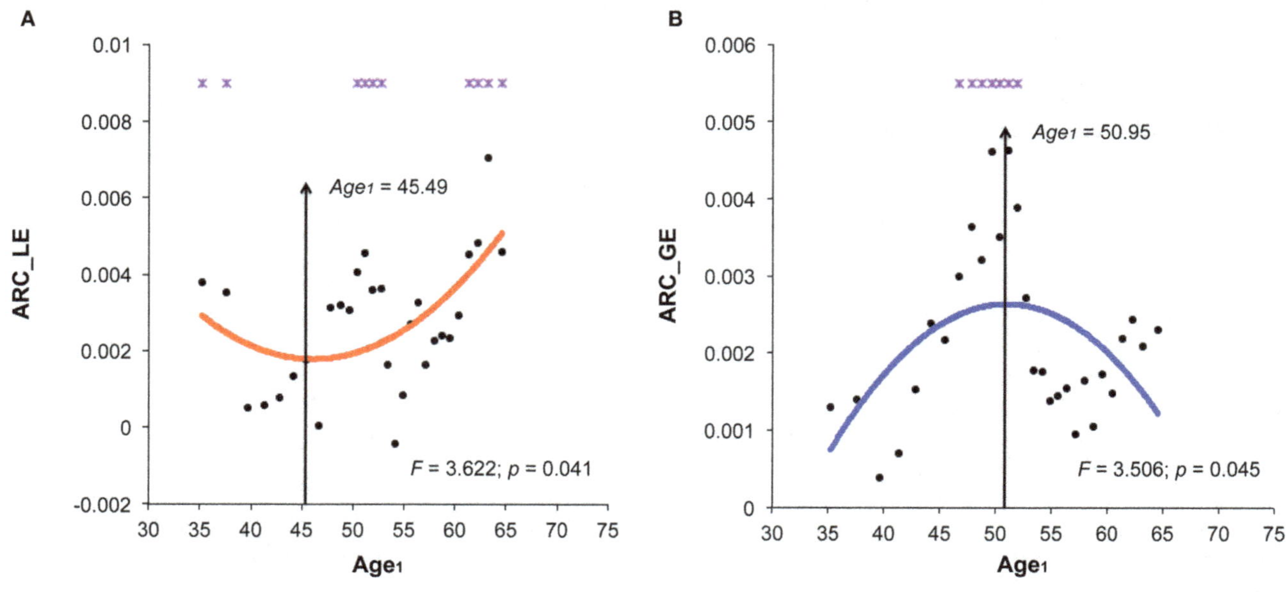

FIGURE 3 | Significant correlations between the annual rate of change in small-world efficiency and the baseline age. (A) Significant positive quadratic correlations between the annual rate of change in local efficiency (*ARC_LE*) and the baseline age (Age_1), peaked at the baseline age of 45.49 years. **(B)** Significant negative quadratic correlations between the annual rate of change in global efficiency (*ARC_GE*) and the baseline age, peaked at the baseline age of 50.95 years. Note that significant differences ($p < 0.05$) in the summary global network properties of the same age group between two scans by the nonparametric permutation test are indicated by violet stars.

Table 2 | Significant negative linear correlation between the annual rate of change in node strength and the baseline age.

System	Lobe	Class	Abbreviation	*F* value
Visual	Occipital	Association	MOG.L	10.416
	Occipital	Association	MOG.R	11.194
	Temporal	Association	ITG.R	21.121
Motor/control	Parietal	Primary	PoCG.L	13.561
	Parietal	Association	SPG.L	14.523
	Frontal	Association	SFGmed.R	17.964
	Frontal	Paralimbic	MCG.R	18.481

The level of significance was set at $p < 0.05$.

significant curvilinear correlations with the baseline age, with a peak at the baseline age of approximately 50. Our results also revealed significant correlations between the *ARC_NS* and the baseline age in many brain regions. Structural brain networks develop into a more distributed organization from young to middle age (approximately 50 years old) and then achieve a localized organization with substantial alterations in old age. Thus, revealing longitudinal changes in the topological properties of structural brain networks may enhance our understanding of the physiology underlying normal aging in the human brain.

ECONOMICAL SMALL-WORLD PROPERTIES AND LONGITUDINAL CHANGES

In this study, the structural brain networks derived from measurements of RGMV in all age-specific groups exhibited the key properties of economical small-world organization. An economical small-world network can provide a topological substrate for both locally specialized processing in the neighborhoods of highly clustered nodes and globally distributed processing on a highly efficient network with short characteristic path lengths (Sporns and Zwi, 2004; Stam, 2004; Achard et al., 2006; Achard and Bullmore, 2007). Our finding of high global and local efficiency in the structural brain networks is consistent with the results of previous functional and structural brain networks studies (He et al., 2007, 2008, 2009; Bassett et al., 2008, 2009; Wang et al., 2009b; Khundrakpam et al., 2012; Wu et al., 2012; Zhu et al., 2012).

We also noted longitudinal changes in small-world efficiency metrics of the structural brain networks. Several age groups in the follow-up scan showed significant higher values in local or global efficiency compared to those in the baseline scan. Moreover, the differences in both local and global efficiency between two scans varied across the age groups and showed significant correlations with the baseline age. *ARC_LE* and *ARC_GE* showed a U-curve and an inverted-U curve trajectory with the baseline age, respectively. In particular, the trajectories of *ARC_LE* and *ARC_GE* peaked at a baseline age of 45.49 and 50.95 years, respectively. These results are consistent with our previous cross-sectional study findings, in which the local and global efficiency showed U-curve and inverted-U curve tendencies, respectively, in young (18–40 years), middle (41–60 years), and old age (61–80 years) groups (the subjects used were from the same dataset of the baseline scan in this study) (Wu et al., 2012).

The longitudinal changes in local and global efficiency could be divided into two processes based on the peaks. First, the period from young to middle age (approximately 50 years old) showed

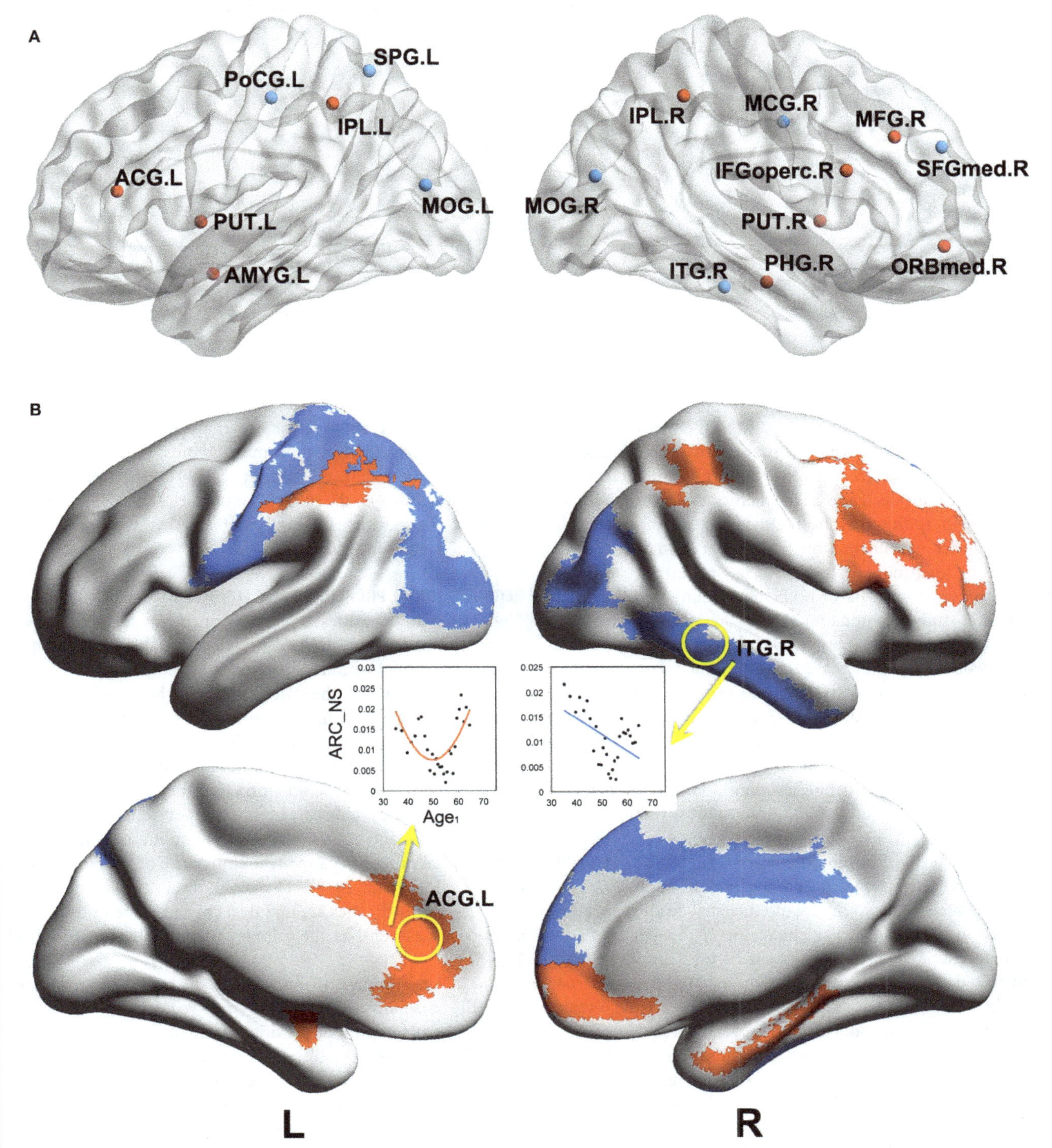

FIGURE 4 | Significant correlations between the annual rate of change in node strength and the baseline age. Significant correlations ($p < 0.05$) are visualized in anatomical space **(A)** and mapped onto the cortical surface **(B)**. Negative linear and positive quadratic correlations are indicated by blue and red colors, respectively. *ARC_NS*: the annual rate of change in node strength; Age_1: the baseline age. Abbreviations are shown in **Table 1**.

decelerated increases in local efficiency and accelerated increases in global efficiency, indicating a fast distribution in the middle age. This period might reflect a maturation process in the structural brain network. A previous study demonstrated that the organization of multiple functional networks shifts from a local anatomical emphasis in children to a more distributed architecture in young adults, indicating the maturation process of the functional systems (Fair et al., 2009). A more recent study on

Table 3 | Significant positive quadratic correlation between the annual rate of change in node strength and the baseline age.

System	Lobe	Class	Abbreviation	*F* value	Peak at the baseline age
Default-mode	Frontal	Paralimbic	ACG.L	8.859	51.17
	Frontal	Paralimbic	ORBmed.R	25.981	53.40
Attention	Frontal	Association	MFG.R	13.169	54.87
	Frontal	Association	IFGoperc.R	18.572	54.15
	Parietal	Association	IPL.L	12.596	51.93
	Parietal	Association	IPL.R	12.521	54.23
Memory	Temporal	Paralimbic	PHG.R	12.612	53.51
	Temporal	Paralimbic	AMYG.L	33.272	52.03
	Subcortical	Subcortical	PUT.L	14.899	52.59
	Subcortical	Subcortical	PUT.R	16.783	53.62

The level of significance was set at $p < 0.05$.

structural brain networks constructed from the measurement of cortical thickness also indicated a more distributed configuration in late childhood, accompanied by significant increases in global efficiency but decreases in local efficiency (Khundrakpam et al., 2012). In addition, white matter plays a vital role in the efficient transfer of information between gray matter regions. Our previous longitudinal study of a large number of healthy subjects (the same datasets of both the baseline and follow-up scans in this study) demonstrated that the white matter ratio increased until approximately age 50 and then decreased in both men and women (Taki et al., 2011a). Several previous studies also indicated that white matter volume seems to increase until the middle age of approximately 45 years and decrease thereafter (Bartzokis et al., 2001; Sowell et al., 2003). Increases in the white matter represent maturational changes, such as myelination that continue until middle adulthood and may, therefore, provide evidence of the maturation of structural brain networks.

Second, the period from middle (approximately 50 years old) to old age showed an accelerated increase in local efficiency and a decelerated increase in global efficiency, leading to a fast localization in the old age. The changes over this period might reflect a degenerative process in the structural brain network with advanced aging. A recent study demonstrated that the structural brain networks in an older cohort (mean age = 66.6 years, range 64–68) had lower global efficiency but higher local efficiency, revealing a more localized configuration compared to the younger cohort (mean age = 46.7 years, range 44–48) (Zhu et al., 2012). Using a sample of 342 healthy individuals aged 72–92 years, a previous DTI tract-derived connectivity study indicated that the global efficiency of the structural brain networks decreased significantly with older age (Wen et al., 2011). It is important to note that a regular configuration with less global integration upsets the optimal balance of a small-world network and is related to many neurological and psychiatric disorders described as dysconnectivity syndromes (Catani and ffytche, 2005). Several previous studies have reported a regular configuration or a reduction in the global efficiency of brain networks in patients with diseases such as AD and amnestic mild cognitive impairment (aMCI, the prodromal stage of AD), providing further support for the characterization of AD and aMCI as dysconnectivity syndromes and indicating the functional basis of cognitive deficits (Stam et al., 2007; He et al., 2008; Bai et al., 2012; Zhao et al., 2012; Wang et al., 2013). Therefore, we speculate that advanced aging is associated with a high risk for dysconnectivity syndromes.

REGIONAL NODAL PROPERTIES AND LONGITUDINAL CHANGES

Node strength measures the interconnectivity of a node with other regions and can be used to determine the relative importance of a node within a network. We identified significant correlations between the *ARC_NS* and the baseline age in many brain regions, mainly consisting of recently evolved association (9/17) and primitive limbic/paralimbic (5/17) regions. Association regions contribute to the integrity of multiple functional systems such as the attention and memory systems, while limbic/paralimbic regions are highly interconnected with the prefrontal regions and subcortical regions and are mainly involved in emotional processing and the maintenance of a conscious state of mind (Mesulam, 1998). Thus, our results support the view that age-related changes are mainly a characteristic of the association cortex rather than the primary cortex (Albert and Knoefel, 1994).

The brain regions showing significant negative correlations with the baseline are primarily involved in the visual and motor/control systems. A previous study of the structural brain networks in elderly subjects using DTI data demonstrated significant positive correlations between the regional nodal efficiency and visuospatial, processing speed, and executive functions in many cortical regions (Wen et al., 2011). Therefore, we speculate that our findings of the decreases of *ARC_NS* with the baseline age in the visual and motor/control systems might be related to the decline of these functions with normal aging. It is well-known that visual abilities decline during normal (non-pathological) aging, and older individuals tend to have reduced visual acuity and contrast sensitivity (Spear, 1993; Owsley, 2011). A recent study using event-related potentials (ERPs) also found that visual acuity declined as a function of age when young adults (18–32 years), young–old adults (65–79 years), and old–old adults (80+ years) performed a visual processing task involving selective attention to color (Daffner et al., 2012). Moreover, normal aging-related degeneration in the brain is accompanied by reduced force control, progressive slowness, and impaired motor ability (Roos et al., 1997; Smith et al., 1999; Krampe, 2002). Worsened task performance (e.g., slower speed with increasing memory load) in old adults (mean age = 71.27) is associated with decreases in the functional network connectivity between components comprising the supplementary motor area and the middle cingulate gyrus and between the precuneus and the middle/superior frontal cortex (Steffener et al., 2012). A previous resting-state fMRI study indicated a significant decrease in the functional connectivity of the motor network in aged subjects (mean age = 61.8) compared to young subjects (mean age = 26.5 years) (Wu et al., 2007). A more recent fMRI study using a visual oddball task also indicated that elderly subjects (mean age = 63.9 years) showed a decrease in connectivity within the somatomotor network compared to younger subjects (mean age = 24.1 years) (Geerligs et al., 2012).

We also found significant quadratic correlations between the *ARC_NS* and the baseline age in many brain regions, predominately from frontal (4/10), temporal (2/10), parietal (2/10), and subcortical (2/10) areas. It is notable that the significant quadratic correlations peaked at a baseline age from 51.17 to 54.87 years. Thus, in these brain regions, the *ARC_NS* increased with the baseline age in the period from middle (approximately 50 years old) to old age. More importantly, the identified brain regions are mainly associated with the default-mode, attention, and memory systems. The scaffolding theory of aging and cognition (STAC) suggests that scaffolding is a normal process present across the lifespan that involves use and development of complementary, alternative neural circuits to achieve a particular cognitive goal and is protective of cognitive function in the aging brain (Park and Reuter-Lorenz, 2009). Thus, our results are in line with the STAC and suggest a compensation mechanism of structural brain network reorganization with advanced aging. It has been indicated that cognitive decline is associated with differences in the structure and function of the aging brain, and it has been suggested that increased activation is either caused by disruption, whether structural or functional, or is a compensatory response to such disruption (Hedden and Gabrieli, 2004; Persson et al., 2006; Grady, 2012). Previous findings from several studies on structural and functional brain networks also support this view. Many brain regions, primarily from the frontal and temporal lobes, show increases in regional nodal efficiency in structural brain networks (Gong et al., 2009). Several regions, mostly in the lateral occipital-parietal junction and the paralimbic/subcortical area, reveal increased node betweenness in old age (Wu et al., 2012). The decrease in visual memory and visuoconstructive functions is strongly associated with the age-dependent enhancement of functional connectivity in both temporal lobes (Schlee et al., 2012). However, a recent study showed reduced structural association in the high-order cognitive networks of older adults compared to young adults, while no differences were observed in the sensorimotor networks (Montembeault et al., 2012). The following possible reasons are given for the discrepancies between this finding and our results: only eight brain regions were included in the previous study, whereas the present study was a whole-brain analysis; furthermore, only a comparison between young (mean age = 23.5 ± 3.1 years) and old (mean age = 67.3 ± 5.9 years) age was analyzed in the previous study, neglecting the other comparisons (young vs. middle; middle vs. old). Moreover, most of the identified brain regions showing positive quadratic correlations with the baseline age are found to be altered in AD patients (Bai et al., 2012; Zhao et al., 2012; Wang et al., 2013). For example, several brain regions (e.g., ACG.L, ORBmed.R, IFGoperc.R, IPL.L, IPL.R, and PUT.R) in AD patients show significant increases in regional nodal properties (e.g., the regional local and global efficiency) (Zhao et al., 2012). Thus, these findings provide further evidence supporting the view that advanced aging confers a high risk for neurodegenerative diseases, such as AD.

METHODOLOGY

Several methodological issues need to be addressed. First, structural brain networks can be constructed in two ways: (1) indirectly from inter-regional correlation of morphological measurements (e.g., cortical thickness, RGMV, and surface area) in sMRI data; (2) directly from characteristics of white matter fibers (e.g., fiber number, fractional anisotropy, apparent diffusion coefficient, or distance) in diffusion tensor imaging (DTI) data (Bassett and Bullmore, 2009; He and Evans, 2010; Lo et al., 2011; Xia and He, 2011). Although there is still no direct proof that correlations of morphological measurements across subjects are indicative of axonal connectivity via white matter tracts, strong correlations between brain regions known to be anatomically connected have been observed in previous optimized voxel-based morphometry studies (Mechelli et al., 2005; Pezawas et al., 2005). Moreover, a recent study indicated that approximately 35–40% of cortical thickness correlations showed convergent diffusion connections across the cerebral cortex and most of them were the positive thickness correlations (Gong et al., 2012). However, the authors also found that almost all of the negative correlations (>90%) did not have a matched diffusion connection, suggesting different mechanisms behind the positive and negative thickness correlations. Since we defined structural connectivity as the absolute value of correlation of RGMV in this study, the association between correlation of RGMV and diffusion connections should be investigated further in future studies. Second, previous studies indicate that different parcellation strategies affect the topological properties (e.g., the local efficiency, global efficiency, small-worldness, and modularity) of structural or functional brain networks (Wang et al., 2009a; Fornito et al., 2010; Zalesky et al., 2010). A previous study also indicates that regional volumes are positively correlated with their mutual information, which measures the functional connectivity between each region and the remaining brain regions (Salvador et al., 2008). Thus, variations in parcellation templates (e.g., AAL used in this study) may affect the network structure of the human brain; future studies should include comparisons of network topology with different parcellation templates. Third, because all of the subjects in this study were over 20 years old, young and adolescent subjects should be included in future studies of brain network development. Finally, further investigations will also examine longitudinal changes in the topological properties of the human brain network using different neuroimaging modalities, such as diffusion tensor imaging, functional MRI, and electroencephalography.

CONCLUSION

In this study, we quantitatively analyzed the topological organization of structural brain networks using a longitudinal design over 6 years. Our results reveal economical small-world properties of structural brain networks and longitudinal changes in both global and regional network properties. The structural brain networks develop into a fast distribution at approximately the age of 50 and then transform into a fast localization with substantial alterations in old age. Our findings may contribute to understanding the mechanism of normal aging in the human brain and help to distinguish neurodegenerative diseases from normal aging.

ACKNOWLEDGMENTS

This study was supported by the 2007 Tohoku University Global Century Centre of Excellence (GCOE) Program (Ministry of Education, Culture, Sports, Science and Technology; MEXT) titled "Global Nano-Biomedical Engineering Education and Research Network Centre." The brain MRI database was constructed at the Aoba Brain Imaging Center with a grant from the Telecommunications Advancement Organization (National Institute of Information and Communications Technology) of Japan.

FUNDING

This study was supported by grants-in-aid from the Ministry of Education, Culture, Sports, Science, and Technology (20790875, 24103701, and 23240056), Japan and Guangdong Natural Science Foundation (S2012040007743), China.

REFERENCES

Achard, S., and Bullmore, E. (2007). Efficiency and cost of economical brain functional networks. *PLoS Comput. Biol.* 3:e17. doi: 10.1371/journal.pcbi.0030017

Achard, S., Salvador, R., Whitcher, B., Suckling, J., and Bullmore, E. (2006). A resilient, low-frequency, small-world human brain functional network with highly connected association cortical hubs. *J. Neurosci.* 26, 63–72.

Akaike, H. (1974). A new look at the statistical model identification. *IEEE Trans. Automat. Contr.* 19, 716–723.

Albert, M., and Knoefel, J. (1994). *Clinical Neurology of Aging, 2nd Edn.* New York, NY: Oxford University Press.

Andrews-Hanna, J. R., Snyder, A. Z., Vincent, J. L., Lustig, C., Head, D., Raichle, M. E., et al. (2007). Disruption of large-scale brain systems in advanced aging. *Neuron* 56, 924–935.

Bai, F., Shu, N., Yuan, Y., Shi, Y., Yu, H., Wu, D., et al. (2012). Topologically convergent and divergent structural connectivity patterns between patients with remitted geriatric depression and amnestic mild cognitive impairment. *J. Neurosci.* 32, 4307–4318.

Bartzokis, G., Beckson, M., Lu, P. H., Nuechterlein, K. H., Edwards, N., and Mintz, J. (2001). Age-related changes in frontal and temporal lobe volumes in men: a magnetic resonance imaging study. *Arch. Gen. Psychiatry* 58, 461–465.

Bassett, D. S., and Bullmore, E. T. (2009). Human brain networks in health and disease. *Curr. Opin. Neurol.* 22, 340–347.

Bassett, D. S., Bullmore, E. T., Meyer-Lindenberg, A., Apud, J. A., Weinberger, D. R., and Coppola, R. (2009). Cognitive fitness of cost-efficient brain functional networks. *Proc. Natl. Acad. Sci. U.S.A.* 106, 11747–11752.

Bassett, D. S., Bullmore, E., Verchinski, B. A., Mattay, V. S., Weinberger, D. R., and Meyer-Lindenberg, A. (2008). Hierarchical organization of human cortical networks in health and schizophrenia. *J. Neurosci.* 28, 9239–9248.

Bullmore, E., and Sporns, O. (2009). Complex brain networks: graph theoretical analysis of structural and functional systems. *Nat. Rev. Neurosci.* 10, 186–198.

Bullmore, E. T., and Bassett, D. S. (2011). Brain graphs: graphical models of the human brain connectome. *Annu. Rev. Clin. Psychol.* 7, 113–140.

Bullmore, E. T., Suckling, J., Overmeyer, S., Rabe-Hesketh, S., Taylor, E., and Brammer, M. J. (1999). Global, voxel, and cluster tests, by theory and permutation, for a difference between two groups of structural MR images of the brain. *IEEE Trans. Med. Imaging* 18, 32–42.

Catani, M., and ffytche, D. H. (2005). The rises and falls of disconnection syndromes. *Brain* 128, 2224–2239.

Daffner, K. R., Haring, A. E., Alperin, B. R., Zhuravleva, T. Y., Mott, K. K., and Holcomb, P. J. (2012). The impact of visual acuity on age-related differences in neural markers of early visual processing. *Neuroimage* 67, 127–136.

Declaration of Helsinki. (1991). *BMJ* 302:1194.

Fair, D. A., Cohen, A. L., Power, J. D., Dosenbach, N. U., Church, J. A., Miezin, F. M., et al. (2009). Functional brain networks develop from a "local to distributed" organization. *PLoS Comput. Biol.* 5:e1000381. doi: 10.1371/journal.pcbi.1000381

Fornito, A., Zalesky, A., and Bullmore, E. T. (2010). Network scaling effects in graph analytic studies of human resting-state FMRI data. *Front. Syst. Neurosci.* 4:22. doi: 10.3389/fnsys.2010.00022

Friston, K. J., Holmes, A. P., Worsley, K. J., Poline, J. P., Frith, C. D., and Frackowiak, R. S. J. (1995). Statistical parametric maps in functional imaging: a general linear approach. *Hum. Brain Mapp.* 2, 189–210.

Geerligs, L., Maurits, N. M., Renken, R. J., and Lorist, M. M. (2012). Reduced specificity of functional connectivity in the aging brain during task performance. *Hum. Brain Mapp.* doi: 10.1002/hbm.22175. [Epub ahead of print].

Gong, G., He, Y., Chen, Z. J., and Evans, A. C. (2012). Convergence and divergence of thickness correlations with diffusion connections across the human cerebral cortex. *Neuroimage* 59, 1239–1248.

Gong, G., Rosa-Neto, P., Carbonell, F., Chen, Z. J., He, Y., and Evans, A. C. (2009). Age- and gender-related differences in the cortical anatomical network. *J. Neurosci.* 29, 15684–15693.

Grady, C. (2012). The cognitive neuroscience of ageing. *Nat. Rev. Neurosci.* 13, 491–505.

Greicius, M. D., and Kimmel, D. L. (2012). Neuroimaging insights into network-based neurodegeneration. *Curr. Opin. Neurobiol.* 25, 727–734.

He, Y., Chen, Z., and Evans, A. (2008). Structural insights into aberrant topological patterns of large-scale cortical networks in Alzheimer's disease. *J. Neurosci.* 28, 4756–4766.

He, Y., Chen, Z. J., and Evans, A. C. (2007). Small-world anatomical networks in the human brain revealed by cortical thickness from MRI. *Cereb. Cortex* 17, 2407–2419.

He, Y., Dagher, A., Chen, Z., Charil, A., Zijdenbos, A., Worsley, K., et al. (2009). Impaired small-world efficiency in structural cortical networks in multiple sclerosis associated with white matter lesion load. *Brain* 132, 3366–3379.

He, Y., and Evans, A. (2010). Graph theoretical modeling of brain connectivity. *Curr. Opin. Neurol.* 23, 341–350.

Hedden, T., and Gabrieli, J. D. (2004). Insights into the ageing mind: a view from cognitive neuroscience. *Nat. Rev. Neurosci.* 5, 87–96.

Hosseini, S. M., Koovakkattu, D., and Kesler, S. R. (2012). Altered small-world properties of gray matter networks in breast cancer. *BMC Neurol.* 12:28. doi: 10.1186/1471-2377-12-28

Jean Talairach, P. T. (1988). *Co-planar Stereotaxic Atlas of the Human Brain.* Stuttgart: Thieme.

Khundrakpam, B. S., Reid, A., Brauer, J., Carbonell, F., Lewis, J., Ameis, S., et al. (2012). Developmental changes in organization of structural brain networks. *Cereb. Cortex.* doi: 10.1093/cercor/bhs187. [Epub ahead of print].

Krampe, R. T. (2002). Aging, expertise and fine motor movement. *Neurosci. Biobehav. Rev.* 26, 769–776.

Lancaster, J. L., Woldorff, M. G., Parsons, L. M., Liotti, M., Freitas, C. S., Rainey, L., et al. (2000). Automated Talairach atlas labels for functional brain mapping. *Hum. Brain Mapp.* 10, 120–131.

Latora, V., and Marchiori, M. (2001). Efficient behavior of small-world networks. *Phys. Rev. Lett.* 87:198701. doi: 10.1103/PhysRevLett.87.198701

Li, Y., Wang, Y., Wu, G., Shi, F., Zhou, L., Lin, W., et al. (2012). Discriminant analysis of longitudinal cortical thickness changes in Alzheimer's disease using dynamic and network features. *Neurobiol. Aging* 33, 427.e15–427.e30.

Liu, Y., Liang, M., Zhou, Y., He, Y., Hao, Y., Song, M., et al. (2008). Disrupted small-world networks in schizophrenia. *Brain* 131, 945–961.

Lo, C. Y., He, Y., and Lin, C. P. (2011). Graph theoretical analysis of human brain structural networks. *Rev. Neurosci.* 22, 551–563.

Maldjian, J. A., Laurienti, P. J., and Burdette, J. H. (2004). Precentral gyrus discrepancy in electronic versions of the Talairach atlas. *Neuroimage* 21, 450–455.

Maldjian, J. A., Laurienti, P. J., Kraft, R. A., and Burdette, J. H. (2003). An automated method for neuroanatomic and cytoarchitectonic atlas-based interrogation of fMRI data sets. *Neuroimage* 19, 1233–1239.

Maslov, S., and Sneppen, K. (2002). Specificity and stability in topology of protein networks. *Science* 296, 910–913.

Mechelli, A., Friston, K. J., Frackowiak, R. S., and Price, C. J. (2005). Structural covariance in the human cortex. *J. Neurosci.* 25, 8303–8310.

Meier, T. B., Desphande, A. S., Vergun, S., Nair, V. A., Song, J., Biswal, B. B., et al. (2012). Support vector machine classification and characterization of age-related reorganization of functional brain networks. *Neuroimage* 60, 601–613.

Mesulam, M. M. (1998). From sensation to cognition. *Brain* 121, 1013–1052.

Meunier, D., Achard, S., Morcom, A., and Bullmore, E. (2009). Age-related changes in modular organization of human brain functional networks. *Neuroimage* 44, 715–723.

Montembeault, M., Joubert, S., Doyon, J., Carrier, J., Gagnon, J. F., Monchi, O., et al. (2012). The impact of aging on gray matter structural covariance networks. *Neuroimage* 63, 754–759.

Owsley, C. (2011). Aging and vision. *Vision Res.* 51, 1610–1622.

Park, D. C., and Reuter-Lorenz, P. (2009). The adaptive brain: aging and neurocognitive scaffolding. *Annu. Rev. Psychol.* 60, 173–196.

Persson, J., Nyberg, L., Lind, J., Larsson, A., Nilsson, L. G., Ingvar, M., et al. (2006). Structure-function correlates of cognitive decline in aging. *Cereb. Cortex* 16, 907–915.

Pezawas, L., Meyer-Lindenberg, A., Drabant, E. M., Verchinski, B. A., Munoz, K. E., Kolachana, B. S., et al. (2005). 5-HTTLPR polymorphism impacts human cingulate-amygdala interactions: a genetic susceptibility mechanism for depression. *Nat. Neurosci.* 8, 828–834.

Risacher, S. L., Shen, L., West, J. D., Kim, S., McDonald, B. C., Beckett, L. A., et al. (2010). Longitudinal MRI atrophy biomarkers: relationship to conversion in the ADNI cohort. *Neurobiol. Aging* 31, 1401–1418.

Roos, M. R., Rice, C. L., and Vandervoort, A. A. (1997). Age-related changes in motor unit function. *Muscle Nerve* 20, 679–690.

Rubinov, M., and Sporns, O. (2010). Complex network measures of brain connectivity: uses and interpretations. *Neuroimage* 52, 1059–1069.

Salvador, R., Martíez, A., Pomarol-Clotet, E., Gomar, J., Vila, F., Sarró, S., et al. (2008). A simple view of the brain through a frequency-specific functional connectivity measure. *Neuroimage* 39, 279–289.

Sanabria-Diaz, G., Melie-Garcia, L., Iturria-Medina, Y., Aleman-Gomez, Y., Hernandez-Gonzalez, G., Valdes-Urrutia, L., et al. (2010). Surface area and cortical thickness descriptors reveal different attributes of the structural human brain networks. *Neuroimage* 50, 1497–1510.

Sato, K., Taki, Y., Fukuda, H., and Kawashima, R. (2003). Neuroanatomical database of normal Japanese brains. *Neural Netw.* 16, 1301–1310.

Schlee, W., Leirer, V., Kolassa, S., Thurm, F., Elbert, T., and Kolassa, I. T. (2012). Development of large-scale functional networks over the lifespan. *Neurobiol. Aging* 33, 2411–2421.

Smith, C. D., Umberger, G. H., Manning, E. L., Slevin, J. T., Wekstein, D. R., Schmitt, F. A., et al. (1999). Critical decline in fine motor hand movements in human aging. *Neurology* 53, 1458–1461.

Sowell, E. R., Peterson, B. S., Thompson, P. M., Welcome, S. E., Henkenius, A. L., and Toga, A. W. (2003). Mapping cortical change across the human life span. *Nat. Neurosci.* 6, 309–315.

Spear, P. D. (1993). Neural bases of visual deficits during aging. *Vision Res.* 33, 2589–2609.

Sporns, O. (2011a). From simple graphs to the connectome: networks in neuroimaging. *Neuroimage* 62, 881–886.

Sporns, O. (2011b). The human connectome: a complex network. *Ann. N.Y. Acad. Sci.* 1224, 109–125.

Sporns, O., Tononi, G., and Kotter, R. (2005). The human connectome: a structural description of the human brain. *PLoS Comput. Biol.* 1:e42. doi: 10.1371/journal.pcbi.0010042

Sporns, O., and Zwi, J. (2004). The small world of the cerebral cortex. *Neuroinformatics* 2, 145–162.

Spreng, R. N., and Schacter, D. L. (2012). Default network modulation and large-scale network interactivity in healthy young and old adults. *Cereb. Cortex* 22, 2610–2621.

Stam, C. J. (2004). Functional connectivity patterns of human magnetoencephalographic recordings: a 'small-world' network? *Neurosci. Lett.* 355, 25–28.

Stam, C. J., Jones, B. F., Nolte, G., Breakspear, M., and Scheltens, P. (2007). Small-world networks and functional connectivity in Alzheimer's disease. *Cereb. Cortex* 17, 92–99.

Steffener, J., Habeck, C. G., and Stern, Y. (2012). Age-related changes in task related functional network connectivity. *PLoS ONE* 7:e44421. doi: 10.1371/journal.pone.0044421

Sun, J., Tong, S., and Yang, G. Y. (2012). Reorganization of brain networks in aging and age-related diseases. *Aging Dis.* 3, 181–193.

Taki, Y., Kinomura, S., Sato, K., Goto, R., Kawashima, R., and Fukuda, H. (2011a). A longitudinal study of gray matter volume decline with age and modifying factors. *Neurobiol. Aging* 32, 907–915.

Taki, Y., Kinomura, S., Sato, K., Goto, R., Wu, K., Kawashima, R., et al. (2011b). Correlation between baseline regional gray matter volume and global gray matter volume decline rate. *Neuroimage* 54, 743–749.

Taki, Y., Kinomura, S., Sato, K., Goto, R., Wu, K., Kawashima, R., et al. (2011c). Correlation between degree of white matter hyperintensities and global gray matter volume decline rate. *Neuroradiology* 53, 397–403.

Taki, Y., Thyreau, B., Kinomura, S., Sato, K., Goto, R., Wu, K., et al. (2012a). A longitudinal study of age- and gender-related annual rate of volume changes in regional gray matter in healthy adults. *Hum. Brain Mapp.* doi: 10.1002/hbm.22067. [Epub ahead of print].

Taki, Y., Thyreau, B., Kinomura, S., Sato, K., Goto, R., Wu, K., et al. (2012b). A longitudinal study of the relationship between personality traits and the annual rate of volume changes in regional gray matter in healthy adults. *Hum. Brain Mapp.* doi: 10.1002/hbm.22145. [Epub ahead of print].

Tzourio-Mazoyer, N., Landeau, B., Papathanassiou, D., Crivello, F., Etard, O., Delcroix, N., et al. (2002). Automated anatomical labeling of activations in SPM using a macroscopic anatomical parcellation of the MNI MRI single-subject brain. *Neuroimage* 15, 273–289.

Uddin, L. Q., Supekar, K., and Menon, V. (2010). Typical and atypical development of functional human brain networks: insights from resting-state FMRI. *Front. Syst. Neurosci.* 4:21. doi: 10.3389/fnsys.2010.00021

Wang, J., Wang, L., Zang, Y., Yang, H., Tang, H., Gong, Q., et al. (2009a). Parcellation-dependent small-world brain functional networks: a resting-state fMRI study. *Hum. Brain Mapp.* 30, 1511–1523.

Wang, L., Zhu, C., He, Y., Zang, Y., Cao, Q., Zhang, H., et al. (2009b). Altered small-world brain functional networks in children with attention-deficit/hyperactivity disorder. *Hum. Brain Mapp.* 30, 638–649.

Wang, J., Zuo, X., Dai, Z., Xia, M., Zhao, Z., Zhao, X., et al. (2013). Disrupted functional brain connectome in individuals at risk for alzheimer's disease. *Biol. Psychiatry* 73, 472–481.

Wang, J., Zuo, X., Gohel, S., Milham, M. P., Biswal, B. B., and He, Y. (2011). Graph theoretical analysis of functional brain networks: test-retest evaluation on short- and long-term resting-state functional MRI data. *PLoS ONE* 6:e21976. doi: 10.1371/journal.pone.0021976

Wang, L., Li, Y., Metzak, P., He, Y., and Woodward, T. S. (2010). Age-related changes in topological patterns of large-scale brain functional networks during memory encoding and recognition. *Neuroimage* 50, 862–872.

Wang, L., Su, L., Shen, H., and Hu, D. (2012). Decoding lifespan changes of the human brain using resting-state functional connectivity MRI. *PLoS ONE* 7:e44530. doi: 10.1371/journal.pone.0044530

Wen, W., Zhu, W., He, Y., Kochan, N. A., Reppermund, S., Slavin, M. J., et al. (2011). Discrete neuroanatomical networks are associated with specific cognitive abilities in old age. *J. Neurosci.* 31, 1204–1212.

Wig, G. S., Schlaggar, B. L., and Petersen, S. E. (2011). Concepts and principles in the analysis of brain networks. *Ann. N.Y. Acad. Sci.* 1224, 126–146.

Wu, K., Taki, Y., Sato, K., Kinomura, S., Goto, R., Okada, K., et al. (2012). Age-related changes in topological organization of structural brain networks in healthy individuals. *Hum. Brain Mapp.* 33, 552–568.

Wu, K., Taki, Y., Sato, K., Sassa, Y., Inoue, K., Goto, R., et al. (2011). The overlapping community structure of structural brain network in young healthy individuals. *PLoS ONE* 6:e19608. doi: 10.1371/journal.pone.0019608

Wu, T., Zang, Y., Wang, L., Long, X., Hallett, M., Chen, Y., et al. (2007). Aging influence on functional connectivity of the motor network in the resting state. *Neurosci. Lett.* 422, 164–168.

Xia, M., and He, Y. (2011). Magnetic resonance imaging and graph theoretical analysis of complex brain networks in neuropsychiatric disorders. *Brain Connect.* 1, 349–365.

Xie, T., and He, Y. (2011). Mapping the Alzheimer's brain with connectomics. *Front. Psychiatry* 2:77. doi: 10.3389/fpsyt.2011.00077

Zalesky, A., Fornito, A., Harding, I. H., Cocchi, L., Yücel, M., Pantelis, C., et al. (2010). Whole-brain anatomical networks: does the choice of nodes matter? *Neuroimage* 50, 970–983.

Zhao, X., Liu, Y., Wang, X., Liu, B., Xi, Q., Guo, Q., et al. (2012). Disrupted small-world brain networks in moderate Alzheimer's disease: a resting-state FMRI study. *PLoS ONE* 7:e33540. doi: 10.1371/journal.pone.0033540

Zhu, W., Wen, W., He, Y., Xia, A., Anstey, K. J., and Sachdev, P. (2012). Changing topological patterns in normal aging using large-scale structural networks. *Neurobiol. Aging* 33, 899–913.

18

Dysregulated but not decreased salience network activity in schizophrenia

Thomas P. White *†, James Gilleen† and Sukhwinder S. Shergill

Department of Psychosis Studies, Institute of Psychiatry, King's College London, London, UK

***Correspondence:**
Thomas P. White, Cognition, Schizophrenia and Imaging Laboratory, Department of Psychosis Studies, PO Box 96, Institute of Psychiatry, King's College London, de Crespigny Park, London, SE5 8AF, UK.
e-mail: thomas.1.white@kcl.ac.uk
† These authors have contributed equally to this work.

Effective estimation of the salience of environmental stimuli underlies adaptive behavior, while related aberrance is believed to undermine rational thought processes in schizophrenia. A network including bilateral frontoinsular cortex (FIC) and dorsal anterior cingulate cortex (dACC) has been observed to respond to salient stimuli using functional magnetic resonance imaging (fMRI). To test the hypothesis that activity in this salience network (SN) is less discriminately modulated by contextually-relevant stimuli in schizophrenia than in healthy individuals, fMRI data were collected in 20 individuals with schizophrenia and 13 matched controls during performance of a modified monetary incentive delay (MID) task. After quantitatively identifying spatial components representative of the FIC and dACC features of the SN, two principal analyses were conducted. In the first, modulation of SN activity by salience was assessed by measuring response to trial outcome. First-level general linear models were applied to individual-specific time-courses of SN activity identified using spatial independent component analysis (ICA). This analysis revealed a significant salience-by-performance-by-group interaction on the best-fit FIC component's activity at trial outcome, whereby healthy individuals but not individuals with schizophrenia exhibited greater distinction between the response to hits and misses in high salience trials than in low salience trials. The second analysis aimed to ascertain whether SN component amplitude differed between the study groups over the duration of the experiment. Independent-samples *T*-tests on back-projected, percent-signal-change scaled SN component images importantly showed that the groups did not differ in the overall amplitude of SN expression over the entire dataset. These findings of dysregulated but not decreased SN activity in schizophrenia provide physiological support for mechanistic conceptual frameworks of delusional thought formation.

Keywords: schizophrenia, salience, cortical networks, fMRI, reward

INTRODUCTION

The finite capacity of our attentional and behavioral resources necessitates that we assign preferential salience to certain environmental stimuli, while limiting responses to others. Appropriately selecting the stimuli to which we assign salience is therefore a key component of adaptive behavior. Relatedly, the allocation of incentive salience to both primary and more abstract rewarding stimuli potently modulates behavior (Robbins and Everitt, 1996).

Electrophysiological recordings from the macaque striatum show that phasic dopaminergic responses to rewarding stimuli temporally mimic the prediction error of reward-value models, implicating this region as the source of a reinforcement signal required to adjust the probability of subsequent action selection (Schultz et al., 1997). Comparable human blood oxygenation-level dependent (BOLD) responses in striatum to novel, aversive and intense stimuli suggest that this response indexes salience-related features such as familiarity, contextual relevance and predictability more generally (Zink et al., 2004). A complementary model of the role of phasic striatal dopamine therefore proposes that the basal ganglia concertedly act as a centralized selection device, allocating attentional resources between competing motor programs in a contextually-relevant manner (Redgrave et al., 1999). The reward findings uphold this model insofar as test animals are generally required to shift attention to rewarding stimuli and carry out a motor program to realize their consumption.

Human BOLD findings also imply an analogous, attention-switching function in a cortical network comprising dorsal anterior cingulate cortex (dACC) and bilateral frontoinsular cortex (FIC), subsuming anterior insula (AI), and inferior frontal gyrus (IFG). These regions are consistently coactive with task-specific regions when stimuli are modulated in terms of cognitive, emotional and homeostatic salience, which implies they fundamentally code salience (Menon, 2011); they also exhibit a temporal signature dissociable from task-specific regions via seed-region correlation and independent component analysis (ICA) suggesting that they represent a salience network (SN; Seeley et al., 2007), Moreover, analyzing Granger-causal relationships from multi-task functional magnetic resonance imaging (fMRI) data, Sridharan et al. (2008) observed that right FIC activity consistently preceded and predicted activity in regions of the default mode network (DMN; medial prefrontal cortex, precuneus and bilateral angular gyrus), where activity is typically greater during times of introspection, and also regions of the central executive network (CEN; bilateral dorsolateral PFC and posterior parietal cortex), where activity is typically greater when attention is focused on environmental stimuli. They suggested that right FIC was therefore crucial in switching between these two contrasting modes of brain function.

The cortical SN appears to be a focus of pathology in schizophrenia. Structurally, these regions are amongst the most consistently observed sites of gray-matter reduction in the disorder (Ellison-Wright et al., 2008), and focal alterations in SN volume are observed to be associated with the severity of reality distortion in schizophrenia (Palaniyappan et al., 2011). Reduced functional connectivity has also been observed within the SN in schizophrenia compared to controls during volitional eye saccades (Tu et al., 2010) and at rest (Tu et al., 2012). However, within-SN dysconnectivity is not unequivocally apparent in schizophrenia. Resting-state connectivity between a FIC seed and other SN constituents was recently reported to be unaffected by schizophrenia, despite significant connectivity reductions in both DMN and CEN (Woodward et al., 2011). Combined assessment of within- and between-network connectivity in schizophrenia as compared with controls has revealed less consistent functional relationships within the SN and between the SN and DMN during passive perceptual stimulation (White et al., 2010a).

The monetary incentive delay (MID) task presents an adaptable framework for assessing SN functional modulation in schizophrenia. Investigating gains (but not losses) Walter et al. (2009, 2010) demonstrated that activity in dACC and a region encompassing AI and ventrolateral prefrontal cortex is more sensitively modulated at outcome in healthy individuals than schizophrenia patients in tasks that vary reward magnitude and those that vary reward probability. Furthermore, Waltz et al. (2010) reported significant group-by-outcome interactions in right FIC and pregenual ACC BOLD responses in a MID task involving both gains and losses, with controls exhibiting greater activity for gains than losses and patients exhibiting greater responses for losses than gains. While these latter findings are in line with anhedonic symptoms of schizophrenia, from a biological perspective salience should be attributed to both positive and negative events—potential rewards and dangers must both be appropriately detected. As a result, salience coding should be expectedly heightened to both positive and negative extremes. Moreover, the success with which potential losses and gains are respectively obtained or avoided should additionally contribute to salience coding to maximally adapt subsequent behavioral output.

The notion that individuals with schizophrenia exhibit not just muted salience attribution to conventionally salient stimuli but also aberrantly excessive salience attribution at other times is central to dominant theories of delusion formation (Kapur, 2003; Kapur et al., 2005). This suggests that attenuated reward signals in cortical SN and striatum (for review, see Heinz and Schlagenhauf, 2010) paint an incomplete picture. Here, we use spatial ICA of fMRI data to identify the cortical SN in individuals with schizophrenia and matched controls during performance of a modified MID task. We present analyses conducted to assess the explicit hypotheses that: (1) cortical SN activity focused in both dACC and FIC will be modulated by the salience of rewarding monetary stimuli at reward outcome in healthy individuals; (2) SN modulation by task and performance will be diminished in schizophrenia; and (3) despite this putative dysregulation in schizophrenia, the cortical SN will be no less evident in these individuals than in healthy controls over the duration of the task.

MATERIAL AND METHODS

PARTICIPANTS

Twenty individuals satisfying DSM-IV criteria for schizophrenia (American Psychiatric Association, 1994) and 13 healthy controls were recruited to take part in the study. All participants were right-handed and groups did not differ significantly in terms of age or intelligence quotient (IQ) assessed using the National Adult Reading Test (NART; Nelson, 1982). Summary demographic and psychiatric-symptom details are provided in **Table 1**.

Diagnosis of schizophrenia was confirmed by assessment of clinical case notes and confirmation of suitability by each individual's consultant psychiatrist. Patients were recruited in a clinically stable condition and were excluded if presenting evidence of comorbid diagnosis or a medical disorder resulting in an IQ of less than 85. Symptom severity and classification were assessed using the Positive and Negative Syndrome Scale (PANSS; Kay et al., 1987). Sixteen patients were receiving treatment with atypical antipsychotic medications: olanzapine ($n = 8$); risperidone ($n = 4$); quetiapine ($n = 2$); clozapine ($n = 1$); and sulpiride ($n = 1$). The remaining four patients were receiving typical antipsychotic medications: zuclopenthixol ($n = 2$); flupentixol ($n = 1$); and chlorpromazine ($n = 1$). Chlorpromazine equivalent doses were computed for oral antipsychotic medications using data presented by Woods (2003). In the case of risperidone Consta injection, 25 mg Consta injection every 14 days was taken to equate to 4 mg oral risperidone per day, in accordance with the British National Formulary recommendation (Joint Formulary Committee, 2008).

Table 1 | Sample details.

Measure	Group	
	Schizophrenia group ($n = 20$)	**Healthy group ($n = 13$)**
(A) GROUP MEAN DEMOGRAPHIC DETAILS. BRACKETED VALUES DENOTE STANDARD DEVIATION		
Age (years)	36.9 (6.95)	31.3 (9.7)
Intelligence quotient (NART)	101.6 (11.62)	106.4 (9.1)
(B) MEAN SCHIZOPHRENIA GROUP PANSS SCORES. BRACKETED VALUES DENOTE STANDARD DEVIATION		
Positive	13.77 (6.92)	
Negative	13.31 (5.92)	
General	26.81 (6.5)	

NART, national adult reading test (Nelson, 1982); PANSS, positive and negative signs and symptoms of schizophrenia (Kay et al., 1987).

The average chlorpromazine-equivalent dose was 292.7 (range: 100–700) mg/day.

Healthy volunteers were recruited by local advertisement and excluded from study if: they reported a personal history of psychiatric or neurological illness or diagnosis of schizophrenia in a first-degree relative; they exhibited an IQ of less than 85; or they had a recent history of illicit substance use.

Ethical approval was provided by Essex 1 Research and Ethic Committee (08/H0301/116). All participants provided informed written consent and were given an inconvenience allowance for study participation plus additional payment proportional to task performance.

EXPERIMENTAL PROCEDURE

Participants performed a modified MID task (Knutson et al., 2001) comprising three 15-min sessions, each containing 48 trials split equally between the different experimental conditions. Participants viewed a screen, onto which visual stimuli were projected, using mirrors mounted on the scanner headcoil. Trials were categorized as either: win trials, in which pressing the button within a target time window resulted in the relevant reward (hit), while failure to do so (miss) resulted in no financial change; or loss trials, in which poor performance (miss) led to loss of the relevant monetary value, while good performance (hit) led to avoidance of this loss. Win and loss trials were further categorized according to the magnitude of their potential financial value (£5, £0.50, and £0). This permitted evaluation of graded incentive salience. As trials with a large potential reward/loss have greater financial implications, they should be considered more salient. Each trial began with a cue notifying trial type (win vs. loss; magnitude of reward), followed by a probe indicating when to perform the right index finger button press and then, following a delay, visual feedback indicating trial outcome. On completion of each trial, participants were required to manually report their feeling of subjective contentment using a visual analog scale (VAS), ranging from satisfied (1) to dissatisfied (9). A schematic representation of an example trial, including the timelines of phase 1 (anticipation to act), phase 2 (anticipation of outcome), and phase 3 (outcome), and the stimuli presented in the experiment is provided in **Figure 1**.

MRI DATA ACQUISITION

Four hundred and forty-eight gradient-echo echo-planar BOLD images (TR/TE: 2000/25 ms, flip angle: 75°, matrix: 64 × 64) were acquired on a 3 Tesla GE Excite II MR scanner (GE Healthcare, USA) during each run of the task. Each whole-brain image contained 38 non-contiguous slices of 2.4-mm thickness separated by a distance of 1 mm, and with in-plane isotropic voxel resolution of 3.4 mm.

BEHAVIORAL DATA ANALYSIS

The time taken to make the button-press response following presentation of probe stimulus (reaction time; RT) was recorded for each trial. To reduce the effects of trials in which no response was made, the within-session median RT was calculated and these values averaged to give subject-specific mean RTs for each condition

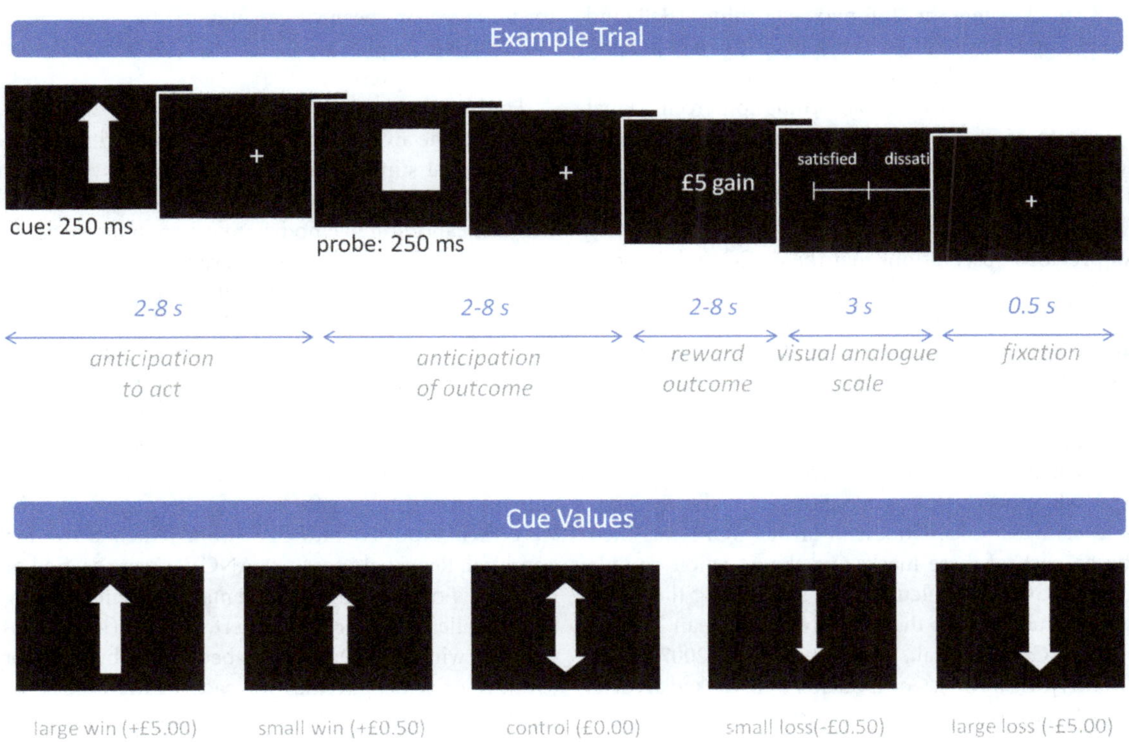

FIGURE 1 | The monetary incentive delay task. Showing an example trial (top) and the various cue values used (bottom).

over the experiment as a whole. A repeated-measures ANOVA test was performed within SPSS (SPSS Inc., USA) to assess differences related to trial valence (win or loss), salience (£5 or £0.50), and group (healthy or schizophrenia). Similarly, the hit rate (percentage calculated on the basis of number of hits and total trials) was calculated for each condition averaged across sessions. Again, a repeated-measures ANOVA was conducted to assess differences relating to trial valence, salience and group. *Post-hoc* T-tests were performed to assess the specifics of significant main effects and between-factor interactions.

fMRI DATA PREPROCESSING AND ANALYSIS

fMRI data were preprocessed using SPM5 (Wellcome Department of Imaging Neuroscience, University of London, UK). Data were realigned to the first image of the series, normalized to a standard-brain template and smoothed using an 8-mm FWHM Gaussian kernel.

Spatial ICA was performed on the pre-processed data using the Group ICA fMRI Toolbox (GIFT; http://icatb.sourceforge.net) within Matlab 7.8 (MathWorks, USA). GIFT uses a temporal concatenation approach during which data reduction is performed via multi-staged principal component analysis (PCA) and aggregation to generate common-group maps. These components are subsequently back-projected onto each individual's data to create subject-specific spatial maps with corresponding time-courses (Calhoun et al., 2008, 2009).

Prior to ICA, data dimensionality was estimated using Minimum Length Description criteria to be 64. Since model order determines network spatial characteristics including subnetwork parcellation, ICA was constrained to produce 64 components. ICA was performed using the Infomax algorithm (Bell and Sejnowski, 1995), and repeated five times with Icasso (Himberg et al., 2004) to maximize the stability of the derived components. Components were also scaled according to percent signal change to facilitate inter-subject comparisons of their time-courses. Back-reconstruction was carried out using GICA3 on the basis of previous empirical support for the accuracy of this method (Erhardt et al., 2011).

In light of previous observations that the dACC and FIC features of the SN are customarily dissociated into separate fMRI spatial components (Sridharan et al., 2008; White et al., 2010a), it was considered appropriate to attempt to identify these SN features independently. To this end, binary masks of (1) the dACC and (2) the FIC, were constructed from a downloadable SN map (http://findlab.stanford.edu/research; Shirer et al., 2012). Each binary mask was dilated by one voxel to favor components whose outside-mask loadings were greater in regions immediately proximate to the specified masks. Goodness-of-fit (GOF) was then assessed between each of these masks and the 64 whole-sample component maps. GOF was calculated by subtracting the mean Z-score of voxel values outside the mask from the mean Z-score of voxels within it (Greicius et al., 2004; Seeley et al., 2007) using Matlab 7.8 (MathWorks, USA). Components were ranked according to GOF and the best-fit component for each binary mask selected for subsequent investigation.

Having identified the two best-fit SN whole-sample components, their voxel-wise robustness was assessed statistically for the whole sample using one-sample T-tests conducted on whole-brain, back-reconstructed loading images for each participant. This identified the voxels with strongest loadings for these components, although it must be stressed that each component is a whole-brain component. To identify regions of strong positive loading, significance was ascribed according to a cluster-level criterion based on the spatial extent of suprathreshold voxel clusters. Voxel-level inclusion of $P < 0.001$ and cluster-level significance of $P < 0.05$ family-wise error corrected were used throughout this work. In addition, two-samples T-tests were performed to investigate between-group differences in the amplitude of expression of the SN components over the entire dataset. Little difference between individuals with schizophrenia and healthy controls was predicted here according to the hypothesis that SN activity is dysregulated rather than diminished.

To investigate modulation of SN activity by task-related events at outcome, first-level GLMs were applied to the back-projected time-courses of the two SN components, with the hypothesis that these events would predict activity less in individuals with schizophrenia than in healthy controls. This technique permits assessment of distributed, event-related brain activity and has advantages over the conventional voxel-wise, mass-univariate approach including: (1) it reduces the chances of Type-1 error inherent to mass-univariate analyses on account of the large number of tests involved in the latter; (2) it reduces the chances of Type-2 error likely in the latter as a consequence of attempts to stringently correct for these multiple tests; and (3) it presents a readily understandable summary statistic for a distributed feature of brain activity, which has been previously identified by virtue of its temporal congruity. The conjoined use of GLMs and ICA has for these reasons been successfully used in wide-ranging settings (for recent examples, see Caulo et al., 2011; Luckhoo et al., 2012; White et al., in press).

For the current GLM-ICA analyses we modeled the time-course of the BOLD response associated with the presentation of the visual stimuli throughout the task, by convolving a vector of delta functions for the onset and durations of these stimuli with the canonical haemodynamic response function. Regressors were included in the GLMs for events split by cue value, performance and phase. This resulted in 30 conditions (5 cue values × 2 performance outcomes × 3 phases) for each of the three sessions. When necessary, regressors were included for void trials during which no button-press response was registered. Session-specific realignment parameters were also included in the GLMs as covariates of no interest. Resulting, individual-specific GLMs were applied to the time-courses of the best-fit FIC and dACC components. Beta coefficients for responses at trial outcome were then exported into SPSS (SPSS Inc., USA) for statistical appraisal. Repeated-measures ANOVAs were carried out to assess the effects on the beta coefficients of within-subjects factors of reward salience (£5 or £0.50), performance (hit or miss) and trial valence (win or loss), and the between-subject factor of group (healthy or schizophrenia) for each of the best-fit components separately. *Post-hoc* confirmatory T-tests were performed to assess the direction of significant effects.

The relationship between psychiatric symptomatology and SN task modulation was assessed in the schizophrenia group using bivariate Pearson correlation between above-calculated beta coefficients and PANNS positive, negative and general psychopathology scores. Similarly, the relationship between antipsychotic medication and SN task modulation was investigated by assessing correlation between beta coefficients and chlorpromazine equivalent dosage in the same individuals. In a further analysis to investigate whether medication class predicted SN modulation, a repeated-measures ANOVA was conducted in the schizophrenia group to assess the effects on beta estimates of salience, performance and trial outcome as in the previous analyses; however, this analysis also included a binary covariate detailing whether each individual had been prescribed typical or atypical antipsychotic medication.

RESULTS

BEHAVIOR

Hit rate and RT results are summarized in **Figure 2**; statistical findings from the repeated-measures ANOVA conducted on these measures is provided in **Table 2**. There was a significant valence-by-salience interaction [$F_{(1,\ 32)} = 9.02$, $P = 0.005$] in RT. Subsequent T-tests demonstrated that while RT was significantly less for large win trials compared to small win trials [$T_{(32)} = 3.76$, $P = 0.001$], no significant difference was observed between large and small loss trials. A valence-by-group interaction [$F_{(1,\ 32)} = 6.57$, $P = 0.015$] was also observed in RT. Patients demonstrated significantly shorter RTs averaged across win trials (246.03 ± 24.07 ms) as compared to loss trials [250.42 ± 23.93 ms; $T_{(19)} = 2.84$, $P = 0.011$]. By contrast, healthy individuals exhibited non-significant differences in RT between these conditions [win trials: 238.82 ± 23.98 ms; loss trials: 235.26 ± 20.58 ms; $T_{(12)} = 1.19$, $P = 0.255$]. There was an additional weak trend toward a group effect in hit rate [$F_{(1,\ 32)} = 2.78$, $P = 0.11$]. This was observed on account of the increased number of void trials, for which no participant response was recorded, in the schizophrenia group as compared to the healthy group [healthy group: 1.33 ± 0.96 %; schizophrenia group: 5.75 ± 7.61 %; $T_{(32)} = 2.07$, $P = 0.05$]. VAS ratings categorized on the basis of trial type and group are presented in **Figure 3**. Main-effect and interaction statistics for VAS measures are shown in **Table 3**.

SN IDENTIFICATION AND CHARACTERISATION

Figure 4 displays GOF scores between the FIC mask and each of the 64 whole-sample components. The GOF score for the best-fit component was 2.87. This Z-score equates to a P-value of 0.004, and as such this component can be confidently declared to focus on FIC regions. A one-sample T-test on individual-specific component maps for the best-fit component demonstrated significant positive clusters in bilateral IFG and anterior insula and is displayed in **Figure 5**. Statistical characteristics of its gray-matter foci are presented in **Table 4(A)**. **Figure 6** displays GOF scores between the dACC mask and each of the 64 whole-sample components. The best-fit dACC component, whose whole-sample

Table 2 | Modulation of hit rate and reaction time.

Measure	Effect	F-value	P-value
Hit rate	V	1.49	0.231
	S	0.41	0.529
	G	2.78	0.105
	V × S	0.01	0.913
	V × G	0.66	0.423
	S × G	0.36	0.551
	V × S × G	1.54	0.224
Reaction time	V	0.72	0.790
	S	3.83	0.059
	G	1.97	0.171
	V × S	9.02	0.005
	V × G	6.57	0.015
	S × G	3.13	0.086
	V × S × G	0.26	0.874

Valence, V; Salience, S; Group, G.

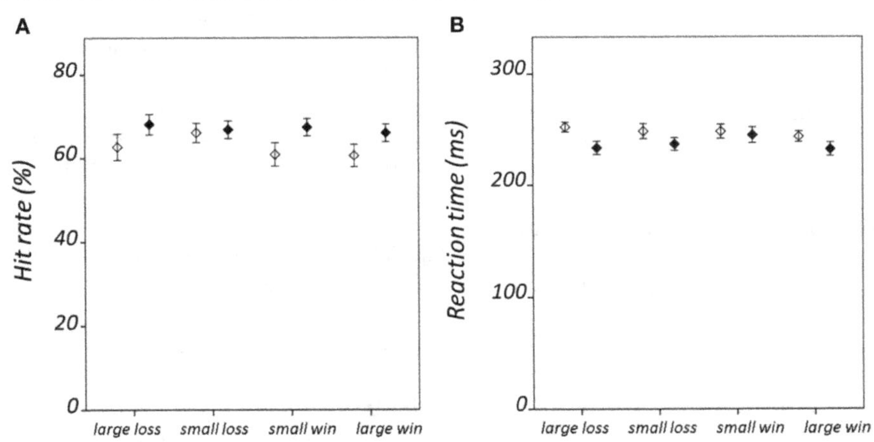

FIGURE 2 | Condition-specific behavioral results. Showing **(A)** hit rate, and **(B)** reaction time. Error bars denote standard error of the mean. Healthy group results are shown in black and schizophrenia group results in white.

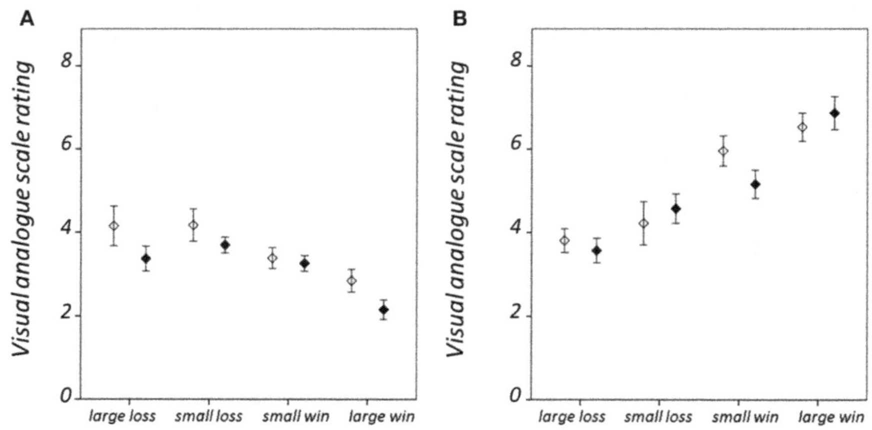

FIGURE 3 | Condition-specific visual analog scale (VAS) rating results. For **(A)** hit trials, and **(B)** miss trials. VAS ratings range between 1 when the participant reported feeling "satisfied" and 9 when "dissatisfied." Error bars denote standard error of the mean. Healthy group results are shown in black and schizophrenia group results in white.

Table 3 | Modulation of visual analog scale ratings.

Effect	*F*-value	*P*-value
V	20.72	7×10^{-5}
S	1.27	0.268
P	34.58	2×10^{-6}
G	1.75	0.20
V × S	5.91	0.021
V × P	49.143	1×10^{-6}
V × G	0.02	0.891
S × P	8.06	0.008
S × G	0.11	0.746
P × G	0.55	0.465
V × S × P	27.14	1×10^{-4}
V × S × G	2.19	0.149
S × P × G	2.00	0.167
V × P × G	0.35	0.561
V × S × P × G	4.29	0.046

Valence, V; Salience, S; Performance, P; Group, G.

GOF with the dACC mask was 1.38 (which equates to a *P*-value of 0.168) and had maximal loadings in medial prefrontal regions. This component is displayed in **Figure 5** and statistics relating to its gray-matter foci are presented in **Table 4(B)**.

BETWEEN-GROUP DIFFERENCES IN SN COMPONENT AMPLITUDE

Whole-brain examination of between-group amplitude differences in the best-fit FIC and dACC components conducted using two-samples *T*-tests revealed no significant clusters (using either an uncorrected or FWE-corrected cluster level of $P < 0.05$ and a voxel-level threshold of $P < 0.001$).

SN ACTIVITY AT REWARD OUTCOME

Figure 7 and **Table 5** present beta coefficients for the best-fit FIC component at time of trial outcome. As is shown in **Table 6**, there was an overall main effect of group [$F_{(1,\ 32)} = 4.82$, $P = 0.036$]. Subsequent independent samples *T*-tests revealed that beta estimates for schizophrenia patients averaged over conditions were significantly smaller than those for healthy individuals. Interestingly, a significant salience-by-performance-by-group interaction was also observed [$F_{(1,\ 32)} = 4.280$, $P = 0.047$]. Healthy individuals displayed a trend toward greater responses for hits compared to misses (across both valences of conditions) in the high salience trials [$T_{(12)} = 2.055$, $P = 0.061$] and a non-significant effect for low salience trials [$T_{(12)} = -1.730$, $P = 0.107$]; by contrast, performance did not significantly modulate FIC response for either high or low salience trials in the schizophrenia group [high salience: $T_{(19)} = 0.483$, $P = 0.634$; low salience: $T_{(19)} = -0.483$, $P = 0.966$]. There was also a highly significant valence-by-salience interaction on FIC activity at reward outcome [$F_{(1,\ 32)} = 11.353$, $P = 0.002$]. A follow-up paired-samples *T*-test of the full study sample revealed that, while there was a non-significant difference in FIC modulation between high and low salience conditions for win trials [$T_{(32)} = 0.944$, $P = 0.352$], high salience loss trials evoked greater responses than corresponding low salience trials [$T_{(32)} = 3.482$, $P = 0.001$]. No other main effects or between-factor interactions were significant for this component. For the best-fit ACC component task modulation at reward outcome is shown in **Figure 8**, and beta estimates summarized in **Table 5**. No main effects or between-factor interactions were significant at conventional statistical thresholds, as is shown in **Table 7**.

RELATIONSHIPS WITH SYMPTOM AND MEDICATION

No statistically significant relationship was observed between SN task modulation and psychiatric symptomatology, medication dosage or medication class.

DISCUSSION

This salience-focused fMRI study of individuals with schizophrenia and matched control subjects employed spatial ICA to identify components of brain activity with maximal spatial correspondence with two principal features of the SN, namely the FIC and

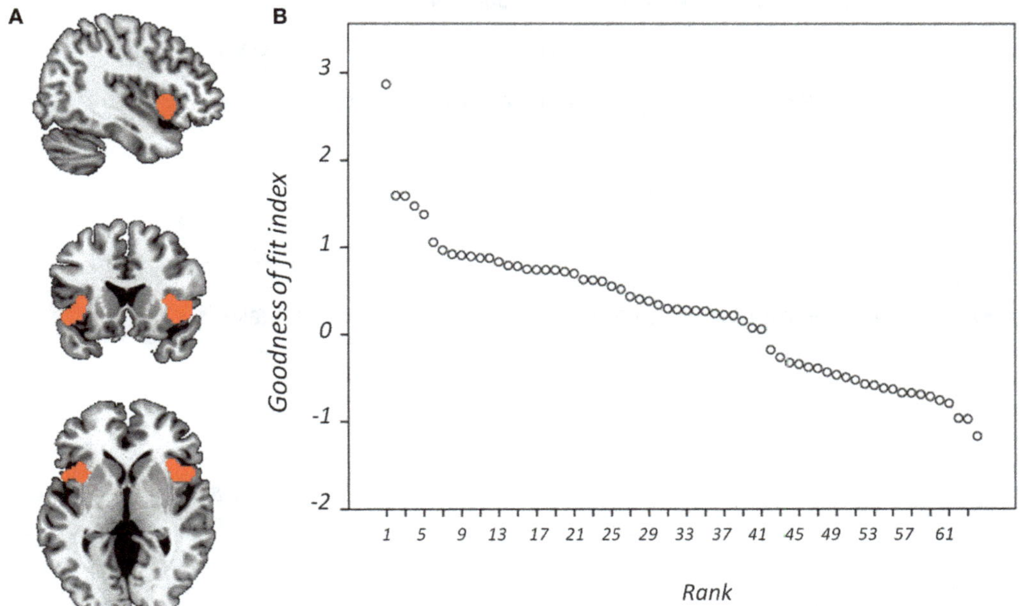

FIGURE 4 | Goodness-of-fit (GOF) with frontoinsular cortex mask. Showing **(A)** the mask is overlaid onto a standardized T_1-weighted image shown according to the neurological convention; and **(B)** GOF with this mask for each component displayed according to rank.

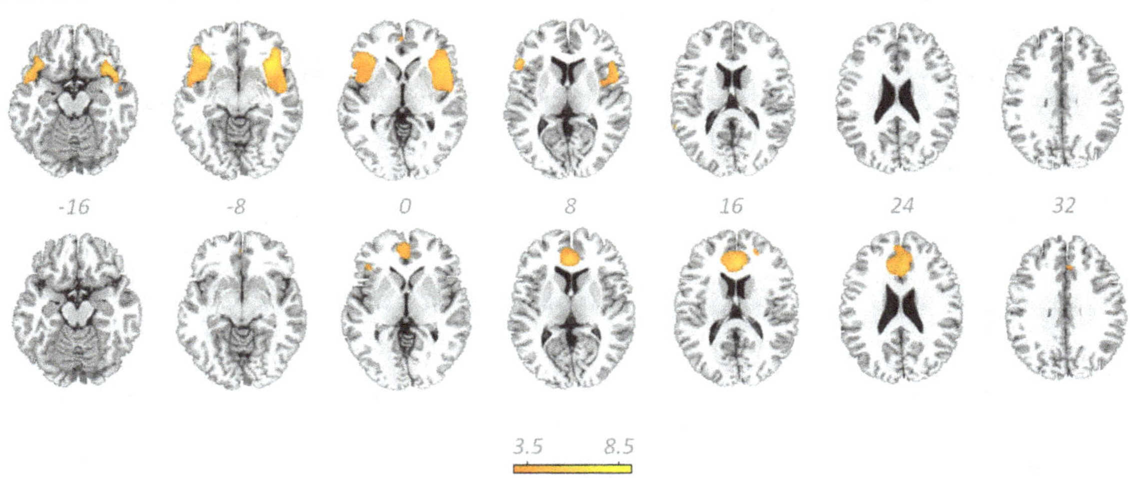

FIGURE 5 | The salience network. Showing the best-fit frontoinsular cortex component (top row) and the best-fit anterior cingulate cortex component (bottom row) overlaid on a standardized T_1-weighted image. Colorbar denotes T-scores from one sample T-tests and relates to both components. These images are thresholded at uncorrected P-threshold of 0.001.

dACC; modulation of the activity of these components at trial outcome was then investigated to test the hypothesis that SN would be temporally dysregulated in schizophrenia.

The best-fit FIC group component exhibited a high GOF with the FIC mask ($Z = 2.87$, $P = 0.004$). It was characterized by maximal positive loadings in bilateral regions principally including AI and IFG, and can therefore be confidently described as exhibiting substantial FIC focus. Its hemispherically bilateral distribution is in accord with numerous fMRI ICA characterizations of the SN (for example, Seeley et al., 2007; Sridharan et al., 2008; White et al., 2010b), although it is noted that right FIC has been ascribed particular, influential roles in cognitive switching (Sridharan et al., 2008). GLM analysis of activity in this component at trial outcome produced findings of amplitude modulation suggestive of its role in salience coding.

A significant salience-by-performance-by-group interaction on FIC component activity was evident at trial outcome. In healthy individuals a trend toward greater responses for hits than misses was observed for high salience trials but less robustly for low salience trials. Since the outcome of a specific trial potentially

Table 4 | One-sample *T*-test results for the best-fit salience network components.

Brain structure (Brodmann area)	MNI coordinates	*T*-value	Cluster size (k_E)
(A) SIGNIFICANT GRAY-MATTER FOCI OF THE BEST-FIT FRONTO-INSULAR CORTEX COMPONENT			
Left inferior frontal gyrus (47)	−34 18 −12	8.11	2641
Left insula (13)	−44 10 −2	5.81	2641
Left superior temporal gyrus (22)	−54 14 −6	5.81	2641
Right inferior frontal gyrus (47)	34 30 −10	5.86	2108
Right superior temporal gyrus (38)	46 10 −10	4.58	2108
Right anterior cingulate gyrus (32)	2 48 0	3.29	76
(B) SIGNIFICANT GRAY-MATTER FOCI OF THE BEST-FIT ANTERIOR CINGULATE CORTEX COMPONENT			
Left anterior cingulate gyrus (24)	−4 32 14	6.60	2053
Right anterior cingulate gyrus (24)	6 28 18	6.45	2053
Right anterior cingulate gyrus (32)	2 48 2	4.61	2053
Right inferior frontal gyrus (47)	46 26 4	4.09	91

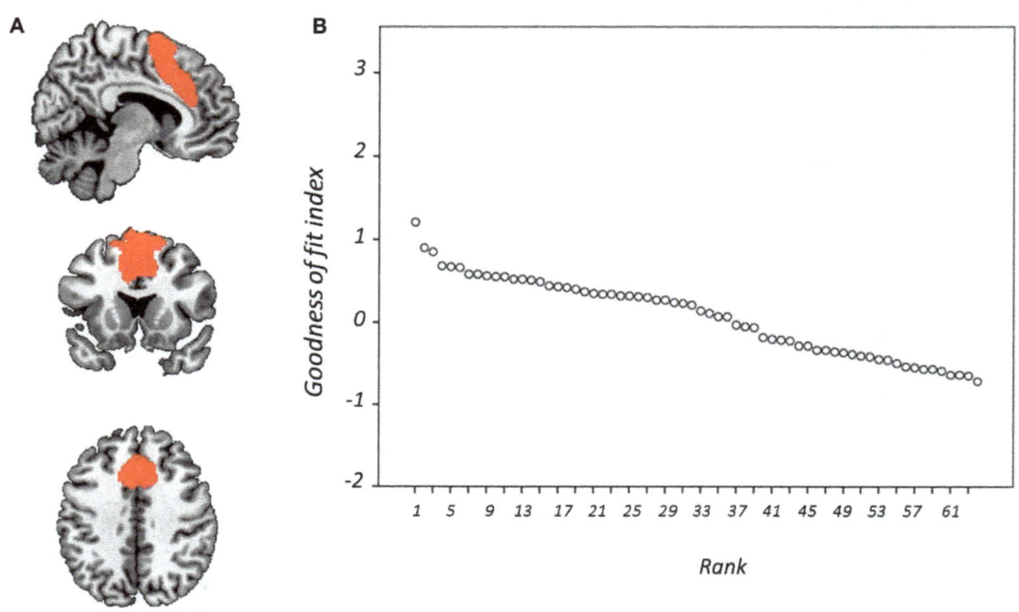

FIGURE 6 | Goodness-of-fit (GOF) with anterior cingulate cortex mask. Showing **(A)** the mask is overlaid onto a standardized T_1-weighted image shown according to the neurological convention; and **(B)** GOF with this mask for each component displayed according to rank.

modulates its financial implications, and the differential consequences of the hit or miss are greater in high salience trials, it is unsurprising that the cortical system purported to encode salience exhibits modulation of activity in this manner in healthy individuals. An interesting addendum here is that FIC responses to hits exceed those to misses across high salience trials of both reward valences. Learning from a large-magnitude failure is an important aspect of adaptive behavior, and is contingent on importance being placed on the event in question; as such, it is somewhat surprising that this is not reflected in FIC activity at reward outcome.

Contrary to the healthy individuals, FIC component activity was not significantly modulated by performance as a function of salience in the individuals with schizophrenia. Non-significant performance effects were observed for both the high and low salience trial types. This demonstrates a functional impairment in FIC regulation in these individuals with potential behavioral repercussions. Efficient reinforcement learning must rely on determination of not only the potential salience of environmental events (as would be demonstrated by a main effect of salience) but also how this salience changes contextually (as would be demonstrated in this instance by a salience-by-performance interaction). That this effect is not evident in individuals with schizophrenia provides further physiological support for reinforcement learning deficits in these individuals (Evans et al., 2011; Maia and Frank, 2011).

There was also a significant salience-by-valence interaction on FIC activity at trial outcome. Across the whole sample, responses for large-loss hits exceeded those for small-loss hits, while the corresponding comparisons for win trials were insignificant. These

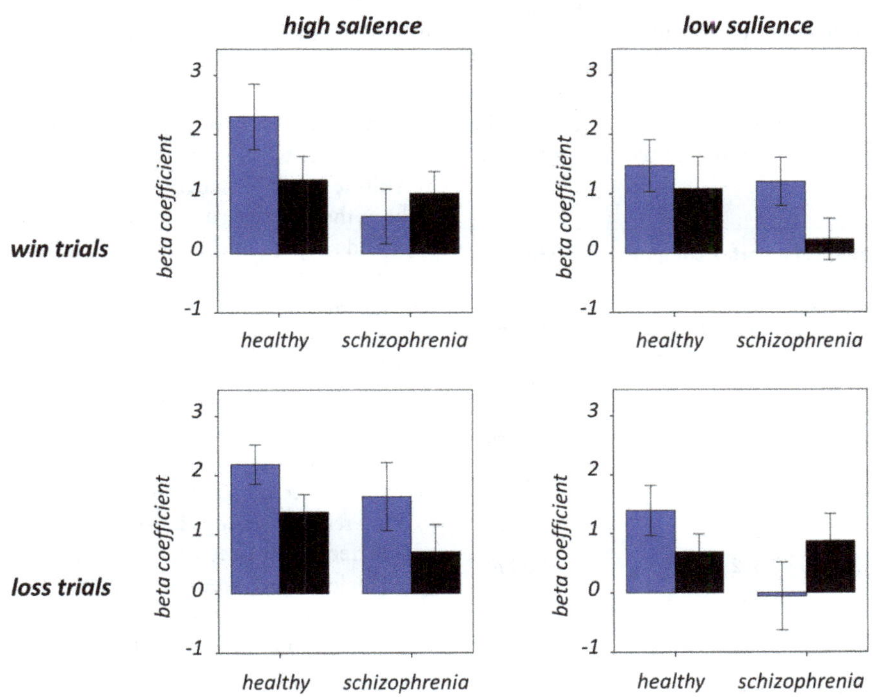

FIGURE 7 | Frontoinsular cortex component activity at trial outcome. Condition-specific beta coefficients are shown, with blue and black bars denoting hit and miss trials, respectively. Error bars denote standard error of the mean.

Table 5 | Beta coefficients for salience network responses at outcome.

Condition	FIC component		ACC component	
	Healthy group	**Schizophrenia group**	**Healthy group**	**Schizophrenia group**
Large win—hit	2.30 (2.07)	0.62 (2.07)	0.87 (1.45)	0.65 (1.51)
Large win—miss	1.24 (1.48)	1.01 (1.64)	0.97 (0.89)	0.71 (1.00)
Small win—hit	1.47 (1.64)	1.20 (1.81)	0.93 (0.47)	0.58 (1.21)
Small win—miss	1.08 (2.00)	0.23 (1.57)	0.83 (0.95)	0.73 (0.92)
Large win—hit	1.39 (1.59)	−0.06 (2.56)	0.81 (0.78)	0.69 (1.12)
Large win—miss	0.69 (1.14)	0.87 (2.06)	1.09 (1.09)	0.87 (0.92)
Large win—hit	2.19 (1.25)	1.64 (2.59)	1.40 (0.98)	0.69 (1.44)
Large win—miss	1.37 (1.12)	0.70 (2.07)	0.71 (0.74)	0.45 (1.07)

Group mean values and their standard deviation in brackets.
Frontoinsular cortex, FIC; Anterior cingulate cortex, ACC.

findings provide a cortical correlate of "loss aversion," by which individuals exhibit increased sensitivity for loss compared to gain (Tversky and Kahneman, 1979). Previous behavioral evidence suggests that this phenomenon is reduced in individuals with schizophrenia (Tremeau et al., 2008), representing a failure in the integration of affective and cognitive systems. Thus, while the current data highlight a finely-tuned aspect of SN function, it appears that the FIC does not act as the physiological substrate for the loss-aversion deficits previously observed in individuals with schizophrenia. Nevertheless, these findings of enhanced FIC sensitivity to negative events are broadly concordant with previous observations that right AI is influential in processing emotionally negative stimuli, such as those evoking feelings of disgust (Phillips et al., 1997).

The responses of the FIC component at trial outcome were consistently smaller in individuals with schizophrenia as compared to healthy individuals, as was demonstrated by the main effect of group in the repeated-measures ANOVA. This finding demonstrates that activity at this time was less tightly linked to the environmental stimuli in these individuals. While this is in itself noteworthy, the importance of this finding is magnified by the concomitant observations that contrasting features of FIC activity remain unchanged in the disorder. Despite the between-group differences in SN task modulation, voxel-wise comparison revealed no significant between-group difference in amplitude of SN expression over the dataset. This result suggests that the SN is similarly active in schizophrenia and that this network is similarly coherent in the disorder, thus acting as an integrated system (as reported by Woodward et al., 2011), despite exhibiting attenuated task-related responses in schizophrenia. In summary, these data suggest that the SN is dysregulated in schizophrenia rather than attenuated *per se*. This work, similarly to EEG reports of increased background oscillatory activity in the face of decreased event-related activity (Winterer et al., 2004), therefore provides evidence of a generalized failure to appropriately recruit task-relevant brain structures in schizophrenia. Unconventional recruitment of SN structures has particular clinical relevance in light of the putative consequences of this aberrance in the formation and shaping of thoughts. According to the aberrant salience hypothesis of psychotic illness (Kapur, 2003; Kapur et al., 2005), salience attribution is not only diminished for events to which salience is usually attributed, but also increased for events to which salience would not normally be assigned. This paper therefore adds a useful extension to the sizeable literature reporting diminished responses during reward (and more generally during salience processing) in regions including FIC and ventral striatum (for review, see Heinz and Schlagenhauf, 2010).

Table 6 | Modulation of frontoinsular cortex component activity by task.

Effect/interaction	*F*-value	*P*-value
V	0.037	0.848
S	1.282	0.266
P	2.467	0.126
G	4.820	0.036
V × S	11.353	0.002
V × P	0.112	0.740
V × G	0.082	0.776
S × P	2.092	0.158
S × G	0.263	0.612
P × G	1.099	0.302
V × S × P	0.584	0.450
V × S × G	0.356	0.555
V × P × G	0.175	0.679
S × P × G	4.280	0.047
V × S × P × G	0.025	0.876

Valence, V; Salience, S; Performance, P; Group, G.

Our results relating to SN activity in ACC are less clear—no main effects or between-factor interactions were significant—but nevertheless raise important methodological issues related to the study of brain networks using ICA. The best-fit ACC component exhibited a GOF of 1.38 with the dACC mask. This value is at the 17th percentile and as such would not permit rejection of the null hypothesis (that the component does not significantly fit the mask) according to conventional statistical thresholds. Nevertheless, this component's global maximal positive loadings were in ACC and its significant positive clusters were limited to ACC and IFG. From this perspective, it can be validly adjudged a reasonable ACC component, albeit one whose ACC focus was

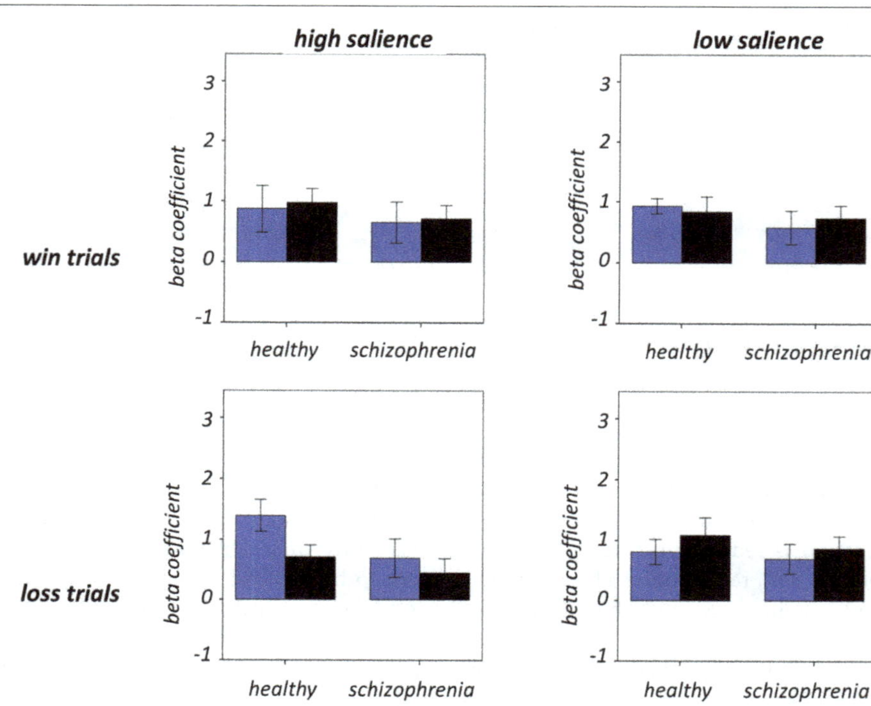

FIGURE 8 | Anterior cingulate cortex component activity at trial outcome. Condition-specific beta coefficients are shown, with blue and black bars denoting hit and miss trials, respectively. Error bars denote standard error of the mean.

Table 7 | Modulation of anterior cingulate cortex component activity by task.

Effect/interaction	*F*-value	*P*-value
V	0.188	0.667
S	0.176	0.678
P	0.073	0.789
G	1.299	0.263
V × S	0.008	0.929
V × P	0.797	0.379
V × G	0.130	0.721
S × P	3.37	0.077
S × G	0.537	0.469
P × G	0.290	0.594
V × S × P	3.247	0.081
V × S × G	0.527	0.473
V × P × G	0.027	0.869
S × P × G	1.055	0.312
V × S × P × G	0.131	0.720

Valence, V; Salience, S; Performance, P; Group, G.

more ventral than is conventional for the SN, given its extension into subgenual regions. The use of objective measures such as the GOF index (Greicius et al., 2004; Petrella et al., 2011) to identify components is preferential to visual inspection but is not without potential pitfall. Lability of distributed large-scale networks should be expected in view of variability of contemporaneous task demands and the psychological processes exercised. On these grounds, if activity in independent networks is coordinated over the course of an experiment they might reasonably be expected to be amalgamated into conglomerate spatial components. Despite the SN being initially identified by procedures such as ICA and seed-region connectivity (Seeley et al., 2007), this problem is particularly likely for networks such as the SN, which are responsible for processing stimuli at a fundamental level and hence likely to be coactive with task-specific regions in numerous tasks.

Antipsychotic medication is a potentially critical confounder of the study of reward salience systems in schizophrenia on account of its dopaminergic mode of action. However, several reports suggest that atypical antipsychotics have a normalizing effect on cerebral activity (for example, Lane et al., 2004). Confounding medication effects cannot be totally discounted in the present study; however, no significant relation was observed between chlorpromazine equivalent dosage or medication class and SN task modulation. While follow-up study in a drug-naïve sample is required to explicitly discount medication confounding effects, it is relevant that aberrant striatal activity during reward processing in schizophrenia has been shown to predate antipsychotic medication treatment (Schlagenhauf et al., 2009).

The application of GLMs to component time-courses lessens the multiple-comparison problem inherent in mass-univariate assessments of whole-brain activity using fMRI. However, a limitation of this procedure is that it does not permit fine-tuned regional inferences, since resultant beta coefficients relate to the component as a whole. As such, their utility depends on the justified selection of meaningful components of activity for GLM assessment. This criterion is met by the current analysis (in particular for the FIC component), given the spatial concordance of the current SN components with previous characterizations of the SN (Sridharan et al., 2008; Shirer et al., 2012).

A further limitation of this work is the employment of uneven sample sizes between the study groups. However, it is not considered that this difference significantly contributed to the findings presented. Since the healthy group sample was sufficient to detect wide-ranging within-group effects at conventional statistical thresholds, it can be reasonably claimed that the healthy group sample characteristics represent a realistic approximation of the population characteristics. Furthermore, our healthy sample was of comparable magnitude to those employed in previous fMRI investigations of abnormal reward processing in schizophrenia (for review, see Heinz and Schlagenhauf, 2010).

This work, in line with recent observations confirms the importance of FIC and to a lesser degree ACC in processing salient stimuli, and presents evidence of SN activity as a useful index of cognitive processes such as loss aversion. SN task modulation is more weakly apparent in schizophrenia as predicted by the considerable literatures of aberrant reward and target processing in the disorder (Kiehl and Liddle, 2001; Walter et al., 2009). The observation that the FIC component is not significantly reduced in amplitude in patients compared to healthy controls, when assessed in its entirety rather than from an event-related perspective, suggests that SN activity is not simply attenuated but rather temporally dysregulated in schizophrenia. This indirectly implies abnormally high SN activity at other times, in line with theories of abnormal salience attribution in the disorder.

REFERENCES

American Psychiatric Association. (1994). *Diagnostic and Statistical Manual of Mental Disorders: DSM-IV, 4th Edn.* Washington, DC: American Psychiatric Association.

Bell, A. J., and Sejnowski, T. J. (1995). An information-maximization approach to blind source separation and blind deconvolution. *Neural Comput.* 7, 1129–1159.

Calhoun, V. D., Kiehl, K. A., and Pearlson, G. D. (2008). Modulation of temporally coherent brain networks estimated using ICA at rest and during cognitive tasks. *Hum. Brain Mapp.* 29, 828–838.

Calhoun, V. D., Liu, J., and Adali, T. (2009). A review of group ICA for fMRI data and ICA for joint inference of imaging, genetic, and ERP data. *Neuroimage* 45, S163–S172.

Caulo, M., Esposito, R., Mantini, D., Briganti, C., Sestieri, C., Mattei, P. A., et al. (2011). Comparison of hypothesis- and a novel hybrid data/hypothesis-driven method of functional MR imaging analysis in patients with brain gliomas. *Am. J. Neuroradiol.* 32, 1056–1064.

Ellison-Wright, I., Glahn, D. C., Laird, A. R., Thelen, S. M., and Bullmore, E. (2008). The anatomy of first-episode and chronic schizophrenia: an anatomical likelihood estimation meta-analysis. *Am. J. Psychiatry* 165, 1015–1023.

Erhardt, E. B., Rachakonda, S., Bedrick, E. J., Allen, E. A., Adali, T., and Calhoun, V. D. (2011). Comparison of multi-subject ICA methods for analysis of fMRI data. *Hum. Brain Mapp.* 32, 2075–2095.

Evans, S., Shergill, S. S., Chouhan, V., Bristow, E., Collier, T., and Averbeck, B. B. (2011). Patients with schizophrenia show increased aversion to angry faces in an associative learning task. *Psychol. Med.* 41, 1471–1479.

Greicius, M. D., Srivastava, G., Reiss, A. L., and Menon, V. (2004). Default-mode network activity distinguishes Alzheimer's disease from healthy aging: evidence from functional MRI. *Proc. Natl. Acad. Sci. U.S.A.*101, 4637–4642.

Heinz, A., and Schlagenhauf, F. (2010). Dopaminergic dysfunction in schizophrenia: salience attribution revisited. *Schizophr. Bull.* 36, 472–485.

Himberg, J., Hyvärinen, A., and Esposito, F. (2004). Validating the independent components of neuroimaging time series via clustering and visualization. *Neuroimage* 22, 1214–1222.

Joint Formulary Committee. (2008). *British National Formulary, 56th Edn.* London: British Medical Association and Royal Pharmaceutical Society of Great Britain.

Kapur, S. (2003). Psychosis as a state of aberrant salience: a framework linking biology, phenomenology, and pharmacology in schizophrenia. *Am. J. Psychiatry* 160, 13–23.

Kapur, S., Mizrahi, R., and Li, M. (2005). From dopamine to salience to psychosis – linking biology, pharmacology and phenomenology of psychosis. *Schizophr. Res.* 79, 59–68.

Kay, S. R., Fiszbein, A., and Opler, L. A. (1987). The positive and negative syndrome scale (PANSS) for schizophrenia. *Schizophr. Bull.* 13, 261–276.

Kiehl, K. A., and Liddle, P. F. (2001). An event-related functional magnetic resonance imaging study of an auditory oddball task in schizophrenia. *Schizophr. Res.* 48, 159–171.

Knutson, B., Fong, G. W., Adams, C. M., Varner, J. L., and Hommer, D. (2001). Dissociation of reward anticipation and outcome with event-related fMRI. *Neuroreport* 12, 3683–3687.

Lane, C. J., Ngan, E. T., Yatham, L. N., Ruth, T. J., and Liddle, P. F. (2004). Immediate effects of risperidone on cerebral activity in healthy subjects: a comparison with subjects with first-episode schizophrenia. *J. Psychiatry Neurosci.* 29, 30–37.

Luckhoo, H., Hale, J. R., Stokes, M. G., Nobre, A. C., Morris, P. G., Brookes, M. J., et al. (2012). Inferring task-related networks using independent component analysis in magnetoencephalography. *Neuroimage* 62, 530–541.

Maia, T. V., and Frank, M. J. (2011). From reinforcement learning models to psychiatric and neurological disorders. *Nat. Neurosci.* 14, 154–162.

Menon, V. (2011). Large-scale brain networks and psychopathology: a unifying triple network model. *Trends Cogn. Sci.* 15, 483–506.

Nelson, H. E. (1982). *The National Adult Reading Test (NART): Test Manual.* Windsor, ON: NFER-Nelson.

Palaniyappan, L., Mallikarjun, P., Joseph, V., White, T. P., and Liddle, P. F. (2011). Reality distortion is related to the structure of the salience network in schizophrenia. *Psychol. Med.* 41, 1701–1708.

Petrella, J. R., Sheldon, F. C., Prince, S. E., Calhoun, V. D., and Doraiswamy, P. M. (2011). Default mode network connectivity in stable vs progressive mild cognitive impairment. *Neurology* 76, 511–517.

Phillips, M. L., Young, A. W., Senior, C., Brammer, M., Andrew, C., Calder, A. J., et al. (1997). A specific neural substrate for perceiving facial expressions of disgust. *Nature* 389, 495–498.

Redgrave, P., Prescott, T. J., and Gurney, K. (1999). Is the short-latency dopamine response too short to signal reward error? *Trends Neurosci.* 22, 146–151.

Robbins, T. W., and Everitt, B. J. (1996). Neurobehavioural mechanisms of reward and motivation. *Curr. Opin. Neurobiol.* 6, 228–236.

Schlagenhauf, F., Sterzer, P., Schmack, K., Ballmaier, M., Rapp, M., Wrase, J., et al. (2009). Reward feedback alterations in unmedicated schizophrenia patients: relevance for delusions. *Biol. Psychiatry* 65, 1032–1039.

Schultz, W., Dayan, P., and Montague, P. R. (1997). A neural substrate of prediction and reward. *Science* 275, 1593–1599.

Seeley, W. W., Menon, V., Schatzberg, A. F., Keller, J., Glover, G. H., Kenna, H., et al. (2007). Dissociable intrinsic connectivity networks for salience processing and executive control. *J. Neurosci.* 27, 2349–2356.

Shirer, W. R., Ryali, S., Rykhlevskaia, E., Menon, V., and Greicius, M. D. (2012). Decoding subject-driven cognitive states with whole-brain connectivity patterns. *Cereb. Cortex* 22, 158–165.

Sridharan, D., Levitin, D. J., and Menon, V. (2008). A critical role for the right fronto-insular cortex in switching between central-executive and default-mode networks. *Proc. Natl. Acad. Sci. U.S.A.* 105, 12569–12574.

Tremeau, F., Brady, M., Saccente, E., Moreno, A., Epstein, H., Citrome, L., et al. (2008). Loss aversion in schizophrenia. *Schizophr. Res.* 103, 121–128.

Tu, P., Buckner, R. L., Zollei, L., Dyckman, K. A., Goff, D. C., and Manoach, D. S. (2010). Reduced functional connectivity in a right-hemisphere network for volitional ocular motor control in schizophrenia. *Brain* 133, 625–637.

Tu, P. C., Hsieh, J. C., Li, C. T., Bai, Y. M., and Su, T. P. (2012). Cortico-striatal disconnection within the cingulo-opercular network in schizophrenia revealed by intrinsic functional connectivity analysis: a resting fMRI study. *Neuroimage* 59, 238–247.

Tversky, A., and Kahneman, D. (1979). Prospect theory: an analysis of decision under risk. *Econometrica* 47, 263–292.

Walter, H., Heckers, S., Kassubek, J., Erk, S., Frasch, K., and Abler, B. (2010). Further evidence for aberrant prefrontal salience coding in schizophrenia. *Front. Behav. Neurosci.* 3:62. doi: 10.3389/neuro.08.062.2009

Walter, H., Kammerer, H., Frasch, K., Spitzer, M., and Abler, B. (2009). Altered reward functions in patients on atypical antipsychotic medication in line with the revised dopamine hypothesis of schizophrenia. *Psychopharmacology (Berl.)* 206, 121–132.

Waltz, J. A., Schweitzer, J. B., Ross, T. J., Kurup, P. K., Salmeron, B. J., Rose, E. J., et al. (2010). Abnormal responses to monetary outcomes in cortex, but not in the basal ganglia, in schizophrenia. *Neuropsychopharmacology* 35, 2427–2439.

White, T. P., Jansen, M., Doege, K., Mullinger, K. J., Park, S. B., Liddle, E. B., et al. (in press). Theta power during encoding predicts subsequent-memory performance and default mode network deactivation. *Hum. Brain Mapp.* doi: 10.1002/hbm.22114

White, T. P., Joseph, V., Francis, S. T., and Liddle, P. F. (2010a). Aberrant salience network (bilateral insula and anterior cingulate cortex) connectivity during information processing in schizophrenia. *Schizophr. Res.* 123, 105–115.

White, T. P., Joseph, V., O'Regan, E., Head, K. E., Francis, S. T., and Liddle, P. F. (2010b). Alpha-gamma interactions are disturbed in schizophrenia: a fusion of electroencephalography and functional magnetic resonance imaging. *Clin. Neurophysiol.* 121, 1427–1437.

Winterer, G., Coppola, R., Goldberg, T. E., Egan, M. F., Jones, D. W., Sanchez, C. E., et al. (2004). Prefrontal broadband noise, working memory, and genetic risk for schizophrenia. *Am. J. Psychiatry* 161, 490–500.

Woods, S. W. (2003). Chlorpromazine equivalent doses for the newer atypical antipsychotics. *J. Clin. Psychiatry* 64, 663–667.

Woodward, N. D., Rogers, B., and Heckers, S. (2011). Functional resting-state networks are differentially affected in schizophrenia. *Schizophr. Res.* 130, 86–93.

Zink, C. F., Pagnoni, G., Martin-Skurski, M. E., Chappelow, J. C., and Berns, G. S. (2004). Human striatal responses to monetary reward depend on saliency. *Neuron* 42, 509–517.

19

Disparity between dorsal and ventral networks in patients with obsessive-compulsive disorder: Evidence revealed by graph theoretical analysis based on cortical thickness from MRI

Seung-Goo Kim[1,2], Wi Hoon Jung[3], Sung Nyun Kim[4], Joon Hwan Jang[4] and Jun Soo Kwon[1,3,4]*

[1] Department of Brain and Cognitive Sciences, Seoul National University, Seoul, South Korea
[2] Research Group for Cortical Networks and Cognitive Functions, Max Planck Institute for Human Cognitive and Brain Sciences, Leipzig, Germany
[3] Clinical Cognitive Neuroscience Center, SNU-MRC, Seoul National University Hospital, Seoul, South Korea
[4] Department of Psychiatry, College of Medicine, Seoul National University, Seoul, South Korea

***Correspondence:**
Jun Soo Kwon, Department of Psychiatry, Seoul National University College of Medicine, 101 Daehak-ro, Jongno-gu, Seoul 110-744, South Korea
e-mail: kwonjs@snu.ac.kr

As one of the most widely accepted neuroanatomical models on obsessive-compulsive disorder (OCD), it has been hypothesized that imbalance between an excitatory direct (ventral) pathway and an inhibitory indirect (dorsal) pathway in cortico-striato-thalamic circuit underlies the emergence of OCD. Here we examine the structural network in drug-free patients with OCD in terms of graph theoretical measures for the first time. We used a measure called efficiency which quantifies how a node transfers information efficiently. To construct brain networks, cortical thickness was automatically estimated using T1-weighted magnetic resonance imaging. We found that the network of the OCD patients was as efficient as that of healthy controls so that the both networks were in the small-world regime. More importantly, however, disparity between the dorsal and the ventral networks in the OCD patients was found in terms of graph theoretical measures, suggesting a positive evidence to the imbalance theory on the underlying pathophysiology of OCD.

Keywords: obsessive-compulsive disorder, magnetic resonance imaging, cortical thickness, structural connectivity, graph theoretical analysis, network efficiency, small-worldness, dorsal-ventral imbalance

1. INTRODUCTION

Obsessive-compulsive disorder (OCD) is an anxiety disorder characterized by intrusive, distressing thoughts and ritualistic, repetitive behaviors (American Psychiatric Association, 1994). The most widely accepted neuroanatomical model of OCD has suggested the involvement of a direct and an indirect cortico-striato-thalamic (CST) pathway (Cummings, 1993; Saxena et al., 1998). In this model, the direct pathway involves in an excitatory input to the internal part of globus pallidus that leads to a disinhibition of thalamus and increased excitation of prefrontal cortex, whereas the indirect pathway involves in an inhibitory input to the external part of globus pallidus that evokes an increased inhibition of thalamus and decreased excitation of prefrontal cortex (Mataix-Cols and van den Heuvel, 2006). Although the over-simplification of the model is questioned (Menzies et al., 2008; Milad and Rauch, 2011), the dichroism has been a well-known basis in approaching the disorder for a long time (Saxena et al., 1998).

Functional studies driven by the CST model have converged on altered activation in patients with OCD in relation to healthy controls in basal ganglia, caudate nucleus, thalamus, orbital frontal cortex, cingulate gyrus, dorsal lateral cortex and parietal regions, using single-photon emission computed tomography (SPECT), positron emission tomography (PET) or functional magnetic resonance imaging (fMRI) (Whiteside et al., 2004; Friedlander and Desrocher, 2006). Despite of the inconsistencies in the literature to some degree, many papers reported higher activations from OCD patients in orbital frontal cortex and basal ganglia, in particular striatum, which have been related to the "hyperactivation of ventral fronto-strital system". In addition, lower activations from OCD patients in dorsal lateral prefrontal cortex and anterior cingulate gyrus, which have been known as the "hypoactivation of dorsal fronto-strital system" (Saxena et al., 1998; Remijnse et al., 2005; Oh et al., 2012; Mataix-Cols and van den Heuvel, 2006).

In relation to the functional findings supporting the CST hypothesis, structural neuroimaging evidences of the abnormalities in OCD patients have been cumulated. Structural alterations were mainly localized in prefrontal regions and basal ganglia. In meta-analyses, gray matter densities in bilateral anterior putamina were found to be higher in OCD patients than healthy controls, and those in dorsal prefrontal regions were found to be lower in OCD patients (Radua and Mataix-Cols, 2009; Rotge et al., 2010). In addition, diffusion tensor imaging (DTI) studies have shown that smaller fractional anisotropy (FA), which has been commonly used to characterize local diffusion and thus to infer white matter integrity (Basser, 1995), were found in clinical population with OCD in the anterior part of cingulum, corpus callosum and other white matter regions in frontal and parietal lobes (Szeszko et al., 2005; Garibotto et al., 2009; Ha et al., 2009;

Bora et al., 2011; Koch et al., 2012; Nakamae et al., 2011; Oh et al., 2012).

It should be noted that the previous structural studies mentioned above have mainly focused on differences in local morphology using massive univariate frameworks such as voxel-based morphometry (VBM; Ashburner and Friston, 2000) or tract-based spatial statistics (TBSS; Smith et al., 2006). Due to its complex nature of brain network, local alterations might not be sufficient to understand the disorder. As needs for investigating connectivities within the CST circuits and between other brain regions have been motivated in the previous literature on OCD (Remijnse et al., 2005; Mataix-Cols and van den Heuvel, 2006; Menzies et al., 2008), a seed-based correlation method (Harrison et al., 2009; Jang et al., 2010) and a whole-brain graph analysis have been used in functional studies (Zhang et al., 2011).

While it is demonstrated that network analyses are capable of investigating the properties of human brains that could not be described using the conventional analyses (Bullmore and Sporns, 2009), relatively new neuroimaging modalities such as DTI and resting-fMRI have been mainly used for the brain connectivity studies. In order to exploit conventional anatomical scans such as T1-weighted MRI, a network analysis based on the correlation of local morphology has been proposed as an alternative framework to examine structural networks in human brains (Worsley et al., 2004; Lerch and Evans, 2005; He et al., 2007; Bernhardt et al., 2011).

In the studies, gray matter is characterized by cortical thickness in a sub-millimeter resolution using cortical surface reconstruction techniques (Dale et al., 1999; Fischl and Dale, 2000; MacDonald et al., 2000). This approach, which only requires T1-weighted MRI, assumes that the positive correlation of cortical thickness may reflect the anatomical connectivity, presumably because of common experiences, shared trophic or maturational influences (Lerch et al., 2008; He et al., 2009; Raznahan et al., 2011). These networks constructed based on cortical thickness have shown their resemblance to DTI-based networks (Gong et al., 2012) and similar modular structures with known functional modules (Chen et al., 2008, 2011). More recently, the cortical thickness-based network in developing brains notably overlapped a functional network known as default-mode-network (DMN; Raznahan et al., 2011).

Here we apply the cortical thickness network analysis on patients with OCD. To our best knowledge, there has been no preceding study to examine graph theoretical measures of brain networks in patients with OCD based on the correlation of cortical thickness so far. As the cortical thickness network analysis has shown its ability to detect reliable and meaningful attributes of human brains in healthy population (He et al., 2007; Chen et al., 2008, 2011; Gong et al., 2009, 2012) and clinical populations with disorders such as multiple sclerosis (He et al., 2009), Alzheimer's disease (He et al., 2008) or temporal lobe epilepsy (Bernhardt et al., 2011), we expect to find alterations in the brain of patients with OCD in terms of network properties, in particular, with a supporting evidence for the dorsal-ventral imbalance in the CST circuits (Saxena et al., 1998; Mataix-Cols and van den Heuvel, 2006), as well as abnormalities in other circuits including dorsal anterior cingulate cortex (Milad and Rauch, 2011) and parietal cortex (Menzies et al., 2008).

Our main contributions include: (1) performing a cortical thickness network analysis on drug-free patients with OCD, (2) investigating graph theoretical measures in the perspective of the major hypothesis of OCD at a network-level (Latora and Marchiori, 2001) and a node-level (Achard and Bullmore, 2007), and finally (3) examining the pathophysiology of OCD in terms of disparity between dorsal and ventral networks, as recently shown as a spatial bias in FA alteration within corpus callosum in OCD patients (Oh et al., 2012).

2. MATERIALS AND METHODS

2.1. PARTICIPANTS

We recruited 32 patients who fulfilled the criteria for OCD in DSM-IV (American Psychiatric Association, 1994) *via* the OCD clinic at Seoul National University Hospital (Seoul, Korea). The patients were diagnosed using the Structured Clinical Interview for DSM-IV (SCID; First et al., 1996). All of the patients with OCD were drug-free: 23 patients were drug-naïve, and the other 9 patients were unmedicated for at least 4 weeks at the time of inclusion. Four patients were assessed to have personality disorders in addition to OCD: three were with obsessive-compulsive personality disorders and one was with schizotypal personality disorder. In addition to the patients, we also recruited 35 age- and gender-matched controls (HC) using the SCID Non-patient Version to confirm that none of the controls was with Axis I psychiatric disorders. The exclusion criteria for both patients and control included lifetime history of psychosis, bipolar disorder, major depressive disorder, substance abuse or dependence, significant head injury, seizure disorder or mental retardation. All participants were right-handed. The severity of depression and anxiety was measured by self-reporting Beck's Depression Inventory (BDI; Beck et al., 1961) and Beck's Anxiety Inventory (BAI; Beck et al., 1988), respectively. The severity of OC symptoms was assessed with clinician-administered Yale-Brown Obsessive-Compulsive Scale (Y-BOCS; Goodman et al., 1989). The institutional review board (IRB) of Seoul National University Hospital (H-1209-025-424) approved the present study. All participants were fully instructed about the procedures of scanning and assessment and then submitted written informed consents.

2.2. IMAGE ACQUISITION AND GRAPH CONSTRUCTION

We obtained magnetic resonance imaging (MRI) using 1.5T MAGNETOM Avanto syngo scanner (Siemens, Erlangen, Germany). T1-weighted 3D images were acquired with the following parameters: TR $=$ 1160 ms, TE $=$ 4.76 ms, FOV $=$ 230 mm, flip angle $= 15°$, voxel size: $0.45 \times 0.45 \times 0.90$ mm, volume dimension: $350 \times 263 \times 350$ mm.

The steps of image analysis are illustrated in **Figure 1**. To compare brain networks between the patients and the controls at the final stage of analysis, we estimated cortical thicknesses from MRIs and constructed brain networks based on them. The detailed steps of the present analysis are explained in the followings. The analysis was carried by custom MATLAB (Mathworks Inc., Natick, MA, USA) codes, if not otherwise specified.

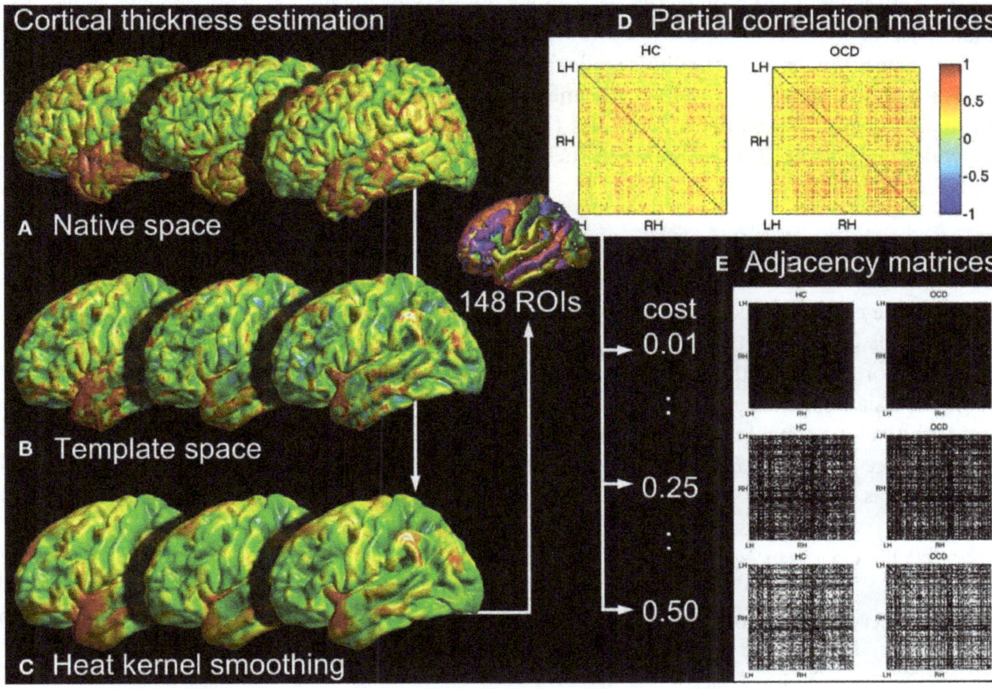

FIGURE 1 | The illustration of analysis steps to construct networks from MRI. The cortical thicknesses are estimated in native spaces (**A**, section 2.2.1), normalized into the template space (**B**, section 2.2.2), and smoothed by a heat kernel based on Laplace-Beltrami eigenfunctions (**C**, section 2.2.3). Partial correlations are computed over 148 ROIs (**D**, section 2.2.4) and binarized to obtain adjacency matrices at a certain rewiring cost (**E**, section 2.2.5).

2.2.1. Cortical thickness estimation

The reconstruction of cortical surfaces and the estimation of cortical thickness were performed using FreeSurfer[1]. As in its standard pipeline (Dale et al., 1999), the intensity of T1-weighted images were normalized and the bias of B0 field was corrected. Then the images were resampled in a unit millimeter isovoxel. An inner cortical surface (the interface between white matter and gray matter) and an outer cortical surface (the interface between gray matter and cerebrospinal fluid) were modeled as triangular tessellation. The cortical thickness was computed by averaging distances from the inner surface to outer surface and the distance from the outer surface to the inner surface (Fischl and Dale, 2000).

2.2.2. Spatial normalization and resampling on a template surface

The estimated cortical surfaces were spatially normalized onto a given template surface, called *"fsaverage6"* with 40962 vertices for each hemisphere, using curvature matching technique to align major sulci patterns (Fischl et al., 1999). Then the cortical thickness was resampled onto the template surface, resulting in the correspondence of measures across all participants. This normalization enables a direct comparison of a vertex or a set of vertices across participants.

2.2.3. Heat kernel smoothing *via* Laplace-Beltrami eigenfunction

Individual cortical thickness maps on the template surface were smoothed using a heat kernel smoothing technique based on Laplace-Beltrami (LB) eigenfunctions (Seo et al., 2010; Kim et al., 2011b; Seo and Chung, 2011). The surface-based smoothing reduces the impact of possible abrupt noise or errors from MRI scanning, surface reconstruction and thickness estimation, thus increases statistical power (Chung et al., 2005; Lerch and Evans, 2005). In addition, due to its analytic formulation, the heat kernel smoothing *via* LB eigenfunctions has a benefit of circumventing numerical errors in conventional smoothing techniques based on iterations. Theoretical details are explained in somewhere else (Seo et al., 2010). In this paper, we used 4000 orthonormal bases of LB eigenfunctions. The measurements were smoothly recovered with the bandwidth parameter σ of 10 mm, using freely available MATLAB codes by Moo K. Chung[2].

2.2.4. Partial correlation between ROIs

Automatic parcellations of gray matter into 74 regions-of-interest (ROIs) per hemisphere were adapted from (Fischl et al., 2004; Destrieux et al., 2010), which was included in FreeSurfer as *"Destrieux 2009 atlas"*. Although the 148 ROIs are less uniform in terms of area (mean area $= 13.73 \pm 9.68\,\text{cm}^2$) than in a high-resolution parcellation with about 1000 ROIs (mean area $\sim 1.5\,\text{cm}^2$ with standard deviation less than $0.15\,\text{cm}^2$) used in Hagmann et al. (2007, 2008), the anatomical significance of the current parcellations assists us in interpreting results while reducing the computational loads in permutation tests as described in

[1] http://surfer.nmr.mgh.harvard.edu

[2] http://brainimaging.waisman.wisc.edu/~chung/lb/

the section 2.4. Thickness measures were averaged in each ROI and used in further analysis.

We computed partial correlation between the ROIs while factoring out the effect of age and gender, as well as the mean of measures, as previous cortical thickness network studies (He et al., 2007, 2008, 2009; Bernhardt et al., 2011). First we fit such a general linear model (GLM) as

$$\mathbf{c}(x) = \beta_0 + \beta_1 \mathbf{a} + \beta_2 \mathbf{g} + \varepsilon, \quad (1)$$

where $\mathbf{c}(x)$ is the vector of the cortical thickness of the x-th ROI for individual participants, $\beta_{k=0,\,1,\,2}$ are unknown parameters to estimate, $\mathbf{a}$ is the vector of ages, $\mathbf{g}$ is the vector of genders and ϵ is the vector of Gaussian random noise. Once we estimated the parameters with the least square method, the residuals $\mathbf{c}(x) - \widehat{\mathbf{c}}(x)$ of the GLM were used to compute a correlation matrix $\mathbf{R} = \left[r_{xy}\right] \in \mathbb{R}^{148\times148}$ as

$$r_{xy} = \mathrm{corr}(\mathbf{c}(x) - \widehat{\mathbf{c}}(x), \mathbf{c}(y) - \widehat{\mathbf{c}}(y)), \quad (2)$$

$\mathrm{corr}(\mathbf{i}, \mathbf{j})$ is the Pearson product of two vectors $\mathbf{i}$ and $\mathbf{j}$ as

$$\mathrm{corr}(\mathbf{i}, \mathbf{j}) = \frac{\sum \mathbf{ij} - \left[\left(\sum \mathbf{i} \sum \mathbf{j}\right)/n\right]}{\left[\mathbf{i}^2 - \left(\sum \mathbf{i}\right)^2/n\right]\left[\mathbf{j}^2 - \left(\sum \mathbf{j}\right)^2/n\right]}, \quad (3)$$

where n is the number of the elements of $\mathbf{i}$ or $\mathbf{j}$. Since we are interested in the anatomical connectivity due to neuronal associations under the same assumptions in the previous network studies based on cortical thickness (He et al., 2007, 2009; Bernhardt et al., 2011), we do not examine anti-correlations in this paper. Although negative association should also be studied in the future to reveal the biological mechanism of the cortical thickness interdependence (Lerch et al., 2008; Raznahan et al., 2011), it would be beyond the scope of the current study.

2.2.5. Network construction for different rewiring costs

For it is known that the *rewiring costs*, or the density, of a network critically affects the graph theoretical properties and topological characteristics of network (Eguíluz et al., 2003; Latora and Marchiori, 2003; Achard et al., 2006; Gong et al., 2009), we controlled the costs to compare the brain networks of the OCD patients with that of the controls. When an undirected and unweighted graph $\mathcal{G}$ is written as a set of two sets as

$$\mathcal{G} = \{\mathcal{V}, \mathcal{E}\}, \quad (4)$$

where $\mathcal{V}$ is the set of vertices and $\mathcal{E}$ is the set of edges, then the cost of a graph $\mathcal{G}$ is given as

$$\mathrm{cost}(\mathcal{G}) = \frac{K}{N(N-1)/2}, \quad (5)$$

where $K = |\mathcal{E}|$ as the number of edges and $N = |\mathcal{V}|$ as the number of vertices in the graph $\mathcal{G}$. Note that $N(N-1)/2$ is the largest number of possible K. Thus the cost equals to zero when there is no connections and the cost equals to one when every node is directly connected to all the other nodes. We binarized the correlation matrices so that they have the equivalent cost, ranging from 0.01 to 0.50 with a step of 0.01. It resulted in 100 (50 costs × 2 groups) adjacency matrices $\mathbf{A}_{g,\,c}$ with the dimensionality of 148 × 148, where g is the group index ($g = 1$ for the controls; $g = 2$ for the OCD patients) and c is the cost ($c = 0.01, 0.02, \ldots, 0.50$). The denser graphs with the cost of more than 0.50 are indistinguishable between the groups and even from the theoretical models (random and lattice), thus we did not include the range over 0.50 in our study. One might note that the selected range of cost is slightly wider than in some previous studies: $0.05 \le c \le 0.40$ (Bernhardt et al., 2011), $0.06 \le c \le 0.40$ (He et al., 2008), but narrower than in another study: $0 < c < 1$ (He et al., 2009). However, determining a threshold for binary graph analysis is no trivial issue, and even selecting multiple thresholds also introduces empirical choices (Langer et al., 2013). It should be noted that using too high threshold (i.e., low cost) has a risk of excluding true connections (false negative) and too low threshold (i.e., high cost) has a risk of including false connections (false positive).

2.3. GRAPH MEASURES: EFFICIENCY AT NETWORK AND NODE LEVELS

In order to characterize the properties of cortical thickness networks, we used *efficiency* in this paper, which measures how efficiently a network exchanges information (Latora and Marchiori, 2001). The efficiency measure is given in two ways: (Latora and Marchiori, 2001): *global efficiency* and *local efficiency*, which are closely related to the *small-worldness* measures such as *characteristic path length* and *clustering coefficients* (Watts and Strogatz, 1998). In contrast to the small-worldness measures are defined only in a network with only one connected component, the efficiency measures are more adoptable for the real-world networks as they are also applicable to disconnected networks.

In addition to the originally proposed network-wise measures for efficiency (Latora and Marchiori, 2001), a node-wise measure has been used in the previous brain connectivity literature (Achard and Bullmore, 2007; He et al., 2009; Wang et al., 2009b; Lo et al., 2010), but only limited to the global efficiency. Combining two levels (network- and node-) and two efficiency measures (global and local), we used four different types of efficiency measures in the paper, as explained in the following subsections.

For the assessment of real-world networks from human brains, we generated cost-matched theoretical networks. The theoretical networks provide benchmarks for a network with a maximal global efficiency [i.e., a random network for unweighted graphs; Latora and Marchiori (2003)] or a network with a high local efficiency (i.e., a regular lattice) under a given constraint of cost. A "economic behavior" of network, or small-worldness, is often used to describe a network with a low characteristic path length, or a high global efficiency, as a random network and a high clustering coefficient, or a high local efficiency, as a regular lattice (Latora and Marchiori, 2003). For each level of cost, 1000 random networks with uniform probability of connections and 1000 lattice networks with the fixed patterns of adjacent connections were synthesized, then the graph measures were averaged over instances. The efficiency measures in the followings were computed using a custom modification of the MATLAB code in Brain Connectivity Toolbox[3].

2.3.1. *Global efficiency*

Global efficiency of a graph $\mathcal{G}$ is given (Latora and Marchiori, 2001) as

$$E_{\mathrm{glob}}(\mathcal{G}) = \frac{1}{(N-1)N} {}_{i\in\mathcal{G}\, j\in\mathcal{G}} \frac{1}{d_{ij}}, \tag{6}$$

where N is the number of nodes in the graph $\mathcal{G}$, the nodes i and j within $\mathcal{G}$ are different, $(i \neq j)$ and d_{ij} is the shortest path length, or geodesic distance (Newman, 2003), between the two nodes. One may note that $E_{\mathrm{glob}}(\mathcal{G})$ quantifies the expectation on how closely a node is connected to all the other nodes in the whole network. It has a clear relation to a graph theoretical measure previously known as *characteristic path length* (Watts and Strogatz, 1998). While the characteristic path length is the arithmetic mean of the shortest path lengths, the E_{glob} is the reciprocal of the harmonic mean of the shortest path lengths (Latora and Marchiori, 2003). The E_{glob} is bounded from 0 to 1. When there are no connections between any nodes, all geodesic distances are equal to infinity then the E_{glob} equals to zero. On the other hand, when the all nodes are directly connected, all distances are equal to one and the E_{glob} also equals to one.

2.3.2. *Local efficiency*

Local efficiency of a network $\mathcal{G}$ is given as the average of the global efficiencies of sub-graphs (Latora and Marchiori, 2001) as

$$E_{\mathrm{loc}}(\mathcal{G}) = \frac{1}{N} {}_{i\in\mathcal{G}} E_{\mathrm{glob}}(\mathcal{G}_i) \tag{7}$$

where $\mathcal{G}_i$ is a sub-graph centering the node i, that is, the set of the node i and its neighbors (the nodes with the distance of a single edge from the node i) and the set of edges between the nodes. As the measure depicts connectivity within local neighbors, Latora and Marchiori (2003) have shown that the $E_{\mathrm{loc}}(\mathcal{G})$ is related to *clustering coefficient* (Watts and Strogatz, 1998). As the $E_{\mathrm{loc}}(\mathcal{G})$ is the average of $E_{\mathrm{glob}}(\mathcal{G}_i)$, the measure is also bounded from 0 to 1. The higher the measure, the more efficiently the nodes within a local network are interconnected.

2.3.3. *Nodal efficiency*

Besides of network-level, we can measure how efficiently an individual node transfer information at node-level as

$$E_{\mathrm{nodal}}(i;\mathcal{G}) = \frac{1}{N-1} {}_{j\in\mathcal{G}} \frac{1}{d_{ij}}, \tag{8}$$

where $j \neq i$. $E_{\mathrm{nodal}}(i;\mathcal{G})$ is known as *nodal efficiency* (Achard and Bullmore, 2007). When the global efficiency $E_{\mathrm{glob}}(\mathcal{G})$ can be understood as "the global efficiency of a network", we can regard the nodal efficiency $E_{\mathrm{nodal}}(i;\mathcal{G})$ as "the global efficiency of a node". Remind that the term "global" or "local" only indicates whether the efficiency measure is computed for the interconnections to the all nodes, i.e., global network, or whether it is for the intra-connections within the neighboring nodes, i.e., local network (Latora and Marchiori, 2003).

2.3.4. *Neighboring efficiency*

The efficiency within the local neighbors of a node is computed as

$$E_{\mathrm{nbr}}(i;\mathcal{G}) = E_{\mathrm{glob}}(\mathcal{G}_i) = \frac{1}{(N_i-1)N_i} {}_{m\in\mathcal{G}_i\, n\in\mathcal{G}_i} \frac{1}{d_{mn}} \tag{9}$$

where N_i is the number of nodes in a sub-graph $\mathcal{G}_i$ and the nodes m and n in $\mathcal{G}_i$ are different $(m \neq n)$. We call this measure $E_{\mathrm{nbr}}(i;\mathcal{G})$ as *neighboring efficiency*, which is a node-level measure of local efficiency, as well as the nodal efficiency $E_{\mathrm{nodal}}(i;\mathcal{G})$ is a node-level measure of global efficiency. By definition, $E_{\mathrm{nbr}}(i;\mathcal{G})$ is given when $N_i \geq 2$, otherwise $E_{\mathrm{nbr}}(i;\mathcal{G}) = 0$ for a node with no connections or only one connection.

2.4. STATISTICAL INFERENCES

We tested the equalities of the expected efficiency measures between the controls and the OCD patients. The null hypotheses of the equality of the expected network-level efficiencies (E_{glob}, E_{loc}) between the networks of the controls ($\mathcal{G}_1$) and that of the OCD patients ($\mathcal{G}_2$) are given as

$$\begin{cases} H_0^{\mathrm{glob}} : \mathbb{E}\left(E_{\mathrm{glob}}(\mathcal{G}_2)\right) - \mathbb{E}\left(E_{\mathrm{glob}}(\mathcal{G}_1)\right) = 0 \\ H_0^{\mathrm{loc}} : \mathbb{E}(E_{\mathrm{loc}}(\mathcal{G}_2)) - \mathbb{E}(E_{\mathrm{loc}}(\mathcal{G}_1)) = 0. \end{cases} \tag{10}$$

For the node-level measures (E_{nodal}, E_{nbr}), the null hypotheses of equality at a node i are given as

$$\begin{aligned} H_0^{\mathrm{nodal}}(i) &: \mathbb{E}\big(E_{\mathrm{nodal}}(i;\mathcal{G}_2)\big) - \mathbb{E}\big(E_{\mathrm{nodal}}(i;\mathcal{G}_1)\big) = 0 \\ H_0^{\mathrm{nbr}}(i) &: \mathbb{E}\big(E_{\mathrm{nbr}}(i;\mathcal{G}_2)\big) - \mathbb{E}\big(E_{\mathrm{nbr}}(i;\mathcal{G}_1)\big) = 0. \end{aligned} \tag{11}$$

We used randomization to compute the exact p-values for the significances of differences (Nichols and Holmes, 2001) in the global, local, nodal and neighboring efficiency as given in section 2.3. The group identifiers ($g = 1, 2$) were randomly permuted for 2000 times and the identical analysis steps were applied to construct graphs and derive efficiency measures. The difference between the two randomly separated groups were used to obtain the null distribution under the hypothesis H_0 that there is no difference between the controls and the OCD patients. The p-values were calculated at each cost as two-tailed p-values.

The significance level is given as 0.05 in this study. We did not apply any multiple comparison corrections in comparing the efficiency measures for each ROI as in the previous brain connectivity studies (Achard and Bullmore, 2007; Wang et al., 2009a), neither for each cost since the networks with the adjacent costs are obviously not independent. The similar relationship between the networks across the costs has been explained

[3] https://sites.google.com/site/bctnet/

by *graph filtration* (Lee et al., 2011), the process in which the succeeding network embeds the preceding network with the decreasing threshold of correlation (or the increasing "epsilon" distance in constructing *Rips complexes* (Ghrist, 2007) in an N-dimensional similarity space). We pursued, however, a persistent group difference over the various costs as well in this study.

3. RESULTS

3.1. DEMOGRAPHIC AND CLINICAL VARIABLES OF PARTICIPANTS

Demographic and clinical variables are tabulated with corresponding statistics and p-values in **Table 1**. There were no significant differences in age ($p = 0.49$), gender ratio ($p = 0.88$), education year ($p = 0.59$) and IQ ($p = 0.49$). BDI and BAI scores in the OCD patients were significantly higher than the controls (BDI, $p < 10^{-7}$; BAI, $p < 10^{-6}$). The mean of total Y-BOCS in the OCD patients was 21.03 with the standard deviation of 6.06.

Out of 32 OCD patients, 13 patients (41%) were with contamination, 8 patients (25%) with checking, 5 patients (16%) with aggressions and 5 patients (16%) with other obsessions of sex, religion, somatic, or a combination of them as their prominent symptoms, as classified with Y-BOCS Symptom Checklist (Goodman et al., 1989). The main symptom of one patient was not determined. No significant differences between the two largest subgroups (contamination *vs.* checking) were found in total Y-BOCS ($p = 0.31$), neither in obsession ($p = 0.10$) nor compulsion ($p = 0.98$) subscores. The equalities across the other subgroups were not tested due to the small sizes of the subgroups. In addition, we did not find the effect of the history of medications on the severity of OCD either; between 23 drug-naïve patients and 8 unmedicated patients, there were no significant differences in total Y-BOCS ($p = 0.25$) and the subscores of obsession ($p = 0.90$) and compulsion ($p = 0.58$).

Table 1 | The summary of demographic and clinical variables.

Variable	Controls ($n = 35$)	OCD patients ($n = 32$)	t-/z-stat.	p-value
Age (year)	23.94 ± 3.60	24.81 ± 6.41	0.69	0.49
Gender (men/women)	24/11	21/11	0.15	0.88
Education (year)	14.03 ± 1.29	14.34 ± 3.23	0.53	0.59
IQ	113.20 ± 9.98	111.40 ± 11.32	−0.69	0.49
BDI	4.26 ± 6.17	17.37 ± 10.71	6.21	$<10^{-7}$
BAI	4.54 ± 5.49	18.72 ± 13.70	5.65	$<10^{-6}$
Y-BOCS				
Obsession	–	11.97 ± 3.49	–	–
Compulsion	–	9.06 ± 4.69	–	–
Total	–	21.03 ± 6.06	–	–

The mean and the standard deviation of the variables are shown except for gender. The IQ was estimated by Korean-Wechsler adult intelligence scale-revised (K-WAIS-R). Abbreviations: BDI, Beck's depression inventory; BAI, Beck's anxiety inventory; Y-BOCS, Yale-Brown obsessive-compulsive disorder Scale.

3.2. NO GROUP DIFFERENCES IN CORTICAL THICKNESS AND CORRELATION COEFFICIENTS

In prior to graph measure analysis, we compared cortical thickness covayring age and gender with multiple comparison correction by SurfStat MATLAB toolbox[4] (Worsley et al., 2009). We found no significant group differences (Figure not shown; corrected $p > 0.56$ in left hemisphere and $p > 0.16$ in right hemisphere). In addition, inter-regional correlations r_{xy} as given in (Equation 2) were compared between groups using Fisher's z-transformation. Due to the substantially large number ($148 \times 147/2$ for all possible pairs) of simultaneous testings, false-discovery-rate (FDR; Benjamini and Hochberg, 1995) is used for this case. Once again, no correlation between the pairs of nodes were found to be significantly different between the patients with OCD and the controls ($q > 0.40$).

3.3. SMALL-WORLDNESS OF THE BRAIN NETWORKS

The global efficiencies and local efficiencies of the brain networks, as well as the random and lattice networks with the matched costs, are given over the varying costs $(0.01, 0.02, \cdots, 0.50)$ in **Figure 2**. We found that the network-level efficiency measures of the brain networks were invariently in-between the cost-matched random and lattice networks as

$$E_{\text{glob}}(\mathcal{G}_{\text{rnd}}) > E_{\text{glob}}(\mathcal{G}_{\text{brain}}) > E_{\text{glob}}(\mathcal{G}_{\text{lat}}) \text{ and}$$
$$E_{\text{loc}}(\mathcal{G}_{\text{lat}}) > E_{\text{loc}}(\mathcal{G}_{\text{brain}}) > E_{\text{loc}}(\mathcal{G}_{\text{rnd}}), \tag{12}$$

except for two extreme cases (cost of 0.01 and 0.50).

These characteristics of inequalities have been typically referred as economic small-world behaviors of networks (Latora and Marchiori, 2003; Achard and Bullmore, 2007). It has been found that many brain networks of clinical populations are still in the small-world regime despite the significantly altered properties of patients in comparison with the healthy populations (He et al., 2007, 2008, 2009; Wang et al., 2009b; Lo et al., 2010). Thus we presume that the cortical thickness network of the OCD patients has the small-world architecture, as well as that of the controls.

3.4. NO GROUP DIFFERENCES IN NETWORK-LEVEL EFFICIENCY

We found significantly smaller global efficiencies in the OCD patients than the controls at the cost of 0.06 ($p = 0.03$), 0.48 ($p = 0.04$) and 0.49 ($p = 0.02$), but found no differences at the other costs. No significant group differences in local efficiency were found at any costs we studied. In addition, the area under curves (AUC) divided by the range of costs, or the mean of efficiencies across the discrete costs, were compared. We found no differences in the mean global efficiency ($p = 0.14$) nor the mean local efficiency ($p = 0.74$). Taken together, we did not find a clear distinction between the OCD patients and the controls in terms of the aggregated network-level efficiency measures.

3.5. GROUP DIFFERENCES IN NODE-LEVEL EFFICIENCY

In contrast to the results of network-level efficiency, we found significant group differences at node-level. The heat maps of

[4] http://www.math.mcgill.ca/keith/surfstat/

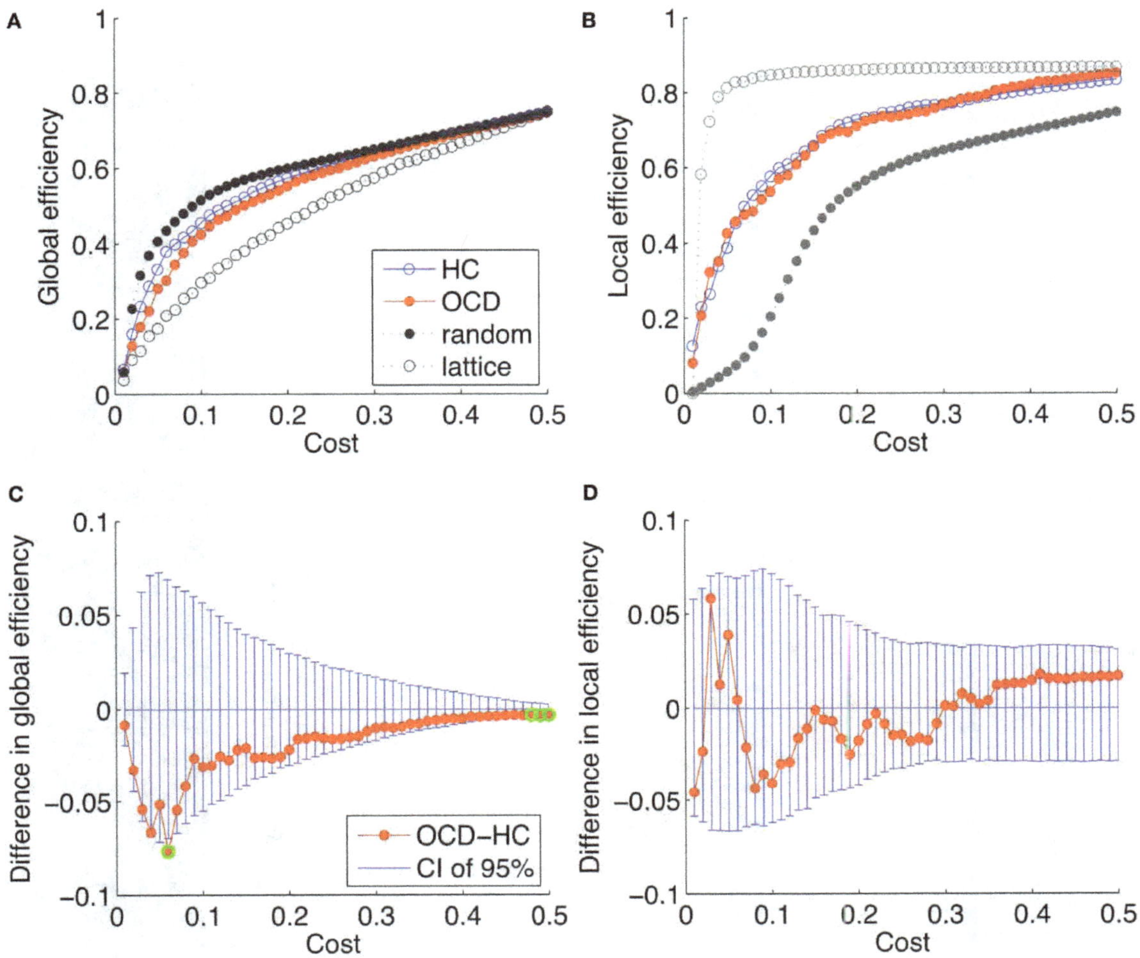

FIGURE 2 | Global efficiencies and local efficiencies of the brain networks of the controls (HC), and the OCD patients (OCD) are plotted over variant rewiring costs with the ones of random and lattice networks with matched costs (A,B). The differences between the OCD patients and controls are plotted with the 95% confidence intervals (CI) of the null distributions obtained from 2000 permutations **(C,D)**. The significantly different points ($F < 0.05$) are marked with green circles **(C)**. Note that no significant differences were found in the local efficiencies.

group-wise nodal efficiency and neighboring efficiency over costs are given in **Figures 3, 4**, respectively. Additionally, the differences in efficiency measures between the groups and the negative logarithm with the base of ten of p-values are also shown together. The logarithmic p-value is signed as positive when the efficiency is greater in the OCD patients than in the controls ($-\log_{10} p > 0$) and as negative when the value is smaller in the patients than in the controls ($\log_{10} p < 0$).

What can be prominently noted from **Figure 3** is that the number of disconnected nodes (the nodes with infinity distance to all other nodes thus zero nodal efficiency; blue pixels in **Figures 3A,B**) at a low cost are larger in the OCD patients than in the controls (e.g., when $c = 0.01$, 74 in OCD, 61 in HC), and that it takes higher costs to be connected to any nodes in the OCD patients ($c = 0.20$) than in NC ($c = 0.15$). Unlike the small-wordness measure (Watts and Strogatz, 1998), which is given for a connected network, the efficiency measure (Latora and Marchiori, 2003) enables the investigation of the disconnected graphs with smaller costs in the present study.

As we have done previously for the network-level efficiency measures, the AUC divided by the range of costs were compared for each node, so that we can compare mean measures across costs. Out of the 148 ROIs, 9 nodes showed significant group differences in nodal efficiencies, while 15 nodes were found to be significantly different in neighboring efficiencies ($p < 0.05$), as summarized in **Table 2**. For frontal regions, left orbital frontal gyrus and right lateral orbital sulcus showed lower neighboring efficiencies in the OCD patients than the controls, while left middle frontal sulcus exhibited smaller nodal efficiency as well. On the other hand, parietal regions such as left postcentral gyrus, right postcentral sulcus, left superior parietal gyrus, and bilateral sulci intermedius primus of Jensen showed higher efficiency measures in the OCD patients. Finally, medial occipito-temporal gyri around parahippocampal gyri bilaterally showed smaller nodal and neighboring efficiencies in the patients with

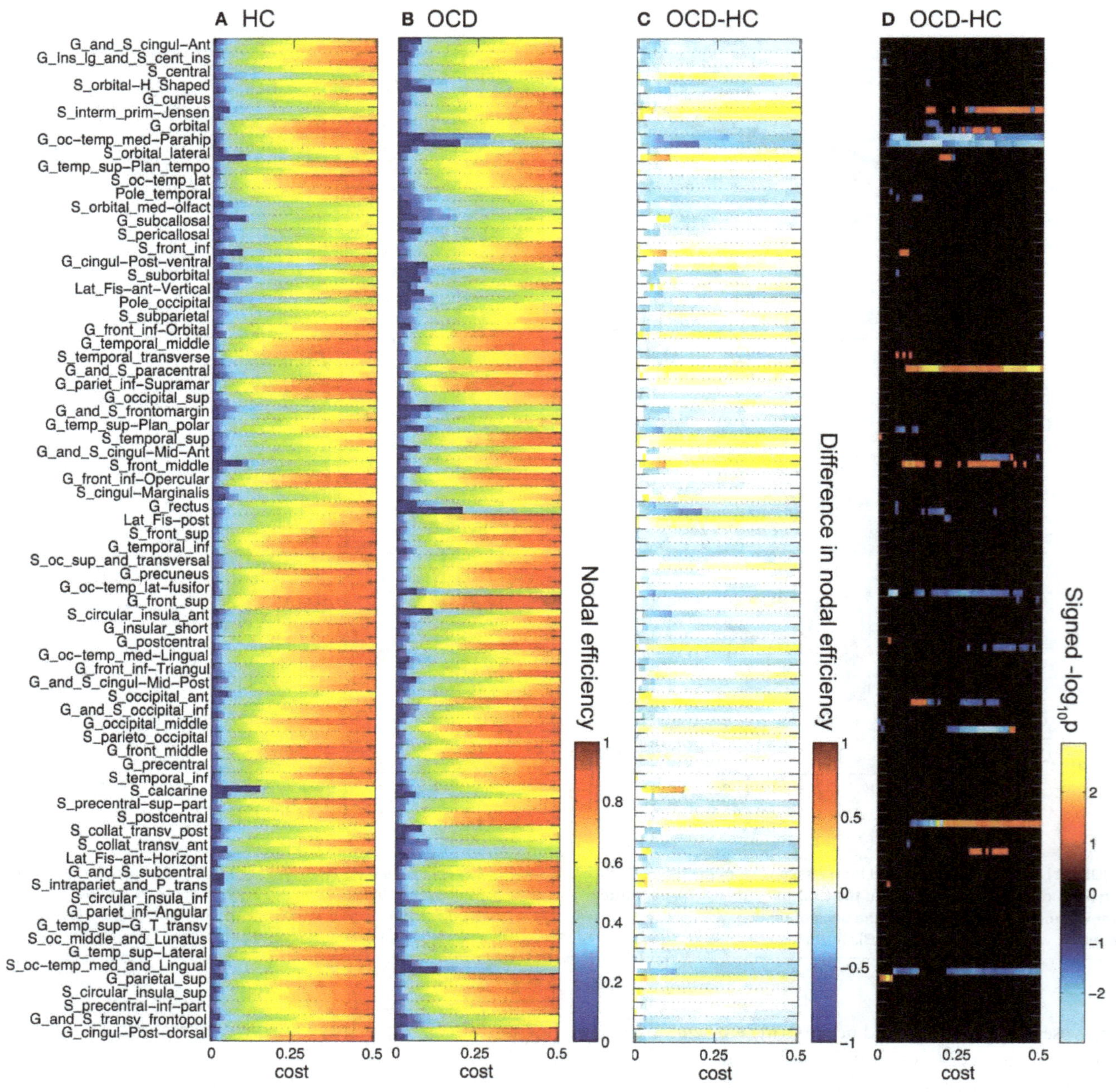

FIGURE 3 | Nodal efficiencies for 148 ROIs are plotted over cost for the controls (HC, A) and the OCD patients (OCD, B). Along the Y-axis, 74 ROI labels are indicated for each set of two rows separated by dashed horizontal lines (upper row for the left hemisphere; lower row for the right hemisphere). See Destrieux et al. (2010) for abbreviation of the ROI labels. The group differences as HC subtracted from OCD are shown **(C)**. The warm color shows higher nodal efficiency in OCD than in HC, and the cool color shows the opposite. The signed logarithmic p-values for the significance of group differences are also given **(D)**. The positive values means higher nodal efficiency in OCD than in HC ($-\log_{10} p > 0$), and vice versa ($\log_{10} p < 0$).

OCD, with smaller nodal efficiency in right lateral and medial occipito-temporal gyri.

3.5.1. Spatial pattern of node-level efficiency differences

Interestingly, the spatial bias of the node-level differences in efficiency measures was found at a large scale (i.e., dorsal *vs.* ventral). For the sake of simplicity, the nodes are classified either as a dorsal or ventral node, based on the Z-coordinate of the center of mass of a ROI, in relation to the median of Z-coordinates of the all ROIs. Mind that this separation based on the Z-coordinate is only for the purpose of a simple comparison of the spatial distribution. Further investigation on community structures based on thickness correlation also might be useful to analyze the distribution of local alterations, but we did not include such an analysis in the present study to keep our focus here to the efficiency of networks. The geometrical distribution of the efficiency measures

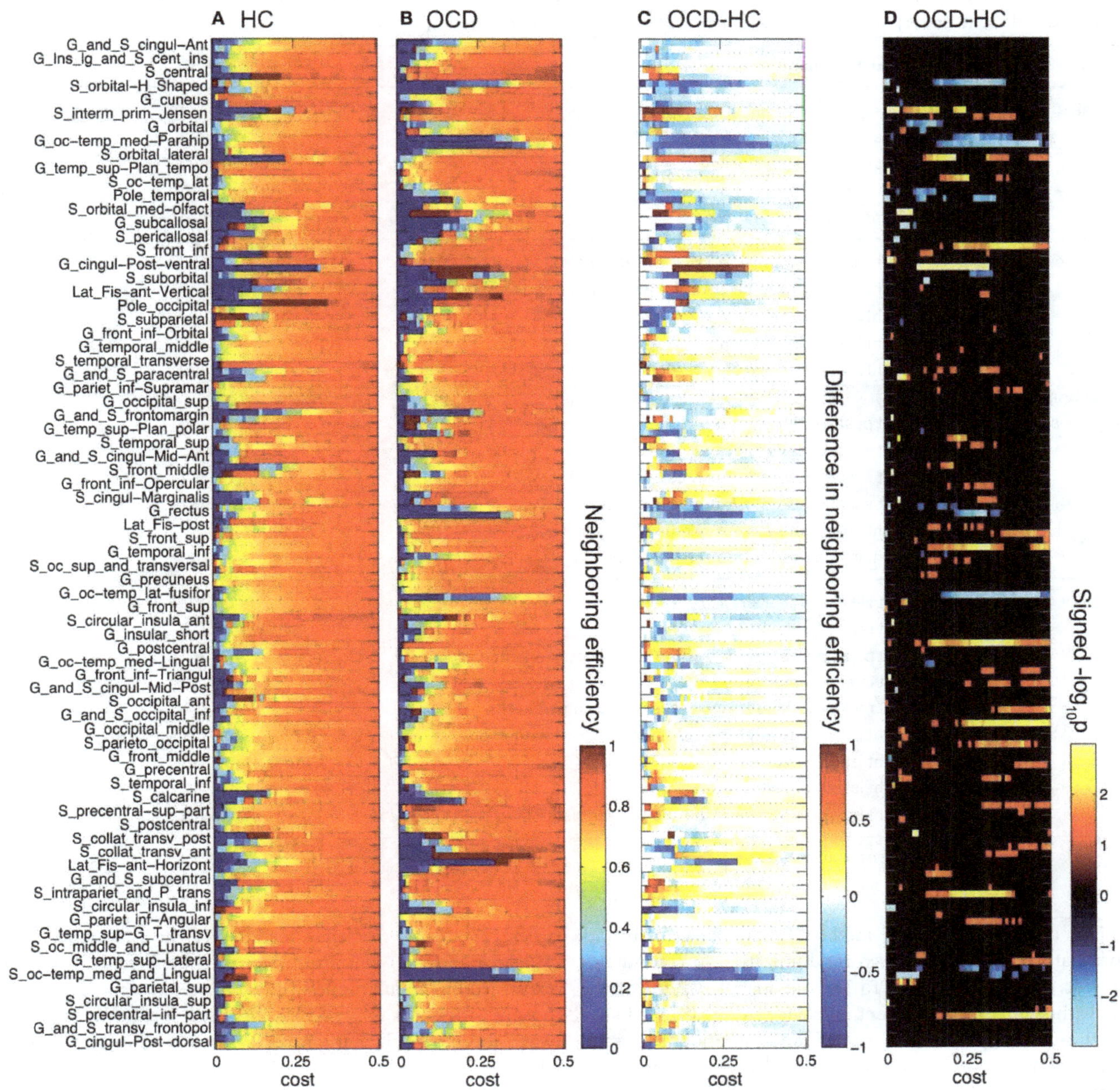

FIGURE 4 | Neighboring efficiencies for 148 ROIs are plotted over cost for the controls (HC, A) and the OCD patients (OCD, B). The group differences as HC subtracted from OCD **(C)** and the signed logarithmic *p*-values **(D)** are also shown. The same graphical scheme is the same as **Figure 3**. The warm color means higher neighboring efficiency in OCD than in HC and the cold color means the opposite **(C,D)**.

and the corresponding binary networks in the template space are visualized in **Figures 5, 6**, for nodal efficiency and neighboring efficiency, respectively. As previously hinted at by **Table 2**, it can be noticed that the efficiency measures of many dorsal nodes are greater in the OCD patients than the controls, and the ones of many ventral nodes are smaller from **Figures 5, 6**. The signed *p*-values of 148 ROIs are summarized while the location (dorsal or ventral) of nodes with significant group differences marked in **Figure 7**. For the nodal efficiency E_{nodal} (**Figure 7A**), all of the 4 nodes with significantly larger values in the OCD patients (nodes above the upper red line) were dorsal without any ventral nodes (100%; green), and all of the 5 nodes with significantly smaller values (nodes under the lower red line) were ventral (100%; magenta). For the neighboring efficiency E_{nbr} (**Figure 7B**), 6 out of 8 nodes with significantly greater values in the OCD patients were dorsal (75%), and all of the 7 nodes with significantly smaller values were ventral (100%).

Although the spatial bias in the present results seems clearly discernible (100%; 100%; 75%; 100%), one may be interested in the stability of the present finding. It can be possible to compute

Table 2 | The summary of the nodes with significant differences in mean efficiency ($p < 0.05$) as the subtraction of controls (HC) from the OCD patients (OCD-HC) with corresponding p-values for nodal efficiency (A) and neighboring efficiency (B).

Location	Structure name	OCD-HC	p-value
A. Nodal efficiency (E_{nodal})			
Dorsal nodes	Paracentral loblue and sulcus	0.1699	0.023
	Left middle frontal sulcus	0.2002	0.037
	Right postcentral sulcus	0.1316	0.034
	Right middle occipital gyrus	0.0944	0.041
Ventral nodes	Left parahippocampal part of the medial occipito-temporal gyrus	−0.2836	0.015
	Right parahippocampal part of the medial occipito-temporal gyrus	−0.3653	0.001
	Right gyrus rectus	−0.2620	0.049
	Right lateral occipito-temporal gyrus	−0.2427	0.034
	Right medial occipito-temporal sulcus and lingual sulcus	−0.2690	0.026
B. Neighboring efficiency (E_{nbr})			
Dorsal nodes	Left postcentral gyrus	0.1208	0.019
	Left superior parietal gyrus	0.0989	0.033
	Left sulcus intermedius primus of Jensen	0.3367	0.014
	Left superior part of the precentral sulcus	0.1552	0.027
	Right sulcus intermedius primus of Jensen	0.1787	0.030
	Right intraparietal sulcus and transverse-parietal sulcus	0.1349	0.024
Ventral nodes	Left H-shaped orbital sulcus	−0.4093	0.004
	Left orbital gyrus	−0.1367	0.032
	Left parahippocampal part of the medial occipito-temporal gyrus	−0.4367	0.015
	Left inferior temporal gyrus	0.0722	0.047
	Left medial occipito-temporal sulcus and lingual sulcus	−0.4374	0.035
	Right parahippocampal part of the medial occipito-temporal gyrus	−0.5707	0.003
	Right lateral orbital sulcus	0.3416	0.028
	Right lateral occipito-temporal gyrus	−0.3742	0.002
	Right horizontal ramus of the anterior segment of the lateral fissure	−0.5793	0.011

Dorsal nodes and ventral nodes are separated for tabulation.

reliability using a resampling method known as jack-knifing. Unfortunately, however, we used randomization to compute p-values for group differences. To see the spatial pattern of the nodes with significantly different efficiency in a resampled subset, each subset requires a new run of randomization and graph measure computation. It renders impractical computational load with the current MATLAB codes. Thus we have not carried out the analysis for this study. We discuss on the spatial bias of node-level efficiency measures between the dorsal and ventral networks from the perspective of the imbalance theory of dorsal-ventral pathways in the OCD patients in the following section.

3.5.2. Altered relationship between node-level efficiency and node centrality

In addition to the spatial pattern, the relationship between the efficiency and centrality are further examined. We used degree, which is the number of connected edges to a node, as a simple measure for node centrality. The mean efficiencies are plotted over degrees in **Figure 8**. The efficiency is fitted using a GLM as

$$E(i) = \beta_0 + \beta_1 D(i) + \beta_2 G(i) + \beta_3 D(i)G(i) + \varepsilon \qquad (13)$$

where $E(i)$ is an efficiency measure of the i-th node, $D(i)$ is a degree and $G(i)$ is a group index. The efficiencies were well explained by the full models (nodal efficiency, $R^2 = 0.98$; neighboring efficiency, $R^2 = 0.50$). We used logarithm of degrees when the model fit is improved as in case of neighboring efficiency (R^2 for the full model with a linear degree measure is 0.39).

The interactions between group index and degree were found to be significant for nodal efficiency ($p < 0.005$) and neighboring efficiency ($p < 0.0005$). The nodes with significantly difference efficiencies seem to be responsible for the interaction, especially for that the nodes with lower efficiency are deviated from the fitting lines. The p-values for the interactions without the nodes with significantly smaller efficiencies were higher than significance level in the study (nodal efficiency, $p = 0.23$; neighboring efficiency, $p = 0.24$). Thus the nodes with significantly smaller efficiencies in patients with OCD seem to be aberrant from the other nodes in the OCD patients. As an illustration for this idea, the degrees and efficiencies of the nodes with the smaller efficiencies from OCD patients are plotted over cost in **Figure 9**. For comparison, the measures of the other nodes with similar degrees from the patients are also given. In the process of graph

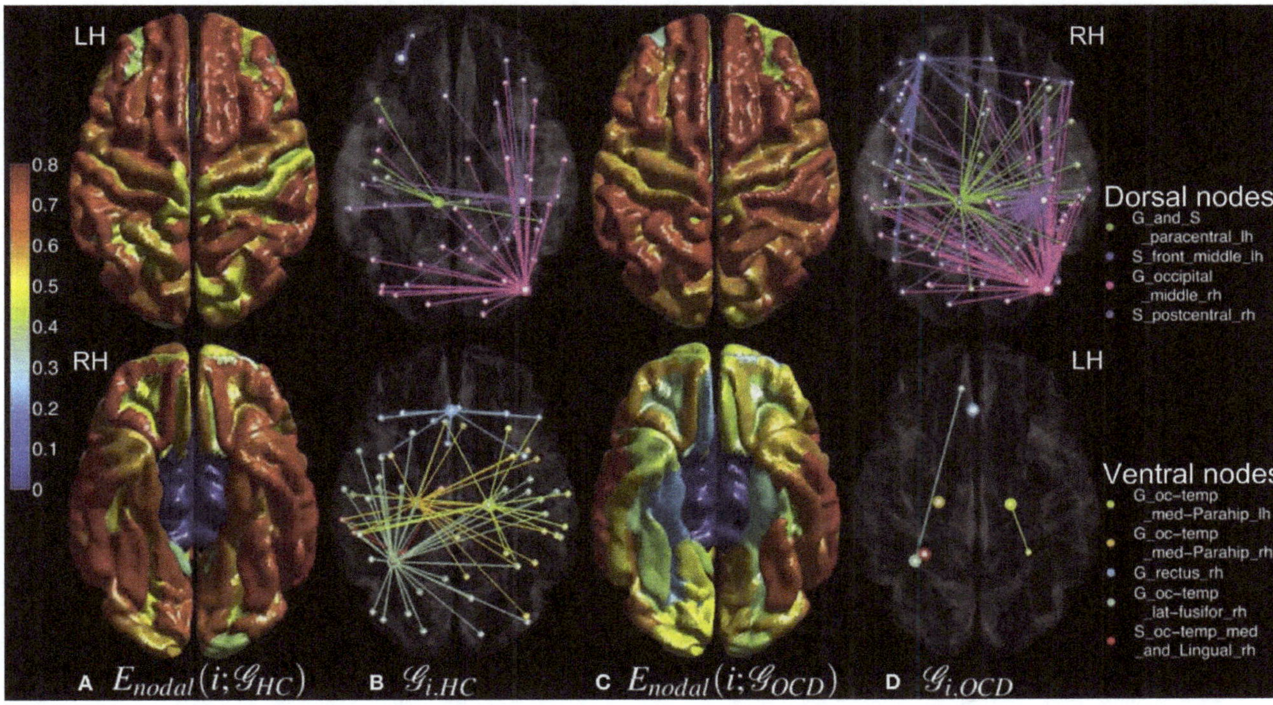

FIGURE 5 | Mean nodal efficiencies across costs are overlaid on the cortical surfaces of the controls (HC, column A) and the OCD patients (OCD, column C) from a dorsal view (upper row) and a ventral view (lower row). See the color bar on the leftmost side for the color coding from 0 to 0.8. The sub-graphs ($\mathcal{G}_i$) of the binary networks at the cost of 0.10 are shown as well for HC (column **B**) and OCD (column **D**). From the nodes that showed significantly different nodal efficiencies (marked by thick circles), their first neighbors are connected in distinct colors which correspond to the ROI legend on the rightmost side.

growth with the increasing cost, the efficiencies of the nodes without significant group differences (gray lines) increase earlier than the nodes with significant group differences (cyan lines). Thus the nodes with group differences have smaller mean efficiency (AUC divided by the range of cost) than the other nodes with similar mean degrees, deviating from the fitting lines in **Figure 8**.

4. DISCUSSION

4.1. THE BRAIN NETWORK OF OCD PATIENTS IN THE SMALL-WORLD REGIME

We found that the brain network of the OCD patients is within the small-world regime as well as that of the controls. The small-worldness of neuronal network has been demonstrated in various scales: the neuronal system of *C. elegans* (Watts and Strogatz, 1998), the brains of cats and macaque monkeys (Hilgetag and Kaiser, 2004; Kaiser, 2007), and that of humans (Sporns et al., 2004; Sporns and Honey, 2006; Achard and Bullmore, 2007; Hagmann et al., 2007; He et al., 2007; Hagmann et al., 2008). Although the network properties were found to be altered to a significant degree, the brain networks of clinical population also exhibited small-worldness distinctively from the cost-matched theoretical networks (He et al., 2008, 2009; Wang et al., 2009a; Bernhardt et al., 2011). In consistence with a previous functional network study on the OCD patients (Zhang et al., 2011), we confirmed that the structural network of the patients shows small-worldness as well in terms of inequality of network-level efficiency measures (Equation 12) as shown in **Figure 2**.

The small-worldness of a network implies the existence of local clusters in relation to its equivalent random counterpart (Kaiser, 2011). As it can be seen in **Figures 1E**, **10**, the cortical thickness networks from both of the OCD patients and the controls remarkably showed the variant degrees of connections across nodes. Regarding that the random and lattice networks are generated to have uniform distributions of degrees, the variety of degrees of the real-world brain networks makes them clearly distinguishable from the theoretical networks. In particular, the pattern of mean degrees showed noteworthy resemblance between the brain networks of the OCD patients and the control as given in **Figure 10**. The correlation of mean degrees between the groups was strongly positive ($r = 0.4969, p < 10^{-9}$). It may imply that the essential structures and functions of brain network are still preserved in the OCD patients, as shown as intact capabilities of basic behaviors and primitive functioning of the patients, though diverse impairment in high level cognitive functioning (Graybiel and Rauch, 2000; Kuelz et al., 2004).

4.2. DORSAL AND VENTRAL DISPARITY IN OCD PATIENTS

The most significant contribution of our present study is detecting the disparity between the dorsal and the ventral networks in

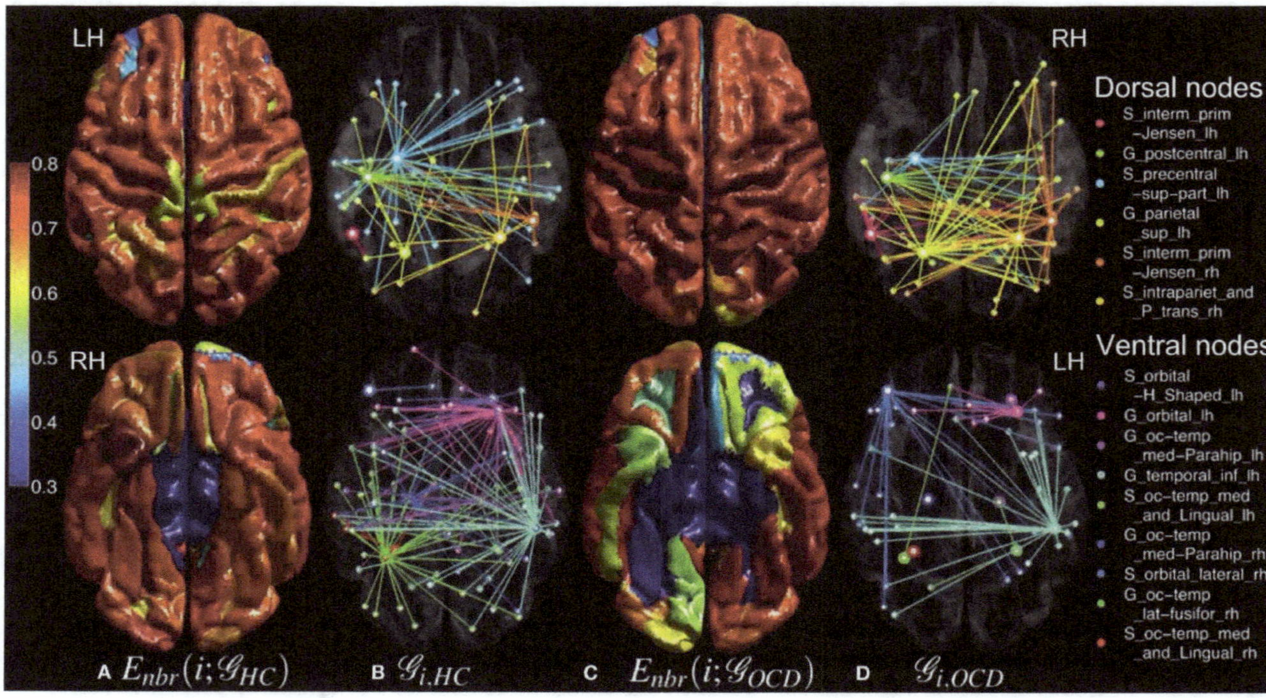

FIGURE 6 | Mean neighboring efficiencies across costs for the controls (HC, column A) and the patients with OCD (OCD, column C) and the sub-graphs ($\mathcal{G}_i$) of the corresponding binary networks at the cost of 0.1 (HC, column B; OCD, column D) are shown in the same graphical scheme as Figure 5, except that the color coding range of neighboring efficiencies is adjusted from 0.3 to 0.8 for a better visualization.

the OCD patients in terms of graph theoretical measures, supporting the hypothesis on "the imbalance of tone" between direct and indirect CST pathways (Saxena et al., 1998, 2001).

Although we could not find any group differences in the mean network-level efficiency measures, we found significant alterations of the node-level efficiency in the OCD patients that were localized with an evident spatial bias as shown in **Figures 5, 6**, which may reflect the imbalance between the dorsal and ventral pathways in the patients. In particular, the topological alterations were particularly localized in sensory-motor regions including paracentral lobule, postcentral regions, parietal cortices and middle frontal cortex as greater nodal or neighboring efficiencies in the OCD patients than the controls, and the aberrations were also detected in the ventral frontal and temporal regions including orbital cortices the parahippocampal cortices as smaller nodal or neighboring efficiencies in the OCD patients. We have shown that the ratios of nodes with significantly greater or smaller efficiency are not equal between the dorsal and ventral nodes, which may reflect the spatial disparity of the subnetworks in the patients with OCD, as shown in **Figure 7**.

Our findings are in accordance with the previous VBM studies those found local alterations of gray matter in parietal cortex (Kim et al., 2001; Valente et al., 2005), middle temporal and occipital cortex (Togao et al., 2010) and orbital frontal cortex (Pujol et al., 2004; Szeszko et al., 2008). Given the neuropathological model (Saxena et al., 2001; Menzies et al., 2008), those regions have been considered as the loci of the abnormalities of OC symptoms such as attention control deficit, excessive anxiety and failure of impulse control (Friedlander and Desrocher, 2006; Menzies et al., 2008).

More interestingly, the present findings seem to be closely related to a multivariate study on the structural network of OCD patients (Menzies et al., 2007), which used a statistical technique called partial least square (PLS; McIntosh et al., 1996). Unlike the massive univariate approaches such as VBM, PLS extracts spatial patterns that optimally correlate with a given measure of interest from the whole image. Thus the ability of PLS to detect a component with covariance is quite similar to that of the cortical thickness network analysis we used in this paper, in the sense of multivariate approaches. Their study showed that higher gray matter density in a "parieto-cingulo-striatal system" and lower gray matter density in a "fronto-temporal system" were correlated with increasing behavioral impairment in OCD patients (Menzies et al., 2007), with a striking congruence with the current findings.

4.3. ABERRANT RELATIONSHIP BETWEEN EFFICIENCY AND CENTRALITY IN OCD PATIENTS

We also found that significant interactions between degree centrality and group on node-level efficiency. The interactions seemed to be driven by the nodes that showed significant group differences, which are deviated even from the other nodes within the patients. In particular, the nodes with smaller efficiency in OCD patients demonstrated different graph growth trajectory with the increasing costs, compared to the other nodes in OCD patients with similar mean degrees. The nodal efficiency of a node can increase without the additional connections to the node but

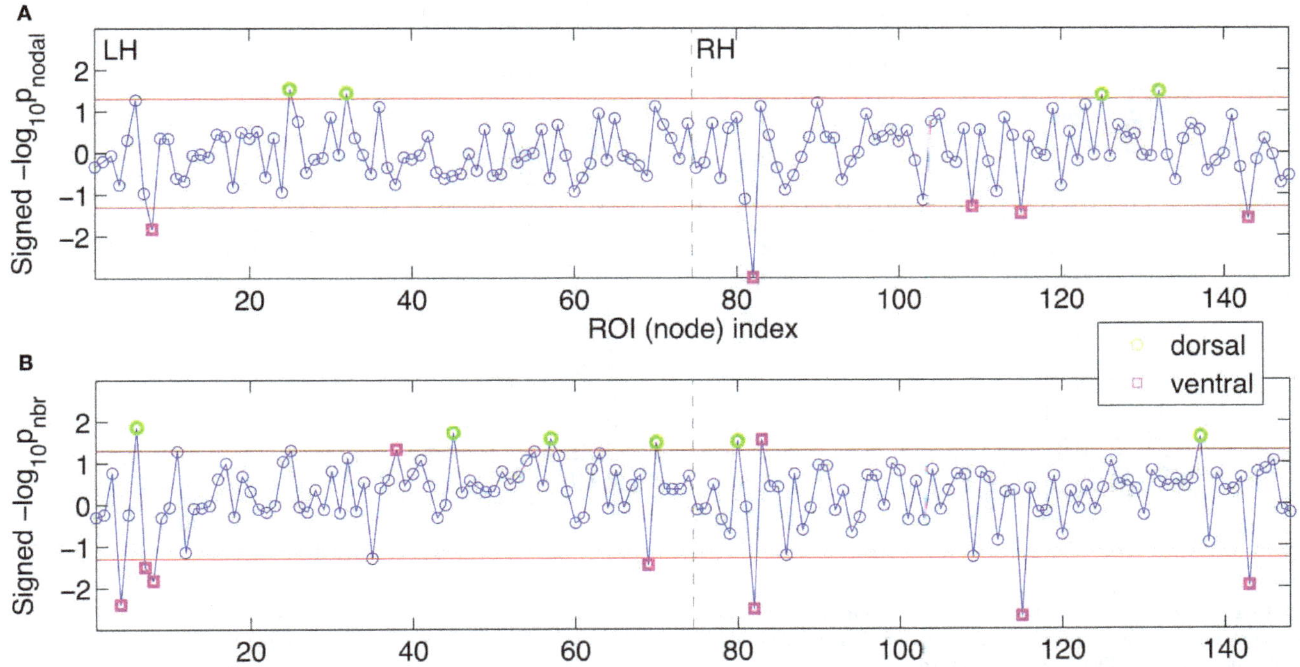

FIGURE 7 | The mean node-level efficiency measures were compared. Signed logarithmic *p*-values for nodal efficiency **(A)** and for neighboring efficiency **(B)** are given. The x-axis indicates the index of the ROI, or the node, from the left hemisphere (LH) to the right hemisphere (RH), which are separated by dashed vertical lines. Along the y-axis, the positive values mean the higher efficiency measures in OCD patients than in controls ($-\log_{10} p > 0$), and the negative values mean lower efficiency measures in OCD patients ($\log_{10} p < 0$). The significance level of $\alpha = 0.05$ are marked with red horizontal lines and the suprathreshold nodes are highlighted by green circles (dorsal nodes) or magenta squares (ventral nodes). See **Table 2** for ROI labels.

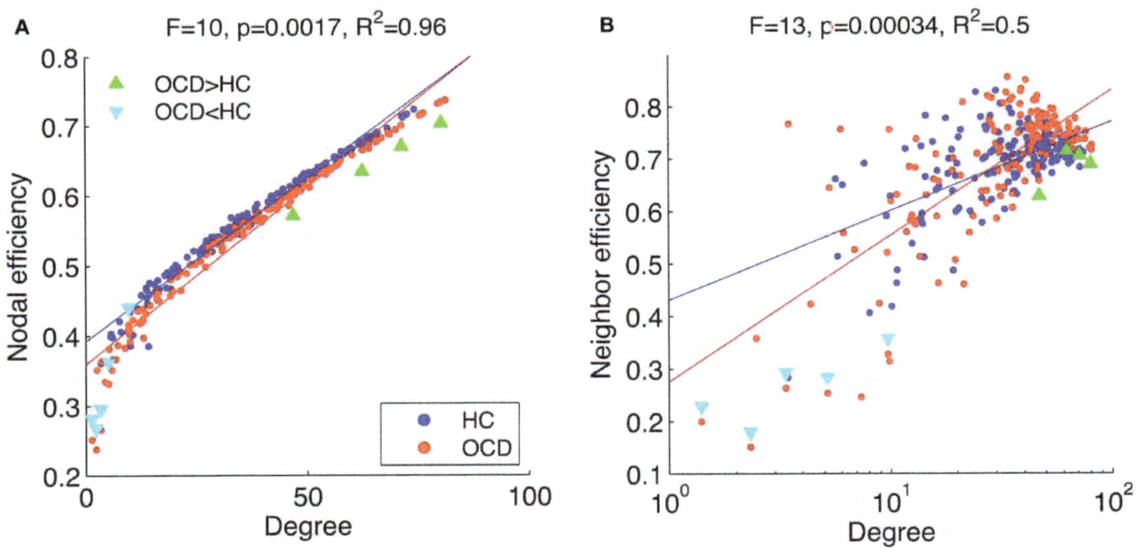

FIGURE 8 | Mean nodal efficiency (A) and neighboring efficiency (B) are shown over mean degrees in a linear (A) and a logarithmic (B) scale. Each point indicate an ROI from the networks of the healthy controls (HC, blue dots) and patients with OCD (OCD, red dots). Specific ROIs with significant group differences in efficiency measures are marked with either green triangles ($E(i; \mathcal{G}_{OCD}) > E(i; \mathcal{G}_{HC})$) or cyan triangles ($E(i; \mathcal{G}_{OCD}) < E(i; \mathcal{G}_{HC})$). Regression lines are given for each group (HC, blue line; OCD, red line). Above panels, *F*-statistic and *p*-value for a GLM testing the interaction between logarithm of degree and group and R^2 for the full model are given.

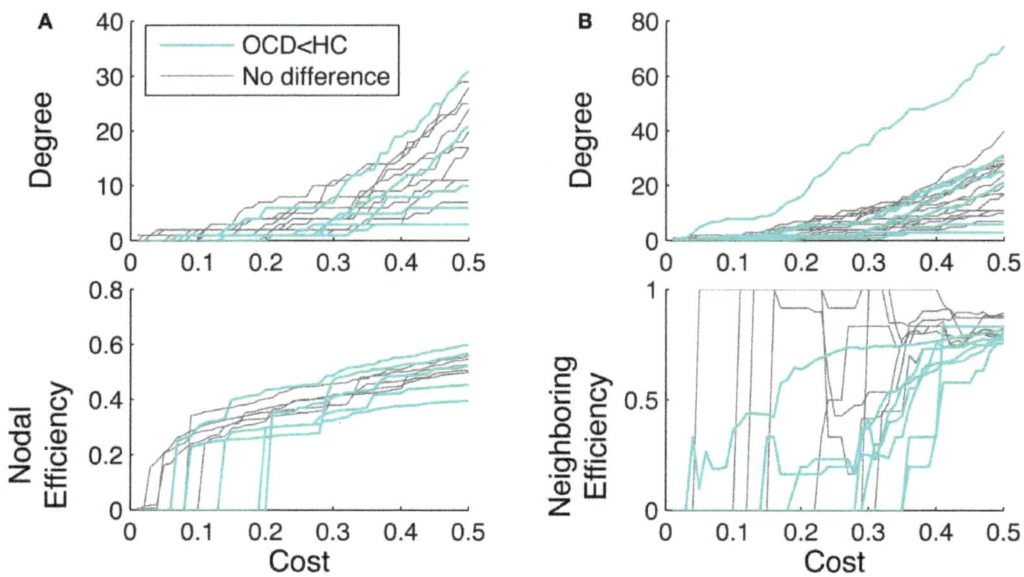

FIGURE 9 | Degree (upper row) and efficiency (lower row) are plotted over cost for the nodes with smaller nodal efficiency (A, cyan) and smaller neighboring efficiency (B, cyan) from OCD patients. For comparison, the measures of the other nodes from the patients with similar mean degrees are also shown (gray). The nodes with smaller efficiency in OCD than healthy controls exhibits different growth of efficiency even though the mean degrees are similar to the other nodes in OCD.

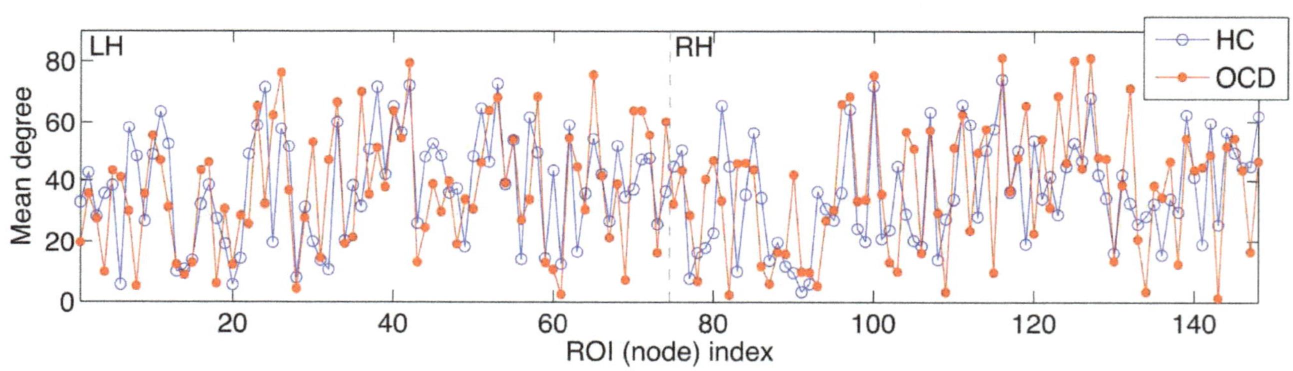

FIGURE 10 | The averaged degrees across costs over 148 ROIs are shown for the controls (HC) and OCD patients (OCD) on the y-axis. Similarly to **Figure 7**, the x-axis indicates the index of the ROI from the left hemisphere (LH) to the right hemisphere (RH), which are separated by dashed vertical lines.

by the additional connections to the other node that is already connected to the node. In other words, a node that is connected to a hub node can have high nodal efficiency even with only 1°. In case of OCD patients in the present study, the nodes without group differences (**Figure 9A**, gray lines) showed abrupt increase of nodal efficiency at a low cost (<0.05) without much increase of degrees. On the other hand, the nodes with group differences (**Figure 9A**, cyan lines) took high costs to have sudden increase of nodal efficiency, which is likely to be the point when the node is connected to the other node with high degrees.

Neighboring efficiency does not monotonously increase by increasing cost, since the measure quantifies the connections between the first neighbors of the node. Thus the neighboring efficiency can suddenly decrease during the graph growth when a new node without any connections to the pre-existing first neighbors is connected. In our case of OCD patients, the nodes without group differences (**Figure 9B**, gray lines) showed sudden increases at low degrees and sudden decrease, while the nodes with group differences (**Figure 9B**, cyan lines) evolved with slowly increasing neighboring efficiency, which means connecting unrelated nodes into its the first neighborhood.

Only 3 nodes out of 24 nodes with group difference in efficiency found to be with significantly different degree between groups ($p < 0.05$). It is presumably because that the nodes with significant group differences showed different trajectory of evolution. Thus the difference in node level efficiency could not be explained solely by degree centrality but also the connectivity of other nodes as well. As an alternative measure for centrality in a close relation with efficiency, *information centrality* has been introduced (Latora and Marchiori, 2004), but further investigation in terms of graph theories remains to pursuit in this paper.

4.4. CORTICAL THICKNESS NETWORK AND THE PATTERN OF FUNCTIONAL ACTIVATIONS IN OCD PATIENTS

The disruption of structural architecture may correlate with the alteration of the functional activation of involved areas. Specifically, the cortical thickness network has demonstrated its spatial correspondence to the DMN in human brains (Raznahan et al., 2011), and the altered relationship between the subcortico-cortical structures in a mouse model of Huntington's disease, in which its subcortical functions were impaired by a gene-knockout (Lerch et al., 2008). Here, the altered efficiency measures at a node level in the cortical thickness network of OCD patients implicate the different pattern of one-to-n similarity of local morphology of a node (nodal efficiency), or the different pattern of n-to-n similarity within the neighbors of the node (neighboring efficiency) in relation to the network of the controls. Although we do not have concurrent functional dataset of the participants, an fMRI meta-analysis using activation likelihood estimation (ALE; Turkeltaub et al., 2002) demonstrated that a greater activation was found in the left inferior parietal cortex in OCD patients than controls and a smaller activation in the left parahippocampal gyrus was found during various tasks (Menzies et al., 2008) in relation to our current findings. However, it would be fair to note that the meta-analysis also reported the foci of abnormal activations that are not clearly relevant to our results, as well as other studies that showed the different patterns of activation in OCD patients, during tasks (Nakao et al., 2005; Han et al., 2011) and using PET at rest (Kwon et al., 2003). Thus the relationship between the patterns of functional activation and the efficiencies of cortical thickness network may not be simply straightforward but manifold due to the complex nature of human brains.

A recent whole-brain analysis on the functional connectivity of OCD patients showed significantly higher or lower inter-regional correlations of activations at rest (Zhang et al., 2011). The spatial patterns of aberrant functional connectivity in their findings were not quantified, but it can be noted that higher correlations were found between parietal nodes, cingulate nodes and dorsal frontal nodes and lower correlations were found between prefrontal nodes and posterior temporal nodes (Zhang et al., 2011). Although a larger number of samples and simultaneous multi-modal data will be beneficial to clarify the interaction between the structural and functional networks, we conjecture that the topological alteration in the structural network in OCD patients would exhibit concurrent deviant patterns of functional activations.

It can be added to discussion, that the resting-state hyperactivity in the ventral networks in OCD patients has been consistently found in terms of greater local activation (Kwon et al., 2003; Friedlander and Desrocher, 2006) and higher cortico-strial functional connectivity of the basal ganglia (Harrison et al., 2009). Intriguingly, it was demonstrated that the ventral network, primarily including orbital frontal cortex, showed smaller deactivation (i.e., the failure of inhibition), responding to the participant's own error, thus resulting in higher activation in OCD patients compared to controls (Stern et al., 2011). The coarse connections and lower efficiency in the ventral network of the OCD patients in our present findings implies that the morphometric similarity of the ventral nodes with other nodes is disturbed. It may reflect the underlying pathology of the dysfunction of inhibitory controls in the OCD patients.

4.5. LIMITATIONS AND FUTURE WORKS

The first methodological limitation of our study is that the current practice of cortical thickness network analysis is restricted to cortical structures. Although the subcortical structures were considered to be highly involved in the pathophysiology of mental disorders including OCD (Cummings, 1993; Saxena et al., 2001), the present technical issues such as MR imaging resolution and tissue contrast still render the surface analysis problematic to the other brain structures than neocortices, despite recent computational advances (Khan et al., 2008; Qiu et al., 2010). Alternatively, the volumetric measure of a subcortical structure may be used along with the cortical thickness (Lerch et al., 2008). In addition, it can also be possible to characterize the covariance structure of local morphology in volumetric space (Kim et al., 2011a; Tijms et al., 2012). It may be useful to adapt and combine those methods to investigate the relationship within and between the cortical and subcortical networks.

The second limitation is that we could not separate the OCD patients by their main symptoms, mainly due to the small size of subgroups. As there have been rich discussions and supporting evidences for the heterogeneity of OCD symptoms (Mataix-Cols and van den Heuvel, 2006; van den Heuvel et al., 2009; Koch et al., 2012), possible subtypes and multi-dimensions of the disorder were discussed in the context of refining the diagnosis criteria in the next generation of DSM (Leckman et al., 2010; Mataix-Cols et al., 2010; Taylor, 2011). Even though we did not carry out the analyses on the subgroups of the OCD patients in this paper, a methodological improvement of the diagnosis and a larger number of samples may resort the inconsistency in the previous findings due to the diversity of OCD.

In relation to heterogeneity, we did not find any group differences in cortical thickness in the current sample. Although we previously reported cortical thinning in other patients with unmedicated OCD (Shin et al., 2007), it was demonstrated that a severity of OCD subtype may be correlated with the cortical thickness (Nakamae et al., 2012). The underlying mechanism of OCD might not be directly reflected in the local morphometry, but rather be manifested in the interaction of complex networks, which motivated the series of graph analysis on human brain including the current study as well.

In conclusion, we have examined the network properties in the patients with OCD based on the cortical thickness for the first time. The anatomical network in the OCD patients was in the small-world regime as well as that of the healthy controls. We found topological alterations in the patients in terms of efficiency at node level and its relation to node centrality. The alteration showed disparity between the dorsal and ventral networks, which may contribute to confirm the dorsal-ventral imbalance hypothesis (Saxena et al., 2001).

ACKNOWLEDGMENTS

The authors would like to thank Dr. Moo K. Chung for methodological consulting. The portion of this work was presented at the 18th Annual Meeting of the Organization for Human Brain Mapping, Beijing, China, June, 2012. This work was supported by the National Research Foundation of Korea grant (2012-0005150) funded by the Ministry of Education, Science and Technology (MEST) of the Republic of Korea.

REFERENCES

Achard, S., and Bullmore, E. (2007). Efficiency and cost of economical brain functional networks. *PloS. Comput. Biol.* 3, 174–183. doi: 10.1371/journal.pcbi.0030017

Achard, S., Salvador, R., Whitcher, B., Suckling, J., and Bullmore, E. (2006). A resilient, low-frequency, small-world human brain functional network with highly connected association cortical hubs. *J. Neurosci.* 26, 63. doi: 10.1523/JNEUROSCI.3874-05.2006

American Psychiatric Association (1994). *Diagnostic and Statistical Manual of Mental Disorders: DSM-IV*. Washington, DC: American Psychiatric Association

Ashburner, J., and Friston, K. (2000). Voxel-based morphometry – the methods. *Neuroimage* 11, 805–821. doi: 10.1006/nimg.2000.0582

Basser, P. J. (1995). Inferring microstructural features and the physiological state of tissues from diffusion-weighted images. *NMR Biomed.* 8, 333–344. doi: 10.1002/nbm.1940080707

Beck, A., Epstein, N., Brown, G., and Steer, R. (1988). An inventory for measuring clinical anxiety: psychometric properties. *J. Consult. Clin. Psychol.* 56, 893–897. doi: 10.1037/0022-006X.56.6.893

Beck, A., Ward, C., Mendelson, M., Mock, J., and Erabaugh, J. (1961). An inventory for measuring depression. *Arch. Gen. Psychiat.* 4, 561–571. doi: 10.1001/archpsyc.1961.01710120031004

Benjamini, Y., and Hochberg, Y. (1995). Controlling the false discovery rate: a practical and powerful approach to multiple testing. *J. Roy. Stat. Soc. B Met.* 57, 289–300.

Bernhardt, B., Chen, Z., He, Y., Evans, A., and Bernasconi, N. (2011). Graph-theoretical analysis reveals disrupted small-world organization of cortical thickness correlation networks in temporal lobe epilepsy. *Cereb Cortex.* 21, 2147–2157. doi: 10.1093/cercor/bhq291

Bora, E., Harrison, B. J., Fornito, A., Cocchi, L., Pujol, J., Fontenelle, L. F., et al. (2011). White matter microstructure in patients with obsessive-compulsive disorder. *J. Psychiatry Neurosci.* 36, 42–46. doi: 10.1503/jpn.100082

Bullmore, E., and Sporns, O. (2009). Complex brain networks: graph theoretical analysis of structural and functional systems. *Nat. Rev. Neurosci.* 10, 186–198. doi: 10.1038/nrn2575

Chen, Z. J., He, Y., Rosa-Neto, P., Germann, J., and Evans, A. C. (2008). Revealing modular architecture of human brain structural networks by using cortical thickness from MRI. *Cereb Cortex.* 18, 2374–2381. doi: 10.1093/cercor/bhn003

Chen, Z. J., He, Y., Rosa-Neto, P., Gong, G., and Evans, A. C. (2011). Age-related alterations in the modular organization of structural cortical network by using cortical thickness from MRI. *Neuroimage* 56, 235–245. doi: 10.1016/j.neuroimage.2011.01.010

Chung, M. K., Robbins, S., Dalton, K. M., Davidson, R. J., Alexander, A. L., and Evans, A. C. (2005). Cortical thickness analysis in autism with heat kernel smoothing. *Neuroimage* 25, 1256–1265. doi: 10.1016/j.neuroimage.2004.12.052

Cummings, J. (1993). Frontal-subcortical circuits and human behavior. *Arch. Neurol.* 50, 873–880. doi: 10.1001/archneur.1993.00540080076020

Dale, A. M., Fischl, B., and Sereno, M. I. (1999). Cortical surface-based analysis – I. Segmentation and surface reconstruction. *Neuroimage* 9, 179–194. doi: 10.1006/nimg.1998.0395

Destrieux, C., Fischl, B., Dale, A., and Halgren, E. (2010). Automatic parcellation of human cortical gyri and sulci using standard anatomical nomenclature. *Neuroimage* 53, 1–15. doi: 10.1016/j.neuroimage.2010.06.010

Eguíluz, V., Chialvo, D., Cecchi, G., Baliki, M., and Apkarian, V. (2003). Scale-free brain functional networks. *Phys. Rev. Lett.* 94:e4. doi: 10.1103/PhysRevLett.94.018102

First, M., Spitzer, R., Gibbon, M., and Williams, J. (1996). *Structured Clinical Interview for DSM-IV Axis I Disorder*. New York, NY: New York State Psychiatric Institute.

Fischl, B., and Dale, A. (2000). Measuring the thickness of the human cerebral cortex from magnetic resonance images. *Proc. Natl. Acad. Sci. U.S.A.* 97, 11050–11055. doi: 10.1073/pnas.200033797

Fischl, B., Sereno, M., Tootell, R., and Dale, A. (1999). High-resolution intersubject averaging and a coordinate system for the cortical surface. *Hum. Brain Mapp.* 8, 272–284. doi: 10.1002/(SICI)1097-0193(1999)8:4<272::AID-HBM10>3.0.CO;2-4

Fischl, B., van der Kouwe, A., Destrieux, C., Halgren, E., Ségonne, F., Salat, D., et al. (2004). Automatically parcellating the human cerebral cortex. *Cereb Cortex.* 14, 11. doi: 10.1093/cercor/bhg087

Friedlander, L., and Desrocher, M. (2006). Neuroimaging studies of obsessive-compulsive disorder in adults and children. *Clin. Psychol. Rev.* 26, 32–49. doi: 10.1016/j.cpr.2005.06.010

Garibotto, V., Scifo, P., Gorini, A., Alonso, C., Brambati, S., Bellodi, L., et al. (2009). Disorganization of anatomical connectivity in obsessive compulsive disorder: a multi-parameter diffusion tensor imaging study in a subpopulation of patients. *Neurobiol. Dis.* 37, 468–476. doi: 10.1016/j.nbd.2009.11.003

Ghrist, R. (2007). Barcodes: the persistent topology of data. *Bull. Am. Math. Soc.* 45, 61–76. doi: 10.1090/S0273-0979-07-01191-3

Gong, G., He, Y., Chen, Z. J., and Evans, A. C. (2012). Convergence and divergence of thickness correlations with diffusion connections across the human cerebral cortex. *Neuroimage* 59, 1239–1248. doi: 10.1016/j.neuroimage.2011.08.017

Gong, G., Rosa-Neto, P., Carbonell, F., Chen, Z., He, Y., and Evans, A. (2009). Age- and gender-related differences in the cortical anatomical network. *J. Neurosci.* 29, 15684–15693. doi: 10.1523/JNEUROSCI.2308-09.2009

Goodman, W., Price, L., Rasmussen, S., Mazure, C., Fleischmann, R., Hill, C., et al. (1989). The Yale-Brown obsessive compulsive scale: I. Development, use, and reliability. *Arch. Gen. Psychiat.* 46, 1006–1011. doi: 10.1001/archpsyc.1989.01810110048007

Graybiel, A., and Rauch, S. (2000). Toward a neurobiology of obsessive-compulsive disorder. *Neuron* 28, 343–347. doi: 10.1016/S0896-6273(00)00113-6

Ha, T. H., Kang, D.-H., Park, J. S., Jang, J. H., Jung, W. H., Choi, J.-S., et al. (2009). White matter alterations in male patients with obsessive-compulsive disorder. *Neuroreport* 20, 735–739. doi: 10.1097/WNR.0b013e32832ad3da

Hagmann, P., Cammoun, L., Gigandet, X., Meuli, R., Christopher J. H., van Wedeen, J., et al. (2008). Mapping the structural core of human cerebral cortex. *PloS Biol.* 6, 1479–1493. doi: 10.1371/journal.pbio.0060159

Hagmann, P., Kurant, M., Gigandet, X., Thiran, P., Wedeen, V., Meuli, R., et al. (2007). Mapping human whole-brain structural networks with diffusion MRI. *PLoS ONE* 2:e597. doi: 10.1371/journal.pone.0000597

Han, J. Y., Kang, D.-H., Gu, B.-M., Jung, W. H., Choi, J.-S., Choi, C.-H., et al. (2011). Altered brain activation in ventral frontal-striatal regions following a 16-week pharmacotherapy in unmedicated obsessive-compulsive disorder. *J. Korean Med. Sci.* 26, 665–674. doi: 10.3346/jkms.2011.26.5.665

Harrison, B., Soriano-Mas, C., Pujol, J., Ortiz, H., López-Solà, M., Hernández-Ribas, R., et al. (2009). Altered corticostriatal functional connectivity in obsessive-compulsive disorder. *Arch. Gen. Psychiat.* 66, 1189–1200. doi: 10.1001/archgenpsychiatry.2009.152

He, Y., Chen, Z., and Evans, A. (2007). Small-world anatomical networks in the human brain revealed by cortical thickness from MRI. *Cereb Cortex.* 17, 2407. doi: 10.1093/cercor/bhl149

He, Y., Chen, Z., and Evans, A. (2008). Structural insights into aberrant topological patterns of large-scale cortical networks in Alzheimer's disease. *J. Neurosci.* 28:4756. doi: 10.1523/JNEUROSCI.0141-08.2008

He, Y., Dagher, A., Chen, Z., Charil, A., Zijdenbos, A., Worsley, K., et al. (2009). Impaired small-world efficiency in structural cortical networks in multiple sclerosis associated with white matter lesion load. *Brain* 132, 3366–3379. doi: 10.1093/brain/awp089

Hilgetag, C., and Kaiser, M. (2004). Clustered organization of cortical connectivity. *Neuroinformatics* 2, 353–360. doi: 10.1385/NI:2:3:353

Jang, J., Kim, J.-H., Jung, W., Choi, J.-S., Jung, M., Lee, J.-M., et al. (2010). Functional connectivity in fronto-subcortical circuitry during the resting state in obsessive-compulsive disorder. *Neurosci. Lett.* 474, 158–162. doi: 10.1016/j.neulet.2010.03.031

Kaiser, M. (2007). Brain architecture: a design for natural computation. *Philos. Trans. R. Soc. A.* 365, 3033–3045.

Kaiser, M. (2011). A tutorial in connectome analysis: topological and spatial features of brain networks. *Neuroimage* 57, 892–907. doi: 10.1016/j.neuroimage.2011.05.025

Khan, A., Wang, L., and Beg, M. (2008). FreeSurfer-initiated fully-automated subcortical brain segmentation in MRI using large deformation diffeomorphic metric mapping. *Neuroimage* 41, 735–746. doi: 10.1016/j.neuroimage.2008.03.024

Kim, J.-J., Lee, M. C., Kim, J., Kim, I. Y., Kim, S. I., Han, M. H., et al. (2001). Grey matter abnormalities in obsessive-compulsive disorder. *Br. J. Psychiatry* 179, 330–334. doi: 10.1192/bjp.179.4.330

Kim, S.-G., Chung, M. K., Hanson, J., Avants, B. B., Gee, J. C., Davidson, R. J., et al. (2011a). "Structural connectivity via the tensor-based morphometry," in *IEEE International Symposium on Biomedical Imaging*, (Chicago, IL), 808–811.

Kim, S.-G., Chung, M. K., Seo, S. H., Schaefer, S. M., van Reekum, C., and Davidson, R. J. (2011b). "Heat kernel smoothing via Laplace-Beltrami eigenfunctions and its application to subcortical structure modeling," in *Pacific-Rim Symposium on Image and Video Technology*, volume 7087 of Lecture Notes in Computer Science, ed Y.-S. Ho (Gwangju, South Korea: Springer), 36–57.

Koch, K., Wagner, G., Schachtzabel, C., Schultz, C. C., Straube, T., Gullmar, D., et al. (2012). White matter structure and symptom dimensions in obsessive-compulsive disorder. *J. Psychiatry Res.* 46, 264–270. doi: 10.1016/j.jpsychires.2011.10.016

Kuelz, A. K., Hohagen, F., and Voderholzer, U. (2004). Neuropsychological performance in obsessive-compulsive disorder: a critical review. *Biol. Psychol.* 65, 185–236. doi: 10.1016/j.biopsycho.2003.07.007

Kwon, J. S., Kim, J.-J., Lee, D. W., Lee, J. S., Lee, D. S., Kim, M.-S., et al. (2003). Neural correlates of clinical symptoms and cognitive dysfunctions in obsessive–compulsive disorder. *Psychiatry Res.* 122, 37–47. doi: 10.1016/S0925-4927(02)00104-X

Langer, N., Pedroni, A., and Jäncke, L. (2013). The problem of thresholding in small-world network analysis. *PLoS One* 8:e53199. doi: 10.1371/journal.pone.0053199

Latora, V., and Marchiori, M. (2001). Efficient behavior of small-world networks. *Phys. Rev. Lett.* 87, 198701.

Latora, V., and Marchiori, M. (2003). Economic small-world behavior in weighted networks. *Eur. Phys. J. B* 32, 249–263. doi: 10.1140/epjb/e2003-00095-5

Latora, V., and Marchiori, M. (2004). A measure of centrality based on the network efficiency. *New J. Phys.* 9, 1–11. doi: 10.1088/1367-2630/9/6/188

Leckman, J., Denys, D., Simpson, H., Mataix-Cols, D., Hollander, E., Saxena, S., et al. (2010). Obsessive–compulsive disorder: a review of the diagnostic criteria and possible subtypes and dimensional specifiers for DSM-V. *Depress. Anxiety* 27, 507–527. doi: 10.1002/da.20669

Lee, H., Chung, M. K., Kang, H., Kim, B.-N., and Lee, D. S. (2011). Computing the shape of brain networks using graph filtration and Gromov-Hausdorff metric. *Med. Image Comput. Comput. Assist. Inter.* 14(Pt 2), 302–309.

Lerch, J., Carroll, J., Dorr, A., Spring, S., Evans, A., Hayden, M., et al. (2008). Cortical thickness measured from MRI in the YAC128 mouse model of Huntington's disease. *Neuroimage* 41, 243–251. doi: 10.1016/j.neuroimage.2008.02.019

Lerch, J. P., and Evans, A. (2005). Cortical thickness analysis examined through power analysis and a population simulation. *Neuroimage* 24, 163–173. doi: 10.1016/j.neuroimage.2004.07.045

Lo, C.-Y., Wang, P.-N., Chou, K.-H., Wang, J., He, Y., and Lin, C.-P. (2010). Diffusion tensor tractography reveals abnormal topological organization in structural cortical networks in Alzheimer's disease. *J. Neurosci.* 30, 16876–16885. doi: 10.1523/JNEUROSCI.4136-10.2010

MacDonald, D., Kabani, N., Avis, D., and Evans, A. (2000). Automated 3-D extraction of inner and outer surfaces of cerebral cortex from MRI. *Neuroimage* 12, 340–356. doi: 10.1006/nimg.1999.0534

Mataix-Cols, D., Frost, R., Pertusa, A., Clark, L. A., Saxena, S., Leckman, J., et al. (2010). Hoarding disorder: a new diagnosis for DSM-V? *Depress. Anxiety* 27, 556–572. doi: 10.1002/da.20693

Mataix-Cols, D., and van den Heuvel, O. (2006). Common and distinct neural correlates of obsessive-compulsive and related disorders. *Psychiatr. Clin. N. Am.* 29, 391–410, viii. doi: 10.1016/j.psc.2006.02.006

McIntosh, A., Bookstein, F., Haxby, J., and Grady, C. (1996). Spatial pattern analysis of functional brain images using partial least squares. *Neuroimage* 3(3 Pt 1), 143–157. doi: 10.1006/nimg.1996.0016

Menzies, L., Achard, S., Chamberlain, S., Fineberg, N., Chen, C.-H., del Campo, N., et al. (2007). Neurocognitive endophenotypes of obsessive-compulsive disorder. *Brain* 130, 3223–3236. doi: 10.1093/brain/awm205

Menzies, L., Chamberlain, S., Laird, A., Thelen, S., Sahakian, B., and Bullmore, E. (2008). Integrating evidence from neuroimaging and neuropsychological studies of obsessive-compulsive disorder: The orbitofronto-striatal model revisited. *Neurosci. Biobehav. R* 32, 525–549. doi: 10.1016/j.neubiorev.2007.09.005

Milad, M., and Rauch, S. (2011). Obsessive-compulsive disorder: beyond segregated cortico-striatal pathways. *Trends Cogn. Sci.* 16, 43–51. doi: 10.1016/j.tics.2011.11.003

Nakamae, T., Jin, N., Sakai, Y., Nishida, S., Yamada, K., Nishimura, T., et al. (2011). Diffusion tensor imaging and tract-based spatial statistics in obsessive-compulsive disorder. *J. Psychiatry Res.* 45, 687–690. doi: 10.1016/j.jpsychires.2010.09.016

Nakamae, T., Narumoto, J., Sakai, Y., Nishida, S., Yamada, K., Kubota, M., et al. (2012). Reduced cortical thickness in non-medicated patients with obsessive-compulsive disorder. *Prog. Neuropsychopharmacol. Biol. Psychiatry.* 37, 90–95. doi: 10.1016/j.pnpbp.2012.01.001

Nakao, T., Nakagawa, A., Yoshiura, T., Nakatani, E., Nabeyama, M., Yoshizato, C., et al. (2005). Brain activation of patients with obsessive-compulsive disorder during neuropsychological and symptom provocation tasks before and after symptom improvement: a functional magnetic resonance imaging study. *Biol. Psychiatry* 57, 901–910. doi: 10.1016/j.biopsych.2004.12.039

Newman, M. E. J. (2003). The structure and function of complex networks. *SIAM Rev.* 45, 167–256. doi: 10.1137/S003614450342480

Nichols, T., and Holmes, A. (2001). Nonparametric permutation tests for functional neuroimaging: a primer with examples. *Hum. Brain Mapp.* 15, 1–25. doi: 10.1002/hbm.1058

Oh, J. S., Jang, J. H., Jung, W. H., Kang, D. H., Choi, J. S., Choi, C. H., et al. (2012). Reduced fronto-callosal fiber integrity in unmedicated OCD patients: a diffusion tractography study. *Hum. Brain Mapp.* 33, 2441–2452. doi: 10.1002/hbm.21372

Pujol, J., Soriano-Mas, C., Alonso, P., Cardoner, N., Menchón, J. M., Deus, J., et al. (2004). Mapping structural brain alterations in obsessive-compulsive disorder. *Arch. Gen. Psychiatry* 61, 720–730. doi: 10.1001/archpsyc.61.7.720

Qiu, A., Brown, T., Fischl, B., Ma, J., and Miller, M. (2010). Atlas generation for subcortical and ventricular structures with its applications in shape analysis. *IEEE Trans. Image Process.* 19, 1539–1547.

Radua, J., and Mataix-Cols, D. (2009). Voxel-wise meta-analysis of grey matter changes in obsessive-compulsive disorder. *Br. J. Psychiatry* 195, 393–402. doi: 10.1192/bjp.bp.108.055046

Raznahan, A., Lerch, J. P., Lee, N., Greenstein, D., Wallace, G. L., Stockman, M., et al. (2011). Patterns of coordinated anatomical change in human cortical development: a longitudinal neuroimaging study of maturational coupling. *Neuron* 72, 873–884. doi: 10.1016/j.neuron.2011.09.028

Remijnse, P. L., van den Heuvel, O. A., and Veltman, D. J. (2005). Neuroimaging in obsessive-compulsive disorder. *Curr. Med. Imag. Rev.* 1, 331–351. doi: 10.2174/157340505774574808

Rotge, J. Y., Langbour, N., Guehl, D., Bioulac, B., Jaafari, N., Allard, M., et al. (2010). Gray matter alterations in obsessive-compulsive disorder: an anatomic likelihood estimation meta-analysis. *Neuropsychopharmacol* 35, 686–691. doi: 10.1038/npp.2009.175

Saxena, S., Bota, R., and Brody, A. (2001). Brain-behavior relationships in obsessive-compulsive disorder. *Semin. Clin. Neuropsychiatry* 6, 82–101. doi: 10.1053/scnp.2001.21833

Saxena, S., Brody, A., Schwartz, J., and Baxter, L. (1998). Neuroimaging and frontal-subcortical circuitry in obsessive-compulsive disorder. *Br. J. Psychiatry Suppl.* 1998, 26–37.

Seo, S. H., and Chung, M. K. (2011). "Laplace-Beltrami eigenfunction expansion of cortical manifolds," in *IEEE International Symposium on Biomedical Imaging*, (Chicago, IL), 372–375.

Seo, S. H., Chung, M. K., and Vorperian, H. (2010). Heat kernel smoothing using Laplace-Beltrami eigenfunctions. *Med. Image Comput. Comput. Assist. Inter.* 13 (Pt 3), 505–512. doi: 10.1007/978-3-642-15711-0_63

Shin, Y. W., Yoo, S. Y., Lee, J. K., Ha, T. H., Lee, K. J., Lee, J. M., et al. (2007). Cortical thinning in obsessive compulsive disorder. *Hum. Brain Mapp.* 28, 1128–1135. doi: 10.1002/hbm.20338

Smith, S., Jenkinson, M., Johansen-Berg, H., Rueckert, D., Nichols, T., mackay, C., et al. (2006). Tract-based spatial statistics: voxelwise analysis of multi-subject diffusion data. *Neuroimage* 31, 1487–1505. doi: 10.1016/j.neuroimage.2006.02.024

Sporns, O., Chialvo, D., Kaiser, M., and Hilgetag, C. (2004). Organization, development and function of complex brain networks. *Trends Cogn. Sci.* 8, 418–425. doi: 10.1016/j.tics.2004.07.008

Sporns, O., and Honey, C. (2006). Small worlds inside big brains. *Proc. Natl. Acad. Sci. U.S.A.* 103, 19219–19220. doi: 10.1073/pnas.0609523103

Stern, E., Welsh, R., Fitzgerald, K., Gehring, W., Lister, J., Himle, J., et al. (2011). Hyperactive error responses and altered connectivity in ventromedial and frontoinsular cortices in obsessive-compulsive disorder. *Biol. Psychiatry* 69, 583–591. doi: 10.1016/j.biopsych.2010.09.048

Szeszko, P. R., Ardekani, B. A., Ashtari, M., Malhotra, A. K., Robinson, D. G., Bilder, R. M., et al. (2005). White matter abnormalities in obsessive-compulsive disorder: A diffusion tensor imaging study. *Arch. Gen. Psychiatry* 62, 782–790. doi: 10.1001/archpsyc.62.7.782

Szeszko, P. R., Christian, C., MacMaster, F., Lencz, T., Mirza, Y., Taormina, S. P., et al. (2008). Gray matter structural alterations in psychotropic drug-naive pediatric obsessive-compulsive disorder: an optimized voxel-based morphometry study. *Am. J. Psychiatry* 165, 1299–1307. doi: 10.1176/appi.ajp.2008.08010033

Taylor, S. (2011). Early versus late onset obsessive–compulsive disorder: evidence for distinct subtypes. *Clin. Psychol. Rev.* 31, 1083–1100. doi: 10.1016/j.cpr.2011.06.007

Tijms, B. M., Seriès, P., Willshaw, D. J., and Lawrie, S. M. (2012). Similarity-based extraction of individual networks from gray matter MRI scans. *Cereb Cortex.* 22, 1530–1541. doi: 10.1093/cercor/bhr221

Togao, O., Yoshiura, T., Nakao, T., Nabeyama, M., Sanematsu, H., Nakagawa, A., et al. (2010). Regional gray and white matter volume abnormalities in obsessive–compulsive disorder: a voxel-based morphometry study. *Psychiatry Res.* 184, 29–37. doi: 10.1016/j.pscychresns.2010.06.011

Turkeltaub, P. E., Eden, G. F., Jones, K. M., and Zeffiro, T. A. (2002). Meta-analysis of the functional neuroanatomy of single-word reading: method and validation. *Neuroimage* 16(3 Pt A), 765–780. doi: 10.1006/nimg.2002.1131

Valente, A. A., Miguel, E. C., Castro, C. C., Amaro, E., Duran, F. L., Buchpiguel, C. A., et al. (2005). Regional gray matter abnormalities in obsessive-compulsive disorder: a voxel-based morphometry study. *Biol. Psychol.* 58, 479–487. doi: 10.1016/j.biopsych.2005.04.021

van den Heuvel, O., Remijnse, P., Mataix-Cols, D., Vrenken, H., Groenewegen, H., Uylings, H., et al. (2009). The major symptom dimensions of obsessive-compulsive disorder are mediated by partially distinct neural systems. *Brain* 132, 853–868. doi: 10.1093/brain/awn267

Wang, J., Wang, L., Zang, Y., Yang, H., Tang, H., Gong, Q., et al. (2009a). Parcellation-dependent small-world brain functional networks: a resting-state fmri study. *Hum. Brain Mapp.* 30, 1511–1523. doi: 10.1002/hbm.20623

Wang, L., Zhu, C., He, Y., Zang, Y., Cao, Q., Zhang, H., et al. (2009b). Altered small-world brain functional networks in children with attention-deficit/hyperactivity disorder. *Hum. Brain Mapp.* 30, 638–649. doi: 10.1002/hbm.20530

Watts, D. J., and Strogatz, S. H. (1998). Collective dynamics of 'small-world' networks. *Nature* 393, 440–442. doi: 10.1038/30918

Whiteside, S., Port, J., and Abramowitz, J. (2004). A meta-analysis of functional neuroimaging in obsessive-compulsive disorder. *Psychiatry Res.* 132, 69–79. doi: 10.1016/j.pscychresns.2004.07.001

Worsley, K., Taylor, J., Carbonell, F., Chung, M., Duerden, E., Bernhardt, B., et al. (2009). Surfstat: a matlab toolbox for the statistical analysis of univariate and multivariate surface and volumetric data using linear mixed effects models and random field theory. *Neuroimage* 47, S102–S102. doi: 10.1016/S1053-8119(09)70882-1

Worsley, K., Taylor, J., Tomaiuolo, F., and Lerch, J. (2004). Unified univariate and multivariate random field theory. *Neuroimage* 23(Suppl. 1), S189–S195. doi: 10.1016/j.neuroimage.2004.07.026

Zhang, T., Wang, J., Yang, Y., Wu, Q., Li, B., Chen, L., et al. (2011). Abnormal small-world architecture of top-down control networks in obsessive-compulsive disorder. *J. Psychiatr. Neurosci.* 36, 23–31. doi: 10.1503/jpn.100006

20

Modular reorganization of brain resting state networks and its independent validation in Alzheimer's disease patients

Guangyu Chen*[1]*, Hong-Ying Zhang*[2,3]*, Chunming Xie*[1,4]*, Gang Chen*[1]*, Zhi-Jun Zhang*[4]*, Gao-Jun Teng*[2]** and Shi-Jiang Li*[1,5]**

[1] *Department of Biophysics, Medical College of Wisconsin, Milwaukee, WI, USA*
[2] *Department of Radiology, Jiangsu Key Laboratory of Molecule Imaging and Functional Imaging, Medical School of Southeast University, Nanjing, PR China*
[3] *Department of Radiology, Subei People's Hospital of Jiangsu Province, Yangzhou University, Yangzhou, PR China*
[4] *Department of Neuropsychiatry, Affiliated Zhong Da Hospital of Southeast University, Nanjing, PR China*
[5] *Department of Psychiatry and Behavioral Medicine, Medical College of Wisconsin, Milwaukee, WI, USA*

Correspondence:
Gao-Jun Teng, Department of Radiology, Jiangsu Key Laboratory of Molecule Imaging and Functional Imaging, Medical School of Southeast University, 87 Dingjiaqiao Road, Nanjing 210009, PR China
e-mail: gjteng@vip.sina.com;
Shi-Jiang Li, Department of Biophysics, Medical College of Wisconsin, 8701 Watertown Plank Road, Milwaukee, WI 53226, USA
e-mail: sjli@mcw.edu

Previous studies have demonstrated disruption in structural and functional connectivity occurring in the Alzheimer's Disease (AD). However, it is not known how these disruptions alter brain network reorganization. With the modular analysis method of graph theory, and datasets acquired by the resting-state functional connectivity MRI (R-fMRI) method, we investigated and compared the brain organization patterns between the AD group and the cognitively normal control (CN) group. Our main finding is that the largest homotopic module (defined as the insula module) in the CN group was broken down to the pieces in the AD group. Specifically, it was discovered that the eight pairs of the bilateral regions (the opercular part of inferior frontal gyrus, area triangularis, insula, putamen, globus pallidus, transverse temporal gyri, superior temporal gyrus, and superior temporal pole) of the insula module had lost symmetric functional connection properties, and the corresponding gray matter concentration (GMC) was significant lower in AD group. We further quantified the functional connectivity changes with an index (index A) and structural changes with the GMC index in the insula module to demonstrate their great potential as AD biomarkers. We further validated these results with six additional independent datasets (271 subjects in six groups). Our results demonstrated specific underlying structural and functional reorganization from young to old, and for diseased subjects. Further, it is suggested that by combining the structural GMC analysis and functional modular analysis in the insula module, a new biomarker can be developed at the single-subject level.

Keywords: Alzheimer's disease, MCI, validation, module analysis, resting-state functional connectivity, brain network, gray matter concentration, graph theory

INTRODUCTION

Alzheimer's disease (AD) is considered a disconnection syndrome (Geschwind, 1965; Delbeuck et al., 2003). Recent studies demonstrated that the underlying neural mechanisms responsible for the disconnection syndrome are involved in the functional disruption in the brain of AD patients (Horwitz et al., 1987; Wada et al., 1998). An increasing number of studies have focused on imaging the default mode network (DMN) in aging and dementia by using intrinsic blood oxygenation level-dependent (iBOLD) signals, acquired by the resting-state functional MRI (R-fMRI) method (Lustig et al., 2003; Greicius et al., 2004; Sorg et al., 2009; Khalili-Mahani et al., 2012). The measurement of functional disruption in the DMN could become a potential clinical diagnostic biomarker for AD because convergent evidence demonstrated that brain atrophy, Aβ-amyloid plaque deposition and metabolic deficits co-occurred in the DMN (Buckner et al., 2009). Several other studies demonstrated that functional disruption also occurred in other areas besides the DMN, such as the hippocampus and the insular networks (Li et al., 2002; Bonthius et al., 2005; Royall, 2008; Xie et al., 2012). However, despite these scientific advancements, efforts to cross-validate the functional disruption trait as a biomarker have been of limited success.

Specifically, several studies provided the diagnostic power of the DMN for AD (Li et al., 2002; Greicius et al., 2004; Fleisher et al., 2009; Koch et al., 2010, 2012), but follow-up studies by other research groups are either lacking (Li et al., 2002; Greicius et al., 2004; Fleisher et al., 2009; Koch et al., 2010, 2012), controversial (Zhang et al., 2009; Yu et al., 2011), or failed to confirm a solid diagnostic value (Prvulovic et al., 2011). As a result, despite the efforts during the past decade, there is no robust biomarker based on R-fMRI technology, which has substantially limited its potential utility value in AD research and treatment. There are several factors that may contribute to the current stagnant status. First, in typical seed-based R-fMRI studies, the group-level t-tests often statistically identified the connectivity maps that highlight voxels where functional connectivity is disrupted. Such a statistical approach often overestimates the diagnostic power, even if the leave-one-out approach or seven-fold cross-validation method is employed (Chen et al., 2011a; Westman et al., 2012a,b). Second, because of compensatory mechanisms or increased activation, brain connectivity may be reorganized along the continuum of disease progression (He et al., 2008; Sanz-Arigita et al., 2010). Not only did the functional connectivity decrease in certain regions, but it also increased in other regions (Zhang et al., 2010). As a result, the summation of the overall connectivity strength may not change significantly. Third, the disconnection syndrome in AD may be the result of the functional and structural disruptions in the large-scale networks; therefore, the seed-based network alone, such as the DMN, may have no sufficient power as a biomarker. As a result, when applying trained classifiers to independent datasets, the specificity and sensitivity were low.

To overcome these shortcomings and to move the research field forward, the present study is focusing on three new approaches. First, we extend the seed-based analysis to the modular analysis method (He et al., 2009; Meunier et al., 2009a,b, 2010) to examine the patterns of brain network reorganization at the large-scale network level to test the hypothesis that the AD network organization is a reconfiguration from CN networks where some subnetworks that are related to cognitive processing may change and others are preserved. A previous study (Faria et al., 2012) addressed the factor that network (or called Atlas)-based analysis can enhance SNR and reproducibility of resting-state functional connectivity. In addition, in using network-based functional connectivity, the number of false positive cross-correlations can be significantly reduced due to the reduced number of the total pairs of correlations. To our knowledge, the applicability of the modular analysis to examine the resting-state functional network reorganization pattern in mild cognitive impairment (MCI) and AD brains has not been demonstrated. Second, based on specific changes in brain reorganization patterns at the module level, an exploratory analysis was performed to evaluate if the changes can be employed as a biomarker for AD. Third, we employed an additional six independent R-fMRI datasets from human subjects to independently cross-validate the module-based biomarker at the single-subject level.

MATERIALS AND METHODS

HUMAN SUBJECTS

A total of 331 subjects in eight groups were employed for this study. Two R-fMRI datasets obtained from the cognitively normal (CN) group ($N = 30$) and the mild AD group ($N = 30$) from the Medical College of Wisconsin (MCW) site (referred to herein as MCW datasets) (**Table 1**) were employed as the testing datasets to identify changes in the modular reorganization patterns occurring in AD brains as a biomarker. We then employed six additional independent R-fMRI datasets to cross-validate the biomarker. Among the six sets of datasets, one was obtained from amnestic mild cognitive impairment (aMCI) subjects ($N = 23$) from the MCW site, three datasets were obtained from a group of 56 elderly subjects from Southeast University, Nanjing, China, comprised of elderly CN subjects ($N = 20$), aMCI subjects ($N = 22$), and AD subjects ($N = 14$) (referred to herein as Nanjing datasets) (**Table 1**) (Zhang et al., 2010). The other two independent R-fMRI datasets are comprised of 192 young subjects; these were downloaded from the 1000 Functional Connectomes Project database (www.nitrc.org/projects/fcon_1000/) from Beijing Zang's datasets (http://www.nitrc.org/frs/shownotes.php?release_id=819) (referred to herein as Beijing datasets) (**Table 1**) (Biswal et al., 2010). All of these subjects were obtained from databanks. For detailed subject information, please refers to originally published papers (Biswal et al., 2010; Zhang et al., 2010; Chen et al., 2011a).

IMAGING ACQUISITION OF MCW DATASETS

Imaging was performed using a whole-body 3T Signa GE scanner with a standard quadrature transmit receive head coil. During the resting-state acquisitions, no specific cognitive tasks were performed, and the study participants were instructed to close their eyes and relax inside the scanner. Sagittal resting-state functional MRI (fMRI) datasets of the whole brain were obtained in 6 minutes with a single-shot gradient echo-planar imaging (EPI) pulse sequence. The fMRI imaging parameters were: TE of 25 ms, TR of 2 s, flip angle of 90°; 36 slices were obtained without gap; slice thickness was 4 mm with a matrix size of 64 × 64 and field of view of 24 × 24 cm. High-resolution SPGR 3D axial images were acquired for anatomical reference. The parameters were: TE/TR/TI of 4/10/450 ms, flip angle of 12°, number of slices of 144, slice thickness of 1 mm, matrix size of 256 × 192. To make sure that cardiac and respiratory frequencies did not account for any significant artifacts in the low-frequency spectrum, a pulse oximeter and respiratory belt were employed to measure these physiological noise sources. Further processing ensured a minimizing of the potential aliasing effects.

IMAGING ACQUISITION OF BEIJING DATASETS

The data was acquired at 3T Siemens Scanner. We used 192 subjects out of a total of 198 young subjects from Beijing Zang's datasets. Six subjects were discarded during the preprocessing procedures for a variety reasons. The imaging acquisition parameters can be found on the website (http://www.nitrc.org).

IMAGING ACQUISITION OF NANJING DATASETS

The data was acquired at 1.5T Philips Scanner. Subjects wore headphones and were instructed to lie in a supine position in a standard head coil of a 1.5-T MR imaging unit (Eclipse; Philips, Best, The Netherlands). Structural images were obtained. Resting-state functional images were acquired by using a gradient-echo EPI sequence (TR/TE, 3000/40 ms; flip angle, 90°, slice thickness, 6 mm; slice gap, 0 mm; field of view, 240 mm; and matrix size, 64 × 64; 18 axial slices and 128 time points). For detailed parameters and demographic information, please refer to previous study (Zhang et al., 2010). All of these studies were conducted with Institutional Review Board approval and were in compliance with Health Insurance Portability and Accountability Act (HIPAA) regulations or similar polices in China.

DATA PREPROCESSING

We used Analysis of Functional NeuroImages (AFNI) software (http://afni.nimh.nih.gov/afni/) and MATLAB (Mathworks) in this study for data processing. The first five volumes of each raw resting-state functional imaging dataset were discarded to allow for T1 equilibration. Interleaved slice acquisition-dependent time shifts were corrected (AFNI command, *to3d -time:zt* nz nt TR tpattern). Spikes in time series data were removed (AFNI command, *3dDespike*). Data were then motion corrected (Six motion parameters, including roll, pitch, in the superior, left and posterior direction displacement were estimated by volume registration of the R-fMRI data, and then, were regressed out by using Afni command 3dDeconvolve to control possible micromovement effects). There was no group difference for movement parameters. Detrend processing procedure using AFNI commands (*3dvolreg and 3dDetrend*) was performed. The reference template in Talairach space, which contained 116 anatomically defined regions of interest (ROIs) (Tzourio-Mazoyer et al., 2002), was transformed and aligned to the SPGR images and EPI resting-state functional images for each subject (AFNI command, *3dfractionize*). This resulted in 116 mapped ROIs. The average time course within each ROI was extracted from the resting-state functional imaging datasets. Averaged white matter signal and cerebrospinal fluid (CSF) signal were extracted using white matter mask (http://afni.nimh.nih.gov/pub/dist/data/TTwm+tlrc) and CSF (http://afni.nimh.nih.gov/pub/dist/data/ TT_csf+tlrc) mask in Talairach space. These two masks were transformed and aligned to the SPGR and echo planar images for each subject (AFNI command, *3dfractionize*). Then, the average time courses within the CSF or the eroded white matter mask, together with global mean signals, were removed as nuisance regressors from the 116 regional time courses with linear regression using Matlab (Mathworks).

POSTPROCESSING

Brain functional network

We constructed a region-wise whole-brain resting-state functional network for each subject. A network size is N (N is the number of Nodes or ROIs, in this study, $N = 116$), there are $N \times (N-1)/2$ possible edges in a fully connected network expressed in a matrix. The weighted strength of each edge between nodes i and j was defined as CC_{ij} (cross-correlation coefficient (**CC**) between two time series of *ROI(i)* and *ROI(j)*). The weighted distance of each edge between a pair of directly connected nodes *ROI(i)* and *ROI(j)* was defined as $d_{ij} = 1 - CC_{ij}$. The adjacent matrix of CC_{ij} represents graph G, such that $G = \{V, S, D\}$, consisting of a set of vertices(Nodes) $V = \{V_1, V_2, \ldots, V_N\}$, a set of edges $S = \{CC_{ij}|i, j = 1, 2, \ldots, N\}$ and a set of associating weighted edge distances D = {1 – CC_i, j|i, j = 1, 2, … ,N} between brain regions *ROI(i)* and *ROI(j)*.

Group network

A group functional network matrix (**A**) is constructed by the ratio of mean to the standard deviation of all individuals' matrices in this group. Each element value of **A** is calculated as follows:

$$a_{ij} = \frac{\frac{1}{n}\sum_{k=1}^{n} CC_{k,i,j}}{\sqrt{\frac{1}{n}\sum_{k=1}^{n}(CC_{k,i,j} - \mu_{ij})^2}} \tag{1}$$

This matrix can reduce the intersubject variation of the functional connectivity especially those connections with large intersubject variation. k is the subject number, n is the number of subjects, i and j are two ROIs of *ROI(i)* and *ROI(j)*. In this study, we only use the positive CC value in group network as previously described (Chen et al., 2011b) for further modular analysis.

Modularity

Module is defined as a community, the inside of which has denser connections than the rest of the network (Newman and Girvan, 2004). Several algorithms have been developed to detect those modules (Clauset et al., 2004; Duch and Arenas, 2005). The basic approach is to measure the maximum modularity value, Q, which is defined as:

$$Q = \frac{1}{2m}\sum_{i,j}\left[a_{ij} - \frac{k_i k_j}{2m}\right]\delta(c_i, c_j). \tag{2}$$

a_{ij} is the adjacent weighted matrix which represents the network, m is the number of connections in the network, and k_i is the degree of node i (Ahnert et al., 2007) and c_i is the module i.

In order to find the communities in the brain functional network, we use the spectral algorithm of Newman (Newman, 2006; Leicht and Newman, 2008), which is implemented in the Brain Connectivity Tool Box (https://sites.google.com/a/brain-connectivity-toolbox.net/bct/Home). This program can find the network organization pattern with the best modularity value (Q).

Quantitative measurement of modular reorganization in AD

Based on our hypothesis that AD may reorganize modular patterns compared to CN, the reorganization pattern may exhibit the disruption properties of the whole-brain function network. In order to quantify the changes in the modular patterns in the subnetworks, we created two functional indices (index A and index B) to measure the inter- and intra-hemisphere connections. Index A measures an average of functional connectivity strength

Table 1 | Summary of demographic information for test and validation groups of subjects.

Groups	Number	Age	Male/Female	MMSE	Education (year)	
CN_3T	30	75.9 ± 6.42	16/14	29.4 ± 1.03	NA	Test group
AD_3T	30	76.7 ± 5.28	17/13	24.8 ± 2.97	NA	
MCI_3T	23	76.1 ± 6.84	11/12	27.83 ± 1.67	NA	Validation group
CN_1.5T	20	68.9 ± 6.44	7/13	28.6 ± 1.05	10 ± 3.71	Validation group
MCI_1.5T	22	71.6 ± 4.95	10/12	27.2 ± 1.4	10.7 ± 3.50	Validation group
AD_1.5T	14	71.3 ± 5.09	5/9	22.2 ± 2.91	9.6 ± 4.96	Validation group
Young 18–22 3T	150	20.4 ± 1.13	59/91	NA	NA	Validation group
Young 23–26 3T	42	23.9 ± 1.02	27/15	NA	NA	Validation group

in homotopic pairs $(ROI\_L(i), ROI\_R(i))$

$$\text{indexA} = \frac{1}{n}\sum_{i=1}^{n} CC\,(ROI\_L(i), ROI\_R(i)) \tag{3}$$

Where $ROI\_L(i)$ and $ROI\_R(i)$ are two corresponding bilateral homotopic regions, and $CC(ROI\_L(i), ROI\_R(i))$ is the two time courses CC value of $ROI\_L(i)$ and $ROI\_R(i)$. The n is the number of pairs of homotopic regions to calculate index A. Index B is used to measure an average of functional connectivity strength within selected unilateral ROIs.

$$\text{indexB} = \frac{1}{n}\left(\sum_{i=1}^{n}\sum_{j=1}^{n} CC\left(ROI\_L(i), ROI\_L(j)\right) + \sum_{i=1}^{n}\sum_{j=1}^{n} CC\left(ROI\_R(i), ROI\_R(j)\right)\right) \tag{4}$$

There are n ROIs from the right hemisphere (ROI_R) and n corresponding homotopic ROIs from the left hemisphere (ROI_L).

Gray matter concentration (GMC)

Besides the functional connectivity, we also calculated the GMC on the AAL template within the regions that showed functional disruption. The gray matter of each subject is segmented by using SPM 8 software (www.fil.ion.ucl.ac.uk/spm/software/spm8/) and then normalized into Talairach space to extract each part of the regions using AFNI and 116 AAL templates. GMC value of each region is the average overall voxel values within those regions involved in modular reorganization.

RESULTS

MAXIMUM MODULARITY VALUE (Q)

The Q is determined with the modular algorithm, which measures how a network can be separated into different subnetworks. With the MCW dataset, **Figure 1** shows the averaged maximum modularity values of individual subjects in each group as a function of number of edges (NE). All subjects in groups CN and AD have larger averaged Q values than their corresponding random networks, indicating that their complex functional networks have a strong ability to form modules, and the module analysis method can be applied to disease populations, such as MCI and AD. There is no group difference in Q value at all different thresholds of NE after the familywise error correction.

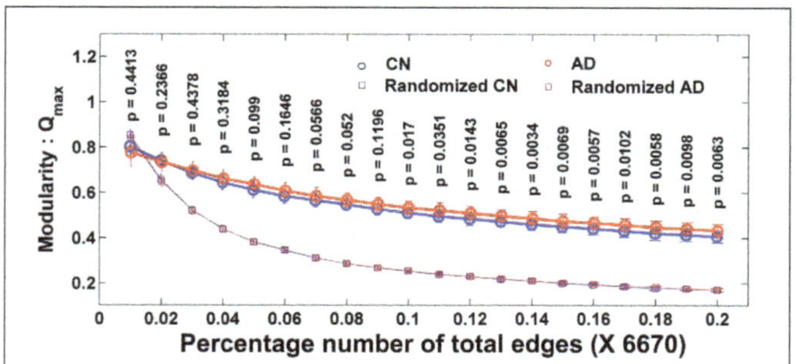

FIGURE 1 | Individual modularity values (Q) distribution of a network as the function of the number of edges and its corresponding random network. Error bar shows the standard deviation. All groups' networks have a significantly larger Q-value than the corresponding random networks. Larger Q shows the ability of a network to form modules.

MODULE STRUCTURES IN THE AD GROUP WERE REORGANIZED, UNLIKE THE CN GROUP

Although the complex functional network of the AD group has the ability to form the modular structures, similar to the CN group, the modular patterns and membership are quite different between the CN and AD groups, and demonstrated network reorganization patterns. The modular structures are expressed into two forms of presentations: the graphic presentation and mapping presentation, as illustrated in **Figures 2A,B** for CN and AD groups, respectively. For the CN group, the brains were organized into seven modules. For the AD group, the brain modules were reorganized into eight modules. The module-reorganization patterns between CN and AD are graphically illustrated in **Figures 2C,D**. The largest module in the CN group (CN-1) was broken down into two separated modules in the AD group (AD-1 and AD-2). The module CN-2 is disrupted into three modules (AD-3, AD-4, and AD-8) and module CN-6 is disrupted into four modules (AD-4, AD-6, AD-7, AD-8).

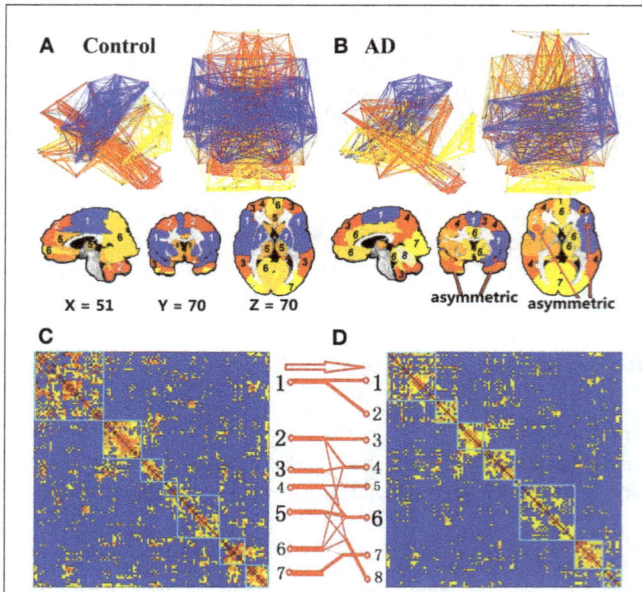

FIGURE 2 | Module of the non-threshold positive group networks of CN and AD at 3T. Color represents the individual community. First row of **(A)** and **(B)** is the network view, the second row of **(A)** and **(B)** shows the brain module organization overlaid in the brain template and the last row (**C** and **D**) is the module reorganization pattern between CN and AD. The label module numbers in the brain views of **(A)** and **(B)** are matched with the module numbers in **(C)** and **(D)**, respectively. Two matrices, **(C)** and **(D)**, show the grouped CC matrix of CN and AD. In **(C)** and **(D)**, numbers along each matrix labeled the module number for each group. Red arrow and red connection lines show the reorganization pattern from CN to AD. The thickness of each line represents the number of members.

To compare the module membership composition between CN and AD groups and identify specific brain regions that disrupted away from the original module, the module CN-1 was cited as an example. As listed in **Table 2**, the module CN-1 contained eight pairs of homotopic brain regions, which are defined as geometrically symmetric across interhemispheric regions. This well-organized module is highly symmetric across hemispheres in the control network (**Figure 2A**). We called this module the "insula module," because its members are involved in saliency, switching, attention and control functions of the insula network (Menon and Uddin, 2010). Noticeably, eight out of 16 homotopic regions were broken in the AD group. The eight regions on the right hemisphere formed a new module in the AD group (AD-2) (labeled in Red bold in **Table 2**). These eight regions are the right opercular part of inferior frontal gyrus, right area triangularis, right insula, right putamen, right globus pallidus, right transverse temporal gyri, right superior temporal gyrus, and right superior temporal pole. The formation of the new module AD-2 not only indicated that the insula module is broken down, but also indicated there is severe disruption between left and right hemisphere communication in the AD brains.

QUANTIFICATION AND VALIDATION OF THE INSULA MODULE IN HEALTHY YOUNG, CN, MCI, AND AD GROUPS

To quantify the insula module disruption between hemispheres, two functional indices were obtained [index A calculated from Equation (3) and index B calculated from Equation (4)]. As illustrated in **Figures 3A,B**, functional connections of the eight pairs of homotopic (contralateral) regions of the insula module were disconnected in the AD group. As shown in **Figure 3C**, index A is significantly ($p < 0.018$) decreased in the AD group compared to the CN group. Index B shows no significant difference related to the AD and CN groups but has increasing trends ($p < 0.12$). To cross-validate the results with indices A and B, we employed six additional independent datasets in order to avoid an *overly optimistic* estimate of the error rate by the *resubstitution method* or the *leave-one-out method*. First, we employed the MCW dataset containing 23 aMCI subjects. As shown in **Figure 3D**, index A, individually calculated from each aMCI subject in the aMCI group, was significantly lower than that in the CN group and index B showed no difference. Second, we employed the Beijing datasets containing the young groups of subjects (group age between 18 and 22 years old, and group age between 23 and 26 years old, total 192 subjects). As shown in **Figure 3D**, index A of young subjects has stronger homotopic connectivity strength than that of the elderly CN subjects and no differences for index B. Third, we further demonstrated that datasets acquired on the 1.5T scanner can be employed to validate our results. With the Nanjing datasets acquired from 1.5T scanner, index A of the MCI and AD groups is significantly reduced compared to the CN group, as shown in **Figure 3E**. These validated results demonstrated that index A as a biomarker can be quantitatively employed for monitoring AD progression in the continuum of disease processes: higher index A in young, decrease in elderly CN groups, and more significantly decreased in the MCI and AD groups.

Table 2 | Regions in the insula module (blue module).

Blue module (insula community)	
Left	**Right**
Left precentral gyrus	Right precentral gyrus
Left opercular part of inferior frontal gyrus	**Right opercular part of inferior frontal gyrus**
Left area triangularis	**Right area triangularis**
Left rolandic operculum	Right rolandic operculum
Left insula	**Right insula**
Left middle cingulate	Right middle cingulate
Left postcentral gyrus	Right postcentral gyrus
Left superior parietal lobule	Right superior parietal lobule
Left inferior parietal lobule	Right inferior parietal lobule
Left supramarginal gyrus	Right supramarginal gyrus
Left paracentral lobule	Right paracentral lobule
Left putamen	**Right putamen**
Left globus pallidus	**Right globus pallidus**
Left transverse temporal gyri	**Right transverse temporal gyri**
Left superior temporal gyrus	**Right superior temporal gyrus**
Left superior temporal pole	**Right superior temporal pole**
	Right supplementary motor area
	Right amygdala

The eight right brain regions (in red bold) are no longer the members of the blue module in the AD brains.

Decreased gray matter concentration (GMC) of these eight pairs of homotopic regions in MCI and AD groups. The disrupted functional connectivity occurred in the eight pairs of homotopic regions in the insula module. In addition, the average gray matter concentration (GMC) of those regions showed significant decrease in the MCI and AD groups in comparison to the CN groups. The GMC decrease in the MCI and AD group was observed, as shown in **Figure 3F**. To determine if the GMC changes affect the calculation of index A, the variance of the GMC factor was controlled out. As shown in **Figure 3G**, index A is still valid in distinguishing between CN from MCI or AD status. These results also indicated that although structural density and functional connectivity decrease may be related, their changes are not necessary proportional (Palop et al., 2006). With this trait, we have combined index A and GMC to examine their diagnostic potential, as described below.

Diagnostic power of index A and GMC as biomarkers to classify CN, MCI, and AD statuses. Through the measurement of index A and GMC on each single subject, we have explored their potential as biomarkers to classify CN, MCI, and AD statuses. As shown in **Figure 4**, the result from testing groups (CN vs. AD) provided 94% of area under the curve (AUC) of the receiver operation characteristic (ROC) curve. The validation results provided 78 and 71% of AUC to classify between CN and AD, and between MCI and AD, respectively. With Nanjing datasets acquired on the 1.5T Siemens scanner, these validation results become 85% (AD vs. CN) and 80% (MCI vs. CN), and 70% (MCI vs. AD). For the young subject groups as the healthiest population, there is a perfect 100% specificity and sensitivity (AUC 100%) in comparison to the AD group.

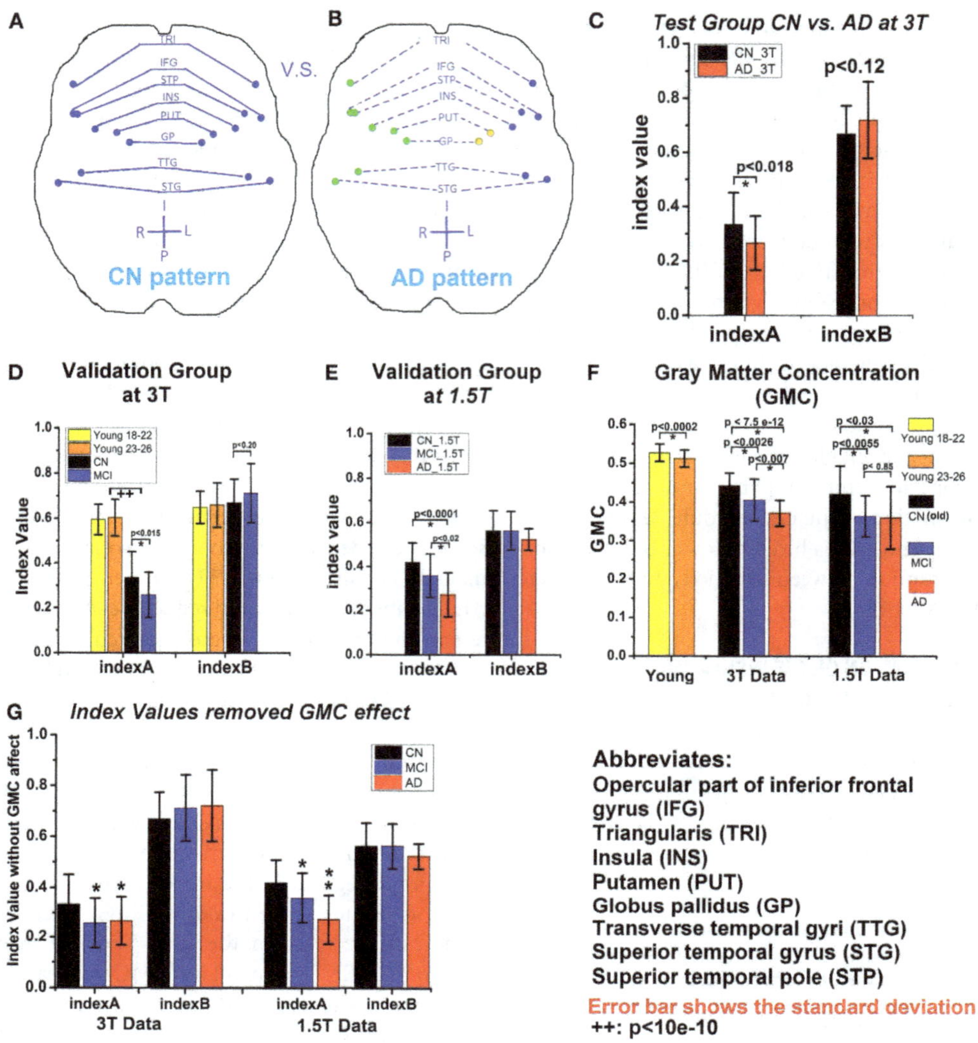

FIGURE 3 | (A) and **(B)** Show the changes of insula module between CN **(A)** and AD **(B)**; each dot is the center of an AAL-based brain region; regions with same color are in the same module, solid line means higher connection, while the dash line represents the weaker connection. **(C)** Two indices (index A and index B) of CN_3T and AD_3T (test groups). **(D)** Two indices of two young subject groups, CN_3T and MCI_3T (validation groups). **(E)** Two indices of CN_1.5T, MCI_1.5T, and AD_1.5T (validation groups). **(F)** The average of GMC of each group. **(G)** The two indices after removal of the GMC effect of each group; where (*) represents the significance ($p < 0.05$) in comparison to CN_1.5T and (**) represents the significance ($p < 0.05$) in comparison to the MCI group. Error bar indicates the standard deviation. (++) represents both young groups have significant larger index A value than the old CN_3T and MCI_3T groups.

DISCUSSION

Several studies have employed the modular analysis method to demonstrate that the brain has modular organization (Hilgetag et al., 2000; Chen et al., 2008; Hagmann et al., 2008). In comparison to small-world metrics, modular analysis can provide detailed network organization patterns as to how the nodes are connected to form subnetworks or communities in a complex network (Hilgetag et al., 2000; Chen et al., 2008; Hagmann et al., 2008). Using this advantage, modular analysis methods have been applied to diseased resting-state brain networks, such as in chronic back pain (Balenzuela et al., 2010) and schizophrenia (Alexander-Bloch et al., 2010; Yu et al., 2011). Using magnetoencephalography (MEG), it was also found that the module strength and the number of modules significantly changed in AD patients (de Haan et al., 2012). Our results are consistent with these findings and demonstrated the applicability of R-fMRI datasets for modular analysis to AD.

In the control network, as expected, module patterns are well organized with symmetric distribution. Each pair of the interhemispheric homotopic regions, for the most part, is in the same communities. Many literature references substantiate that the brain functional network forms an interhemispheric symmetric pattern with highly consistent functional connectivity between homotopic regions (Zuo et al., 2010). A high degree of symmetry in the motor cortex of resting-state functional connectivity has been reported (Biswal et al., 1995; Van den Heuvel and Hulshoff

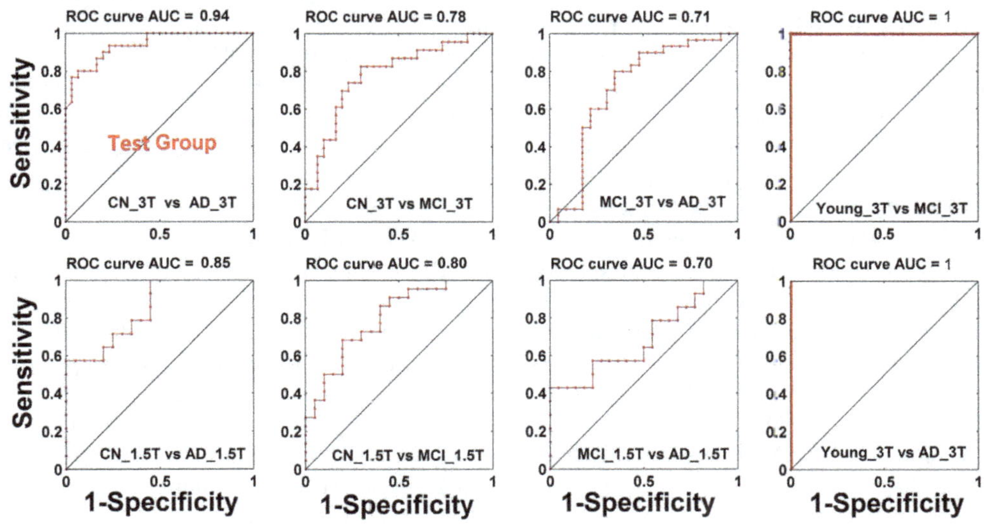

FIGURE 4 | Classification power (ROC curve) when both biomarkers of GMC and index A are combined.

Pol, 2010). The well-known DMN (Raichle et al., 2001; Greicius et al., 2004) has a symmetric, well-organized pattern. Similar to the module method, Mezer (Mezer et al., 2009) used the clustering method and discovered a symmetric pattern of clusters between the two hemispheres. This was true not only in the human brain, but also in the rat brain. The highest values of functional connectivity exist between interhemispheric homotopic regions (Pawela et al., 2008, 2010). However, not all the interhemispheric homotopic regions are symmetric, only some regions and their homotopic regions belong to different communities. This may be due to the dynamic changes of the functional connectivity (Chang and Glover, 2010).

As expected in mild AD group, some of the communities lost symmetric properties. There are more single regions whose homotopic regions are in different communities. For example, module 1 (blue module in **Figure 2A**) in the control group is very symmetric, while it is separated into two modules in the AD group (blue and brown modules in **Figure 2B**). Decreased symmetric properties or functional connectivity between interhemispheric homotopic regions have been found in many diseased functional networks. In behavioral research, Yamina (Lakmache et al., 1998) found that AD subjects performed normally when using intrahemispheric processing, but did poorly when interhemispheric communication was required. For instance, in imaging research, EEG studies (Locatelli et al., 1998; Babiloni et al., 2004) of AD found decreased coordination between interhemispheric networks. In the cocaine-dependent group, Kelly (Kelly et al., 2011) investigated the interhemispheric homotopic connections using the Voxel-Mirrored Homotopic Connectivity method, and found the striking cocaine-dependence-related reduction in interhemispheric resting-state functional connectivity among nodes of the dorsal attention network. Also, decreased interhemispheric functional connectivity in subjects with impaired awareness were found (Ovadia-Caro et al., 2012). Therefore, this phenomenon of losing symmetric properties may reflect the cognitive decline and unbalanced state in the functional network of the diseased brain.

The most significant finding of this module study is the interrupted integration of insula module in AD group. Anatomically, the insula is a crucial hub in the human brain network; it is widely connected to the cortical, limbic, and paralimbic structures. Functionally, it is involved in high-order cognition, emotion, autonomic, and sensory process (Naqvi et al., 2007; Allen et al., 2008). The previous study has shown that the insula was affected in AD and its atrophy was significantly decreased from the normal population (Fan et al., 2008). The seed-based functional connectivity of the insular regions was discovered to be significantly decreased in the regions that functionally connected with insula. This disruption was associated with episodic-memory deficits in aMCI patients (Xie et al., 2012). Our results are not only consistent with these previous findings, they indicate a disruption between the insula and other brain regions. Also, we detected the breakdown of the insula module in the AD group, which is a possible neural underpinning of AD dementia.

Our findings demonstrated that the specific reorganized modular patterns can be quantified with index A in the CN, MCI, and AD groups. Unlike biomarkers with inverse U-shape patterns, such as the fMRI method due to the compensatory mechanisms (Dickerson and Sperling, 2009), index A is a monofunction with the disease progression of AD. Index A of aMCI and AD subjects is significantly lower than that of CN and young subjects. Because the biggest risk factor of AD is aging, the congruency between the changes in the index A value, and changes in age, demonstrated the potential of index A to serve as a biomarker. This characteristic of the monofunction of index A with age is very important for diagnostic accuracy by decreasing false positive and negative errors.

We showed the potential of using structural changes (GMC) and functional disruption in the insula module (index A) as a biomarker for AD. Recent revision of the NINCDS-ADRDA

(National Institute of Neurological and Communicative Disorders and Stroke and the AD and Related Disorders Association [now known as the Alzheimer's Association]) criterion for the diagnosis of AD suggested adding abnormal biomarkers, such as MRI, positron emission tomography (PET), CSF, and brain atrophy to strengthen their roles (Kohannim et al., 2010; Nettiksimmons et al., 2010; Walhovd et al., 2010; McKhann et al., 2011; Zhang et al., 2011; Dai et al., 2012; Ewers et al., 2012; Westman et al., 2012b). The effective combination of these biomarkers can clinically provide more diagnostic power than using a single biomarker. In this study, we found that the combination of MRI atrophy biomarker and the R-fMRI biomarker of insula module could enhance the classification of AD and monitor the progression along the continuum of AD development both in the test and validation group. Our results demonstrated the great feasibility of combining both MRI-based biomarkers of the insula module in AD diagnosis.

In summary, with the modular analysis, we demonstrated the ability of index A and GMC of the insula module in distinguishing MCI and AD from old and young, healthy CN subjects, and its power of cross-validation with six independent datasets. The combination of the MRI-based structural biomarker and functional biomarker will significantly enhance the diagnostic power. Further studies will be needed to characterize the relationships between different biomarkers for AD (Sperling et al., 2009; Kohannim et al., 2010; Nettiksimmons et al., 2010; Sheline et al., 2010a,b; Walhovd et al., 2010; Zhang et al., 2011; Ewers et al., 2012; Johnson et al., 2012).

ACKNOWLEDGMENTS

Dr. Gao-Jun Teng has full access to all of the study data and took responsibility for the integrity of the data and the accuracy of the data analysis. The authors thank Ms. Carrie M. O'Connor, M.A., for editorial assistance, and Mr. B. Douglas Ward, M.S., for discussions related to the statistical analysis. This work was supported by National Natural Science Foundation of China (30825014, 30870704, 30971016, 81061120529 (Zhi-Jun Zhang); 81171323 (Chunming Xie); 91132727 (Xiangyong Zhang); 81171021 (Yongmei Shi); National Institutes of Health grants: RO1 AG20279 (Shi-Jiang Li), the DANA Foundation (Shi-Jiang Li). Social Development and Scientific and Technology Project of Yangzhou (YZ2011087).

REFERENCES

Ahnert, S. E., Garlaschelli, D., Fink, T. M., and Caldarelli, G. (2007). Ensemble approach to the analysis of weighted networks. *Phys. Rev. E Stat. Nonlin. Soft Matter Phys.* 76:016101.

Alexander-Bloch, A. F., Gogtay, N., Meunier, D., Birn, R., Clasen, L., Lalonde, F., et al. (2010). Disrupted modularity and local connectivity of brain functional networks in childhood-onset schizophrenia. *Front. Syst. Neurosci.* 4:147. doi: 10.3389/fnsys.2010.00147

Allen, J. S., Emmorey, K., Bruss, J., and Damasio, H. (2008). Morphology of the insula in relation to hearing status and sign language experience. *J. Neurosci.* 28, 11900–11905. doi: 10.1523/JNEUROSCI.3141-08.2008

Babiloni, C., Miniussi, C., Moretti, D. V., Vecchio, F., Salinari, S., Frisoni, G., et al. (2004). Cortical networks generating movement-related EEG rhythms in Alzheimer's disease: an EEG coherence study. *Behav. Neurosci.* 118, 698–706. doi: 10.1037/0735-7044.118.4.698

Balenzuela, P., Chernomoretz, A., Fraiman, D., Cifre, I., Sitges, C., Montoya, P., et al. (2010). Modular organization of brain resting state networks in chronic back pain patients. *Front. Neuroinform.* 4:116. doi: 10.3389/fninf.2010.00116

Biswal, B. B., Mennes, M., Zuo, X. N., Gohel, S., Kelly, C., Smith, S. M., et al. (2010). Toward discovery science of human brain function. *Proc. Natl. Acad. Sci. U.S.A.* 107, 4734–4739. doi: 10.1073/pnas.0911855107

Biswal, B., Yetkin, F. Z., Haughton, V. M., and Hyde, J. S. (1995). Functional connectivity in the motor cortex of resting human brain using echo-planar MRI. *Magn. Reson. Med.* 34, 537–541. doi: 10.1002/mrm.1910340409

Bonthius, D. J., Solodkin, A., and Van Hoesen, G. W. (2005). Pathology of the insular cortex in Alzheimer disease depends on cortical architecture. *J. Neuropathol. Exp. Neurol.* 64, 910–922. doi: 10.1097/01.jnen.0000182983.87106.d1

Buckner, R. L., Sepulcre, J., Talukdar, T., Krienen, F. M., Liu, H., Hedden, T., et al. (2009). Cortical hubs revealed by intrinsic functional connectivity: mapping, assessment of stability, and relation to Alzheimer's disease. *J. Neurosci.* 29, 1860–1873. doi: 10.1523/JNEUROSCI.5062-08.2009

Chang, C., and Glover, G. H. (2010). Time-frequency dynamics of resting-state brain connectivity measured with fMRI. *Neuroimage* 50, 81–98. doi: 10.1016/j.neuroimage.2009.12.011

Chen, G., Ward, B. D., Xie, C., Li, W., Wu, Z., Jones, J. L., et al. (2011a). Classification of Alzheimer disease, mild cognitive impairment, and normal cognitive status with large-scale network analysis based on resting-state functional MR imaging. *Radiology* 259, 213–221.

Chen, G., Xie, C., and Li, S. J. (2011b). Negative functional connectivity and its dependence on the shortest path length of positive network in the resting-state human brain. *Brain Connect.* 1, 195–206.

Chen, Z. J., He, Y., Rosa-Neto, P., Germann, J., and Evans, A. C. (2008). Revealing modular architecture of human brain structural networks by using cortical thickness from MRI. *Cereb. Cortex* 18, 2374–2381. doi: 10.1093/cercor/bhn003

Clauset, A., Newman, M. E., and Moore, C. (2004). Finding community structure in very large networks. *Phys. Rev. E Stat. Nonlin. Soft Matter Phys.* 70:066111.

Dai, Z., Yan, C., Wang, Z., Wang, J., Xia, M., Li, K., et al. (2012). Discriminative analysis of early Alzheimer's disease using multi-modal imaging and multi-level characterization with multi-classifier (M3). *Neuroimage* 59, 2187–2195. doi: 10.1016/j.neuroimage.2011.10.003

de Haan, W., van der Flier, W. M., Koene, T., Smits, L. L., Scheltens, P., and Stam, C. J. (2012). Disrupted modular brain dynamics reflect cognitive dysfunction in Alzheimer's disease. *Neuroimage* 59, 3085–3093. doi: 10.1016/j.neuroimage.2011.11.055

Delbeuck, X., Van der Linden, M., and Collette, F. (2003). Alzheimer's disease as a disconnection syndrome. *Neuropsychol. Rev.* 13, 79–92. doi: 10.1023/A:1023832305702

Dickerson, B. C., and Sperling, R. A. (2009). Large-scale functional brain network abnormalities in Alzheimer's disease: insights from functional neuroimaging. *Behav. Neurol.* 21, 63–75.

Duch, J. A., and Arenas, A. (2005). Community detection in complex networks using extremal optimization. *Phys. Rev. E Stat. Nonlin. Soft Matter Phys.* 72, 027104–027107. doi: 10.1103/PhysRevE.72.027104

Ewers, M., Insel, P., Jagust, W. J., Shaw, L., Trojanowski, J. J., Aisen, P., et al. (2012). CSF biomarker and PIB-PET-derived beta-amyloid signature predicts metabolic, gray matter, and cognitive changes in nondemented subjects. *Cereb. Cortex* 22, 1993–2004. doi: 10.1093/cercor/bhr271

Fan, Y., Resnick, S. M., Wu, X., and Davatzikos, C. (2008). Structural and functional biomarkers of prodromal Alzheimer's disease: a high-dimensional pattern classification study. *Neuroimage* 41, 277–285. doi: 10.1016/j.neuroimage.2008.02.043

Faria, A. V., Joel, S. E., Zhang, Y., Oishi, K., van Zjil, P. C., Miller, M. I., et al. (2012). Atlas-based analysis of resting-state functional connectivity: evaluation for reproducibility and multi-modal anatomy-function correlation studies. *Neuroimage* 61, 613–621. doi: 10.1016/j.neuroimage.2012.03.078

Fleisher, A. S., Sherzai, A., Taylor, C., Langbaum, J. B., Chen, K., and Buxton, R. B. (2009). Resting-state BOLD networks versus task-associated functional MRI for distinguishing Alzheimer's disease risk groups. *Neuroimage* 47, 1678–1690. doi: 10.1016/j.neuroimage.2009.06.021

Geschwind, N. (1965). Disconnexion syndromes in animals and man. I. *Brain* 88, 237–294. doi: 10.1093/brain/88.2.237

Greicius, M. D., Srivastava, G., Reiss, A. L., and Menon, V. (2004). Default-mode network activity distinguishes Alzheimer's disease from healthy aging: evidence from functional MRI. *Proc. Natl. Acad. Sci. U.S.A.* 101, 4637–4642. doi: 10.1073/pnas.0308627101

Hagmann, P., Cammoun, L., Gigandet, X., Meuli, R., Honey, C. J., Wedeen, V. J., et al. (2008). Mapping the structural core of human cerebral cortex. *PLoS Biol.* 6:e159. doi: 10.1371/journal.pbio.0060159

He, Y., Chen, Z., and Evans, A. (2008). Structural insights into aberrant topological patterns of large-scale cortical networks in Alzheimer's disease. *J. Neurosci.* 28, 4756–4766. doi: 10.1523/JNEUROSCI.0141-08.2008

He, Y., Wang, J., Wang, L., Chen, Z. J., Yan, C., Yang, H., et al. (2009). Uncovering intrinsic modular organization of spontaneous brain activity in humans. *PLoS ONE* 4:e5226. doi: 10.1371/journal.pone.0005226

Hilgetag, C. C., Burns, G. A., O'Neill, M. A., Scannell, J. W., andYoung, M. P. (2000). Anatomical connectivity defines the organization of clusters of cortical areas in the macaque monkey and the cat. *Philos. Trans. R. Soc. Lond. B Biol. Sci.* 355, 91–110.

Horwitz, B., Grady, C. L., Schlageter, N. L., Duara, R., and Rapoport, S. I. (1987). Intercorrelations of regional cerebral glucose metabolic rates in Alzheimer's disease. *Brain Res.* 407, 294–306. doi: 10.1016/0006-8993(87)91107-3

Johnson, K. A., Fox, N. C., Sperling, R. A., and Klunk, W. E. (2012). Brain imaging in Alzheimer disease. *Cold Spring Harb. Perspect. Med.* 2:a006213.

Kelly, C., Zuo, X. N., Gotimer, K., Cox, C. L., Lynch, L., Brock, D., et al. (2011). Reduced interhemispheric resting state functional connectivity in cocaine addiction. *Biol. Psychiatry* 69, 684–692. doi: 10.1016/j.biopsych.2010.11.022

Khalili-Mahani, N., Chang, C., van Osch, M. J., Veer, I. M., van Buchem, M. A., Dahan, A., et al. (2012). The impact of "physiological correction" on functional connectivity analysis of pharmacological resting state fMRI. *Neuroimage* 65, 499–510. doi: 10.1016/j.neuroimage.2012.09.044

Koch, W., Teipel, S., Mueller, S., Benninghoff, J., Wagner, M., Bokde, A. L., et al. (2012). Diagnostic power of default mode network resting state fMRI in the detection of Alzheimer's disease. *Neurobiol. Aging* 33, 466–478. doi: 10.1016/j.neurobiolaging.2010.04.013

Koch, W., Teipel, S., Mueller, S., Buerger, K., Bokde, A. L., Hampel, H., et al. (2010). Effects of aging on default mode network activity in resting state fMRI: does the method of analysis matter. *Neuroimage* 51, 280–287. doi: 10.1016/j.neuroimage.2009.12.008

Kohannim, O., Hua, X., Hibar, D. P., Lee, S., Chou, Y. Y., Toga, A. W., et al. (2010). Boosting power for clinical trials using classifiers based on multiple biomarkers. *Neurobiol. Aging* 31, 1429–1442. doi: 10.1016/j.neurobiolaging.2010.04.022

Lakmache, Y., Lassonde, M., Gauthier, S., Frigon, J. Y., and Lepore, F. (1998). Interhemispheric disconnection syndrome in Alzheimer's disease. *Proc. Natl. Acad. Sci. U.S.A.* 95, 9042–9046. doi: 10.1073/pnas.95.15.9042

Leicht, E. A., and Newman, M. E. (2008). Community structure in directed networks. *Phys. Rev. Lett.* 100:118703.

Li, S. J., Li, Z., Wu, G., Zhang, M. J., Franczak, M., and Antuono, P. G. (2002). Alzheimer Disease: evaluation of a functional MR imaging index as a marker. *Radiology* 225, 253–259. doi: 10.1148/radiol.2251011301

Locatelli, T., Cursi, M., Liberati, D., Franceschi, M., and Comi, G. (1998). EEG coherence in Alzheimer's disease. *Electroencephalogr. Clin. Neurophysiol.* 106, 229–237. doi: 10.1016/S0013-4694(97)00129-6

Lustig, C., Snyder, A. Z., Bhakta, M., O'Brien, K. C., McAvoy, M., Raichle, M. E., et al. (2003). Functional deactivations: change with age and dementia of the Alzheimer type. *Proc. Natl. Acad. Sci. U.S.A.* 100, 14504–14509.

McKhann, G. M., Knopman, D. S., Chertkow, H., Hyman, B. T., Jack, C. R., Jr., Kawas, C. H., et al. (2011). The diagnosis of dementia due to Alzheimer's disease: recommendations from the National Institute on Aging-Alzheimer's Association workgroups on diagnostic guidelines for Alzheimer's disease. *Alzheimers Dement.* 7, 263–269.

Menon, V., and Uddin, L. Q. (2010). Saliency, switching, attention and control: a network model of insula function. *Brain Struct. Funct.* 214, 655–667. doi: 10.1007/s00429-010-0262-0

Meunier, D., Achard, S., Morcom, A., and Bullmore, E. (2009a). Age-related changes in modular organization of human brain functional networks. *Neuroimage* 44, 715–723.

Meunier, D., Lambiotte, R., and Bullmore, E. T. (2010). Modular and hierarchically modular organization of brain networks. *Front. Neurosci.* 4:200. doi: 10.3389/fnins.2010.00200

Meunier, D., Lambiotte, R., Fornito, A., Ersche, K. D., and Bullmore, E. T. (2009b). Hierarchical modularity in human brain functional networks. *Front. Neuroinform.* 3:37. doi: 10.3389/neuro.11.037.2009

Mezer, A., Yovel, Y., Pasternak, O., Gorfine, T., and Assaf, Y. (2009). Cluster analysis of resting-state fMRI time series. *Neuroimage* 45, 1117–1125. doi: 10.1016/j.neuroimage.2008.12.015

Naqvi, N. H., Rudrauf, D., Damasio, H., and Bechara, A. (2007). Damage to the insula disrupts addiction to cigarette smoking. *Science* 315, 531–534. doi: 10.1126/science.1135926

Nettiksimmons, J., Harvey, D., Brewer, J., Carmichael, O., DeCarli, C., Jack, C. R. Jr., et al. (2010). Subtypes based on cerebrospinal fluid and magnetic resonance imaging markers in normal elderly predict cognitive decline. *Neurobiol. Aging* 31, 1419–1428. doi: 10.1016/j.neurobiolaging.2010.04.025

Newman, M. E. J. (2006). Modularity and community structure in networks. *Proc. Natl. Acad. Sci. U.S.A.* 103, 8577–8582. doi: 10.1073/pnas.0601602103

Newman, M. E., and Girvan, M. (2004). Finding and evaluating community structure in networks. *Phys. Rev. E Stat. Nonlin. Soft Matter Phys.* 69, 026113–026127. doi: 10.1103/PhysRevE.69.026113

Ovadia-Caro, S., Nir, Y., Soddu, A., Ramot, M., Hesselmann, G., Vanhaudenhuyse, A., et al. (2012). Reduction in inter-hemispheric connectivity in disorders of consciousness. *PLoS ONE* 7:e37238. doi: 10.1371/journal.pone.0037238

Palop, J. J., Chin, J., and Mucke, L. (2006). A network dysfunction perspective on neurodegenerative diseases. *Nature* 443, 768–773. doi: 10.1038/nature05289

Pawela, C. P., Biswal, B. B., Cho, Y. R., Kao, D. S., Li, R., Jones, S. R., et al. (2008). Resting-state functional connectivity of the rat brain. *Magn. Reson. Med.* 59, 1021–1029. doi: 10.1002/mrm.21524

Pawela, C. P., Biswal, B. B., Hudetz, A. G., Li, R., Jones, S. R., Cho, Y. R., et al. (2010). Interhemispheric neuroplasticity following limb deafferentation detected by resting-state functional connectivity magnetic resonance imaging (fcMRI) and functional magnetic resonance imaging (fMRI). *Neuroimage* 49, 2467–2478. doi: 10.1016/j.neuroimage.2009.09.054

Prvulovic, D., Bokde, A. L., Faltraco, F., and Hampel, H. (2011). Functional magnetic resonance imaging as a dynamic candidate biomarker for Alzheimer's disease. *Prog. Neurobiol.* 95, 557–569. doi: 10.1016/j.pneurobio.2011.05.008

Raichle, M. E., MacLeod, A. M., Snyder, A. Z., Powers, W. J., Gusnard, D. A., and Shulman, G. L. (2001). A default mode of brain function. *Proc. Natl. Acad. Sci. U.S.A.* 98, 676–682. doi: 10.1073/pnas.98.2.676

Royall, D. R. (2008). Insular Alzheimer disease pathology and the psychometric correlates of mortality. *Cleve. Clin. J. Med.* 75(Suppl. 2), S97–S99.

Sanz-Arigita, E. J., Schoonheim, M. M., Damoiseaux, J. S., Rombouts, S. A., Maris, E., Barkhof, F., et al. (2010). Loss of 'small-world' networks in Alzheimer's disease: graph analysis of FMRI resting-state functional connectivity. *PLoS ONE* 5:e13788. doi: 10.1371/journal.pone.0013788

Sheline, Y. I., Morris, J. C., Snyder, A. Z., Price, J. L., Yan, Z., D'Angelo, G., et al. (2010a). APOE4 allele disrupts resting state fMRI connectivity in the absence of amyloid plaques or decreased CSF Abeta42. *J. Neurosci.* 30, 17035–17040.

Sheline, Y. I., Raichle, M. E., Snyder, A. Z., Morris, J. C., Head, D., Wang, S., et al. (2010b). Amyloid plaques disrupt resting state default mode network connectivity in cognitively normal elderly. *Biol. Psychiatry* 67, 584–587.

Sorg, C., Riedl, V., Perneczky, R., Kurz, A., and Wohlschlager, A. M. (2009). Impact of Alzheimer's disease on the functional connectivity of spontaneous brain activity. *Curr. Alzheimer Res.* 6, 541–553. doi: 10.2174/156720509790147106

Sperling, R. A., Laviolette, P. S., O'Keefe, K., O'Brien, J., Rentz, D. M., Pihlajamaki, M., et al. (2009). Amyloid deposition is associated with impaired default network function in older persons without dementia. *Neuron* 63, 178–188.

Tzourio-Mazoyer, N., Landeau, B., Papathanassiou, D., Crivello, F., Etard, O., Delcroix, N., et al. (2002). Automated anatomical labeling of activations in SPM using a macroscopic anatomical parcellation of the MNI MRI single-subject brain. *Neuroimage* 15, 273–289. doi: 10.1006/nimg.2001.0978

Van den Heuvel, M. P., and Hulshoff Pol, H. E. (2010). Specific somatotopic organization of functional connections of the primary motor network during resting state. *Hum. Brain Mapp.* 31, 631–644.

Wada, Y., Nanbu, Y., Koshino, Y., Yamaguchi, N., and Hashimoto, T. (1998). Reduced interhemispheric EEG coherence in Alzheimer disease: analysis during rest and photic stimulation. *Alzheimer Dis. Assoc. Disord.* 12, 175–181. doi: 10.1097/00002093-199809000-00009

Walhovd, K. B., Fjell, A. M., Brewer, J., McEvoy, L. K., Fennema-Notestine, C., Hagler, D. J., et al. (2010). Combining MR imaging, positron-emission tomography, and CSF biomarkers in the diagnosis and prognosis of Alzheimer disease. *AJNR* 31, 347–354. doi: 10.3174/ajnr.A1809

Westman, E., Aguilar, C., Muehlboeck, J. S., and Simmons, A. (2012a). Regional magnetic resonance imaging measures for multivariate analysis in alzheimer's disease and mild cognitive impairment. *Brain Topogr.* 26, 9–23. doi: 10.1007/s10548-012-0246-x

Westman, E., Muehlboeck, J. S., and Simmons, A. (2012b). Combining MRI and CSF measures for classification of Alzheimer's disease and prediction of mild cognitive impairment conversion. *Neuroimage* 62, 229–238.

Xie, C., Bai, F., Yu, H., Shi, Y., Yuan, Y., Chen, G., et al. (2012). Abnormal insula functional network is associated with episodic memory decline in amnestic mild cognitive impairment. *Neuroimage* 63, 320–327. doi: 10.1016/j.neuroimage.2012.06.062

Yu, Q., Plis, S. M., Erhardt, E. B., Allen, E. A., Sui, J., Kiehl, K. A., et al. (2011). Modular organization of functional network connectivity in healthy controls and patients with schizophrenia during the resting state. *Front. Syst. Neurosci.* 5:103. doi: 10.3389/fnsys.2011.00103

Zhang, H. Y., Wang, S. J., Liu, B., Ma, Z. L., Yang, M., Zhang, Z. J., et al. (2010). Resting brain connectivity: changes during the progress of Alzheimer disease. *Radiology* 256, 598–606. doi: 10.1148/radiol.10091701

Zhang, H. Y., Wang, S. J., Xing, J., Liu, B., Ma, Z. L., Yang, M., et al. (2009). Detection of PCC functional connectivity characteristics in resting-state fMRI in mild Alzheimer's disease. *Behav. Brain Res.* 197, 103–108. doi: 10.1016/j.bbr.2008.08.012

Zhang, Y., Schuff, N., Ching, C., Tosun, D., Zhan, W., Nezamzadeh, M., et al. (2011). Joint assessment of structural, perfusion, and diffusion MRI in Alzheimer's disease and frontotemporal dementia. *Int. J. Alzheimers Dis.* 2011:546871. doi: 10.4061/2011/546871

Zuo, X. N., Kelly, C., Di Martino, A., Mennes, M., Margulies, D. S., Bangaru, S., et al. (2010). Growing together and growing apart: regional and sex differences in the lifespan developmental trajectories of functional homotopy. *J. Neurosci.* 30, 15034–15043. doi: 10.1523/JNEUROSCI.2612-10.2010

Permissions

All chapters in this book were first published by Frontiers; hereby published with permission under the Creative Commons Attribution License or equivalent. Every chapter published in this book has been scrutinized by our experts. Their significance has been extensively debated. The topics covered herein carry significant findings which will fuel the growth of the discipline. They may even be implemented as practical applications or may be referred to as a beginning point for another development.

The contributors of this book come from diverse backgrounds, making this book a truly international effort. This book will bring forth new frontiers with its revolutionizing research information and detailed analysis of the nascent developments around the world.

We would like to thank all the contributing authors for lending their expertise to make the book truly unique. They have played a crucial role in the development of this book. Without their invaluable contributions this book wouldn't have been possible. They have made vital efforts to compile up to date information on the varied aspects of this subject to make this book a valuable addition to the collection of many professionals and students.

This book was conceptualized with the vision of imparting up-to-date information and advanced data in this field. To ensure the same, a matchless editorial board was set up. Every individual on the board went through rigorous rounds of assessment to prove their worth. After which they invested a large part of their time researching and compiling the most relevant data for our readers.

The editorial board has been involved in producing this book since its inception. They have spent rigorous hours researching and exploring the diverse topics which have resulted in the successful publishing of this book. They have passed on their knowledge of decades through this book. To expedite this challenging task, the publisher supported the team at every step. A small team of assistant editors was also appointed to further simplify the editing procedure and attain best results for the readers.

Apart from the editorial board, the designing team has also invested a significant amount of their time in understanding the subject and creating the most relevant covers. They scrutinized every image to scout for the most suitable representation of the subject and create an appropriate cover for the book.

The publishing team has been an ardent support to the editorial, designing and production team. Their endless efforts to recruit the best for this project, has resulted in the accomplishment of this book. They are a veteran in the field of academics and their pool of knowledge is as vast as their experience in printing. Their expertise and guidance has proved useful at every step. Their uncompromising quality standards have made this book an exceptional effort. Their encouragement from time to time has been an inspiration for everyone.

The publisher and the editorial board hope that this book will prove to be a valuable piece of knowledge for researchers, students, practitioners and scholars across the globe.

List of Contributors

Marcus Kaiser
School of Computing Science, Newcastle University, Newcastle upon Tyne, UK
Institute of Neuroscience, Newcastle University, Newcastle upon Tyne, UK
Department of Brain and Cognitive Sciences, Seoul National University, Seoul, South Korea

René C.W. Mandl, Hugo G. Schnack, René S. Kahn and Hilleke E. Hulshoff Pol
Department of Psychiatry, Brain Center Rudolf Magnus, University Medical Center Utrecht, Utrecht, Netherlands

Marcel P. Zwiers
Radboud University Nijmegen, Donders Institute for Brain, Cognition and Behaviour Centre for Cognitive Neuroimaging, Nijmegen, Netherlands

Barry Horwitz
Brain Imaging and Modeling Section, National Institute on Deafness and Other Communication Disorders, National Institutes of Health, Bethesda, MD, USA

Chuhern Hwang
Brain Imaging and Modeling Section, National Institute on Deafness and Other Communication Disorders, National Institutes of Health, Bethesda, MD, USA
National Institute of Biomedical Imaging and Bioengineering, National Institutes of Health, Bethesda, MD, USA
Department of Biomedical Engineering, University of Virginia, Charlottesville, VA, USA

Jeff Alstott
Section on Critical Brain Dynamics, National Institute of Mental Health, National Institutes of Health, Bethesda, MD, USA
Brain Mapping Unit, Behavioural and Clinical Neuroscience Institute, University of Cambridge, Cambridgeshire, UK

Angelica De La Fuente
Ferkauf Graduate School of Psychology, Albert Einstein College of Medicine, Yeshiva University, Bronx, NY, USA

Shugao Xia
Gruss Magnetic Resonance Research Center, Albert Einstein College of Medicine, Yeshiva University, Bronx, NY, USA

Craig Branch
Gruss Magnetic Resonance Research Center, Albert Einstein College of Medicine, Yeshiva University, Bronx, NY, USA
Department of Radiology, Albert Einstein College of Medicine, Yeshiva University, Bronx, NY, USA

Xiaobo Li
Gruss Magnetic Resonance Research Center, Albert Einstein College of Medicine, Yeshiva University, Bronx, NY, USA
Department of Radiology, Albert Einstein College of Medicine, Yeshiva University, Bronx, NY, USA
Department of Neuroscience, Albert Einstein College of Medicine, Yeshiva University, Bronx, NY, USA
Department of Psychiatry and Behavioral Sciences, Albert Einstein College of Medicine, Yeshiva University, Bronx, NY, USA

SeokJun Hong, Andrea Bernasconi and Neda Bernasconi
Neuroimaging of Epilepsy Laboratory, Montreal Neurological Institute and Hospital, McGill University, Montreal, QC, Canada

Boris C. Bernhardt
Neuroimaging of Epilepsy Laboratory, Montreal Neurological Institute and Hospital, McGill University, Montreal, QC, Canada
Department of Social Neuroscience, Max Planck Institute for Human Cognitive and Brain Sciences, Leipzig, Germany

G. E. Anna-Jasmijn Hoff, Manon J. N. L. Benders, Karina J. Kersbergen and L. S. De Vries
Department of Neonatology, Wilhelmina Children's Hospital, University Medical Center Utrecht, Utrecht, Netherlands

M. P. Van den Heuvel
Department of Psychiatry, Brain Center Rudolf Magnus, University Medical Center Utrecht, Utrecht, Netherlands

Zhang Chen, Min Liu and Christian Beaulieu
Department of Biomedical Engineering, Faculty of Medicine and Dentistry, University of Alberta, Edmonton, AB, Canada

Donald W. Gross
Division of Neurology, Department of Medicine, Faculty of Medicine and Dentistry, University of Alberta, Edmonton, AB, Canada

K. Kollndorfer, G. Kasprian, D. Prayer and V. Schöpf
Department of Radiology, Division of Neuro- and Musculoskeletal Radiology, Medical University of Vienna, Vienna, Austria

F. Ph. S. Fischmeister
Department of Neurology, Study Group Clinical fMRI, Medical University of Vienna, Vienna, Austria

Xin Di, Suril Gohel, Eun H. Kim and Bharat B. Biswal
Department of Biomedical Engineering, New Jersey Institute of Technology, Newark, NJ, USA

Diana M. E. Torta, Tommaso Costa and Franco Cauda
Department of Psychology, Università di Torino, Torino, Italy
CCS fMRI-Brain Connectivity and Complex Systems Unit, Koelliker Hospital, Torino, Italy

Sergio Duca
CCS fMRI-Brain Connectivity and Complex Systems Unit, Koelliker Hospital, Torino, Italy

Peter T. Fox
Research Imaging Institute, University of Texas Health Science Center at San Antonio, San Antonio, TX, USA

Qing Gao
School of Mathematical Sciences, University of Electronic Science and Technology of China, Chengdu, China

Qiang Xu, Xujun Duan, Wei Liao, Jurong Ding and Huafu Chen
Key Laboratory for Neuroinformation of Ministry of Education, School of Life Science and Technology, University of Electronic Science and Technology of China, Chengdu, China

Zhiqiang Zhang and Guangming Lu
Department of Medical Imaging, Jinling Hospital, Clinical School, Medical College, Nanjing University, Nanjing, Jiangsu, China

Yuan Li
School of Politics and Public Managements, University of Electronic Science and Technology of China, Chengdu, China

Ariana Anderson and Mark S. Cohen
Department of Psychiatry and Biobehavioral Sciences, Center for Cognitive Neuroscience, University of California Los Angeles, Los Angeles, CA, USA

Annina Visuri
Department of Neurology, Institute of Clinical Medicine, University of Oulu, Oulu, Finland

Riikka Rytty and Liisa Paavola
Department of Neurology, Institute of Clinical Medicine, University of Oulu, Oulu, Finland
Department of Neurology, Oulu University Hospital, Oulu, Finland

Virpi Moilanen
Department of Neurology, Oulu University Hospital, Oulu, Finland

Juha Nikkinen, Ahmed Abou Elseoud, Osmo Tervonen and Vesa Kiviniemi
Department of Radiology, Institute of Clinical Medicine, University of Oulu, Oulu, Finland

Alan E. Renton and Bryan J. Traynor
Neuromuscular Diseases Research Unit, Laboratory of Neurogenetics, National Institute on Aging, National Institutes of Health, Bethesda, MD, USA

Anne M. Remes
Department of Neurology, Institute of Clinical Medicine, University of Eastern Finland, Kuopio, Finland
Department of Neurology, Kuopio University Hospital, Kuopio, Finland

Marie-Christine Ottet
Departement of Psychiatry, Office Médico-Pédagogique (OMP), University of Geneva School of Medicine, Geneva, Switzerland
Signal Processing Laboratory (LTS5), Swiss Federal Institute of Technology (EPFL), Lausanne, Switzerland

Leila Cammoun and Jean-Philippe Thiran
Signal Processing Laboratory (LTS5), Swiss Federal Institute of Technology (EPFL), Lausanne, Switzerland

Marie Schaer
Departement of Psychiatry, Office Médico-Pédagogique (OMP), University of Geneva School of Medicine, Geneva, Switzerland
Department of Psychiatry, Stanford Cognitive and System Neuroscience Laboratory, Stanford University, Palo Alto, CA, USA

Martin Debbané
Departement of Psychiatry, Office Médico-Pédagogique (OMP), University of Geneva School of Medicine, Geneva, Switzerland
Adolescence Clinical Psychology Research Unit, University of Geneva, Geneva, Switzerland

Fang Pu, Yubo Fan and Deyu Li
Key Laboratory for Biomechanics and Mechanobiology of Ministry of Education, Department of Biomedical Engineering, School of Biological Science and Medical Engineering, Beihang University, Beijing, China

Stephan Eliez
Departement of Psychiatry, Office Médico-Pédagogique (OMP), University of Geneva School of Medicine, Geneva, Switzerland
Department of Genetic Medicine and Development, University of Geneva School of Medicine, Geneva, Switzerland

Xinwei Li, Haijun Niu and Shuyu Li
State Key Laboratory of Software Development Environment, Beihang University, Beijing, China
Key Laboratory for Biomechanics and Mechanobiology of Ministry of Education, Department of Biomedical Engineering, School of Biological Science and Medical Engineering, Beihang University, Beijing, China

Zaixu Cui, Suyu Zhong, Pengfei Xu, Yong He and Gaolang Gong
State Key Laboratory of Cognitive Neuroscience and Learning, Beijing Normal University, Beijing, China

Kazunori Sato and Hiroshi Fukuda
Department of Nuclear Medicine and Radiology, Institute of Development, Aging and Cancer, Tohoku University, Sendai, Japan

Kai Wu
Department of Nuclear Medicine and Radiology, Institute of Development, Aging and Cancer, Tohoku University, Sendai, Japan
Department of Biomedical Engineering, School of Materials Science and Engineering, South China University of Technology, Guangzhou, China

Yasuyuki Taki
Department of Nuclear Medicine and Radiology, Institute of Development, Aging and Cancer, Tohoku University, Sendai, Japan
Division of Medical Image Analysis, Department of Community Medical Supports, Tohoku Medical Megabank Organization, Tohoku University, Sendai, Japan
Division of Developmental Cognitive Neuroscience, Institute of Development, Aging and Cancer, Tohoku University, Sendai, Japan

Ryuta Kawashima
Division of Developmental Cognitive Neuroscience, Institute of Development, Aging and Cancer, Tohoku University, Sendai, Japan
Smart Ageing International Research Centre, Institute of Development, Aging and Cancer, Tohoku University, Sendai, Japan
Department of Functional Brain Imaging, Institute of Development, Aging and Cancer, Tohoku University, Sendai, Japan

Haochen Qi
Department of Biomedical Engineering, School of Materials Science and Engineering, South China University of Technology, Guangzhou, China

Thomas P. White, James Gilleen and Sukhwinder S. Shergill
Department of Psychosis Studies, Institute of Psychiatry, King's College London, London, UK

Seung-Goo Kim
Department of Brain and Cognitive Sciences, Seoul National University, Seoul, South Korea
Research Group for Cortical Networks and Cognitive Functions, Max Planck Institute for Human Cognitive and Brain Sciences, Leipzig, Germany

Wi Hoon Jung
Clinical Cognitive Neuroscience Center, SNU-MRC, Seoul National University Hospital, Seoul, South Korea

Sung Nyun Kim and Joon Hwan Jang
Department of Psychiatry, College of Medicine, Seoul National University, Seoul, South Korea

Jun Soo Kwon
Department of Brain and Cognitive Sciences, Seoul National University, Seoul, South Korea
Clinical Cognitive Neuroscience Center, SNU-MRC, Seoul National University Hospital, Seoul, South Korea
Department of Psychiatry, College of Medicine, Seoul National University, Seoul, South Korea

Guangyu Chen and Gang Chen
Department of Biophysics, Medical College of Wisconsin, Milwaukee, WI, USA

Gao-Jun Teng
Department of Radiology, Jiangsu Key Laboratory of Molecule Imaging and Functional Imaging, Medical School of Southeast University, Nanjing, PR China

Hong-Ying Zhang
Department of Radiology, Jiangsu Key Laboratory of Molecule Imaging and Functional Imaging, Medical School of Southeast University, Nanjing, PR China
Department of Radiology, Subei People's Hospital of Jiangsu Province, Yangzhou University, Yangzhou, PR China

Zhi-Jun Zhang
Department of Neuropsychiatry, Affiliated Zhong Da Hospital of Southeast University, Nanjing, PR China

Chunming Xie
Department of Biophysics, Medical College of Wisconsin, Milwaukee, WI, USA
Department of Neuropsychiatry, Affiliated Zhong Da Hospital of Southeast University, Nanjing, PR China

Shi-Jiang Li
Department of Biophysics, Medical College of Wisconsin, Milwaukee, WI, USA
Department of Psychiatry and Behavioral Medicine, Medical College of Wisconsin, Milwaukee, WI, USA

Index

A

Alzheimer's Disease, 15, 22-24, 61, 63, 71, 99, 114, 134, 142-143, 163, 181, 190-192, 203, 221, 223, 230-232

Amygdala, 27, 31-32, 39-40, 80, 99, 101-102, 113-114, 134, 183, 185, 191, 227

Anatomical Connectivity, 14-15, 17-18, 21, 52-53, 55-56, 88, 154, 159, 206, 220, 232

Anterior Cingulate Gyrus, 183, 185, 200

Auditory Network, 66, 70

Axial Diffusivity, 61, 167

B

Beck's Depression Inventory, 135, 206, 210

Blood Oxygenation Level Dependent, 24

Brain Disorders, 1-3, 14-15, 17-19, 21-22

C

Calcarine Gyrus, 68

Cerebellum, 26, 28, 46-47, 75, 77-78, 83-84, 103, 114

Cingulate Cortex, 26, 30, 46, 48, 88-90, 92-101, 103, 115, 134, 141, 156, 158, 160-161, 164, 181, 193, 199-204, 206

Cognitive Dysfunction, 66, 71, 152

Corpus Callosum, 9, 23, 29, 34, 88, 173, 175, 206

Correlation Maps, 66-67, 156

Correlation Matrix, 80-81, 104, 106, 182-183

Cortical Thickness, 28, 31-35, 38-39, 41, 52, 59-60, 62-63, 142, 154, 159-160, 162, 182, 188-191, 205-207, 210, 219-221, 230

D

Default Mode Network, 20, 24-25, 59-60, 65, 70, 73, 80, 118, 142, 162-163, 181, 204, 223, 231

Diffusion Magnetic Resonance Imaging, 166

Diffusion Spectrum Imaging, 16, 24, 60

Diffusion Tensor Imaging, 2, 5, 12, 14, 24-26, 29, 40-42, 52, 62-63, 152, 154, 176, 189-190, 205, 221-222

Disease Progression, 3-4, 223, 229

Dorsal-ventral Imbalance, 205-206

Dorsolateral Prefrontal, 26, 46, 92, 114, 144, 150, 158-160, 164-165

Dynamic Connectome, 1

E

Echo-planar Imaging, 53, 66, 224

Entorhinal Cortex, 31-32, 34-35, 38-40, 162

Event-related Potentials, 30

F

Fractional Anisotropy, 5, 12, 27, 30, 33-34, 52, 62, 163, 166, 189, 205

Functional Connectivity, 13-24, 26-31, 34-37, 39-43, 45, 49-51, 62, 65-73, 79, 83, 85-86, 89, 98-104, 106, 113-122, 125-129, 133-136, 138-143, 154-155, 161-162, 181, 189, 191-192, 194, 204, 219-221, 223-231

Functional Magnetic Resonance Imaging, 1, 24-25, 79, 102, 116, 193

Fusiform Gyrus, 22, 55, 68-69, 102, 164, 183

G

General Linear Model, 6, 55, 61, 154, 171

Global Efficiency, 27, 52, 54, 56, 59, 64, 79-83, 145-147, 150, 171-173, 175, 181, 183-189, 209-210

Graph Theoretical Analysis, 4, 29, 36, 38, 52, 57, 102, 104, 106, 114, 183, 191-192, 205

Gray Matter, 5, 7-8, 30-31, 33, 35-36, 39, 48, 52, 80, 90, 114, 134-136, 138, 140, 144-146, 148-149, 152, 154, 162-163, 165, 169, 181-184, 188, 191, 205-207, 216, 221-223, 226-227

H

Heat Kernel Smoothing, 207, 220

Hippocampus, 31-33, 38-40, 43, 75, 77-78, 103, 140, 145, 148, 151, 162, 183, 223

I

Inferior Parietal Lobule, 83, 139, 183, 185, 227

L

Laplace-beltrami Eigenfunction, 207, 221

Local Efficiency, 27, 52, 54, 56, 64, 83, 98, 144-147, 150-151, 154, 160, 171-173, 175, 183-188, 209-210

M

Magnetic Resonance Imaging, 1, 12-14, 23-25, 29, 39-40, 50, 72-73, 79, 88, 102, 113, 116-117, 129, 142, 144, 154, 163, 166, 182, 192-193, 204-206, 231-232

Magnetoencephalography, 3

Mean Diffusivity, 27, 34, 61-62, 166

Meta-analytic Clustering, 88-89

Meta-analytic Parcellation, 88

Middle Frontal Gyrus, 55, 103, 139, 183, 185

Morphology, 3, 12, 45-46, 152, 154, 162, 206, 219

N

Neural Activity, 16-18, 21, 35, 117

Neural Modeling, 14-15, 17-21

Neuroplasticity, 17, 20-21, 162, 231

Node Strength, 59, 183-188

Non-invasive Neuroimaging, 3, 31

O

Obsessive-compulsive Disorder, 205, 210, 220-222

Orbitofrontal, 26, 28, 32, 34-35, 56, 59-60, 62, 102, 114, 140, 145-147, 158, 164, 183, 185

P

Paracentral Lobule, 55, 68, 183, 227

Parahippocampal Gyrus, 46, 55, 83, 140, 183, 185

Pipeline For Analyzing Brain Diffusion Images, 167

Pipeline System For Octave And Matlab, 166

Positron Emission Tomography, 24, 101, 103, 118, 163, 205, 230

Postcentral Gyrus, 55, 67, 69-70, 140, 183, 185, 214, 227

Posterior Cingulate Cortex, 26, 46, 48, 88, 92, 134, 141, 156, 158, 164, 181

Precentral Gyrus, 26, 55, 69, 102-103, 140, 156-157, 160, 164, 183-184, 227

Precuneus, 20, 24, 29, 46, 52, 55, 67-68, 70-72, 75-78, 83-84, 103, 134, 138, 140, 148, 151, 156, 183, 189, 194

Prefrontal Cortex, 15-16, 24, 26, 43, 46-47, 70, 86, 99, 102-103, 134, 144, 150, 156, 158-160, 165, 194, 205

R

Radial Diffusivity, 61, 167

Reading Network, 65, 70

Region Of Interest, 24, 26, 88, 117, 159-160

Regional Cerebral Blood Flow, 15, 24, 103, 163

Regional Gray Matter Volume, 181-182, 184

Repetition Time, 24, 91, 170

Rolandic Operculum, 55, 183, 227

S

Schizophrenia, 2-4, 18, 20-23, 37-39, 43, 49, 113-114, 116-123, 127-129, 144-145, 149-153, 182, 190-191, 193-204, 228, 230, 232

Sensorimotor Network, 47, 66, 70

Standard Deviation, 54, 92, 104, 106, 139, 147, 182, 194, 201, 207, 210, 225-226, 228

Statistical Parameter Map, 6, 9

Structural Covariance Networks, 36, 39, 154, 159-160, 164

Structural Equation Modeling, 20, 24, 118

Superior Frontal Gyrus, 55, 103, 139, 183, 185

Supplementary Motor Area, 55, 69, 146-147, 158-159, 161, 183, 227

T

Temporal Lobe Epilepsy, 31, 33-34, 38-44, 206, 220

Tractography, 4, 10, 16, 28, 31-35, 37-38, 40-42, 50, 52-55, 57, 61-63, 86, 88, 146, 149, 151-152, 163, 166-170, 173, 175-176, 178, 180, 221

V

Visual Network, 47, 65, 70, 138

Voronoi Tessellation, 90, 92, 97

W

White Matter, 5, 7-12, 26, 33, 35, 40-43, 45, 52, 54-55, 58, 63-64, 80, 104, 106, 144, 146, 149-150, 152, 154, 163, 166, 169, 175-176, 182, 188-191, 205, 207, 220-222, 225

www.ingramcontent.com/pod-product-compliance
Lightning Source LLC
LaVergne TN
LVHW082150200926
848484LV00008B/2135
* 9 7 9 8 8 8 7 4 0 3 1 0 6 *